"This is truly the Bible on women's health! It has been completely revised and updated for a new generation of women who will need its guidance more than ever as they attempt to take control of their health."

—Susan Love, M.D.
Author, *Dr. Susan Love's Breast Book* and *Dr. Susan Love's Menopause and Hormone Book*

"Within these pages, you will find the voice of a women's health movement that is based on shared experience. Listen to it—and add your own."

—Gloria Steinem
Cofounder of *Ms. Magazine* and author, *Outrageous Acts and Everyday Rebellions*

"This wonderful new edition presents up-to-the-minute medical information in a way that is honest, accessible, and affirming of a diverse range of women's experiences. A vital resource for all women."

—Karen Carlson, M.D.
Deputy Director, Center of Excellence in Women's Health, Harvard Medical School

"If only every little girl were born with a copy of *Our Bodies, Ourselves* in her hands, we would raise a society filled with healthy, confident young women. And if women could have only one book on their shelves, let it be this classic tome filled to the brim with practical and empowering information."

—Toni Weschler, M.P.H.
Author, *Taking Charge of Your Fertility*

"*Our Bodies, Ourselves* was first published when my daughter was one year old. Now her daughter is one year old. She will be the third generation of my family to be grateful for this book and the good it does, for all of our sakes."

—Linda Ellerbee
Journalist, author, and feminist

"What has made each generation of women rejoice in discovering themselves in *Our Bodies, Ourselves* is that it still emanates from women's experiences as faithfully as ever."

—Helen Rodriquez-Trias
Former President of the American Public Health Association

"*Our Bodies, Ourselves* is an invaluable resource—just the kind of book that I fear could become harder and harder to find—and one we desperately need. *Our Bodies, Ourselves* is a completely trustworthy source of solid, reliable information about women's health—not just a dependable reference about our physical health, but a wellspring of stamina for our embattled psyches. In an age when women are still being dismissed, regimented, or held in contempt, *Our Bodies, Ourselves* does the simplest and most vital thing: It tells us the truth."

—Dorothy Allison
Author, *Bastard Out of Carolina* and other titles

Other major books by members of the Boston Women's Health Book Collective

Changing Bodies, Changing Lives

Ourselves and Our Children

The New Ourselves, Growing Older

OUR BODIES, OURSELVES

A New Edition for a New Era

The Boston Women's Health Book Collective

Many thanks to Brigham and Women's Hospital for a generous grant and to the Boston University School of Public Health for generous support to produce this revised edition.

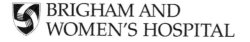

A TOUCHSTONE BOOK
Published by Simon & Schuster
New York London Toronto Sydney

35th Anniversary Edition

This publication contains the opinions and ideas of its author. It is intended to provide helpful and informative material on the subjects addressed in the publication. It is sold with the understanding that the author and publisher are not engaged in rendering medical, health, or any other kind of personal professional services in the book. The reader should consult his or her medical, health, or other competent professional before adopting any of the suggestions in this book or drawing inferences from it.

The author and publisher specifically disclaim all responsibility for any liability, loss, or risk, personal or otherwise, which is incurred as a consequence, directly or indirectly, of the use and application of any of the contents of this book.

TOUCHSTONE
Rockefeller Center
1230 Avenue of the Americas
New York, NY 10020

Copyright © 1984, 1992, 1998, 2005 by the Boston Women's Health Book Collective
All rights reserved,
including the right of reproduction
in whole or in part in any form.

TOUCHSTONE and colophon are registered trademarks
of Simon & Schuster, Inc.

Designed by Katy Riegel

Manufactured in the United States of America

ISBN 0-7432-5611-5

■ CONTENTS

INTRODUCTION

Welcome to *Our Bodies, Ourselves,* the classic book about women's health and sexuality that is written by women, for women. Since its first newsprint version in 1970, *Our Bodies, Ourselves* has been created and revised by women speaking from our own research and experiences about our bodies, health, and medical care.

This edition reflects the work of more than four hundred women—and quite a few men—who share both personal stories and health information based on the latest scientific evidence. The result is a new *Our Bodies, Ourselves,* rewritten for today's realities.

CHANGING TIMES, CONTINUING NEED

Much has changed since the late 1960s and early 1970s, when the group that became the Boston Women's Health Book Collective first started to meet. Abortion is now legal (though threatened), and birth control options have increased; the AIDS epidemic has made safer sex a subject of public discussion; and lesbian and gay couples have the right to marry, at least in Massachusetts. Many groups, including an active movement of women with breast cancer, have drawn new attention to environmental factors in disease and to the politics of research funding. More health care providers are women now, and doctors and medical researchers of both sexes tend to be more sensitive to and knowledgeable about women's concerns than doctors of an earlier generation. Information on women's health is widely available.

But the need for a book like *Our Bodies, Ourselves* remains. Too much medical care still focuses on the expensive "solutions" of drugs and surgery, rather than on prevention or management strategies such as good food and exercise, a clean environment, and safe working conditions. Too often, women's life experiences, from childbirth to menopause, are seen as diseases to be treated rather than natural, healthy processes that sometimes have problems. And too many of us still don't have the knowledge and resources to participate effectively in maintaining our health.

SELF-HELP AND BEYOND

This book offers individual women the tools to take care of ourselves, from eating well and becoming more physically active to learning how to cope better with stress. It provides helpful, clear information about substance abuse, heart disease, eating disorders, and many other conditions that women confront. A new chapter, "Navigating the Health Care System," provides practical advice for getting the best care possible.

Yet *Our Bodies, Ourselves* is about more than self-help. Many aspects of our health, from workplace safety to sexual violence, are often beyond an individual's control. Therefore, this book addresses the political, economic, and social factors that affect our health and medical care: the industrial plants spewing pollution, the fast-food giants pushing junk food, the pharmaceutical companies unethically promoting drugs, the government dismantling our social safety net. We can change these conditions only by working together, sharing our stories with

MORE ON THE WEB

With this edition, the print version of *Our Bodies, Ourselves* is for the first time accompanied by a website that provides more detailed and updated information, longer resource lists, and links to other helpful sites. This new feature was developed to respond to the rapidly changing world of women's health.

Throughout the book, you will see references to the companion website, which can be found at www.ourbodiesourselves.org. To find the material referenced, type the title of the website material, or the corresponding number code, into the "search" box. For example, if you read "For more information, see 'Women and Alcohol Use' (W6) on the companion website, www.ourbodiesourselves.org," you can type in either **Women and Alcohol Use** or **W6.** You can also select a particular chapter to see all of its website content.

You will also come across many references to the "Resources," comprehensive lists of trustworthy organizations, books, and other materials related to the many topics covered in this book. You can find the top ten resources for each chapter at the back of the book. Longer lists, including web links, are posted on the companion website.

other women, and advocating for policies and programs that protect the health of our families, our communities, and the world.

MANY WOMEN'S VOICES

Despite some changes, this edition retains one of the distinctive traits of *Our Bodies, Ourselves:* the use of real women's voices. These first-person stories, set off in italicized passages throughout the text, have been collected from conversations, letters, and e-mail messages that spanned the globe.

Diverse voices are also embodied in the all-embracing "we" of this book. When the Boston Women's Health Book Collective first wrote about "our bodies," the "we" reflected the white, mostly middle-class, well-educated background of many of its founding members. But as more diverse women have helped revise the book, the "we" has grown to include a greater variety of experiences.

MAKING CHANGES TOGETHER

No matter who we are, we often need both information and support to make healthy changes. If we are trying to get more exercise, for example, inviting a friend to share a morning walk may make it more fun. Similarly, if we are feeling overwhelmed as new mothers, we may want to join a play group with other families in the neighborhood. The same principle extends to issues beyond our individual well-being: By working together, we can bring about change and improve the health of our communities.

This new edition of *Our Bodies, Ourselves* serves as a first step on such paths, offering information, stories, and resources so that we can take care of ourselves—and one another.

Heather Stephenson, managing editor
For the Boston Women's Health Book Collective
July 2004, Boston

While the information contained in *Our Bodies, Ourselves* is meant to empower you and give you useful tools and ideas, this book is not intended to replace professional health and medical care.

A LETTER FROM FOUNDERS OF THE BOSTON WOMEN'S HEALTH BOOK COLLECTIVE

It's hard to believe that thirty-five years have passed since we first gathered around our kitchen tables to create *Our Bodies, Ourselves (OBOS)*. These early meetings took place in Boston at the end of the 1960s into the early 1970s, at a time when women throughout the United States and the world were meeting to share experiences and expose the injustices in women's lives. We talked about our bodies, health, and sexuality. In recounting our life stories and health care experiences, we discovered with surprise that many of us shared the same frustrations and misinformation. However, we learned together to trust what we knew about ourselves. In the months and years that followed, we wove our own experiences and the experiences of many diverse women, along with the health and medical in-

formation we carefully researched and a political critique of the profit-oriented medical system, into a dynamic, useful, women-centered body of knowledge.

By disseminating women's experience and knowledge as valid information, *OBOS* challenged the paternalistic medical system. What we couldn't have foreseen then was that our book would help create a women's health movement and radically change the way many people think about health care. Nor could we have known that the book's great success would generate a need for an ongoing women's health organization in which, over the next three decades, some of us would remain active as board or staff members.

Hundreds of women (and some men) have, with care and passion, contributed work, time, and money to keep the organization and the book alive and responsive to women's needs. In its more than twenty translations and adaptations, the book has reached into many corners of the earth, connecting with an ever-growing network of activists throughout the world.

As older women who have struggled for women's rights, written numerous editions of OBOS, and mentored many other health activists and publications, we know that each new generation of women must define and grapple with its own issues in its own cultural and political context. Young women face as many challenges as we ever did. Their activism helps us all maintain the vitality of the women's health movement. With them, we continue to work for the creation of economic and social conditions that ensure good health and good health care, for the right to control our reproductive and sexual lives, including access to excellent birth control, abortion, and maternity care services, and the free expression of our sexuality as heterosexual, lesbian, bisexual, or trans women.

We must never take for granted any rights already won. We must maintain, expand, and protect them, creating for everyone the opportunity to live in a just world that recognizes women's needs and celebrates women's voices.

This latest edition of OBOS has been coordinated by the OBOS staff and written by many new women as well as some founders and other long-time authors of the book. We hope that it will promote dialogue and stimulate activism around women's health issues; that it will offer continuity and a community of effort among and between the generations, acknowledge our similarities and differences, and help forge a shared vision of humane health care for now and decades to come.

Ruth Bell Alexander, Pamela Berger, Vilunya Diskin, Joan Ditzion, Paula Doress-Worters, Nancy Miriam Hawley, Elizabeth MacMahon Herrera, Pamela Morgan, Judy Norsigian, Jane Pincus, Wendy Sanford, Sally Whelan *

* To read more about the founders and the earlier editions of *Our Bodies, Ourselves*, see "History of *Our Bodies, Ourselves* and the Boston Women's Health Book Collective" (W1) on the companion website, www.ourbodiesourselves.org.

Taking Care of Ourselves

CHAPTER 1

For women, life can often seem like a beauty pageant. Throughout every phase of our lives, from childhood to maturity, our appearance is judged and critiqued. Our looks are compared to those of our peers, our sisters, the women in the media, or imaginary ideals. We're rated pretty, ugly, plain—or just plain average. No one has ever asked us if we want to compete in this lifelong beauty contest. Being born female automatically makes us contestants, whether we like it or not.[1]

From the moment we are a *pretty little girl* in a *cute dress*, and our brother is a *big, strong boy* who is *smart*, we learn what society expects from us.[2] We internalize the message that as women, we are defined by our looks, not by our actions, character, or brainpower. These messages surround us in the media, in our communities, and sometimes in our own homes.

Our individual experiences also affect how we feel about our bodies. If we have experienced violence or abuse, we may feel unsafe in our bodies. If we have experienced racism, been ridiculed because we're in a wheelchair, or been made fun of because we have a "big" nose, we may dislike, mistrust, or even hate our bodies. We may respond to hurtful experiences by wanting a "perfect" body, thinking that if we looked like a supermodel, we would be shielded from discrimination, become successful, and find true love. Or we may respond by abusing our bodies with promiscuous sexual behavior, excessive exercise, alcohol or drugs, binging on junk food, or starving ourselves.

VULVA CHIC

Bikini waxing—removing pubic hair that grows outside the swimsuit line—has been around for decades and seems rather quaint compared to what we must contend with now. Brazilian bikini waxing removes every wisp of hair from the genital *and* anal areas, leaving only a tiny decorative pouf at the top. Female celebrities and average women alike gush about the transformative power of going bare.

In many countries, a flash of pubic hair on the beach is considered no big deal, but women in North and South America are, in general, very squeamish about exposing hair *down there*. Today's craze for totally hairless crotches is due largely to the popularity of thongs, which leave little to the imagination. Once the domain of strippers, thongs are now so mainstream that the corner drugstore sells thong-shaped panty liners.

What often goes unsaid in discussions of waxing (blame the ickiness factor) is that as a result of removing all the hair from the pubic region, grown women resemble prepubescent girls, and this is considered erotic. The popular online magazine *Salon* published an essay by a woman who wrote about her first Brazilian bikini wax: "I feel like a 12-year-old, but a naughty, Lolita kind of 12-year-old. This is hot." She quotes a man whose girlfriend got a Brazilian as saying that the "little girl eroticism" of a bare vulva turns him on.[4]

The effort to make our private parts seem younger and more appealing is not limited to waxing alone; increasingly, women are turning to cosmetic surgery. Some women have their inner vaginal lips cut and shortened to make them smaller or more symmetrical through a surgery called labiaplasty. Others undergo surgical tightening of the vagina, which may be stretched by childbirth; such "vaginal rejuvenation" is touted to increase sexual pleasure. Anecdotal evidence suggests that some men are pressuring their female partners to have surgery so they more closely resemble the women in pornographic movies.[5]

The growing popularity of techniques that sculpt and style our vulvas and vaginas makes it clear that no part of our bodies—no matter how intimate—can escape society's critical eye.

How do we nurture a positive body image while we're constantly being judged, while women's bodies are turned into sex objects, and while violence against women pervades our society? What if we are not the current ideal woman, tall and thin with large breasts and a fair complexion? What if we are women of color; what if we are fat, disabled, or super-skinny? While there are many things that divide us as women, the fact that our bodies are never good enough unites us all. We hope this chapter will help you opt out of the beauty contest by understanding how cultural forces have encouraged us to hate our bodies. By examining these external pressures, we can begin to love ourselves and feel comfortable in our own skin. One of the most radical things a woman can do is love her body.[6]

BEAUTY FOR SALE

Our physical characteristics are, for the most part, beyond our control. But many of us have difficulty accepting our bodies, and we spend a tremendous amount of time and money battling nature. For Americans, "self-improvement" rarely means building our character or increasing our contributions to the world; rather, improving ourselves usually means altering our appearance. Many of us believe that by losing weight or getting a face-lift, we can become better people. We spend billions of dollars in the hope that we can transform ourselves from the outside in.

If we want to spend our time and money trying to achieve an impossible beauty ideal, plenty of corporations and medical professionals will help us try. While it is normal to want to look good, magazine publishers and the cosmetics, fashion, and diet industries adeptly exploit the message that we must conform to the current ideal of beauty to be valued as women. Through their relentless ads and articles, they define what the "look" is and ensure that we feel insecure about our ability to meet it. The cosmetics and beauty products industry makes over $43 billion a year,[7] and it spends $1.5 billion on advertising everything from hair dyes to cellulite cream.[8] But what if we can't achieve the right look through cosmetics and dieting alone? Never fear, plastic surgeons are available to alter us, too.

The days when the "makeovers" on television consisted of changing one's appearance through hair, makeup, and clothes are long gone. Today participants have their faces and bodies permanently altered through plastic surgery, right on national TV, without any discussions of the health and psychological risks. No longer only for the rich, plastic surgeons target middle-class people; in the United States, 86 percent of their patients are women.[9] To obtain the "ideal" yet mythical 36–24–36 measurements (a size 10 in the bust, 2 in the waist, 4 in the hips) promoted in the media, most of us would need to submit to the scalpel. Since breasts are made primarily of fat, slim women rarely have large breasts. To achieve the "curvaceously thin" body type—which is unusual in real life—we would not only need to starve ourselves, as do many movie stars, models, and pop singers; we also would need to turn to a combination of liposuction and breast augmentation.[10] (For more about breast implants, see p. 613 in Chapter 28, "Unique to Women.")

Americans are raised to believe that with hard work, anything is possible. The idea that we can transform ourselves is powerful and uniquely American, and it may blind us to the fact that a woman standing 5'4" and weighing 150 pounds will never be able to turn herself into a 5'11", 117-pound supermodel, no matter how hard she tries.

All too often, the beauty ideal embraced by our culture is a white ideal. As early as the 1850s, skin bleaching and hair straightening were pitched to African-Americans as ways to obtain

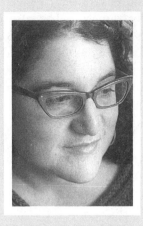

"I LIKE THE WAY MY NOSE MARKS ME"

LISA JERVIS

As an ethnic Jew of a very specific variety—a godless New York City-raised neurotic upper-middle-class girl from a solidly liberal-Democrat family who observed only one Jewish ritual: going out for Chinese food and a movie on Christmas Day—I've had a standing offer for a nose job from adolescence on. "It's not such a big deal," my mom would say. "Doctors do such individual-looking noses these days. It'll look really natural." "It's not too late, you know," she would add in the years after I flat-out refused to let someone break my nose, scrape part of it out, and reposition it into a smaller, less obtrusive shape. "I'll still pay." As if money were the reason I was resisting.

Mainly, I didn't want to be that vain and shallow, and I didn't want scalpels anywhere near my face. But my queasy feelings about plastic surgery aside—the risks, the expense, the frivolity, the blood, the sheer visceral creepiness—I'd have wanted to keep my prominent, bump-adorned honker anyway. Oddly, given how I've felt about my body at various times in my life, I've always been pretty happy with my (dare I say it) God-given nose.

Of friends my own age who've had nose jobs, most didn't want them but were coerced or shamed into it by older Jewish female relatives: mothers, grandmothers, aunts (an experience I'm eternally grateful my mother spared me). Though in this day and age, the lust for a button nose is more a desire for a typical pretty femininity than for any specific de-ethnicizing, when we scratch the surface of what "prettier" means, we find that we might as well be saying "whiter" or "gentile."

I like the way my nose marks me. The first time I met another Jewish feminist writer with whom I would end up working, she asked if I was a member of the tribe. "With this nose, and this hair, you gotta ask?" I replied, laughing. "No," she confessed, "but I figured it was only polite." One WASPy coworker, when I mentioned an upcoming trip to see my family, asked, "So, are your parents just like people in Woody Allen movies?" While his comment sparked some insecurity ("Am I that neurotic?" I thought), I've always appreciated that there's a part of my identity that's instantly recognizable to those who know where to look.

the privileges of white society.[11] Today many Mexican immigrant women in the United States suffer from mercury poisoning as a result of using skin-whitening creams containing mercury. Mercury poisoning can cause neurological and kidney damage, as well as psychiatric disorders. Women of color around the world apply such creams regularly either to lighten or even our complexions, jeopardizing our health.[12]

While we may know that beauty is skin-deep, society still responds differently to people considered physically beautiful. Studies show that people assume attractive women and men are more sexually alluring, sociable, and smart, and that women considered attractive have better-paying jobs and more opportunities for advancement. Research has shown that elementary school teachers often give special treatment to children they find cute, and "good-looking" criminals often get lighter sentences.[13]

Given such evidence, you would think that people who are considered extremely attractive would be much happier than everyone else, but studies show this is not the case. Happiness is more likely the result of a positive outlook, high self-esteem, and nurturing relationships with other people.[14] More disturbing research points to the fact that our quest for beauty can cover up

deeper psychological issues. Finnish researchers found that women who received breast implants for cosmetic reasons were three times more likely to commit suicide than the general population.[15]

HE LOVES ME, HE LOVES ME NOT

For many women, the main reason to "improve" our appearance is to attract and win the approval of men. We have been conditioned to think we must compete with each other for male attention—and to get attention and provoke envy in other women. Many feminists believe this is a consequence of living in a patriarchal society. Women are judged intensely on our looks because men have a disproportionate amount of power and control; in patriarchal societies, women gain status through relationships with men, and appearance serves as a measure of our desirability as sexual partners.[16]

The message that we should keep quiet and look sexy for men is so deeply woven into the fabric of our society that we barely notice it. The pornography industry is focused almost entirely on men's sexual pleasure. "Adult" entertainment means entertainment for men, not for women. And thanks in large part to the Internet, video

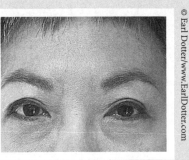

"I THOUGHT SHE WAS ERASING HER CULTURAL INTEGRITY"

EUGENIA SUNHEE KIM

When my sister had her eyelids "done" in Korea, I thought she was a traitor. She had sold out to the Western notion of beauty. "Everybody's doing it," she said.

True, the International Society of Aesthetic Plastic Surgery reports that blepharoplasty (the procedure that cuts eyelids, scrapes away fat, and adds an exaggerated crease to make eyes look bigger) is the most popular plastic surgery in South Korea and Japan. In 2002 it accounted for over 62 percent of all plastic surgery in those nations, a dramatic increase from 12 percent the previous year. In Korea, the procedure is now more common than orthodontic braces. In the United States, it's the most common aesthetic procedure performed on Asian individuals.

My sister thought nothing of the surgery's ethnic implications. She hoped only to improve her looks. I thought she was erasing her cultural integrity.

Then, in my late forties, I had to get surgery to correct a drooping eyelid. The procedure would result in a creased eyelid. I opted to have both eyes done so that they would match.

During surgery, my doctor told me that my right eye had lazy tendencies, like the left. Despite the throbbing pain, I was glad to hear this news, as if I had been medically absolved of the sin of double eyelids.

Two years later, my eyes match and appear more open. I'm glad for that. But those noticeable lids add a foreignness to my face—a subtle difference that makes me blink to recognize the me in the mirror it took so much to learn to love—and I find myself trying to mask the obvious creases with makeup.

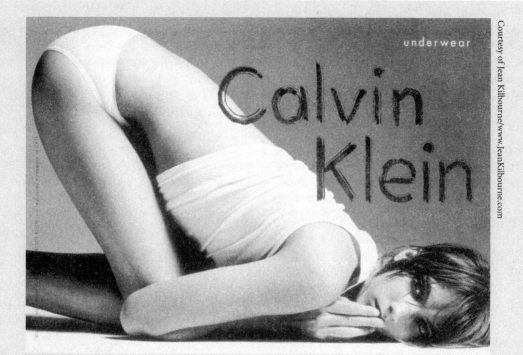

"Calvin Klein is known for provocative and quasi-pornographic ads, such as this one showing a woman in a classic submissive pose," says Jean Kilbourne, author of *Can't Buy Me Love: How Advertising Changes the Way We Think and Feel.* "As is typical in ads featuring young women, her fingers cover her mouth, another sign of submission and a symbol of voiceless-ness. Her eye makeup is so dark and heavy that her eyes seem bruised, blackened. She is powerless but seductive, inviting attention and, as is often the case in the world of porno-graphic fantasy, clearly asking for whatever happens to her. She is simply an object to be used.

"She is also, of course, very young and very thin, as are virtually all models in ads regard-less of the target audience. The adolescent girl, often with a body more like that of an adolescent boy, is the ideal. Signs of maturity, such as a wisp of body hair or any hint of wrin-kles, are erased. This contributes to an infantilization of women in our culture, as well as to a fear of powerful and mature women. Of course, this has a negative effect on female self-esteem. It also affects how men feel about the real, unairbrushed, grown-up women in their lives."

games, and music videos, pornography is now mainstream. Hard-core pornography is never further away than a few clicks of a computer mouse. As a result, much of popular culture now mirrors pornography. Television—from the music videos to the reality shows—features young women submitting to male desires nearly twenty-four hours a day, in what is often little more than soft-core porn. One result of this per-vasive imagery is that a whole generation of boys and girls is learning how women should look and act by viewing submissive and objectified women in the media.

We have been told that men are biologically programmed to be turned on by sexual imagery because they are naturally more visual than women. But researchers have found that women are not necessarily less visual than men, and are no less turned on by visual sexual stimuli. Rather, we have been socialized to behave differently. Considering that pornography and much of our popular culture degrades women, it's not surprising that most women—and many men— are turned off by it.[17]

Obsessing over our appearance is an issue not only for women who want to attract men. All of us must contend with the constant onslaught of media and cultural messages telling us that we need to improve our appearance. Researchers have found that the more we identify with what are considered negative "feminine" traits, like passivity, dependence, and unassertiveness, the more likely we are to suffer from body image problems and disordered eating, regardless of our sexual orientation or gender identity.[18]

Although most of us understandably want to be attractive to others, it can be a challenge to do this without harming our health or buying into stereotypes that undermine our sense of self-worth.

THE MEDIA LIES

Researchers have found that ongoing exposure to certain ideas can shape and distort our perceptions of reality. How many naked bodies do most of us view on a regular basis in real life— not counting what we see in the media? Very few. But if women or men consume a steady diet of fashion magazines or pornography, they encounter more naked or semi-naked female bodies than they would otherwise—female bodies

that just happen to be airbrushed and plastic-surgery-enhanced. It's not surprising that in our media-driven culture, our views of what women should look like are warped.[19] Real women with pubic hair and breasts that aren't perfect round orbs begin to seem unnatural compared to the altered images we see in the media.

It's hard to imagine a world where idealized female imagery is not plastered everywhere, but our current situation is a relatively new phenomenon. Before the mass media existed, our ideas of beauty were limited to our own communities. Until the advent of photography in 1839, people were not exposed to real-life images of faces and bodies. Most people did not even own mirrors.[20]

Most of the women we see in the media are young and white. Hollywood movies rarely feature women over forty, and the older women we do see represented in the media, from movie stars to news anchors and even politicians, look much younger, thanks to plastic surgery. As a result, those of us who choose to age naturally, without the aid of plastic surgery, are sometimes seen as "letting ourselves go."

The image of "perfection" we see in the

MYTH OR REALITY?

- *Most women can obtain the "ideal" body type portrayed by models through diet and exercise.*

Myth. The average American woman will never be able to turn herself into a 5'11", 117-pound supermodel, no matter how hard she tries. To achieve the "curvaceously thin" body type—which is rarely seen in real life— we would not only need to starve ourselves, we would have to resort to risky liposuction and breast implants.

media excludes women with disabilities. This almost total lack of representation means that the lives of disabled women remain a mystery to many able-bodied people. Disabled women are often portrayed as helpless victims who need protection, or as heroines who have beaten the odds. Because women with bodies that are disabled, fat, or old are seen as deviating from what is "normal" and desirable, we are often presented as stereotypes, rather than as real people. The crotchety old woman, the loudmouthed fat woman, and the disabled woman with a heart of gold are widespread clichés in the media. Rarely is our beauty recognized or acknowledged, and we are almost never portrayed as sexual beings.

Living with a physical disability, I have learned from the dominant messages in society that I am not like other women. In fact, for the most part, I'm actually not considered a woman at all.

The small percentage of women of color represented in the media usually conforms closely to the white beauty ideal. As one woman wrote,

As a teenager, I was obsessed with achieving the "white girl" look: slim hips, perky breasts, flat

Kinky or relaxed, in cornrows or in dreads, black women's hair gets a lot of attention, and it is not all positive. On average, African-American women spend 2 percent of our income on our hair, compared to .8 percent for white women. This isn't about vanity; it's a reasonable response to a society ruled by a white aesthetic. Black women have been fired from jobs for wearing ethnic styles like braids and cornrows to the workplace. Every day, little girls have harmful chemicals slathered on their naturally curly locks because someone has convinced their caregivers that relaxed ("straight") hair is the only acceptable option in America.

Because the beauty industry is still highly segregated, mainstream America does not know what African-American women deal with when it comes to our hair. Thankfully, as we've entered the twenty-first century, our crowning glories are no longer subjected to such rigid views. Creativity, flexibility, and pride are reentering the conversations surrounding black hair. Styles that once were deemed taboo are now being applauded and even appropriated by mainstream culture.

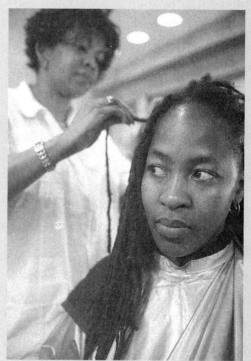

© Tanit Sakakini

A woman gets her hair braided at Quetele's Place of Beauty in Cambridge, Massachusetts.

stomach. I hated that I didn't look like white models in my magazines.

Commercial media must create a fantasy world that we hope, in some way, can become ours. Consequently, magazines, television, movies, and advertisements rarely feature women of color as their stars or on their covers: In a society that is still racist, magazine editors and Hollywood executives know that white women do not, in general, fantasize about looking Latina, black, or Asian.

Although advertising, the most powerful arm of the mass media, is all around us, many of us believe we are immune from its effects. This mistaken belief is one of the reasons it is so effective. The average American sees three thousand ads per day.[21] Almost all commercial media aimed at women are supported by advertising revenue from the fashion, beauty, diet, and food industries, and their survival depends on their ability to please their sponsors. Magazine editors, in a fierce competition for readers, know that to make a sale, they need only play on our doubts or create new ones, making us think we have "problems" that don't really exist ("What's He *Really* Thinking When He Sees You Naked?"). Every part of the female body is picked apart and scrutinized, with most articles telling us outright which products we should buy to fix—or at least camouflage—our numerous "flaws."

I believe that every woman is utterly and completely beautiful. That said, when I find myself faced with produced images of beauty in magazines or billboards, I still can't help but wish I looked like them.

In trying to understand the media's objectification of women and how it makes us feel, it can help to think of the camera lens as a white male eye. Have you noticed that the covers of women's *and* men's magazines are almost always female? The female stars of mainstream movies and TV shows not only look sexy but often behave in the

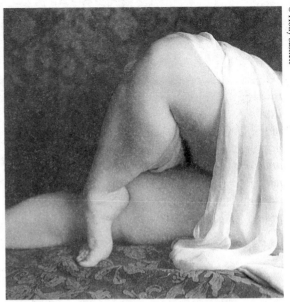

This photo was taken as part of the photographic series *Body Revisited*, a project that helps women with eating disorders gain a different perspective on their bodies. "Because I don't photograph faces, the women can step back and view themselves a little differently," says photographer Holly Sasnett.

kind of subservient, helpless way that many men find appealing. The camera eye is usually focused on women who look and act in a way that pleases men; men look (active), and women receive their gaze (passive). The media's gaze is essentially a male gaze.[22] We are so accustomed to seeing things through the dominant male perspective that we might not even notice the dynamics at play.

The media eye, in its many different forms, objectifies all of us. The result? Many of us begin to objectify ourselves. When you're in an intimate moment with your partner, do you imagine what you look like from the outside rather than focus on the sensations that you feel *inside*? When you walk down the sidewalk, are you thinking about how you appear—about how big your butt looks—instead of thinking about the beauty or stimuli around you? Self-objectification can lead to feeling self-conscious and humiliated, and it can make us believe that our bodies exist only for the pleasure of others.[23]

While making love with my partner I worried that he would see a hair here, or a flabby spot there, and be turned off. I noticed that he was never self-conscious about a skin blemish or when he gained a few pounds. So I started copying him and concentrated more on the sexual pleasure I felt. I began enjoying sex a lot more, and he noticed. He said it made him more excited, and the result? A great new circle of passion and sex.

DO I LOOK FAT?

One could sadly joke that there are two kinds of women in the United States: those who are fat, and those who are afraid of becoming fat. Our self-worth is often tied to the numbers on the bathroom scale. Since mainstream culture tells us that fat women are undesirable to men and to society in general, most of us will do anything to be thin.

Despite our national brainwashing, there is nothing inherently repulsive about fat. On the contrary, fat is inextricably linked to the female form; breasts and hips—two unmistakably female attributes—are made of fat. Women need more body fat than men, and women who are too thin do not menstruate and cannot bear children. In many cultures across the world, fat is a powerful symbol of fertility, and fat women are preferred over thin women. In the United States, men who are attracted to fat women often find themselves ridiculed.

The American obsession with thin women can be linked in many ways to women's burgeoning rights. During the 1800s, women were expected to be slightly plump.[24] But during the twentieth century, this began to change. As American women made great strides in obtaining equal rights, the pressure to be thin grew. In

the 1920s, after women gained the right to vote and were given more access to birth control, the flapper ideal took hold. Flappers dieted their way to a "boyishly slim" figure and bound their breasts to appear flat-chested.[25] The 1960s mirrored this era. As women shed the oppressiveness of the 1950s and fought for their rights, an extremely thin figure once again became popular. Epitomized by the British model Twiggy, the ideal figure was extremely thin and flat-chested.[26] The emphasis on extreme thinness persisted into the 1970s, coexisting with the feminist movement. As women seized opportunities and competed in traditionally male arenas for the first time, female characteristics like hips and breasts were deemphasized.[27]

As we've gained more rights, the cultural focus on our bodies has only grown more intense. The message seems to be that our power as women may increase, but our physical bodies must shrink. One need only call an accomplished woman "fat" to put her in her place. Making us afraid to be fat is a form of social control; we must diet and live in constant terror that we'll gain weight, or else we'll be ostracized from society. Fear of fat robs us of our pride and energy, causes conflict between women, and undermines our self-confidence.

Our current notions about weight are so pathological that even some of us who are pregnant, our bellies bulging with a growing fetus, think of ourselves as fat. Many women risk our lives to lose weight by undergoing dangerous weight loss surgery or consuming untested dietary supplements. In an attempt to shed pounds, nearly half of us are on a diet on any given day, spending almost $40 billion a year on diets that fail 95 percent of the time.[28] In one poll, over half of the women said they would rather get run over by a truck than gain 150 pounds.[29]

Girls learn quickly that fat is the ultimate F-word. Dieting and disordered eating are widespread among adolescent girls.[30] Because the thin ideal is promoted in the media primarily through images of white women, many believe that women of color do not feel the pressure to be thin, and must not suffer from poor body image. Some studies suggest that many black women and girls experience higher levels of body confidence than do women of other races.[31] Other research shows that poor body image and eating disorders affect women of all races. (For more on dieting, weight loss, and eating disorders, see Chapter 2, "Eating Well.")

African-American and Latino men seem more appreciative of bigger thighs and rounded buttocks, but beyond that, their preference for thin women seems similar to that of white men.
My female peers (black, middle-aged, and middle-class) are all on diets. They're all obsessed with weight and hair length and the importance of those things in getting a man.

Asian-American women must contend with the widespread belief that we come in only one size: petite. Another woman writes,

Many of my friends weigh less than 100 pounds and keep losing weight, yet nobody calls that anorexia because Asian women are supposed to be tiny. Doctors are subject to these stereotypes too. At my last physical I weighed 112 pounds; the doctor was shocked, as if I were fat.

Because of the intense cultural focus on body size, our feelings about our weight often get tangled up with how we feel about ourselves. "Do I look fat?" is a mantra uttered by many women, yet beneath the surface, it has little to do with weight. Researchers have found that young women often express themselves through what is called "fat talk." In such conversations, girls use self-disparaging body talk as a way to bond with their peers, with talk about weight substituted for talk about feelings. "I'm so fat" often translates to "I'm depressed" or "My life is out of control." In return, friends will usually assure the girl that she is thin, thus boosting her self-esteem. Such talk can drive some borderline girls to develop full-blown eating disorders.[32]

Though we live in a time of great sensitivity to minority concerns, blatant discrimination and ridicule of fat people is one of the last tolerated prejudices. Our national weight obsession is often cast in moral terms, making bias against fat people acceptable. Thin people are virtuous, credited with the Puritan values of self-control and self-sacrifice, while fat people are slovenly, gluttonous, and lazy.[33] Many fat people internalize these kinds of stereotypes.

Our society assumes that if we're fat, we must desperately want to be thin. Inside every fat person, it is believed, there is a thin person dying to be set free. But many women take pride in being fat and are fighting the anti-fat forces that teach us beauty comes in only one size.

I choose not to spend my life obsessing about my size. I choose not to give my money to the weight loss industry. I choose not to panic over what I eat. I choose to live.

GIRL *POWER*?

Adolescent girls are particularly susceptible to cultural messages because we are learning what it is to be adults. The combination of self-consciousness and spending power makes young people easy prey for corporations. And the beauty industry lures us when we are young—for instance, placing the same ads in *Cosmo-GIRL!* that they put in *Cosmopolitan*. During adolescence, girls gain an average of twenty-five pounds of body fat, which is necessary for proper development.[34] But in a thin-obsessed culture, it's not surprising that most teenage girls experience body anxiety and go on diets.

HOW PARENTS CAN HELP

While a certain amount of body angst is normal for all adolescents, parents can play an active role in nurturing positive body image.

- Observe your own behavior. What we teach our daughters about body image influences them more than media messages. The sad truth is that many girls learn to hate their bodies by watching and listening to their mothers diet and talk about their bodies.

- Analyze media images with your children and help them to recognize when the camera is being used as a male fantasy lens.

- Teach your daughter that power is about what dreams and goals she accomplishes, not about her looks. Help her define and act on her values and interests.

- Help girls focus on health rather than weight. Encourage fun physical activities, and cook and plan healthy meals together. Don't talk about dieting, and be aware that terms like "healthy" and "fit" are often experienced as code words for "thin."

For more tips, see "How Parents Can Help" (W2) on the companion website, www.ourbodiesourselves.org.

A clever advertising tactic that has become mainstream is to manipulate the message that many feminists have tried to promote: that girls have the power to be anything we want, including the president, if only we use our voice and ideas. Advertisers and other media have reinterpreted this idea as "Girl Power," which tells girls we can wear anything we want and no one can tell us otherwise. In this interpretation, power has nothing to do with character or achievement but is instead the result of having a perfect body and not being afraid to show it off.

Many movies and television shows feature "powerful" characters that are in-your-face, aggressive, kick-butt women. But these action heroines dress in skintight clothes, if they bother to wear any, and are almost all white and thin with big breasts. They are nothing more than male fantasy objects that Hollywood constructed, cleverly co-opting the language of feminism. The notion that sexuality and promiscuity equal power and control is particularly perilous for girls navigating our way to adulthood.

OUR BODIES GROWING OLDER

Aging is similar to adolescence in some ways. Our bodies undergo a process of transformation that is beyond our control, fraught with hormonal and physical changes. As the body we have grown comfortable with begins to gradually change, our sense of self and our body image are shaken up.

Everybody has to age, but you never realize it until it sneaks up on you and throws you for a loop. Those reading glasses are not as cute as you once thought they were when you didn't need them all the time. You find yourself inhabited by frequent feelings of invisibility in our sad, sick culture, just because you're not twenty anymore. On some days your hormones grab you by the throat and fling you around the room just for fun. But aside from all this, I must admit, I'm having a blast.

We might be surprised to learn that the body angst we thought we had left behind as a teenager has returned. The lines on our face may cause anxiety not simply because of vanity but because they force us to contemplate our changing bodies and mortality. Although many of us have spent the better part of our lives trying to avoid pregnancy, the loss of our fertility can be difficult. And sadly, many doctors are seeing an increase in eating disorders and compulsive exercise among women at midlife.[35]

Many cultures around the world value the aging process. For example, in China, the word for "teacher" translates to "old master," regardless of her age. In America, however, a youth fixation pervades our society. In a young nation obsessed with self-reinvention and all things *new*, aging is seen as a disease that must be cured—and the medical establishment and the beauty industry are only too happy to promote this idea. Ageism

BUILDING A BETTER BODY IMAGE

- If you do not see images of beauty that resemble your looks, look elsewhere. Try to travel to places where your ancestors came from, or find books, videos, or movies about those places.

- When you find yourself criticizing your looks, compliment yourself on something positive you did recently.

- If you feel the need to alter your appearance in some way, ask yourself if it is what *you* want, or if you are remaking yourself to please others.

- Cut the fat soundtrack that often accompanies meals with women. If you want a piece of chocolate cake, dig in without announcing that you'll have to go to the gym to make up for it.

- Experiment with what weight feels comfortable for you, rather than trying primarily to be thin. (For detailed information about dieting, weight, and eating disorders, see Chapter 2, "Eating Well.")

- Examine how your own behavior encourages the media's tactics. Would you buy a bottle of expensive perfume if the woman in the advertisement weren't beautiful? Do you buy video games for boys that degrade women?

- Rather than being a passive media consumer, use your purchasing power. After popular clothing retailer Abercrombie & Fitch began selling thong underwear for preteen girls, protests and threats of boycotts made them rethink their plans. Refuse to buy products from companies that exploit women and girls in their ad campaigns. Boycott movies with leading men who are twenty years older than their love interests.

- Take up a sport or other activity you've never tried before. By being physically active, we can begin to appreciate what our bodies can *do*, instead of focusing on how we *look*.

- Celebrate who you are—just the way you look!

To read more about how to construct a positive and nurturing body image, see "Building a Better Body Image" (W3) on the companion website, www.ourbodies ourselves.org.

and age discrimination are real concerns, prompting some of us to attempt to preserve a youthful appearance no matter what the cost.

As we grow older, we may feel we're becoming invisible in such a youth-obsessed culture. But if we refuse to keep quiet and play the role that society has given us, our culturally imposed attitudes about aging can evolve into something positive. As one middle-aged woman writes,

I will never lie about my age. Never. I often tell younger women how old I am, especially those who express fear about aging. I feel a responsibility to show them that I'm proud of who I am and what I've achieved in my life.

As we grow through midlife and into our later years, we may embrace the changes rather than resist them.

I look in the mirror and am always a little surprised that with my graying hair and some new wrinkles, I don't feel what I'm "supposed" to be feeling. If I were not constantly bombarded from reading, media, and society in general with reminders that now I'm supposed to be in crisis, withdrawing, feeling depressed, isolated, incapable, or ashamed, these ideas wouldn't occur to me. . . . I am, as always, energetic and involved. . . . I feel that if I dislike my aging looks, I'm denying all the wonderful parts of my life. I don't want to do that.

TAKING BACK OUR BODIES

You get only one body. Take a look at your hands, your feet, your stomach. Close your eyes and feel your breath flow in and out. This is the body that you were born with, and this is the body that you'll die with. There's no escaping it.

Observe the real-life women around you. The tremendous diversity of the female form is breathtaking. We are tall or short, lanky or curvaceous; our eyes vary in color and shape; our skin color ranges from ebony to deep brown to copper to olive to pink; our hair is many-colored and has an almost infinite range of textures.

Very few of us will ever be able to live up to the impossible standards of beauty embraced by our culture. In this way, we are all "different" from what society wants us to be, whether we are disabled or able-bodied, young or old, fat or thin. Learning to accept and love ourselves in our bodies is an important ongoing struggle and a political statement. It can take time to embrace our own beauty, or even to recognize it. The self-loathing that many of us live with each day eats away at our well-being.

I've been fat my whole life. Throughout my childhood, my teens and twenties, I hated myself. When I turned thirty, something changed in me. I decided to accept my body for what it is. Do I wish I were thinner? Yes. But I must play the cards I'm dealt. Once I decided to stop wasting so much time hating myself, I literally felt a huge weight being lifted from my shoulders. I'm much happier now.

We need to do more than love ourselves. To make change, to produce a world in which all of us are accepted, we must see ourselves as part of a community of women and how the personal decisions we make—such as whether to diet or dye our hair or get a face-lift—can affect other women. Our mission, should we accept it, is to create a future in which every woman can experience the joy of being valued completely for who she is—and what she looks like.

NOTES

1. Nancy Etcoff, *Survival of the Prettiest: The Science of Beauty* (New York: Anchor Books, 1999), 68.

2. "Past the Pink and Blue Predicament: Freeing the Next Generation from Sex Stereotypes." Girls, Inc.: 1992.

3. *The American Heritage Dictionary of the English Language,* 4th ed., 2000.

4. Christina Valhouli, "Faster Pussycat, Wax! Wax!," Salon .com (September 2, 1999).

5. Sandy Kobrin, "More Women Seek Vaginal Plastic Surgery," *Women's eNews,* November 14, 2004.

6. "One of the most radical things a woman can do is love her body." Conversation with Catherine Steiner-Adair, March 2004.

7. Euromonitor International, *Consumer USA,* 7th ed. (London: 2003), table 3.567.

8. U.S. Census Bureau, *Statistical Abstract of the United States,* 123rd ed., Washington, D.C., 2003, 794.

9. American Society of Plastic Surgeons (www.plastic surgery.org), statistics for 2003.

10. Kristen Harrison, "Television Viewers' Ideal Body Proportions: The Case of the Curvaceously Thin Woman," *Sex Roles* 48, nos. 5/6 (March 2003): 255–64.

11. Kathy Peiss, *Hope in a Jar: The Making of America's Beauty Culture* (New York: Henry Holt, 1998), 41–42.

12. Dr. S. Allen Counter, "Whitening Skin Can Be Deadly," *The Boston Globe,* December 16, 2003: C12.

13. Ed Diener, Brian Wolsie, Frank Fujita, "Physical Attractiveness and Subjective Well-Being," *Journal of Personality and Social Psychology* 69, no. 11 (July 1995): 120–29.

14. Ibid.

15. Eero Pukkala, Ilona Kulmala, Sirpa-Liisa Hovi, Elina Hemminki, Ilmo Keskimaki, Loren Lipworth, John D. Boice, Jr., and Joseph K. McLaughlin, "Causes of Death Among Finnish Women with Cosmetic Breast Implants, 1971–2001," *Annals of Plastic Surgery* 51, no. 4 (October 2003): 339–42.

16. Based on the author's interview with Alice Eagly, professor of psychology, Northwestern University.

17. Sarah K. Murnen and Mary Stockton, "Gender and Self-Reported Sexual Arousal in Response to Sexual Stimuli: A Meta-Analytic Review," *Sex Roles* 37, nos. 3/4 (August 1997): 135–51.

18. Jacqueline Lakkis, Lina A. Ricciardelli, Robert J. Williams, "Role of Sexual Orientation and Gender-Related Traits in Disordered Eating," *Sex Roles* 41, nos. 1/2 (July 1999): 1–16.

19. Etcoff, *Survival of the Prettiest,* 51.

20. Peiss, *Hope in a Jar,* 45–47.

21. Jean Kilbourne, *Deadly Persuasion: Why Women and Girls Must Fight the Addictive Power of Advertising* (New York: The Free Press, 1999), 27, 58.

22. Laura Mulvey, *Visual and Other Pleasures* (Houndsmills, Basingstroke, Hampshire: Macmillan, 1989), 19.

23. Kathrine D. Gapinski, Kelly D. Brownell, Marianne LaFrance, "Body Objectification and 'Fat Talk': Effects on Emotion, Motivation, and Cognitive Performance," *Sex Roles* 48, nos. 9/10 (May 2003): 377–78.

24. Laura Fraser, *Losing It: False Hopes and Fat Profits in the Diet Industry* (New York: Penguin, 1998), 21.

25. Ibid., 32–40.

26. Ibid., 43.

27. Ibid., 43–44.

28. National Eating Disorders Association, www.national eatingdisorders.org, accessed September 23, 2004.

29. Fraser, *Losing It,* 47.

30. John P. Foreyt, Walker S. Carlos Poston II, and G. Ken Goodrick, "Future Directions in Obesity and Eating Disorders," *Addictive Behaviors* 21, no. 6 (November–December 1996): 767–78.

31. Mimi Nichter, *Fat Talk: What Girls and Their Parents Say About Dieting* (Cambridge, MA: Harvard University Press, 2000), 159–80.

32. Mimi Nichter and Nancy Vuckovic, "Fat Talk: Body Image Among Adolescent Girls," in Nicole Sault, ed., *Many Mirrors: Body Image and Social Relations* (Piscataway, NJ: Rutgers University Press, 1994), 109–31. Also: Gapinski, Brownell, and LaFrance, "Body Objectification and 'Fat Talk' ": 378–79.

33. Fraser, *Losing It,* 53.

34. Nichter, *Fat Talk,* 7.

35. Ginia Bellafante, "When Midlife Seems Just an Empty Plate," *The New York Times,* March 9, 2003, Section 9, 1.

CHAPTER 2

Food touches every aspect of our lives. Our physical health depends on it; we cannot grow, heal, or function without it. It plays a central role in our social lives, connecting us to friends, family, history, and culture. It ties in to our emotions, nurturing as it nourishes, comforting us with memories we have attached to certain tastes. We might view food as an expression of love—a gift we give to those we cherish. Or we might see it as our enemy, a source of extra pounds that pile on with stress and fear.

Step into any standard grocery store, and you may find it hard to locate any fresh food at all. The produce section, all the way on the outside aisle, is the only place you might find food that is not in some way packaged and processed. Even in that section, your apple may have traveled thousands of miles to get to your "local" grocery store. The cornmeal you buy for your bread may or may not be genetically engineered, but since there is no mention of it on the label, you have no choice in the matter. Produce may contain harmful pesticide residues that could adversely affect your health. Since testing and oversight of pesticides are poor, you may not know the safety of the food you and your family are eating. Combine that with heaps of advertising of processed foods, all kinds of conflicting information about what constitutes a healthy diet, and constant cultural pressure to lose weight, and it becomes very difficult to separate fact from fad.

Generally, food passes from the farmer, to a distributor, to a processor, to a large grocery chain, to you. The multiple steps separate us physically and psychologically from the production of food, so we are unaware of farming practices, and it is easier to ignore the consequences of our food choices. Today under 2 percent of the population of the United States is involved in farming. This is a great change from a hundred, even fifty, years ago.[1] We may still imagine small family farms as the most important producers of food when, in fact, most of our food is produced on large factory farms by agribusiness corporations that often exploit the soil and the workers, and potentially endanger the health of their surrounding communities. Considering how fundamental food is to our lives, our lack of knowledge about its production is shocking.

In addition, due to increased international trade, more of our food is coming from other countries. Because of limitations imposed by such global entities as the World Trade Organization, some countries, including the United States, may be importing foods that do not meet existing standards, including food inspection rules (to avoid contaminated products), limits on pesticide levels, limits on the use of hormones in animals raised for meat and poultry

MYTH OR REALITY?

- *I should cut all fat from my diet because it's bad for my health.*

Myth. Fat is an important dietary nutrient. Our bodies need fat for vitamin absorption, healthy nerve development, hormonal balance, and sustained energy. Trans-fatty acids, however, are not healthy for us, and we should avoid them when possible. You can tell if a food has trans-fatty acids by looking at the ingredient list for "hydrogenated" or "partially hydrogenated" fats.

products, and similar regulations designed to reduce our exposure to harmful substances.*

Even when we know how to make good choices, we may not have enough money to eat well, or nutritious foods may be difficult to find. Many low-income communities and communities of color have fast-food restaurants and a convenience store that carries a few staples, but the nearest grocery store may be a long bus ride away. Food at the fast-food restaurants and convenience stores is usually less nutritious and more expensive than at a grocery store. This is a particular burden for families in which both parents are working long hours to make ends meet.

In addition, our increasingly complex world demands more and more time for work, leaving less time for shopping, cooking, and eating. Many of us eat on the run, relying on prepared meals, fast food, and vending machines. But our hectic lifestyles can have drastic effects on our

* For more details about this problem, see "The WTO Comes to Dinner. U.S. Implementation of Trade Rules Bypasses Food Safety Requirements," at www.citizen.org/documents/PCfoodsafety.pdf (by Public Citizen's Global Trade Watch, 2003).

health. Diabetes rates have more than doubled since 1980,[2] and many women continue to die of heart disease. It may be surprising to hear that in a country that has high rates of obesity, many people are undernourished. This happens because even though we may eat a large enough *quantity* of food, the *quality* is so poor that our bodies become deficient in the nutrients we need for good health.

We can take action to protect our own health, but it takes time, energy, and resources to make good choices about what we eat.

My biggest challenge is finding enough time in the day to get food that is healthy, prepare it, and then to remember it's in my fridge! I cope with this by simplifying: If I don't have time to make a salad, I just put all the ingredients in a bag and take it with me.

As an institutional chef at a home for troubled teenagers, I feel a profound sadness that people don't know what food tastes like anymore. People's taste buds have been poisoned by growing up eating exclusively processed and fast foods; they are trained to only appreciate neon-flavored reformulated meat foods like chicken nuggets. My understanding is that all the natural flavors and vitamins are lost in the industrial cooking process, and they are added back in with varying degrees of success. I no longer understand the nutritional value of things like this that are called food.

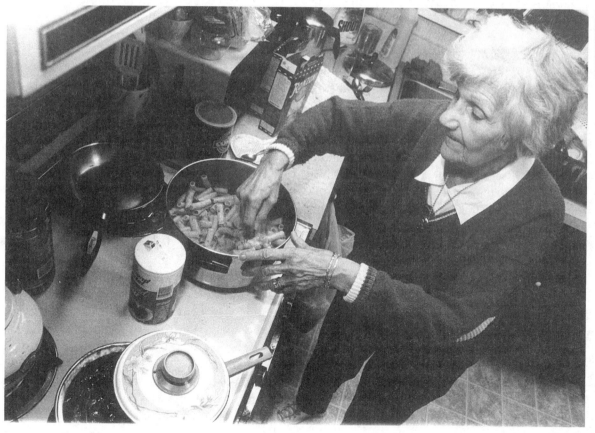

© Donna Alberico

WHAT IS A HEALTHY DIET?

In these times, there seem to be as many "healthy diets" as there are experts. While our specific dietary needs may vary according to our individual body types, metabolisms, and genetics, there are some basic guidelines that can be useful in determining which foods are nutritious and which are not.

1. *Eat whole foods.* A whole food is a plant or animal product that remains as close as possible to its natural state. It is unprocessed, unrefined, and contains greater nutritional value than its factory-made alternatives. For instance, a piece of fresh fruit offers fiber that is missing from fruit juice or sugary fruit drinks; real cheddar is a great source of calcium without the unhealthy additives and colorings of processed American cheese.

A perfect example of the difference between whole and processed foods is the case of whole-grain wheat versus white flour. To make the white flour you see in white bread and most baked goods, the manufacturer takes a whole-wheat berry through a series of steps. First, machines strip the germ and the bran from the outer section of the grain, removing fiber, B vitamins, and other important nutrients. The remaining part of the grain—the nutritionally poor endosperm—is then milled into flour, which removes further nutrients in the process. Humans need these nutrients to digest and absorb vitamins and minerals; when we don't get them from our food, we take them from our bodies' reserves. Because extreme deficiencies of certain B vitamins are associated with diseases of malnutrition, the manufacturers "enrich" the flour by adding back synthetic versions of a few selected nutrients, like thiamine (vitamin B_1), riboflavin (vitamin B_2), and folic acid. But these nutrients alone may not be enough to keep our bodies strong, and eventually, the reserves can become depleted.

Whole foods are also an excellent source of potassium, a mineral that works together with sodium to maintain balanced fluid levels in our cells. To do this properly, our bodies must always have anywhere from two to six times as much potassium as sodium (experts disagree on the precise ratio). All fresh fruits and vegetables contain high levels of potassium. Because it is found abundantly in almost all whole foods, our bodies have evolved to easily process and excrete potassium. Sodium, on the other hand, is hard to come by in whole foods (have you ever eaten a salty apple?). As a result, our bodies have evolved to hoard sodium. Food processing almost always increases sodium and decreases potassium. Thus, a diet heavy in processed foods can threaten our sodium/potassium balance, which can lead to high blood pressure, edema, kidney disease, and low energy.

Now that I'm in my eighties I want to try to be well. I'm very keen on soups these days. I make my own so I can control the sodium content. When I use canned soup I add an equal amount of water to reduce the sodium in each portion.

2. *Emphasize fruits and vegetables.* Fruits and vegetables are high in antioxidants—nutrients that help neutralize toxins in the body. Generally, brightly colored fruits and vegetables contain the highest levels of antioxidants: for example, yellow, orange, and dark green vegetables; citrus fruits; and cruciferous vegetables (those in the cabbage family, such as broccoli, cauliflower, Brussels sprouts, and cabbage). While taking antioxidants in supplement form can be beneficial, those found in foods are much more powerful.

Fruits and vegetables are also high in other vitamins and minerals. Vitamin C, which is supportive to the immune system, is abundant in strawberries, oranges, and bell peppers. Carrots, sweet potatoes, and winter squash are a powerhouse of beta-carotene, which is important for vision. Green leafy vegetables support the health of our bones and teeth, among other things, with high levels of calcium, magnesium, and vitamin K.

In addition to the protection they offer us from disease, fruits and vegetables are essential for our daily bodily functions. Fiber from fruits, vegetables, grains, and legumes helps us digest and move food through our system. The amount of time this takes is called *bowel transit time* (BTT). The ideal BTT is a point of disagreement among experts, but eighteen to thirty hours is considered safe and healthy. A transit time that is too short may not allow your body to absorb nutrients adequately, while a BTT that is too long will allow your body to reabsorb toxins and used hormones that were on the way out. These toxins and hormones then return to your bloodstream and may cause problems, from joint and muscle pains to hormone imbalances. It is normal to have one to three bowel movements per day. If you are not having at least one bowel movement per day, you should consider increasing your fiber intake through the foods mentioned above. (If you are having more than three bowel movements per day, this may be a sign of a serious condition; consult your health care provider.)

Some helpful guidelines to follow: Eat two to four pieces of fresh fruit daily, and fill half your plate with vegetables at any given meal. The graphic on this page may help you to envision what that looks like.

3. *Eat the amount and combination of whole foods that make you feel best.* There are many different approaches to healthy eating. If you feel good eating a high-protein diet with lots of nonstarchy vegetables and few carbohydrates, it may be the best diet for you. However, if you feel best

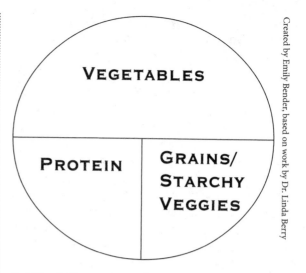

Created by Emily Bender, based on work by Dr. Linda Berry

By filling half your plate with vegetables at meals, in addition to including protein, carbohydrates, and fats, you ensure that you are getting enough vegetables without having to count servings. Well-balanced meals will also help you maintain steady blood sugar throughout the day.

eating a diet high in grains, vegetables, and beans, that may be the best diet for you.

I was a vegetarian for 12 years, thinking that it was the best thing for my health. By the end of that time I was sick and depleted. I reluctantly added meat back into my diet, little by little. It made such a difference, but I still felt sick a lot of the time. I found out that I was sensitive to gluten, so I eliminated that, which helped more, but I still had lots of intestinal discomfort. A couple of years ago I started trying the specific carbohydrate diet, which has totally changed my life. Eliminating all grains, sugar, and some other starchy foods, and focusing my diet on organic meats, cheeses, and lots of fruits and veggies made my intestinal pain disappear within a week. It was miraculous.

4. *Eat local, seasonal organic foods if possible.* The cost and availability of organic foods varies widely depending on your geographic location, so this is not an option for everyone. However, if

organic foods are available, they are almost always a healthier option. Organic farmers constantly replenish the nutrients in their soil to maintain the health and disease resistance of their plants. This allows them to avoid using potentially harmful chemicals, and as a result, their fruits and vegetables contain higher levels of nutrients and fewer toxic chemicals such as pesticides.[3] Buying fruits and vegetables that are local and seasonal is also a wise food choice, for several reasons. The money you spend supports local farmers and stays in the local economy. Knowing where your food comes from and how it is grown gives you safer food choices. And because locally grown produce is generally picked at the peak of ripeness and eaten soon afterward, it is packed with nutrients and tastes great. Look for a local farmers' market in your area by going to www.ams.usda.gov/farmersmarkets/. (For more information, see "Supporting Better Farming Practices" [W4] on the companion website, www.ourbodiesourselves.org.)

Animals that are grass-fed and/or raised on organic foods (and all the products those animals produce) seem to have superior nutritional profiles.[4] In addition, studies have shown that children who grow up eating organic foods have lower levels of toxic chemicals in their bodies than those raised eating conventional foods.[5]

If finances prevent you from choosing all organic foods, you might simply make organic substitutes for the foods most likely to contain pesticide residues: meat, eggs, and dairy products, all of which contain fat. Most pesticides are made from petroleum, which is an oil, and therefore dissolve and store most easily in fats (they are fat-soluble). For more information on pesticides and hormone-disrupting chemicals in the food supply, see Chapter 7, "Environmental and Occupational Health." In addition, the Environmental Working Group (www.ewg.org), a nonprofit advocacy group, found that the following fruits and vegetables contain the highest residues: apples, bell peppers, blueberries, celery,

cherries, grapes (imported), nectarines, peaches, pears, potatoes, red raspberries, spinach, and strawberries. Conversely, the following foods were found to have the lowest pesticide residue levels: asparagus, avocados, bananas, broccoli, cauliflower, corn (sweet), kiwi, mangoes, onions, papaya, pineapples, and peas (sweet).

THE MACRONUTRIENTS

To better understand how the body uses foods, it is helpful to know how the various components of food function to keep us going.

A NOTE ABOUT FISH

Fish and shellfish can be an important part of a healthy diet, since they contain high-quality protein and beneficial fats. The omega-3 fatty acids found in cold-water fish are called *essential fatty acids*—we need to get them from foods because our bodies cannot manufacture them. Unfortunately some fish also contain high levels of mercury and other toxins. The U.S. Environmental Protection Agency (www.epa.gov/waterscience/fishadvice/advice.html) advises women of childbearing age and young children to abstain from shark, swordfish, king mackerel, and tilefish to avoid mercury poisoning. Fresh tuna also contains high levels of mercury. Canned tuna should be eaten no more than once a week; light tuna often has less mercury than albacore. Mercury can cross the placenta of pregnant women and affect the neural development of the fetus. In addition, it can be passed to an infant through breast milk. The Environmental Working Group website www.ewg.org provides an excellent and more comprehensive list of fish that may be unsafe to eat.

Macronutrients—namely proteins, carbohydrates, and fats—are our bodies' basic building blocks. We need them in large quantities simply to survive.

PROTEIN

Proteins are composed of molecules called amino acids, which, when joined in different combinations, make up most of the tissues in our bodies: muscles, organs, skin, nails, and hair, for example. They also make up many of the biochemicals, like enzymes and hormones, which help our bodies grow, heal, digest, and detoxify. There are twenty-three amino acids in the human body, nine of which are essential. Animal sources of protein—such as eggs, dairy products, and meat—contain all nine essential amino acids. Plant sources of proteins—such as beans, nuts, and seeds—lack some of the essential amino acids. Eating a variety of plant proteins throughout the day can assure that our bodies obtain all the essential amino acids we need. Individual needs for protein can vary greatly depending on age, activity level, genetics, or chronic/acute illness. Those of us who do not meet our bodies' need for protein through our diet can experience symptoms of protein deficiency, which include: weakness, poor muscle tone, fatigue, dry and brittle hair and nails, slow wound healing, weakened immune system, blood sugar imbalances, and even depression.

CARBOHYDRATES

Carbohydrates provide the most direct energy to our cells. They can be simple (as in sugars) or complex (as in vegetables and grains) and are readily broken down into glucose, the energy for our cells. Whole-carbohydrate foods such as fruits, vegetables, and whole grains are also good sources of fiber; refined carbohydrates in products made with white flour or white sugar, such as cookies, crackers, bagels, or pasta, do not con-

ENJOY YOUR EGGS!

Although eggs used to be considered an ideal protein source, in the past three decades they have been wrongly accused of contributing to heart disease. As a result, some people have switched to eating only low-fat egg whites or using egg substitutes. Here's why people in good general health can go ahead and eat the whole egg, up to about seven eggs a week:

- Eggs are a nutrient-dense food, providing high levels of nutrients relative to the number of calories.

- Egg yolks are one of the only food sources of vitamin D.

- Egg yolks contain significant amounts of vitamin A, riboflavin, phosphorus, folic acid, selenium, and calcium. They also provide zinc, iron, vitamin B_6, vitamin B_{12}, and vitamin E.

- Egg yolks from free-range chickens fed organic diets high in essential fatty acids contain heart-healthy omega-3 fatty acids—more than eggs from chickens in conventional factories.

- Egg yolks also contain choline, which contributes to healthy brain development *in utero.*[6]

tain fiber. They do, however, provide quick sources of concentrated energy. The problem is that eating refined carbohydrates (in the form of sugar or starch) causes blood sugar to spike quickly, which prompts your body to release insulin, a hormone that escorts the blood sugars into the cells for energy. You may then feel a "crash" within one to three hours. Symptoms of low blood sugar can include fatigue, difficulty concentrating, anxiety, depression, headaches, and feeling shaky or irritable. Any energy that is not used right away is stored in the body as fat. In addition, as blood sugar falls, the body craves more sugar to keep going. Eating more carbohydrates to fill this craving begins the cycle again. Over time, this cycle can lead to insulin resistance, in which the cells become less sensitive to insulin, which in turn leads to weight gain, because the body cannot efficiently use the foods we eat. More body fat can lead to even more insulin resistance, which is a precursor to diabetes and is associated with cardiovascular disease.

FATS

Fats have been much maligned in the past thirty years, but they are essential nutrients. Fat makes you feel full, and it makes things taste good. In addition, our bodies need the fat in foods to absorb vitamins like vitamin A for healthy skin and eyes; vitamins D and K for healthy bones and blood; and vitamin E for its antioxidant properties. Fats from whole foods—such as those found in dairy products, nuts, seeds, meats, and fish—contribute to healthy nerve development, hormonal balance, and sustained energy.

There are three main types of natural fats: saturated, monounsaturated, and polyunsaturated. These names come from the fats' chemical structures; fat molecules are called *saturated,* or chemically complete, when all the carbon molecules in a chain are bonded with hydrogen molecules. *Monounsaturated fats,* such as olive and canola oils, have only one open space where a hydrogen atom could have bonded. *Polyunsaturated fats,* such as corn, safflower, sunflower, and soybean oils, have many open spaces in their chemical structure.

One kind of fat that we know is unhealthy is trans-fatty acid, also known as hydrogenated fat. Trans fats are unsaturated fats with hydrogen molecules synthetically added to their chemical structure to increase their shelf life and solidify them at room temperature. In the process, the fat molecules take on a chemical shape that the body is unable to recognize, process, and digest. Thus, the trans-fatty acids circulate in the body and cause damage. Like natural fats, these trans fats can become part of our cell walls, creating rigid and unhealthy cells. Trans-fatty acids are frequently found in commercial baked goods and processed foods. It is best to avoid foods that list "hydrogenated" and "partially hydrogenated" in the ingredients list.

Standard nutritional advice recommends limiting saturated fats, because they are believed to contribute to high blood cholesterol levels, which are linked to heart disease. However, most studies that have shown a connection between saturated fats and heart disease did not distinguish between saturated fats and trans fats, which we now know are damaging to health. Further research is needed to fully understand the dietary risk factors for heart disease.

DIFFERENT MODELS FOR HEALTHY EATING

THE USDA FOOD GUIDE PYRAMID

Because some of the most common diseases in the United States are associated with diet, the government has developed guidelines for healthy eating. They are commonly displayed in the simple graphic "The USDA Food Guide Pyramid."

The pyramid is based on the USDA publication "Nutrition and Your Health: Dietary Guidelines for Americans." This document is updated every five years, most recently in 2000. Here are the guidelines:

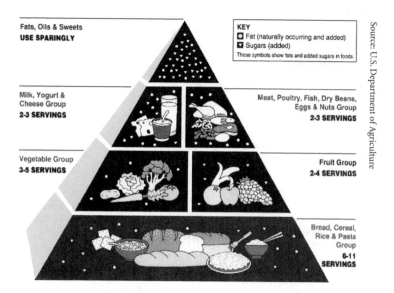

Source: U.S. Department of Agriculture

USDA Food Guide Pyramid

1. *Aim for fitness*
   a. Aim for a healthy weight.
   b. Be physically active each day.

2. *Build a Healthy Base*
   a. Let the pyramid guide your food choices.
   b. Choose a variety of different grains daily, especially whole grains.
   c. Choose a variety of fruits and vegetables daily.
   d. Keep foods safe to eat.

3. *Choose Sensibly*
   a. Choose a diet that is low in saturated fat and cholesterol and moderate in total fat.
   b. Choose beverages and foods to moderate your intake of sugars.
   c. Choose and prepare foods with less salt.
   d. If you drink alcoholic beverages, do so in moderation.

PROBLEMS WITH THE USDA MODEL

The food guide pyramid offers consumers an easy-to-read graphic that encourages a healthy diet and regular exercise. However, it falls short in a number of areas. To begin with, it does not separate whole foods from processed foods; nor does it distinguish between different kinds of fats. Equating natural fats and oils with sugary dessert foods in the "eat sparingly" section at the top of the pyramid is misleading: Dessert and sugar are optional treats, while fat is an essential nutrient. Second, the amount of fruits and vegetables listed is only the minimum one needs. The pyramid does not acknowledge that some individuals may both need, and thrive upon, a diet that contains the same ingredients in differing proportions. Finally, the guidelines on fitness fail to acknowledge that one can be healthy at many different weights. The group that creates guidelines is heavily lobbied by representatives from the food industry, which tries to influence the process to maximize profits.

At this writing, the committee revising the 2005 guidelines is still at work. The proposed revisions suggest that Americans should be including more fish and fiber in our diets and

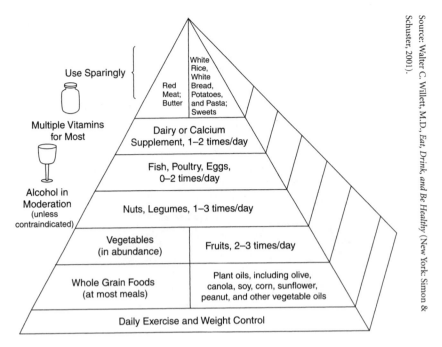

Source: Walter C. Willett, M.D., *Eat, Drink, and Be Healthy* (New York: Simon & Schuster, 2001).

Healthy Eating Pyramid

should focus on exercise. They suggest eating more dark green and orange vegetables and more whole grains, and increasing intake of vitamins A, C, D, and E, as well as folate, calcium, magnesium, potassium, and zinc.[7] For the most up-to-date version of the USDA Food Guide Pyramid, go to www.usda.gov/cnpp/dietary_guidelines.html.

THE HEALTHY EATING PYRAMID

Many highly regarded organizations and professionals have criticized the USDA's recommended eating guidelines. Primary among them is a group of nutritionists at the Harvard School of Public Health, who developed their own pyramid from evidence-based lab studies and research on how people eat in the real world. This Healthy Eating Pyramid offers a significant improvement over the USDA guidelines. The main components are listed in ascending order up the pyramid:

1. Exercise and weight management
2. Whole-grain foods at most meals
3. Plant oils
4. Vegetables in abundance and fruits 2–3 times per day
5. Fish, poultry, and eggs 0–2 times per day for protein
6. Nuts and legumes 1–3 times per day
7. Dairy or a calcium supplement 1–2 times per day
8. Red meat and butter (use sparingly)
9. Refined grains, flours, sugars, and sweets (use sparingly)

In addition, this pyramid cites practices that can increase health: taking multivitamins to assure adequate nutrient intake and drinking alcohol in moderation. (Please note that if you have or a family member has a history of alcoholism, alcohol should be consumed with caution or not at all.)

This pyramid clarifies the importance of

whole foods and fruits and vegetables in maintaining good health. In addition, it acknowledges the importance of fats in the diet, although it recommends restricting the use of saturated fats such as red meat and butter. Unfortunately, the pyramid lists weight management as the first item, which implies that we should prioritize weight loss over other goals such as healthy food choices.

MAKING CHANGES

Changing our diets can be challenging. Some of us can make quick, drastic changes, but most of us need to take smaller steps to assure that we stick with them. Here are some tips that may help you to make changes in your eating patterns.

1. *Practice first.* For example, when you're making oatmeal for the first few times, have a favorite alternative around, in case the oatmeal doesn't come out to your liking. Learning how to cook a new food may take some trial and error.

2. *Eat breakfast.* Eating a substantial breakfast may prevent the midmorning crash that can set off the cravings for sugar and stimulants like coffee. Try whole-grain breads and cereals, free-range eggs, greens, fresh fruits, yogurts, and nuts and seeds. This may require some additional planning, but the food doesn't have to take a long time to prepare. If you make a pot of whole grains—such as brown rice, quinoa, or rye—when you have time to cook, make enough to last three meals. Then all you have to do is heat up the grains in the morning and add some nuts or seeds, milk, yogurt, fruit, etc.

3. *Modify your snacks.* Many of us get hungry midmorning or midafternoon when there is no provision for a meal. If we don't plan for these cravings, then when we *are* hungry and our en-ergy flags, we reach for the most convenient choices: baked goods made with refined flour, candy bars, coffee. None of these foods gives us the sustained energy or the nutrients we need to get through the day. Try planning ahead, and have some nutritious snacks available: a sandwich on whole-grain bread, celery, carrots or apples with nut butter, or plain yogurt with fruits and nuts.

4. *Plan lunch and dinner.* You can begin by doing this just once a week. Plan for a vegetable, a protein food, a starchy vegetable or whole grain, and maybe some nuts and seeds or cheese to add some healthy fat.

5. *After you have practiced and made the above changes, stock your kitchen with fewer processed*

YOUR WHOLE-FOODS
SHOPPING LIST

Grains—try some new ones: brown basmati rice, amaranth, quinoa, kasha (buckwheat)

Lentils and beans

Fresh fruits

Fresh vegetables

Frozen vegetables for when fresh ones aren't available

Poultry, fish

Beef, pork, lamb, buffalo, ostrich, duck, and other meats

Seeds, nuts, and nut butters

Dairy products—cheese, yogurt, milk, etc.

Free-range eggs

SHOPPING WISELY

Supermarkets plan their layouts to slow you down and encourage buying. If you understand how stores are laid out, it can help you be a wise shopper.

1. Outside aisles carry the freshest, most healthy food items; inside aisles carry the more processed, high-sugar, high-fat items.
2. End-of-aisle displays—great savings items—can entice you to buy less nutritious foods.
3. Products advertised most often are less nutritious.
4. Expensive, low-nutrient choices are placed at eye level to catch your attention.

foods. When your pantry and refrigerator contain whole grains, beans, lentils, whole-grain breads, dried fruits, nuts and seeds, broths, fresh fruits and vegetables, unprocessed meats, organic dairy products, and eggs, anything you grab will serve you nutritionally.

VEGETARIANISM

Vegetarian diets exclude meat, fish, and poultry. The most popular version is the lacto-ovo vegetarian diet, which includes dairy products (*lacto*) and eggs (*ovo*). Another is the vegan diet, which eliminates all types of animal products, including dairy products and eggs. A well-planned, varied vegetarian diet can support healthy body functioning.

I've eaten a low-carb vegetarian diet for the last five years. It has helped me regulate my hypo-

READING LABELS

1. Read the ingredients. The ingredients are listed by weight in order of the amounts used in preparation: Products use the greatest quantity of the first ingredient and the least of the last. Most packaged foods are now required to have full ingredient labeling.
2. Check the serving size. All of the nutrient information on the label is based on the serving size, so if you eat the equivalent of two servings, you will receive double the amount of nutrients listed on the label.
3. *Percent daily value* guidelines are determined by the FDA specifically for use on food labels. They tell us the percent of a day's worth of fat, sodium, etc., provided by the food in the context of a 2,000-calorie diet. Simple advice: If a food has 20 percent or more of the daily value, it is high in that nutrient; "low" means no more than 5 percent. There are many nutrients not included on this list, since it is only a simple guidance tool.
4. *Calories from fat* helps you determine the fat content of a food. Fat, saturated fat, and fiber are listed in grams and as a percent daily value; sugars are listed in grams only.
5. *Enriched* means that some of the nutrients removed during processing have been replaced to approximate the levels found in the original food.[8] However, other vitamins and minerals and fiber in whole grains are not restored to such foods as enriched flour, breads, and pasta.
6. *Fortified* means that nutrients have been added. These nutrients, such as

iodine in salt or calcium in fruit drinks, may not normally be found in the food. They may be added in amounts greater than those that naturally occur, such as the large quantities of synthetic vitamins and minerals added to breakfast cereals.

7. Although the labeling must be truthful, a product's advertising can be misleading. Nutrient content descriptions such as "free," "low," "lean," or "light" require a bit of research to interpret correctly. In addition, "cholesterol-free," "light," or "100 percent natural" on a label may disguise that the product is still high in trans fats and sugar.

8. On cans, look at how weight is listed. "Net weight" includes any liquid used for packing. "Drained" or "filled" weight tells you what the actual food weighs.

9. Check the date to see how fresh the food is.

10. If you need more information, write to the manufacturer or distributor. The name and address must be on the label.

glycemia, improve my brainpower, and have more energy.

I don't feel like my health has changed since I became vegan. The hardest thing about it is how so many meat eaters feel compelled to pick fights with me—even though I never bring the subject up.

Those of us who are vegetarians must pay special attention to our intake of two essential nutrients: protein and vitamin B_{12}. Eating a variety of foods, with a focus on protein-rich plant foods such as beans, lentils, nuts, and seeds, as well as dairy and eggs for the non-vegan, will help assure that we get enough protein.[9] Foods from plant sources contain limited amounts of any one essential amino acid. For instance, beans are low in the essential amino acid methionine but high in lysine, while rice is high in methionine but low in lysine. Eating a range of these foods throughout the day increases their protein quality. Vitamin B_{12} is not found in plant products. Women who eat few or no animal products should take a supplement containing vitamin B_{12} to prevent deficiency.

Most children, adolescents, pregnant women, and nursing mothers need to be especially careful to get enough nutrients—particularly protein, calcium, zinc, folic acid, and iron—and sufficient calories to support their special developmental and growth needs. Depending on our individual nutritional needs, metabolism, and genetics, some of us may need animal products to feel our best. If you are concerned that your diet is not meeting your needs, consult a nutritionist or other person knowledgeable about vegetarianism or veganism.

NUTRITIONAL SUPPLEMENTS

Whole foods are always the best sources of nutrients in their most absorbable form. Supplements, however, may be useful.

Commercial agricultural practices and factory farming in the past fifty to sixty years have depleted our soil of vital nutrients. Since the foods we eat derive their nutrients from the soil, it is harder than ever to get all the nutrients we need from food. As mentioned earlier, organically grown foods provide higher nutrient values, but even those foods may not be as nutritious as they once were due to long-term soil depletion. Add to that the thousands of miles many foods travel before they reach our tables. Most fruits and vegetables begin to lose nutritional value soon after they are harvested. For this rea-

WHAT ARE THE RDIS AND WHAT DO THEY MEAN?

The U.S. RDI (reference daily intake), the new name for the U.S. RDA (recommended daily allowance) for vitamins and minerals, was developed to help people avoid diseases of malnutrition like scurvy and rickets. With the exception of calcium, the RDIs for nutrients are the *minimum, not the optimal* amounts required to prevent those diseases. In most cases, there is no danger in eating greater levels of nutrients than those defined in the RDI. In fact, getting your nutrients from foods almost never causes harm.

There are cases in which taking a very high dose of a nutrient in supplement form can be dangerous, such as birth defects caused by pregnant women taking more than 10,000 IUs of *supplemental* vitamin A; but most nutrients are safe in doses higher than the RDI.

Because we know so much about the importance of calcium for building healthy bones, the RDI reflects an amount closer to the optimal intake of this mineral.

son, taking a daily multivitamin can help you get the optimal amounts of nutrients in your body.

There is a dizzying array of nutritional supplements available to consumers in health food stores, grocery stores, pharmacies, and directly from health care providers. Each woman has individualized needs for nutrients at different times in her life: During pregnancy, for example, women have increased needs for most nutrients, especially iron, folic acid, and calcium. The best way to choose nutritional supplements is to consult a nutritionist or a dietitian who is knowledgeable about supplements.

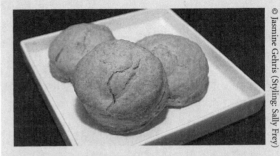

Whole-grain scone

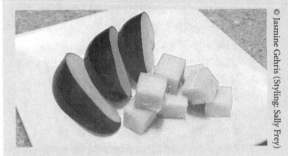

Apple slices and cheese

WHICH SNACK IS HEALTHIER?

Around three P.M., with lunch a distant memory, many of us reach for a snack to quell our hunger pains and give us energy. While both of the snacks pictured above would be a healthier choice than a bag of potato chips or a doughnut, the apple slices with cheese are the better option of the two. The whole-grain scone may seem healthy on the surface, but it actually provides little to no protein, lots of sugars, few vitamins and minerals, and possibly even hydrogenated fats. The apple slices and cheese, on the other hand, provide fiber, vitamins, and minerals from the apple, and protein and fat from the cheese. It's the kind of snack that keeps your blood sugar balanced and provides you with the nutrients you need to get through the day.

There are many types of supplements available. Some people may benefit from supplements made from whole-food concentrates, with all the synergistic food factors still intact. Look for supplements that do not contain sugars, starches, artificial colors and flavors, or other unnecessary ingredients.

HELPING KIDS EAT WELL

In our busy lives we may think that fast foods are the only way to provide our children with quick and convenient meals and snacks. In addition, children are constantly bombarded with advertising images of highly processed, less nutritious foods. Creating appealing alternatives can be a challenge.

Though we do not have a television, other kids at school talk about prepared foods that are "cool." These foods are enticing at times to my son, but he enjoys his healthy lunch with all-organic foods, whole fruit, a sandwich on whole-grain bread with a good source of protein, and a health bar.

When my kids want to eat candy, I look at the ingredients. If it has synthetic colors, I say. "That has paint in it," and they say, "Yuck!" or I'll say, "That's the kind of food that makes your tummy ache."

The most important step we can take in encouraging our children to eat well is to eat well ourselves. Stock your kitchens with nutritious choices: fresh fruits and vegetables, nut butters, hummus, yogurt, cheeses, whole-grain breads, and the like. Children appreciate the opportunity to make their own choices about food. If all the choices available are healthy, children have lots of autonomy when it comes to eating what they like. You can also make healthy foods more fun by preparing them creatively. For example, cutting vegetables into interesting shapes and

EASY, NUTRITIOUS SNACKS FOR KIDS—AND ADULTS, TOO

Peanut butter and banana sandwich on whole-grain bread

Celery with almond butter and raisins

Granola with plain yogurt or milk

Apple slices with slices of cheese

Smoothies with yogurt and fruit

Leftover chicken with crunchy veggies

Nuts and dried fruits

serving them with a yogurt-based dip makes them seem like a fun food adventure. Many children enjoy eating with their fingers, and fresh fruits and veggies make great finger food.

It is important to let kids decide when they are hungry and when they are full, so they learn to trust their own sense of hunger and satiety. Helping them to trust themselves teaches them an important lesson they can use in regulating their eating throughout their lives.

Talking to your kids about food and involving them in growing, buying, and preparing foods can develop their interest in the foods they eat. Have them read product labels for you in the supermarket. Try to find a small space, even if you are in the city, to grow something. Have older kids take turns at cooking meals. Even a three-year-old can chop soft vegetables with a table knife, spread nut butters, help mix batters, or add ingredients to almost any recipe.

At dinnertime we have a ritual of saying something we appreciate about the day. We often recognize the farmer, the animal, the land, and the water for making it possible for us to have this nourishing food.

FOOD AT SCHOOL

Once children are in school, what they eat is influenced by what is available in the school cafeteria and what other children bring in their lunches. In 1996 the U.S. Department of Agriculture (USDA) mandated that school meals meet new dietary guidelines: Each meal should consist of no more than 30 percent overall fat and 10 percent saturated fat, and should contain reduced amounts of salt and sugar. There is no emphasis, however, on whole foods.

One of the most disturbing trends in the past decade is the infiltration of fast-food and soda companies into the schools. Many schools have accepted lucrative contracts for soda and snack vending machines and fast-food lunches in their cafeterias. In addition, twelve thousand schools nationwide have adopted Channel One, a twelve-minute news program by Primedia that contains two minutes of advertisements, largely for candy, soda, and other processed and packaged foods.[10]

Grassroots efforts nationwide are promoting more nutritious school lunches. One way to influence the selection of foods offered in your child's school is to become involved in school activities, and to advocate for healthy foods at school events, fundraisers, and in vending machines. Some schools have found that implementing healthier nutrition policies reduces behavior problems and improves academic performance.[11] The Centers for Disease Control and Prevention (CDC) has developed a guide for schools to help them develop schoolwide nutrition policies. Both the USDA and CDC guidelines are available on the Internet: www.fns.usda.gov/tn/Healthy/changing.html and www.cdc.gov/nccdphp/dash/SHI/index.htm.

I tell my four-year-old that some foods help him grow better than others, and he wants to grow as fast as he can.

DIETING

Television, billboards, fashion magazines, and even medical information often encourage us to internalize weight-based stereotypes. Modeling agencies consider size 10 to be "plus size," though the average American woman wears a size 12. We often hear advertisements enticing us to be good (eat salad) or be bad (eat cake), as if our worth as individuals can be measured by the foods we choose. Even medical and insurance charts listing heights and weights do not take into consideration the natural variations in body size. As a result, food often elicits feelings of guilt, indulgence, and fear.

Whenever someone brings cupcakes or doughnuts into the office, none of the women can eat without saying "I'm so bad" or "I didn't have lunch today, so I'm really hungry" or "I'll have to go to the gym tonight!" Why must we always comment on food? Men don't do that.

Commercial diet schemes prey on Americans' obsession with weight, often targeting—and perpetuating—women and young girls' body image insecurities. The over $40 billion diet industry[12] is based on failure; the more we flounder, the more likely we are to purchase another product, book, or diet scheme. Nonetheless, 50 million Americans are dieting at any given moment.[13] (For more information on dieting and body image, see Chapter 1, "Body Image.")

LOW-CALORIE DIETING

This is the most well known and most practiced of all the diets out there. It is also one of the most unhealthy. Used by women on our own and by well-known diet companies such as Weight Watchers, Jenny Craig, and the Diet Center, this method of calorie deprivation sometimes borders on starvation and cannot be sustained over a long period of time. In their attempt to hook customers, many diet programs create very low-calorie food plans that result in drastic weight loss within the first few weeks. Our bodies interpret this as famine and slow down metabolism so that we can survive on fewer calories. Therefore, when we start eating a normal number of calories again, we process them more slowly and actually gain weight. This, in turn, can lead to a dangerous cycle of yo-yo dieting—further caloric restriction, more slowing of metabolism, and even greater weight gain. This leaves us feeling as if we have failed, and can make us fatter than we would have been if we had never dieted at all.

HIGH-CARBOHYDRATE, LOW-FAT DIETS

This style of eating without caloric restriction may be healthy for some individuals who can tolerate high amounts of carbohydrates in their diets. As with any nutritious diet, the carbohydrates should come primarily from fruits, vegetables, and whole grains. Often, however, people attempt to replace fats with highly refined, sugar-containing foods. Instead of eating two eggs, greens, and whole-wheat toast with butter for breakfast, we might go for a white-flour bagel with jam. The bagel breakfast may be lower in calories and provide for quick energy, but it lacks the nutrient value and sustaining power of the egg breakfast.

HIGH-PROTEIN, LOW-CARB DIETS

A high-protein, low-carbohydrate diet will usually promote weight loss without calorie restriction. However, many people take the "I can eat as much protein and fat as I want" message to mean: "I can eat nothing but bacon and steak and be healthy." Every diet needs to include lots of fruits and vegetables to be healthy. In fact, many people who benefit from these high-protein diets might feel just as good by simply eliminating the refined and processed foods without cutting *all* carbohydrates. Beware of the aggressive marketing of certain brands of nutrition bars and cookies and mixes that claim to be healthy for these high-protein diets. The majority of these products contain synthetic nutrients, hydrogenated oils, and artificial flavoring, coloring, and sweeteners.

Many people believe that weight loss is just a

ARTIFICIAL "FOODS"

In our quest to eat less sugar, less fat, fewer carbs, or fewer calories, many of us turn to artificial sweeteners and fake fats. Products such as Nutrasweet (aspartame), Splenda (sucralose), and Olestra (an artificial fat) have all been approved by the FDA under great pressure from the food industry, at least once against expert recommendation. Because they have been used for such a short time, we really don't understand their long-term effects on human health. For more information, see "Fake Sugars and Fake Fats" (W5) on the companion website, www.ourbodiesourselves.org.

matter of calories eaten versus calories burned, but actually, our weights are determined by a complex web of factors. Our genetic makeup, food allergies, and the quality of the food we eat all play a role in our weight.

GENETIC MAKEUP

Human beings naturally vary in body shape and size. Some of us have large frames, while others of us have small frames. If most of the women in our family are heavy, we may have a genetic predisposition to be larger.

I am a large woman, and I come from a family of generally large women. My mother was heartbroken that I was following in the family tradition of obesity and did everything she could to "help," one year giving me a blender and Slim-Fast for Christmas.

The foods that our ancestors ate may offer some interesting clues to an appropriate diet for our personal health. Ancestry is a factor in the high incidence of certain diet-related chronic illnesses, such as diabetes and alcoholism, among Native Americans in the U.S. Poverty has forced many Native American families to eat nontraditional, unhealthy foods, such as white flour and sugar. Research has shown that biological factors play a role in alcoholism and diabetes rates: Because fermented foods were not a part of the traditional diet, many Native Americans typically lack the enzyme to process alcohol and other sugars.[14]

ALLERGIES

If we are sensitive or allergic to a food, our bodies have trouble processing it. When we continue to eat that offending food, it may compromise our digestive systems, making it difficult for them to work efficiently. In some cases, weight gain can result.

There are two types of food intolerances: true allergies and food hypersensitivities. A true allergic reaction occurs when the immune system reacts to a food protein as if it were a damaging foreign body. It can cause any number of reactions, from a mild rash to a dangerous swelling of the air passages. The most violent responses are called anaphylactic reactions; even a small taste of the allergen, skin contact, or, in some cases, environmental exposure will shut down bodily functions within seconds. These reactions occur most often from peanuts, tree nuts, and shellfish. If you or your child has ever had a severe allergy reaction to a food, it should be carefully avoided, as this type of reaction may get worse with each subsequent exposure. Carrying a portable epinephrine shot prescribed by a doctor is an important safety measure that could save your life or your child's.

When my daughter entered kindergarten, I took her to the supermarket to show her what would make her sick. We also practiced using her epinephrine shot together by sticking an old expired shot into an apple. I didn't want her to be scared of her condition, but I needed her to know how serious it could be. She was only five, and she couldn't read ingredients, so she had to know what to look for.

Food hypersensitivity, though not life-threatening, can be much harder to pin down than allergies. Symptoms are as diverse as muscle and joint pain, congestion, rashes or eczema, migraines, fatigue, intestinal distress, and even depression. To further complicate matters, this type of reaction can show up as many as seventy-two hours after eating a food. The most common food sensitivities are to milk, eggs, seafood, wheat, nuts, seeds, chocolate, oranges, and tomatoes. Corn, soy, gluten, and yeast are also common allergens. The best way to determine if a food is causing symptoms is to do what is called an elimination diet. This involves removing the foods most likely to cause your symptoms for ten to fourteen days. Then you can reintroduce the foods one by one. Keep in mind that sometimes the body will not react until you have a certain amount of a food in your system. So if you don't have a reaction at first, but you begin to have symptoms when you return to eating a food regularly, try eliminating it again. This can be a grueling process, and you might want the support of a nutritionist, who may also be able to help identify foods that are problematic for you.

Breast-feeding is protective against developing food allergies in children.[15] The American Academy of Pediatrics recommends breast-feeding exclusively until babies are six or seven months old, by which time their intestines are mature enough to properly digest solid foods. For further information, see Chapter 23, "The First Year of Parenting."

FOOD QUALITY

Fruits, vegetables, and other whole foods provide nutrients the body needs to digest and function efficiently. Refined and processed foods merely offer "empty calories" lacking high nutritional value. Over time, the body will lose digestive and metabolic capacity. In addition, many of us still feel hungry after we have eaten processed foods, even though we have consumed substantial calories.

OTHER DIET-RELATED HEALTH ISSUES

WEIGHT AND HEALTH

Many of us struggle endlessly with our weight. Approximately 61 percent of American adults are considered overweight or obese, regardless of age, gender, race, and ethnicity. An adult is called obese if her body mass index is 30 or higher.*

The sedentary American lifestyle and the abundance of junk foods often contribute to unhealthy weight gain. Fast-food chains most negatively affect low-income communities. Women of lower socioeconomic status are 50 percent more likely to be above a recommended weight than women of higher socioeconomic status, and women of color are more likely to be above a recommended weight than non-Latina white women.[16] Organic whole foods are often not an option for those on a tight budget.

Studies abound that link health problems to weight gain. According to the U.S. surgeon general, three hundred thousand Americans die each year from obesity-related problems, including heart disease, stroke, high blood pressure, diabetes, and cancer. The Nurses Health Study at Harvard Medical School followed 115,000 nurses for nearly 20 years starting in 1976, and found that women who gained between 11 and 18 pounds over that time had a 25 percent increase in heart disease.[17]

Maintaining a healthy weight, particularly minimizing weight gain, is important for our overall well-being. However, the dangers of being fat may be overstated. Health problems may have as much to do with overall fitness as with weight. Few studies have controls for fat people who exercise regularly, or account for the stress on the body of yo-yo dieting.

The common prescription for being fat is to diet. However, weight loss diets are notoriously unsuccessful; the vast majority of people who lose weight regain it. Therefore, it is best to focus on eating well, exercising, and generally taking good care of yourself, regardless of what the

* To calculate your body mass index, multiply your height in inches by your height in inches. Now divide this number into your weight in pounds. Next multiply this number by 703. This number is your body mass index.

scale says or how you compare to models in a magazine.

EATING PROBLEMS

In the United States, an estimated 5 million girls and women each year suffer from eating disorders—psychological illnesses with serious mortality rates.[18] In Singapore and Tokyo, where as many as one in thirty-six people have eating disorders, the statistics rival those in the United States.[19] In South Africa, a study recently revealed that black South African students in Zululand were abusing laxatives, fasting, and using appetite suppressants to lose weight.[20]

Most of us, at one time or another, have used food to numb or deny our feelings, to comfort ourselves, or to put some order in our lives. Who among us hasn't at one time either binged or felt nauseated when scared, angry, depressed, lonely, or sad? However, when we let food become the major outlet for expressing our feelings, we risk damaging our physical and emotional health. Eating this way is a common strategy for many women to cope with a variety of issues: family problems, stress, anger, verbal and physical abuse, racism, sexism, homophobia, and general feelings of inadequacy. Though disordered eating is often seen as the main problem, it may be a symptom of these other, deeper emotional issues and deflect attention from them.

In the Caribbean, thick, full-figured women are admired, and I was always complimented on my full hips and butt as a child. When I migrated to Boston to study at a major university, I felt as though I was thrown in some twilight zone, where the skinnier you were, the more beautiful and complete you were considered. I unconsciously started purging my food, and thought that I was sick. It was after I lost a lot of weight and received numerous compliments that I willfully started to throw up my food.

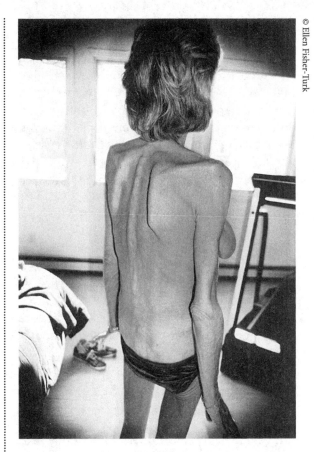

© Ellen Fisher-Turk

Photo therapist Ellen Fisher-Turk works with women who suffer from eating disorders. As women like this forty-six-year-old are photographed almost naked, "their emotional defenses are stripped away along with their clothing," says Fisher-Turk. "When they look at the photos, they can see their denial and their defenses, which is what keeps an eating disorder going."

Experts have identified three major categories of eating disorders:

- *Anorexia nervosa* is characterized by the incessant pursuit of thinness, an intense fear of gaining weight, a distorted body image, and a refusal to maintain a normal body weight. Two types of anorexia nervosa exist. Those suffering from the restricting type severely limit caloric intake by extreme dieting or fasting; they may also exercise excessively. Those of the binge-eating/purging type exhibit the same restricting behavior but also engage in bouts of gorging, followed by vomiting and/or abuse of laxatives or diuretics.

- *Bulimia nervosa* consists of episodes of binge eating and purging that occur an average of twice a week for at least three months. Binge eaters devour an excessive amount of food in a brief period of time, often feeling out of control and unable to stop. A characteristic binge might include a pint of ice cream, a bag of chips, cookies, and large quantities of water or soda, all consumed in a short time. Again, purging behavior such as vomiting, abusing laxatives or diuretics, and/or excessive exercise occurs after the binge in an effort to get rid of any digested calories.

- *Binge-eating disorder* (BED) is a more recently described disorder that comprises bingeing similar to bulimia, but without the purging behavior used to avoid gaining weight. As among bulimics, those experiencing BED feel a lack of control and engage in bingeing an average of twice a week.

Other disordered eating behaviors exist, but they have not been officially categorized as psychiatric illnesses.

Girls and women are much more likely to develop eating problems than our male counterparts and account for 90 percent of all diagnosed eating disorders. As women, we are taught to see ourselves in relation to others, to avoid confrontation, and to conform to societal ideals regarding thinness.[21] We often compare ourselves to other women—even if we never admit it—and model ourselves according to what we think men find attractive. The media's constant pounding of a Western feminine ideal of thinness is evident in magazines, billboards, television sitcoms, and pop icons. This tacit weightism, along with the more direct messages that children (and even adults) send through weight-based taunts and prejudice, contributes to body dissatisfaction and eating disorders. A recent study by researchers at the University of Minnesota found that teasing about body weight was consistently associated with low self-esteem and depression, regardless of the subjects' weight.[22]

When I first started college, it seemed like all of the girls in my dorm gained the Freshman 15. But by sophomore year, a lot of the girls were on a diet and exercising. It soon became the race for the perfect body.

Eating disorders are also affecting girls and women of color globally at an alarming rate. Here is a snapshot of what is going on internationally:

- Fiji, a nation that has traditionally cherished the fuller figure, has witnessed a surge in eating disorders since the arrival of television in 1995.[23]
- India, a country known for its beauty pageant industry and glitzy version of Hollywood (known as Bollywood), has noted a sharp increase in anorexia cases.[24]
- In South Africa, researchers have found that since the abolition of apartheid, girls are developing eating disorders because they believe that they do not fit the Western ideal promoted in the media.[25]

The reality is that no ethnic or socioeconomic group is immune to the dangers of disordered eating. Unfortunately, previous studies did not include ethnically diverse populations; therefore, cases among these groups went unreported.[26]

In the United States, some people believe that African-American and Latino cultures are more accepting of diverse body sizes and a broader beauty ideal. While this may have been true in the past, research demonstrates that binge eating and purging is at least as common among African-American women as among white women.[27] Latina high school students have also been found to have rates of bulimia comparable to those of whites.[28]

I receive funny looks when I tell people that I had an eating disorder. By the age of sixteen I was prepared to be thin and die. Unlike the . . . white dancers in my dance studio, I was curvaceous and filled out. The difference in skin color and hair texture was more than enough for me. I couldn't pull out my hair or scratch off my skin, but I could throw up the guilt that was food, because my goal was to be 100 pounds or less.[29]

Black and Latina stars such as Halle Berry and Christina Aguilera are just as thin as their white counterparts. The influence of these role models may be contributing to body dissatisfaction and weight control behaviors among girls of color.[30]

The way that the media equates thinness with beauty and success further exacerbates the problem. A recent study revealed that Navajo girls suffering from anorexia were more likely to come from upwardly mobile families who moved off the reservation.[31] Asian girls who are recent immigrants to the United States are also falling victim to eating problems. Asian-Americans are often perceived as "model minorities" and expected to be successful and high-achieving. The drive to become the "ideal Asian woman" can lead to perfectionism, which is linked to eating disorders, particularly anorexia.[32]

Eating problems are treatable and preventable. The sooner these problems are diagnosed

POSSIBLE SIGNS OF DISORDERED EATING

- *Change in personality or behavior:* more withdrawn, secretive, depressed, or irritable; spends a great deal of time alone or in the bathroom; prone to tantrums; shoplifts or takes money from friends and family members to meet food needs; denies there is a problem

- *Unusual eating habits:* stops eating with family and/or friends; is eating amounts larger or smaller than normal; stops eating entirely; engages in vomiting or uses laxatives, diet pills, diuretics, or rigorous dieting or fasting to lose or maintain weight

- *Compulsive exercising* to the point of exhaustion

- *Physical symptoms:* failure to gain weight during expected periods of growth (i.e., adolescence); extreme weight change; fine, downy hair growth on the body; insomnia; constipation; skin rash and dry skin; loss of hair and poor nail quality; dental cavities; cessation of or delay in the menstrual cycle; extreme sensitivity to cold; inability to think clearly; irrational thinking; chronic fatigue

If you are concerned that you or someone you care about may have an eating disorder, seek help from a knowledgeable person such as a school nurse, counselor, or health care provider. For a listing of groups that have information on eating disorders and treatment, see "Resources."

and treated, the better the outcomes are likely to be. Due to their complexity, eating problems require a comprehensive treatment plan involving medical care and monitoring, psychosocial interventions, and nutritional counseling.

Prevention, however, is always the most effective measure. Parents, teachers, and peers should not tolerate harassment or teasing about another person's body weight or shape. Well-researched, upbeat prevention programs and curriculums that enhance self-esteem can make a difference in girls' lives. If young girls and teens are provided with positive images, support, and information about healthy minds and bodies, they are much less likely to develop eating problems. An educational program called Full of Ourselves, created by Catherine Steiner-Adair and Lisa Sjostrom, helps to decrease girls' vulnerability to the development of body preoccupation and eating disorders by working to increase girls' self-esteem, promoting body acceptance, providing leadership opportunities, and teaching strategies to resist the cultural emphasis on unhealthy eating and dieting behaviors. The best way to prevent your child from developing an eating disorder is to stop dieting yourself. Children with parents who constantly diet are much more likely to diet themselves and

USING NUTRITION TO ADDRESS OUR HEALTH ISSUES

Tooth and Gum Decay

Without our teeth, we cannot eat many foods that provide important nutrients. Teeth are alive. Your saliva nourishes them through tiny passageways in the tooth. The mouth is, in many ways, a visible part of the inside of your body, reflecting its strengths and weaknesses. Gum disease is associated with cardiovascular disease, and many nutrients, such as coenzyme Q10, zinc, folate, vitamin C, magnesium, and calcium, are important for both gum health and heart health.

Certain types of bacteria found in saliva use sugar in food to create plaque, a sticky coating that helps the bacteria cling to and destroy our teeth. Avoid sticky sweets that stay in your mouth a long time, and whenever possible, eat foods with fiber that scrape off plaque, acting as a toothbrush (raw carrot sticks, apples, celery sticks, whole grains, etc.).

The least cavity-causing way to eat sweets is to have them with meals and not between. The number of times you eat sweets, rather than the total amount, determines how much acid the bacteria produce. Of course, it is also important to brush and floss our teeth daily and to get regular dental cleanings.

Intestinal Problems

Women have higher rates of intestinal disorders, such as irritable bowel syndrome (IBS), Crohn's disease, and ulcerative colitis, than men. While these disorders are often affected by diet and stress, most medical doctors manage them using steroid medications and surgery.

Many women with IBS benefit from eating a diet high in fiber-rich foods, such as beans and whole grains. Others, however, find the most healing diet to be relatively low in starchy foods and high in protein and vegetables. Some people are helped by the Specific Carbohydrate Diet, which is completely grain-free, as detailed in the book *Breaking the Vicious Cycle* by Elaine Gottschall.[33]

In addition, different people can react to different types of fiber in various ways. Soluble fibers like those found in apples and oat bran may cause problems for some people who might be fine with insoluble fibers such as rice bran, or vice versa. Try different types to see what works for you.

Migraines

Migraines can be set off by foods containing tyramine, phenathylamine, monosodium glutamate, or sodium nitrate. Common foods that contain these are chocolate, aged cheeses, sour cream, red wine, pickled herring, chicken livers, avocados, ripe bananas, cured meats, and many Asian and prepared foods.

Osteoporosis

Osteoporosis, a disease caused by the thinning of bones, is responsible for more than 1.5 million fractures each year.[34]

Women are often encouraged to make sure we get enough calcium in our diets to help prevent bone loss and osteoporosis. Unfortunately, there is little proof that increasing calcium intake prevents fractures. Women in other cultures who consume far less calcium than American women have lower rates of osteoporosis. This points to a more complex picture.

Weight-bearing exercises such as walking, running, or lifting weights can increase bone density. A whole-foods diet rich in calcium, magnesium, vitamin D, and vitamin K may also have a preventative effect.

If you want to take a calcium supplement, look for calcium that is *chelated*—bonded to a molecule that will take it where it needs to go. Good choices are calcium citrate, calcium malate, or calcium lysinate. A calcium/vitamin D combination is often best, because many women do not get enough vitamin D. The most common form of calcium is calcium carbonate, which is also the most difficult to absorb. (For more information on osteoporosis, see p. 564 in Chapter 27.)

to become overly concerned with body image. Chronic dieting creates malnutrition and deficiencies that can alter brain chemistry and set the stage for developing an eating disorder. Learning to respect your body and to nourish it with whole foods is one of the best lessons you can ever teach your children.

CHANGES

This is an exciting time in the field of nutrition, but also a time in which our healthful food supply is increasingly at risk. The role of food in promoting health is being studied more than ever, providing reams of new information but making it more difficult to sort through and understand it all. The organic and whole-foods movements are blossoming at the same time that agribusiness corporations are gaining ground and pushing questionably safe, inadequately tested genetically modified foods on the public at home and abroad. As consumers of food, we have the power to influence what happens to our food supply. By supporting small, local farms and buying organic foods, we can help bring about an overall improvement in the food industry.

One of the most exciting and optimistic trends of the twenty-first century so far is the rise of community-supported agriculture (CSA). In this system, nonfarmers "subscribe" to a small farm to support the work of the farmer. In return, subscribers get a weekly box of farm-fresh produce. Subscription prices vary, but most are in the $15-to-$25-per-week range. This is an affordable way to get the healthiest, freshest food available while supporting small farms. It exemplifies the nutritional values that have been emphasized here: Eat whole foods, eat organic when possible, and support your local farmers. For information on how to join a CSA in your area, go to www.nal.usda.gov/afsic/csa/csastate.htm.

NOTES

1. Food and Agriculture Organization of the United Nations, as reported by World Resources Institute: http://earthtrends.wri.org/text/pop/variables/205.htm.

2. Statistics from the National Center for Chronic Disease Prevention and Health Promotion (www.cdc.gov/diabetes/statistics/prev/national/figpersons.htm), accessed September 23, 2004.

3. Studies from the *Journal of Agricultural and Food Chemistry* and *The European Journal of Nutrition* as cited by Marian Burros, "Is Organic Food Probably Better?," *The New York Times*, July 16, 2003, F1.

4. Dr. Joseph Mercola, "Why Grassfed Animal Products Are Better for You: A Quick Review of the Fats That Make Up Your Body," Mercola.com, 2004.

5. Cynthia L. Curl, Richard A. Fenske, Kai Elgethun, "Organophosphorus pesticide exposure of urban and suburban preschool children with organic and conventional diets," *Environmental Health Perspectives: Journal of the National Institute of Environmental Health Sciences* III, no. 3 (March 2003): 377–82. Accessed September 23, 2004 at ehp.niehs.nih.gov/docs/2003/5754/abstract.html.

6. Art Ulene, *The Nutribase Nutrition Facts Desk Reference* (New York: Avery, 1995), 630. Elizabeth Applegate, "Introduction: Nutrition and Functional Roles of Eggs in the Diet," *Journal of the American College of Nutrition* 19, no. 5, 495S–98S.

7. Kim Severson, "New Dietary Guidelines from Feds Expected to Focus on Exercise," *San Francisco Chronicle,* May 28, 2004.

8. W. H. Sebrell, "A Fiftieth Anniversary—Cereal Enrichment," *Nutrition Today* (January/February 1992): 20–21.

9. V. Messina and M. Messina, *The Vegetarian Way: Healthy Eating for You and Your Family* (New York: Crown, 1996), 76–85.

10. Gary Ruskin, "The Fast Food Trap: How Commercialism Creates Overweight Children," *Mothering,* no. 121 (November/December 2003): 40.

11. J. Klotter, "Nutrition Learning and Behavior," *Townsend Letter for Doctors and Patients* (October 2003): 37–38.

12. MarketData Enterprises, The U.S. Weight Loss and Diet Control Market, 2002: www.marketresearch.com/product/display.asp?ProductID=819147. Updated statistic from personal correspondence with Richard Cleland, an assistant director for the Federal Trade Commission's Division of Advertising Practices.

13. FDA/CFSCAN, "The Facts About Weight Loss Products and Programs": http://vm.cfsan.fda.gov/~dms/wgtloss.html.

14. C. L. Ehlers, C. Agneta, M. Betancourt, P. Duro, D. A. Gilder, L. Harris, J. W. Havstad, P. Lau, S. L. Lopez, E. Phillips, J. Roth, T. L. Wall, "Laboratory of Clinical Neurophysiology and San Diego Native American Project," TSRI Scientific Report, the Scripps Research Institute, 2002: www.scripps.edu/research/sr2002/np07.html.

15. "Outcomes of Breastfeeding Versus Formula Feeding," compiled by Jon Ahrendsen, M.D., FAAFP, updated March 2004 by Ginna Wall, M.N., IBCLC: www.lalecheleague.org/chi/Biospec.htm.

16. "Overweight and Obesity at a Glance." U.S. Department of Health and Human Services, www.surgeongeneral.gov/topics/obesity/calltoaction/fact_glance.htm, accessed September 2004.

17. JoAnn E. Manson, et al., "Body Weight and Mortality Among Women," *New England Journal of Medicine* 333, no. 11 (September 14, 1995): 677–85.

18. Eating Disorders Awareness, Prevention, and Education Act of 2003.

19. Jessi Hempel, "Eating Disorders Grow Among Hong Kong Women," *Women's ENews* (September 8, 2002).

20. Kami-Leigh Agard, "Dying to Be Thin," *Woman2 Woman* (March 2003): 40.

21. Jeremy B. Frank and Cheryl D. Thomas, "Externalized Self-perceptions, Self-silencing, and the Prediction of Eating Pathology," *Canada Journal of Behavioral Science* (2003): 219.

22. "Pediatric Obesity: Adolescents Teased About Their Weight May Be More Likely to Be Suicidal," *Medical Letter on the CDC and Atlanta* (August 31, 2003).

23. "TV Brings Eating Disorders to Fiji," BBC News, May 20, 1999.

24. "Anorexia Takes Hold in India," BBC News, June 17, 2003.

25. "Eating Disorders Rise in Zulu Women," BBC News, November 4, 2002.

26. U.S. Department of Health and Human Services, *Body-Wise Handbook* (Office on Women's Health, November 2000). Accessed at www.4woman.gov/BodyImage/bodywise.cfm in November 2003.

27. R. Striegel-Moore and L. Smolak, "The Influence of Ethnicity on Eating Disorders in Women," in R. M. Eisler and M. Hersen, eds., *Handbook of Gender, Culture and Health* (Manhaw, NJ: Lawrence Erlbaum Associates, 2000), 227–53.

28. J. Z. Dounchis, H. A. Hayden, and D. E. Wilfley, "Obesity, Eating Disorders, and Body Image in Ethnically Diverse Children and Adolescents," in J. K. Thompson and L. Smolak, eds., *Body Image, Eating Disorders, and Obesity in Children and Adolescents: Theory, Assessment, Treatment and Prevention* (Washington, D.C.: American Psychological Association, 2000), 67–98.

29. Agard, *Dying to Be Thin,* 40.

30. A. J. Pumariega, C. R. Gustavson, J. C. Gustavson, P. S. Motes, and S. Ayers, "Eating Attitudes in African-American Women: The *Essence* Eating Disorders Survey," *Eating Disorders: The Journal for Treatment and Prevention* 2 (1994): 5–16.

31. U.S. Department of Health and Human Services, *Body-Wise Handbook.* Accessed at www.4woman.gov/Body Image/bodywise.cfm in November 2003.

32. Ibid.

33. Elaine Gottschall, *Breaking the Vicious Cycle* (Baltimore, Ontario: Kirkton Press, 1994). Diet for Crohn's disease, ulcerative colitis, celiac disease, and chronic diarrhea: www.breakingtheviciouscycle.info.

34. Walter C. Willet, *Eat, Drink, and Be Healthy* (New York: Simon & Schuster, 2001), 138–47.

Alcohol, tobacco, and other mood-altering drugs touch the lives of most girls and women. We may have a drink once in a while, or we may drink every day. We may not drink, smoke, or take drugs, but perhaps we share our lives with people who do. We may know someone whose use of alcohol, tobacco, and other drugs hurts them and makes them untrustworthy or abusive. We may need to use drugs because we suffer from chronic pain, illness, or disability, and we might wonder if those drugs are habit-forming. We may live in a community assaulted by poverty and racism, where neighbors and family turn to tobacco, alcohol, and other drugs for relief, but where little is done by society to make help available.

DRUGS WOMEN AND GIRLS USE

Women in the U.S. largely use and abuse legal drugs, such as alcohol, tobacco, and prescription drugs. Despite the attention given to illegal drugs, far fewer women use them.

ALCOHOL

Alcohol is the most common drug used by women (used by 45 percent of girls and women over the age of twelve). Fifteen percent of women in this age range report current binge drinking (five or more drinks on one occasion), and 3 percent report even heavier alcohol use.[1]

TOBACCO

About 21 percent of women smoke, but this can vary depending on age, race/ethnicity, income, education, occupation, sexual orientation, and mental and physical ability.[2]

MOOD-ALTERING PRESCRIPTION DRUGS

Medications such as pain relievers, sedatives, stimulants, and tranquilizers can be used in nonmedical ways. A 2002 survey found that almost 3 percent of girls and women in the U.S. aged twelve or older had used mood-altering prescription drugs for nonmedical reasons in the previous month.[3]

ILLEGAL DRUGS

In 2002, 6 percent of girls and women in the U.S. aged twelve or older were current users of illegal drugs. Marijuana is the most commonly used illegal drug: 4 percent of girls and women over the age of twelve reported current use of marijuana. Under 1 percent of girls and women re-

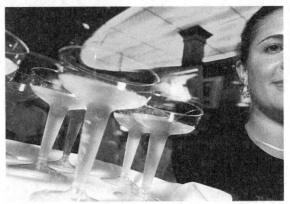

ported being current users of cocaine, Ecstasy, heroin, and other illegal drugs.[4]

This chapter discusses issues, trends, and health effects of the three substances women most commonly abuse—alcohol, tobacco, and tranquilizers—as well as Ecstasy, a drug used by many younger women. It also describes promising treatments and how we can help make positive changes for ourselves and others. (For resources on smoking, alcohol and drug use, and treatment, see the companion website, www .ourbodiesourselves.org.)

HOW SUBSTANCE ABUSE AFFECTS OUR HEALTH

ALCOHOL

One former drinker says,

You think your alcohol use is no big deal—I mean, everyone does it—and then you find yourself driving under the influence, sick with liver problems, isolated from your family—and you think, "How could this have happened?"

We often ignore the harmful effects of alcohol use, mistakenly seeing it as having a lesser effect than other drugs. The short-term effects of alcohol can be pleasurable, but heavy use and abuse can have devastating effects on our bodies:[5]

- Alcohol can diminish motor coordination, judgment, emotional control, and reasoning power, increasing our risk of accidents and injuries and our vulnerability to violence.
- Even low-level alcohol use can disrupt normal menstrual cycles; alcoholic women are known to have a variety of menstrual and reproductive disorders.
- Drinking can increase the risk of mouth, esophageal, and liver cancer, major depression, epilepsy, hemorrhagic stroke, and cirrhosis of the liver. Women develop alcohol-related liver disease after a comparatively shorter period of heavy drinking than do men.
- Other alcohol-related health risks that are higher for women include hypertension (high blood pressure), particularly for African-American women, and an increased risk of osteoporosis (thinning of bones), breast cancer, gastric ulcers, and alcoholic hepatitis.
- Drinking during pregnancy may cause a range of permanent birth defects and developmental disabilities in our children, referred to as fetal alcohol spectrum disorder. These can include learning difficulties and problems with memory, attention, reasoning, and judgment during childhood and beyond. Children born to mothers who drink heavily during pregnancy also may have other physical birth defects. There is no known safe level of alcohol use during pregnancy.
- Drinking at an early age increases our risk for osteoporosis and later addiction problems.

(For more information, see "Women and Alcohol Use" [W6] on the companion website, www.ourbodiesourselves.org.)

TOBACCO

Smoking has extremely serious consequences for our health. The 2001 U.S. Surgeon General's report on women and smoking includes a wealth of information on the health effects of smoking for women. Here is a summary of the findings, with some updates:[6]

- Nearly 178,000 U.S. women die from smoking-related diseases each year.

MYTH OR REALITY?

- *Alcohol is the least harmful of drugs.*

Myth. Alcohol can have dangerous effects on motor coordination, judgment, emotional control, and reasoning power, increasing the risk of accidents and injuries. The bottom line: Alcohol is not harmless, so drink in moderation and don't assume you're sober enough to drive.

- *I should not use birth control pills if I smoke.*

Reality. Women who use oral contraceptives and who also smoke have a substantially increased risk of suffering a heart attack and perhaps a stroke compared to women who do neither.

- *Smoking "light" or low-tar cigarettes will reduce my risk of smoking-related illness.*

Myth. A study released by the National Cancer Institute in 2001 found that "light" and low-tar brands are no less harmful than other brands and do not reduce a smoker's health risks.

- Smokers are twice as likely to have heart attacks and strokes, which are the leading killers of women in the U.S.
- Smoking causes almost 90 percent of all lung cancer deaths in women.
- Smoking increases the risk of cervical cancer.
- In women, smoking causes 90 percent of lung diseases, including emphysema, asthma, and chronic bronchitis.
- Women who use oral contraceptives and smoke have greater risk for heart attacks and strokes than women who do not smoke or do not use birth control pills.
- Women who smoke may have more trouble becoming pregnant, start menstruating earlier, have more period problems, and go into menopause earlier.
- Smoking increases the risk of ulcers, cataracts, and osteoporosis.
- Smoking during pregnancy can pass chemicals found in the tobacco smoke to the fetus. This may result in miscarriage, premature delivery, and slower growth rates of the fetus.
- Newborns in homes where people smoke may be more likely to die of sudden infant death syndrome.
- More and more studies are linking smoking with breast cancer, but further research is needed in this area.
- Quitting smoking *at any age* can slow or reverse the harmful effects of smoking. The earlier one stops, the greater the benefit.

EXPOSURE TO SECONDHAND SMOKE

A waitress who filmed ads for Canadian television to warn others of the dangers of secondhand smoke said:

I've been a waitress for forty years to earn a decent living for my daughter and myself. My doctor told me I had a smoker's tumor, and therefore I'm dying. I never smoked a day in my life.

Exposure to secondhand smoke is a health hazard. Although there is a growing movement to pass laws that eliminate smoking in all public places, many of us are still exposed to secondhand smoke in our homes, our worksites, and public places such as restaurants. Women who work in service and blue-collar jobs are more likely to be around people who smoke on the job.

Regular exposure to secondhand smoke causes lung and heart disease, including lung cancer, in adults who don't smoke; and pneumonia, bronchitis, asthma, and chronic ear infections in children. The Centers for Disease Control estimates that thirty-six thousand adults die each year as a result of exposure to secondhand smoke. Many childhood deaths are also likely caused by this exposure.

(For more information, see "Women and Smoking" [W7] on the companion website, www.ourbodiesourselves.org.)

TRANQUILIZERS (BENZODIAZEPINES)

Prescription mood-altering drugs, such as anti-anxiety agents, antidepressants, and sedatives, have long been marketed to women. Benzodiazepines are one category of prescribed mood-altering drugs, commonly referred to as tranquilizers. Doctors have prescribed them widely, especially to women, since the 1960s—for short-term relief of anxiety and sleeping problems, as well as to ease withdrawal from other drugs. Common tranquilizers are Valium (diazepam), Ativan (lorazepam), Serax (oxazepam), Xanax (alprazolam), and Klonopin (clonazepam). Even short-term use of tranquilizers can harm memory and reasoning, balance and coordination. And there are more serious effects from longer-term use of tranquilizers, including feeling dull, suicidal, and anxious.[7] Like alcohol, tranquilizers can be especially dangerous for women who are pregnant or elderly.

Health professionals have known for twenty-five years that tranquilizers can be addictive—even at standard doses—if taken for more than several weeks, yet these drugs are still prescribed for even much longer periods. Neither health care providers nor women are generally aware of the wide range of withdrawal symptoms associated with stopping tranquilizer use. When we try to stop, we may have any of a long list of problems: increased anxiety and panic attacks, flu-like symptoms, hypersensitivity to light, depression, restlessness, poor memory and concentration, dizziness, weakness, tremors, heart palpitations, sweating, nausea, indigestion, bodily pains. These symptoms may come and go over months, and we may feel we need to resume taking the drug for relief.

A woman who was prescribed benzodiazepines said of the withdrawal experience:

I will never touch another benzo again as long as I live. I would rather die than go through what I did on it and the horrible withdrawal.

If you decide to cut back or stop using tranquilizers, work with your doctor to taper off slowly.[8] (Tapering off means taking a little less, then staying at that dose for a couple of days, then dropping to a lower dose, waiting, and then taking even less, until you're off the drug.) It can be a long process, but it might help you avoid or minimize the worst of the symptoms and help you stay off.

(For more information, see "Women and Tranquilizers" [W8] on the companion website, www.ourbodiesourselves.org.)

ECSTASY

An Ecstasy user says,

Playing with life and death can be a bit of a thrill until you realize that sometimes you cannot be in control of your own body because of what you've put in it.

Use of Ecstasy, an illegal drug, has been rising steadily since 1992. Ecstasy (also called MDMA) is a synthetic combination drug that has both stimulant and hallucinogenic effects. Despite its positive relaxing and social effects, it can be dangerous. We might feel anxiety, paranoia, and depression from use of Ecstasy in the short term; in the long term, Ecstasy can cause serious impairment in mental function and memory. Using Ecstasy in settings such as raves can cause severe dehydration, heat exhaustion, and liver malfunction, all of which can lead to death. As with many drugs, women seem to be more sensitive to the effects of Ecstasy than men.[9] We may experience more intense perceptual changes and suffer more long-term effects, such as depression, mood swings, paranoia, and anxiety. (For more information, see "Women and Ecstasy and Other Illegal Drugs" [W9] on the companion website, www.ourbodiesourselves.org.)

INFLUENCES ON OUR USE AND MISUSE OF SUBSTANCES

Although we might be aware of the risks involved with using alcohol, tobacco, and other drugs, we may still use them. Why? There are three major influences on us: how the drugs are promoted; the personal and social pressures we feel; and the fact that these substances can all be addictive.

PROMOTION OF PRODUCTS

One of the most compelling influences on us is the media's relentless promotion of alcohol, tobacco, and other drugs. Ads, movies, and television shows try to make us think that these substances will bring us health, happiness, success, sophistication, and freedom—the very things that their use can, in reality, diminish and destroy.

The tobacco industry has a long history of marketing to women and girls, dating back to the 1920s. Tobacco companies began marketing brands specifically designed for women in the 1960s and 1970s, with advertising that equated smoking with independence, sophistication, and beauty. The marketing of brands called "slims" and "thins" played into the social pressures on women to control weight. More recent campaigns have carried themes of rebelliousness (an ad for Winston cigarettes proclaims, "Yeah, I have a tattoo and no, you can't see it") and have reflected the movement toward individual expression (an example is the Virginia Slim's "Find Your Voice" campaign, with pictures of women of color and text in Spanish and Swahili).

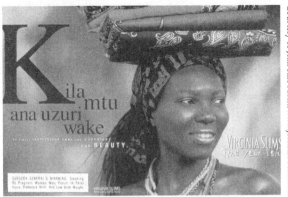

Virginia Slim's "Find Your Voice" advertising campaign features women of color and text in Spanish and Swahili, making their cigarettes seem multicultural and hip. The ads link smoking with individuality and women's freedom.

THE MYTH OF LIGHT AND LOW-TAR CIGARETTES

As women's concerns about the health risks of smoking grew, tobacco companies began in the 1970s to promote "low tar" or "light" cigarettes as a "safer" option, even though the companies knew this wasn't true. Many people believed the claims. However, studies have shown that the introduction of light cigarettes not only did not improve public health but also may have contributed to an increase in smoking-related disease.[10] The National Cancer Institute has found that light and low-tar brands are no less harmful than other brands and do not reduce a smoker's health risks. Studies show that the tobacco industry deliberately marketed these cigarettes to prevent smokers from quitting.[11] Tobacco companies are using similar tactics today by introducing flavored cigarettes and looking for other ways to lure girls and women to smoking.

(For more information on the manipulative promotion of tobacco, see "Our Health vs. Their Profits: The Lure of Smoking Continues for Girls" [W10] on the companion website, www.ourbodiesourselves.org.)

PERSONAL AND SOCIAL PRESSURES

We have never been short of reasons to smoke, drink, and use drugs. Here are some of them: to organize our social relationships, to carve out time for ourselves, to control our emotions, to create an image, and to have a source of comfort and dependability in our lives.[12] Here's what some women have said about their smoking:

The advantage to this is that people are out there [smoking outside] from all different departments . . . and decisions actually get made out there.[13]

I've felt very much at war with that role [mothering] since day one. [I was] using cigarettes to create a sense of space around myself . . . to mark time out for myself.[14]

A lot of my drinking and drug use has to do with childhood issues. I would just drink to numb the feelings for the day. I was so depressed, it was easier to drink than to find the energy and confidence to seek help.

I just wanted to be cool; being cool was always important to me in the rebel part of me. It was also wrong, so I did it.[15]

As far as I can see, you can't count on a guy, because they are not always there, kids aren't always there . . . they [cigarettes] are always there.[16]

ADDICTION

Another reason we use drugs is addiction. We may be afraid to stop, or we may not be able to give them up. We may not know where or how to get help; there may not be an available drug or alcohol program. For ideas on how to stop, see the sections on support and treatment later in this chapter.

Many obstacles can get in the way of finding the support and treatment we need. These may be related to depression, or not having people in our lives who support our desire to get well, or having friends who use. Those of us who are mothers often fear we will lose custody of our children when we seek help. Many of us deny that our substance use is a problem. We may be punished or blamed for the consequences of our use, and our guilt and shame can immobilize us. Many women feel that giving up substance use is like losing a friend. Some of us may want to get help but are afraid we'll be rejected because of being lesbian or transgender.

We shouldn't give up hope. Girls and women do work through these barriers and report that supportive relationships with professionals, family, and friends were the key to getting help. Seeking help sooner, rather than later, also makes the journey easier.

REDUCING THE RISKS

TOBACCO

No level of smoking is considered safe, and the symptoms of addiction can appear within weeks of beginning even occasional smoking.[17] It is also important to avoid being around others who smoke.

DRINKING GUIDELINES FOR WOMEN

The U.S. guideline for moderate drinking by women is to have no more than one drink a day. Canadian guidelines are similar, recommending no more than nine drinks a week for women.[18] It is not wise to drink in these situations:

- If you are pregnant or breast-feeding
- Before you drive or perform tasks that pose a risk to the safety of yourself or others
- If you are taking medication that reacts negatively with alcohol
- If you have medical problems that are likely to get worse if you drink alcohol
- If you have problems with addiction.[19]

WAYS TO REDUCE HARM FROM ALCOHOL AND OTHER DRUG USE

Here are some ways to reduce the risks of drug use:

- *Know the drug(s) you are taking.* Be aware of the potential short- and long-term effects of any drug you take.
- *Don't take drugs* at parties or clubs. If you choose to drink (even water), know where your cup is at all times; you don't want any drugs added to it.
- *Don't mix drugs.* Mixing can dangerously multiply the effects. It's particularly danger-

ous to mix alcohol with other depressants, such as tranquilizers, opiates, and narcotics (pain medicine).

- *Know your body's limits and reactions.* Don't try to gauge the amount you take by what others take, or even by what you were able to consume on other occasions.
- *NEVER share needles* or other injection equipment. Using unclean equipment can spread many diseases, including HIV/AIDS and hepatitis.
- *Be aware of how your choices may influence other key areas of your life.* Ask yourself whether your use of alcohol or other drugs is affecting your finances, your relationships and family life, and your work; ask yourself whether you could get into legal trouble because of the drugs you use.

- *Find other ways* to reduce stress, cope with life, heal, and have fun.

RECOGNIZING A PROBLEM

WHAT DO HARMFUL USE AND DRUG DEPENDENCE LOOK LIKE?

The term *addiction* usually refers to both psychological and physical dependence on a drug, including alcohol. Signs of dependence include withdrawal symptoms (such as depression, anxiety, irritability, cramps, nausea, sweating, and sleeping problems) when we stop using a substance. Another sign is being preoccupied with continuing to use the substance in spite of its negative effect. A third sign is tolerance—the

SOME QUESTIONS THAT MAY HELP YOU IDENTIFY HARMFUL USE OR ADDICTION

- When faced with a problem, do you often turn to alcohol, tobacco, or drugs for relief?
- Do you find that you have to take increasing amounts of alcohol, tobacco, or drugs to achieve the same effects?
- Do you drive when under the influence of alcohol or drugs?
- Has your alcohol, tobacco, or drug use caused any problems in relationships with family, friends, or coworkers?
- Are you sometimes unable to meet home or work responsibilities because of drugs or alcohol?
- Have you had distressing physical or psychological reactions when you've tried to stop using alcohol, tobacco, or drugs?

- Has someone close to you expressed concern about your use of alcohol, tobacco, or drugs?
- Have you—or has anyone else—ever needed medical attention because of your drinking, smoking, or drug use?
- Have you ever tried to stop or cut down on alcohol, tobacco, or drugs and not been able to?
- Do you find yourself spending a lot of time thinking about when and where you will get the next drink or use cigarettes or other drugs again?

If you answered yes to any of these questions, your smoking, drinking, or drug use may be interfering with your life in ways serious enough for you to seek help. Remember, we can make changes in our use long before we become addicted or hit bottom.

need to use more and more to achieve the same effect.

FINDING HELP FOR HARMFUL USE AND ADDICTION

A serious alcohol or drug problem does not go away overnight, but with time, perseverance, self-care, and lots of support, we can recover our lives.

WHAT KINDS OF SUPPORT AND TREATMENT EXIST?

Treatment can take many forms; no one method works for everyone. Programs that provide assistance in all aspects of our lives—physical, emotional, and spiritual—as well as help us heal from past traumas can be particularly useful. As one woman wrote:

With the help of staff and my peers [in the treatment program], I have learned more truth about myself than I have in forty-one years. This info I will use and continue to add to and build upon. I have found so much joy being in the company of women. I have a whole new outlook, and that will affect all aspects of my life.

The following are some of the ways you can meet the challenges of recovering from problems with alcohol, tobacco, and other drugs.

QUITTING TOBACCO USE

Quitting smoking is probably the best thing we can do for our health and the health of those around us. Nearly three out of every four smokers want to quit, but it usually takes several attempts to be successful. Try not to get discouraged by temporary relapses.

There are many different and effective ways for women to stop smoking. You have the best chance if you use a combination:

- Quitting on your own ("cold turkey")
- Using self-help materials available on the Internet (see links on companion website, www.ourbodiesourselves.org)
- Attending classes or support groups
- Calling "quit lines"
- Receiving counseling from health care providers or other trained counselors
- Taking medication, such as nicotine replacement (patch, gum, or lozenge, all available over the counter) or a prescription nasal inhaler or spray, or an antidepressant (Zyban)

The most important thing to know about quitting smoking is that there is no right or wrong method, though using some form of assistance increases the chance of success.[20] Women seem to do best with a combination of methods, including social support, counseling, and medication. These treatments are available through public programs, telephone quit lines, clinics, and hospitals and will double or triple the chances of quitting permanently. If you menstruate, it may be easier to quit during the first half of your menstrual cycle. You may also want to try quitting during a time when you are not feeling overly stressed.

There are many resources to help you stop smoking. Look for them at your workplace, your health care provider, community organizations such as the American Lung Association (see www.lungusa.org), and on the Internet. A national program called Circle of Friends helps women quit smoking and empowers nonsmokers to support women who choose to quit. Their toll-free telephone number (1-800-243-7000) provides information on how to quit smoking. Their website (www.join-the-circle.org) has information for women smokers and nonsmokers.

SELF-HELP GROUPS

A woman in recovery says,

My support group is my lifeline, my "family," and my foundation. No addict should go without this feeling of connectedness—it's the biggest need of all.

When we face our problems with alcohol, tobacco, or other drugs, probably the greatest support comes from others who have been there. There are many self-help groups, with varying approaches, including Alcoholics Anonymous, Women for Sobriety, 16 Steps for Discovery and Empowerment, SMART Recovery, and Secular Organizations for Sobriety.

Other self-help groups on related topics, such as self-esteem and experience of trauma, can be helpful in combination with these recovery groups. It's worth putting some effort into finding the right combination of supports in the areas important to you; they can be critical to getting well.

MANAGING WITHDRAWAL

For those of us who have been using alcohol and/or other drugs heavily or for a long time, it's best to have supervision and support from health care providers when withdrawing. We often need help to relieve withdrawal symptoms and to reestablish sleep patterns, as well as to get treatment for a range of medical problems. A hospital or recovery center can be the best place to get this help. Pregnant women and those with HIV who are going through withdrawal from specific drugs, such as opiates and tranquilizers, may need further specialized care. Withdrawal symptoms are temporary, and they subside once the body gets used to the absence of the substance, though the desire for the substance may last for a long time.

TREATMENT FOR ADDICTION

Learning to live without drugs is not about willpower; it's about finding the personal support and nurturance you need, and redefining your life without the drugs by making changes in your habits, friends, and other aspects of your life. One woman in a women's treatment program wrote:

This [recovery program] is the greatest gift I have ever given myself or allowed myself to receive. I love myself, and I am so excited about reintroducing myself to my daughter and teaching and raising her in a healthy environment that I didn't have the opportunity to be raised in! I am the solution!

More than 2 million Americans over the age of twelve (1 percent of the population) receive some kind of special care each year for substance abuse. Another 20 million people—8.7 percent of the population—probably need such attention but don't receive it.[21]

Formal treatment programs provide medical care, individual and group counseling, and a range of other support services to help you quit, cope better, and create support networks. It may be particularly helpful to look for programs that focus on the specific needs of women.

WORKING TOGETHER ON PREVENTION, TREATMENT, AND POLICY

Alcohol, tobacco, and other drugs take a tremendous toll on our health and lives. Because so much emphasis is placed on the dangers of illegal drug use, we lose sight of the fact that legal substances cause the most damage to women as individuals and to society. In fact, tobacco use alone kills many more women than alcohol and all other drugs put together. And during pregnancy, alcohol has a more damaging effect on the fetus than illegal drugs such as cocaine.

Policies that address substance abuse often affect us differently than they do men. For instance, although men still far outnumber women in arrests for drug-related crimes, increasing numbers of women are being imprisoned for drug offenses. Some women who have used drugs during pregnancy have faced legal charges.

Women must be involved in shaping the policies and programs that are created to help us break our substance abuse habits. We must ensure that programs are designed to meet our needs and that policy makers consider how new policies will affect women and girls, as Canada has done with policies addressing tobacco use.[22]

PROMISING POLICY AND TREATMENT INITIATIVES

There are some promising initiatives to improve policy and treatment for people with drug problems and to respond specifically to the needs of girls and women with substance use problems:

- The Drug Policy Alliance is a leading U.S. organization working toward "new drug policies based on science, compassion, health and human rights, and a just society in which the fears, prejudices and punitive prohibitions of today are no more." (For more information on their work, see www.drugpolicy.org/home page.cfm.)
- Some policies have proved effective in reducing smoking and improving the public health. These include implementing clean-indoor-air laws or ordinances that make all workplaces (including bars and restaurants) smoke-free; increasing the excise tax on tobacco, which encourages smokers, especially young people and pregnant women, to quit; ensuring that private insurers and Medicaid provide coverage for services, including counseling and medication, to help people stop smoking; and implementing prevention programs that educate young people and motivate them not to start smoking. (For more information, or to become involved in these efforts, contact Americans for Non-Smokers' Rights, www.no-smoke.org, and the Campaign for Tobacco-Free Kids, www.tobaccofreekids.org.)

- Treatment providers have been working to design comprehensive trauma, mental health, and substance use programs that address women's needs for safety and healing. Seeking Safety (www.seekingsafety.org) and Community Connections (www.communityconnectionsdc.org/trauma_services.htm) are two examples of this work.

- To learn more about international issues regarding women and smoking, check out INWAT, the International Network of Women Against Tobacco (www.inwat.org). Using Women (www.usingwomen.org.uk) is also working on the international level to encourage public involvement in finding alternatives to imprisoning women for drug use.

Our understanding of treatment for and policy related to substance use continues to change. Pressures on us to use alcohol, tobacco, and other mood-altering drugs are stronger than ever. Yet there are promising advances that address the health problems associated with women's substance use. We have much to accomplish in research, policy, enforcement, and treatment to improve the lives of girls and women at risk of or involved in substance abuse, but this work is well under way.

NOTES

1. U.S. Department of Health and Human Services, Substance Abuse and Mental Health Services Administra-

tion, Office of Applied Statistics, "Results from the 2002 National Survey on Drug Use and Health (NSDUH)," accessed December 15, 2003, at www.samhsa.gov/oas/NHSDA/2k2NSDUH/Results/2k2results.htm#toc.

2. Ibid.

3. Ibid.

4. Ibid.

5. Information on alcohol's effects was retrieved from *Alcohol Research and Health: The Journal of the National Institute on Alcohol Abuse and Alcoholism* 26, no. 4, online at www.niaaa.nih.gov/publications/arh26-4/toc26-4.htm, and from J. Rehm, R. Room, K. Graham, M. Monteiro, G. Gmel, and C. T. Sempos, "The Relationship of Average Volume of Alcohol Consumption and Patterns of Drinking to Burden of Disease: An Overview," *Addiction* 98, no. 4, 1209–1228.

6. U.S. Department of Health and Human Services, *Women and Smoking: A Report of the Surgeon General* (Rockville, MD: Office of the Surgeon General, 2001).

7. J. C. Currie, "Manufacturing Addiction: The Overprescription of Benzodiazepines and Sleeping Pills to Women in Canada" (Vancouver, BC: British Columbia Centre of Excellence for Women's Health, 2003).

8. H. Ashton, *Benzodiazepines: How They Work and How to Withdraw* (Newcastle, UK: University of Newcastle), 2002. See www.benzo.org.uk/manual/index.htm.

9. M. E. Liecht, A. Gamma, and F. X. Vollenweider, "Gender Differences in the Subjective Effects of MDMA," *Psychopharmacology (Berl)* (2001) 154, no. 2, 161–68.

10. National Cancer Institute, *Risks Associated with Smoking Cigarettes with Low Machine-Measured Yields of Tar and Nicotine*, Smoking and Tobacco Control Monograph No. 13 (Bethesda, MD: U.S. Department of Health and Human Services, National Institutes of Health, National Cancer Institute, NIH Pub. No. 02-5074, October 2001).

11. Ibid.

12. L. Greaves, *Smoke Screen: Women's Smoking and Social Control* (Halifax, Canada: Fernwood Publishing, 1996).

13. Ibid., 39.

14. Ibid., 47.

15. Ibid., 50.

16. Ibid., 65.

17. M. A. Russell, "The Nicotine Addiction Trap: A 40-Year Sentence for Four Cigarettes," *British Journal of Addiction* 85, no. 2, (February 1990): 293–300.

18. M. Sanchez-Craig, *A Therapist's Manual: Secondary Prevention of Alcohol Problems* (Toronto, ON: Centre for Addiction and Mental Health, 1996).

19. Ibid.

20. U.S. Department of Health and Human Services, *Treating Tobacco Use and Dependence*, Clinical Practice Guideline (Rockville, MD: Public Health Service, June 2000).

21. U.S. Department of Health and Human Services, "Results from the 2002 National Survey on Drug Use and Health (NSDUH)."

22. L. Greaves, V. Barr, and Women and Tobacco Working Group, *Filtered Policy: Women and Tobacco in Canada* (Vancouver, BC: British Columbia Centre of Excellence for Women's Health, 2000).

CHAPTER 4

Our bodies were designed to move. Physical activity—that is, play, exercise, and other movement—is not just for athletes and sports enthusiasts. It is important for all of us.

In the past, women working on farms, in factories, and in the home doing domestic labor led such physically demanding lives that "exercise" for its own sake was a meaningless idea. Today many of us lead much more sedentary lives, and we have to work at getting the kinds of physical activity that a healthy body, mind, and spirit need.

Studies show that 72 percent of women in the United States get no regular exercise,[1] and nearly half of Americans between twelve and twenty-one years old do not exercise daily.[2] The health consequences of our sedentary lifestyles are devastating.

But physical activity can be an enjoyable part of our everyday lives. We might walk to work, play outside, garden, dance, stretch, clean our houses, make love, run. Even a regular brisk walk with a friend or family member can be both healthy for our bodies and good for our souls.

THE HEALTH BENEFITS OF EXERCISE

A growing body of evidence suggests that regular exercise can help us maintain a healthy weight and decrease the risk of high blood pressure, stroke, Type 2 diabetes, and breast cancer.[3] Even light to moderate activity (twenty minutes of walking three times a week) can help reduce blood pressure, lessen the risk of stroke, mitigate chronic pain, and improve heart and lung functions.

Heart disease—the leading cause of death in women over the age of fifty and a disproportionate threat to African-American women—can often be reduced and managed through diet and exercise. Sedentary women are twice as likely to die from heart attacks or strokes as women who are active.

After four heart attacks and a pacemaker placement, exercise has become more important to me than ever. Walking on the treadmill makes me feel like I am actively contributing to my healthy state. I have a genetic problem with cholesterol, but my doctors are convinced that being an active woman of healthy weight has helped me pull through this tremendous amount of surgery.

Loss of bone mass usually begins around the age of thirty-five, but regular weight-bearing "strength training" exercise can slow this process. One example of strength training is lifting several-pound weights. For women who are not

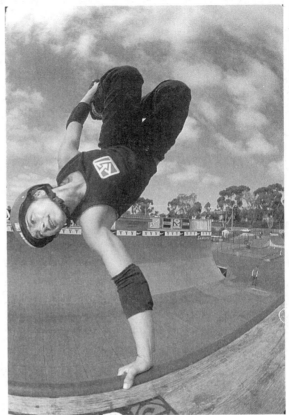

able to use weights, swimming can be a good way to build bone density.

Exercise can also help to reduce or eliminate depression and insomnia.

HOW EXERCISE MAKES US FEEL

Many of us feel anxious and stressed sometimes. Exercise can help us to cope. It can create great connections with our bodies, friends, and community, leading to better physical *and* mental health.

I love the way exercise makes me feel—strong, confident, and relaxed. It is a fun activity for me, allowing me to let out tension and just go "nuts." It raises my spirit on days when I'm feeling

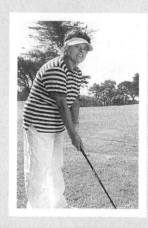
© R. A. McBride

"I HAVE MUCH MORE ENERGY"

RAJINDER KAUR SINGH

I was born in Lahore, India, one of seven children. There was no organized play when I was very young, but starting in the fifth grade, we would follow morning prayer with a half hour of exercises. The students—all girls—would stretch and do jumping jacks. I don't think we ever actually sweated! It was more like waking you up for class. This continued until the tenth grade, and then it stopped.

After that, we didn't even hear about exercise. I think our housework was basically our exercise—we would knead dough for roti, clean the house, bathe the buffalo. It's tiring to bathe the buffalo! The boys played cricket, football, hockey, but the girls didn't do those things. Some girls rode their bikes to college, but I didn't.

After I married and we immigrated to Toronto and then California, my exercise was still pretty much housecleaning: vacuuming. When my youngest son was born, I wanted to lose the baby weight, so I tried to do aerobics. I bought a tape by Kathy somebody and did it for fifteen to twenty minutes at a time. I did that for a few years. I even tried biking a little bit. I didn't have a weight problem or anything, so I guess I wasn't very worried.

Maybe five years ago, I decided to learn to play golf so that I could play with my husband. A year later, I was diagnosed with Type 2 diabetes. Diabetes runs in my family. I decided to control it by monitoring my diet and weight instead of taking a lot of medication. I changed the way I shop, the way I cook, the way I eat. And I made sure I was active in some way every day: daily walks, a lot of gardening, but not enough golf.

I lost twelve pounds, and my sugar is under control. I have much more energy, so I have become even more active. When I go back to India to visit my family, I teach them what I've learned about diabetes and exercise. I hand out pamphlets I wrote in Punjabi, telling people about it. I encourage them to eat in moderation and to at least take a walk every day. Even if it's just to the temple after dinner, I stress that it is important for both men and women to keep their bodies moving.

down and gives me a physical boost when I'm tired.

After being diagnosed with diabetes, and learning that the disease is one of the top killers of Black women, I decided to take control over my life with exercise. Today I am fit, in control of my diabetes, and educating other women about the importance of fitness.

I have always had a poor body image. I have been on some weight loss scheme or another since age ten. Exercise has given me the power to actually enjoy listening to my muscles and inner rhythms.

After exercising, a huge sense of optimism overcomes me.

GETTING STARTED

We all know that exercise is good for us. We start out with the best intentions, but finding the time, energy, facilities, child care—whatever we need to exercise—is often difficult.

After separating from the father of my children, I found solace in food and taking care of my children. As a single parent, who has the time or money to start exercising?

Be patient and diligent—the results won't come right away—but if you stick to it, you'll soon no-

tice the difference. Don't, however, beat yourself up if you skip a workout. It is important to love and accept yourself no matter what stage you are at. . . . You are the only you that you've got, so be kind and gentle to yourself while you push your limits and stretch beyond what's comfortable.

Exercise doesn't have to be hard, expensive, or time-consuming. There are lots of little things that you can do. Get off the bus two or three stops early or park at the far end of the parking lot and walk the rest of the way. Take the stairs instead of the elevator, or go for a walk at lunch. Keep a set of hand weights by the phone and lift them while waiting for the next available sales representative, or do push-ups and crunches while watching TV. Better yet, turn off the TV, put on some music, and dance.

For a structured home workout, check out Miriam Nelson's book *Strong Women Stay Young* (or her website, www.strongwomen.com). Her basic, effective at-home exercise program requires a minimum of time (twenty minutes twice a week) and equipment (a chair, a towel, ankle weights, and dumbbells).

Some exercise is better than no exercise. The American College of Sports Medicine recommends exercising three to five times a week for twenty to thirty minutes, but once or twice a week is better than no exercise at all. Moderate exercise, like walking or dancing, done in five-to-ten-minute increments for a total of thirty minutes, is also effective.

Choose an activity that looks like fun. "I've always wanted to row crew, play squash, do yoga, run a road race, ride a bike, learn to skate, dance the tango . . ." Whatever it is, here's your chance. Look around; use what's close at hand. Do you live next door to a bowling alley? Is there a park with jogging paths down the street? Do you pass by a municipal swimming pool on your way to work? Did a Brazilian dance studio recently open in your neighborhood? Has one of your friends just taken up t'ai chi? Join in. Look for community centers and public recreational facilities. The YWCA and YMCA are low-cost alternatives to commercial health clubs, and most offer financial assistance. Take a lesson. Try something out.

Make exercise convenient. Eliminate as many barriers as possible between you and your workout. Take your gym bag to work—if you go home to change, you may not make it back out the door. Try working out first thing in the morning: Your sense of accomplishment and well-being may stay with you throughout the day.

For those of us who are mothers, finding time for enjoyable exercise may be harder. If you have a young child, try walking at a brisk pace with the baby in a stroller. If you're a runner, a three-wheeled jogging stroller, though expensive, is a worthwhile investment. Or check out a program like Stroller Strides, a fitness program for new mothers. Many gyms have child care services for children as young as six months. Try bartering babysitting time with another new

There are three major kinds of physical activity that contribute to overall fitness—cardiovascular, strength and flexibility.

TYPE OF ACTIVITY	HEALTH BENEFITS
Cardio training: walking, jogging, running, aerobics, dancing, skipping rope, rowing, biking, cross-country skiing, in-line skating, boxing, basketball, soccer, swimming	Improves blood circulation and lung capacity; reduces hypertension (high blood pressure) and increases good cholesterol; burns calories, relieves stress, and improves overall endurance
Strength training: free weights, weight machines (Universal and Nautilus), resistance training	Boosts metabolism; improves muscle tone; strengthens bones, which decreases the risk of osteoporosis later in life
Flexibility training: stretching, yoga, t'ai chi, dance, Pilates, climbing, fencing, gymnastics	Reduces risk of injuries; improves agility, balance, and range of motion; relieves stress

A good fitness plan includes all three types of training. By mixing it up (focusing on cardiovascular work one day and flexibility the next), you'll increase your overall fitness.

parent or, if you are part of a two-parent household, ask your partner to cover child care so you can exercise.

With my second child, I wasn't as nervous about leaving him with a friend while I went to the gym. I realized by then that infants are tougher than they look! Being able to work out—and having some "alone time" to boot—made me feel much healthier, both mentally and physically.

As the kids get older, you can play catch or tag with them. Take them for a walk or a bike ride. Show them how to shoot hoops or take them canoeing. Kids learn by example. If they see you being active and having fun, they are more likely to do the same.

I get up early in the morning before my family and do yoga for fifteen to twenty minutes. I usually fit in an aerobic and Nautilus workout twice a week during my lunch hour (I work near the Y). My daughter is taking a kids' class at the Y, so I'm here on Saturdays, too.

WAYS TO KEEP GOING

- Balance your workouts to include cardio, strength, and flexibility.
- Vary the intensity of your workouts.
- Set short-term, reachable goals.
- Keep a fitness log to chart your progress.
- Find a workout buddy: It's harder to back out if someone is waiting for you.
- Take a lesson.
- Read up on history and technique.
- Train for a specific event.
- Exercise to music.
- Try something new.
- Remember to have fun.

Make exercise a priority, and don't let minor things interfere with your workout.

I put it in my date book and treat it like any other meeting—no canceling.

Don't let any excuse you can fabricate stop you. The benefits outweigh any argument you can conjure up not to exercise. Last year I had a revelation and just changed my life through nutrition and exercise. I educated myself about food and committed myself to exercise. I had a lot of support, but I did it for myself.

Even with a tight schedule, my motto is: You make time for what is important to you.

TEAM SPORTS

Team sports are wonderful. I've been seriously playing sports since high school. I've been rowing for eight years now. It gives me a close working bond with the other women on my team. It makes me feel that my body is a tool rather than an ornament.

Some of us love the excitement and satisfaction that comes from being part of a team. The skills that team sports teach can go far beyond the playing field. If you want to join a team, look for one that is right for you. Some are very competitive, while others are more fun-oriented and give every woman a chance to play. Try talking to the coach or watching a practice to get a sense of the team's style before joining.

Some team sports give your body a well-rounded workout, but others do not. If you play a sport where you spend much of your time standing around waiting for the ball to come to you, a separate cardiovascular activity would be a good addition. Pregame warmups and proper conditioning (building up to strenuous sports) can help you avoid injury.[4]

CARING WHAT OTHER PEOPLE THINK

"I can't do *that*, I'm too weak . . . too slow . . . too fat . . . too skinny . . . too clumsy . . ." "No one will think I'm sexy with muscles that show." "People will call me a dyke if I join that team."

Negative assumptions can keep us from exercising, but old notions about women and sports are changing. Women's wrestling is now an Olympic sport. Strong female athletes such as Mia Hamm, Michelle Wie, and Venus and Serena Williams are superstars. Still, body image sensitivity, homophobia, and other pressures hold some of us back from enjoying exercise. Rather than conforming to social expectations, women need to be comfortable being who we are, so that we can play our best.

EXERCISE, AGE, AND (DIS)ABILITY

Whatever our abilities, it's important to find ways to move our bodies. This may mean participating in adaptive sports programs, or organizing and participating in community events such as walkathons, wheelchair basketball games, and wheelchair dances. For others, it may involve doing a small range of motion exercises while in bed. For those of us with chronic illnesses such as fibromyalgia, chronic fatigue syndrome, and lupus, it can be difficult to find the fine line between gently moving our bodies as much as we're able and pushing too hard and suffering a relapse.

Due to multiple sclerosis, I haven't been able to run off stress in the conventional manner for a

year. But I have discovered a substitute that works for me. I have a motorized scooter, and when the old urge to go for a run hits me, I get on my scooter and ride at high speed around the block a few times. The fresh air on me has the feel of running and is a great stress buster.

Exercise can be an important part of recovering from surgery or a long illness.

I had a mastectomy four years ago and found the weights very important in gaining back my arm strength and sensation.

I have a mental disability (depression, trauma). With exercise, I feel that I have more power over my life; I'm less depressed and hopeless. Physically, I'm stronger, more toned.

Research shows that physical activity can significantly improve our health at any age.[5] It can make us feel better physically and emotionally, supporting other positive changes in our lives.

INJURIES AND SAFETY

To enjoy the benefits of regular exercise, pay attention to your body's signals and don't push too hard. If you are just starting, take a day or two off between workouts to give your body a chance to recover, especially if you are doing a lot of running and jumping.

Always stretch before you start cardio work, but don't stretch a cold muscle. Warm up with a few minutes of light aerobic exercise like walking. Hold the stretch; don't bounce. (You could pull the muscle if you bounce.) Stretch until you feel a little tension, then hold for ten to fifteen seconds, breathing slowly.

Pace yourself during cardio exercises. Listen to your body—if it feels comfortable and not too

1. Balance all three types of fitness: cardio, strength, and flexibility.
2. Stretch out, warm up, and gradually increase the pace.
3. Drink plenty of water.
4. Use the proper equipment for your activity.
5. Slow down, cool off, and stretch to maximize flexibility.
6. Rest between sets and take a day off now and then.
7. Listen to your body.

When treating a sprain, think RICE:

- **Rest:** Avoid activities that use the affected body part.
- **Ice:** Decreases swelling, bleeding, pain, and inflammation. Apply 2-3 times a day, 10-20 minutes, for up to 72 hours after an injury.
- **Compress:** Direct external pressure will decrease hemorrhaging and bleeding. Elastic wraps can be worn throughout the day and removed at night.
- **Elevate:** Raise the injured area to decrease bleeding and prevent fluid accumulation.

hard, then you're on target. Move at a pace that allows you to carry on a conversation. If you are huffing and puffing, slow down. You may also want to learn how to monitor your heart rate by taking your pulse or wearing a monitor. Start your workout by warming up for five minutes, spend fifteen minutes working out, and then cool down for five minutes.

If you're outdoors, remember: Be safe, be seen. Walk and run against the traffic; bike with it. Be aware of your surroundings, move with confidence, and carry a whistle or a cell phone. Use all the safety equipment recommended for your activity (helmets for biking; helmets, wrist, and knee pads for in-line skating).

TOO MUCH EXERCISE?

Some of us exercise to an extreme that actually undermines our health. While we want exercise to be a habit, it can sometimes become an addiction. We may use exercise to numb our feelings or avoid problems such as a faltering relationship or a bad work situation. Or we may become obsessive in the pursuit of a "perfect" body, keeping track of every ounce of weight and every inch of muscle and fat. Too much exercise can have severe health consequences.

I became a serious runner in my late teens, and as the pounds fell away and my timings improved, my pursuit of the perfect runner's form began. I stopped menstruating at twenty-one. I didn't miss it much—it was convenient, for an athlete. I carried my obsession with running and my weight well into my thirties, restricting my diet and setting higher and higher distance goals for myself. I'm thirty-six now, haven't menstruated in fifteen years, suffer constant stress fractures, and have osteopenia. I'm finally facing the facts, but there's not much I can do to reverse the damage. My orthopod says I have a great runner's body— for a sixty-six-year-old.

In the late 1990s, health care professionals identified the female athlete triad as a syndrome with three interrelated components: disordered eating, amenorrhea, and osteoporosis. A significantly restricted diet reduces the body's metabolism and causes changes in the musculoskeletal, cardiovascular, endocrine, and reproductive systems. Low body weight and body fat can lead to amenorrhea (missing three or more consecutive menstrual periods). Amenorrhea has been linked to premature loss of bone mineral density, which can result in osteoporosis.

The female athlete triad is most often experienced by women who participate in sports where performance is subjectively scored (such as gymnastics, dance, and figure skating); endurance sports that emphasize low body weight (distance running, cycling); sports in which participants wear contour-revealing clothes (volleyball, swimming, cross-country skiing, cheerleading); and sports that use weight categories (horse racing, wrestling, rowing).

Amenorrhea is the most recognizable symptom of the female athlete triad. Going without your period is not normal. Proper nutrition and safe training practices are essential for both performance and health.[6]

WHO'S ON THE WHEATIES BOX?: THE POLITICS OF SPORTS

Title IX of the Education Amendments of 1972 mandated that U.S. educational institutions that receive federal funds provide opportunities for women to participate in sports equal to those available for men. Since then, generations of women have come of age playing team sports in school.

Yet in many instances, women are still denied opportunities or treated as second-class citizens. According to the Women's Sports Foundation, U.S. men receive $133 million more in college athletic scholarships then women.[7] Professional tennis players who are female make thirty-seven cents for every dollar their male peers earn. Only 16 percent of collegiate athletic directors are women, and 8 percent of media coverage of

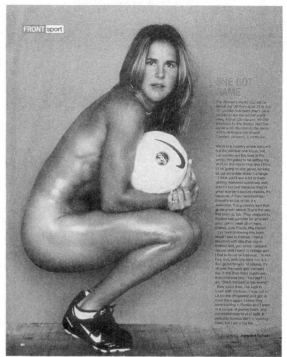

Courtesy of Sarai Walker

Olympic gold medalist Brandi Chastain shows her stuff in this photograph for *Gear* magazine, a classic example of the media's love affair with female athletes who mix strength and sex appeal.

sports focuses on women.[8] Some high schools schedule girls' basketball games on weekday afternoons and the boys' games on Friday at eight P.M. If you want to advocate for change, the Women's Sports Foundation is an excellent resource.

Female athletes are successful thanks to what their bodies can *do,* not how their bodies *look.* But all too often the mainstream media portray sportswomen as sex objects. While male athletes are more likely to be photographed in sporty action shots, female athletes might pose in revealing outfits—or nothing at all.[9] The media fall in love with female athletes who are sexy or who are willing to vamp for the camera; these women, not surprisingly, get more news coverage and endorsements, even if they aren't the best in their field.

This fact was not lost on Sepp Blatter, president of the international soccer governing body known as FIFA (Federation Internationale de Football Association). He suggested that female soccer players wear tighter uniforms to attract more television viewers, as well as fashion and beauty advertisers.[10] The Ladies' Professional Golf Association gave their players makeovers for similar reasons.[11]

It's not news that sex sells, especially images of sexy women. But our culture's attempt to turn female sports stars into pinups might also be due to discomfort with strong women. When soccer player Brandi Chastain posed naked for *Gear* magazine, with only a well-placed ball for cover, male readers may have felt more turned on than threatened by the fact that she could beat them at soccer.

The WNBA, women's World Cup soccer, and the success of individual female athletes represent great strides toward equality. But as women's sports increase in popularity, some questions remain. Who gets the product endorsements—the out lesbian tennis professional or the elfin gymnast? Is it significant that Viagra is a sponsor of the National Football League? Why does a Major League Baseball player make $25 million? And why are many of us happy to watch women's elite sports competitions from the comfort of our couch, but unlikely to exercise regularly ourselves?

These questions give us much to think about when we lace up our shoes and go for a run or start the next set of bench presses.

NOTES

1. Jane E. Brody, "Exercise Is a Habit; Here's Why to Pick It Up," *The New York Times,* September 16, 2003, D7.
2. American Diabetic Association, www.diabetes.org.
3. Michael Waldholz, "Teen Exercise May Prevent Breast Cancer," *The Wall Street Journal,* December 23, 2003, D1.
4. John O'Neil, "Finding Just the Right Cast, as Fractures Increase," *The New York Times,* September 23, 2003, D6.
5. U.S. Department of Health and Human Services, *Physical Activity and Health: A Report of the Surgeon General* (Atlanta, GA: Centers for Disease Control and Prevention, National Center for Chronic Disease Prevention and Health Promotion, 1996).
6. "American College of Sports Medicine Position Stand on the Female Athlete Triad," *Medicine and Science in Sports and Exercise* 29, no. 5 (1997): i–ix.
7. 1999–2000 NCAA Gender-Equity Report, Women's Sports Foundation calculation. Accessed at Women's Sports Foundation's website "About Us" page, www.womenssportsfoundation.org.
8. Ibid.
9. Glenda Crank Holste, "Women Athletes Often Debased by Media Images," *Women's eNews,* October 17, 2000.
10. "Brief Loss of Blatter Control," *The Washington Post,* January 17, 2004, D2.
11. Ian O'Connor, "LPGA Is Going for the Pinups," *USA Today,* July 24, 2002, 3C.

CHAPTER 5

Women have long used massage, herbal medicine, and other methods to heal ourselves, soothe members of our families, assist birth, and tend the ill. Many women continue to use traditional healing methods, which range from ginger tea for a cold to entire medical systems—such as traditional Chinese medicine and ayurvedic medicine—that have their own diagnostic techniques and treatments.

These healing methods are diverse, yet most are rooted in the following principles:

- Health is not merely the absence of disease but a state of well-being in which the body, mind, and spirit are balanced.
- Disease and treatment affect the whole body, not just one part.

- Human energy flow (variously called *chi* or *qi*, *prana*, life force, or vital energy) can be affected by disease or treatment.
- Each person has a great capacity for self-healing.

In North America, holistic health care practices are usually called complementary and alternative medicine, sometimes referred to as CAM. Complementary health practices include both practitioner-administered therapies—such as acupuncture, chiropractic, and massage—and self-care practices, such as meditation and visualization.

Until recently, there was little scientific evidence about the safety and efficacy of many complementary health practices. This began to change in 1992, when the U.S. National Institutes of Health established the Office of Alternative Medicine. Once tiny, this office is now the National Center for Complementary and Alternative Medicine, a $117 million agency[1] whose mission is to fund research and evaluate complementary therapies. The World Health Organization has also gotten involved; in 2002 it launched its first comprehensive traditional medicine strategy. Its main objectives include gathering more evidence on the safety, efficacy, and quality of traditional medicine and complementary and alternative medicine; ensuring the availability and affordability of such medicine, including essential herbal medicines; and documenting traditional medicines and remedies. As more and better research is done, we will have a clearer idea of what complementary therapies are helpful and safe to use.

TRADITIONAL HEALING PRACTICES

In much of the world, traditional healing methods or practices are not alternatives but rather the most commonly used methods of healing. They do not necessarily work as well as some conventional medical therapies, such as treatments for HIV infection. Sometimes we mistakenly romanticize the widespread use of such folk and holistic practices rather than focusing on the absence of useful, more recent medical therapies in poorer regions of the world. In such places, there are often inadequate choices, with the most effective types of interventions out of reach due to high cost.

Although conventional Western medicine is available to most people in North America, many immigrant women continue the healing traditions of our mothers. Some African-Americans still practice rootwork, and many Native American peoples have maintained traditional healing methods. Other traditional healing practices include Puerto Rican *espiritismo*, Mexican-

---

MYTH OR REALITY?

- *Drinking cranberry juice helps prevent urinary tract infections.*

Reality. Unsweetened cranberry juice makes your urine more acidic and prevents bacteria from sticking to the lining of your bladder, so you may be less likely to get a UTI.

- *Herbal remedies are safe.*

Myth. Many popular medicinal herbs are benign, but some are not, so it's a good idea to learn as much as you can about herbs that you take. For example, St. John's wort can decrease levels of many conventional drugs, and when combined with birth control pills, can result in accidental pregnancies.

American *curanderismo*, Haitian *vodoun*, and Hmong folk practices.

When I was a kid, I would always remember my mother boiling a big pot of herbs on the stove. I recall her telling me that many of the roots she knew in Puerto Rico didn't exist here, but there were a few she did know. We would search in local lots, and she would find what we needed for an herbal bath, a cold, or just to keep us away from the "wrong" folk. These are the lessons and early foundations of self-care I will never forget and that I strive to keep alive.

WHY WE CHOOSE COMPLEMENTARY HEALTH THERAPIES

More women than men use complementary health therapies.[2] We choose such alternatives for many reasons, including the belief that these therapies are gentler, safer, more effective, or less expensive than conventional medicine. (These assumptions may or may not be true for particular therapies.) Many women combine complementary health practices with more conventional ones.

How do I integrate different health care models in my life? I go to MDs mostly, but I understand their limits. I've done "talk" therapy and get (and give) massages. I take baths for aching muscles—water relaxes. Once in a while, I experiment with herbs. I think about the food I eat, take some vitamins, and have done some work with the Alexander Technique, which has helped chronic back and shoulder aches.

Many of us with chronic illnesses or disabilities may not find a cure to our diseases or conditions, but certain complementary practices may help us feel better.

I grew up with Crohn's disease and spent way too much time in doctors' offices and in hospitals. When I was older, I began exploring alternative medicine, really hoping to find new ways of taking care of myself. I had a couple of lousy experiences at first—one practitioner told me that I had to just learn to relax and love myself and then my body would heal, and a supposed nutrition specialist had me take massive doses of vitamins that ended up irritating my colon even further. But eventually, I found a great naturopath who has helped me tremendously. She has taken the time to really get to know my body and has supported me as I have experimented with different supplements, kinds of bodywork, and other holistic treatments. I still have a chronic illness—which I hate—but finding a practitioner who is smart and creative and supportive has helped me accept the limitations of my body and feel as well as I can within them.

Many complementary methods encourage self-care and prevention rather than focusing solely on treatment, as conventional Western medicine often does. Some of us choose complementary practices because they offer more possibilities for participation in our own healing. Ideally, holistic health care takes into account the whole woman and includes our relationships with our families and our communities.

TRADITIONAL AND COMPLEMENTARY APPROACHES

This section describes some of the most widely used complementary healing approaches. (For more information on the following practices, see "Resources" on the companion website, www.ourbodiesourselves.org.)

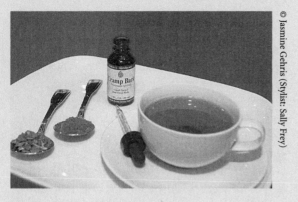

Cramp bark (*Viburnum opulus*)

© Jasmine Gehris (Stylist: Sally Frey)

Dried cramp bark is used to treat many kinds of muscle cramps, including menstrual cramps. Take an infusion three times daily, or take ten to thirty drops daily of a one-to-one fluid extract. To make an infusion, pour two cups of boiling water over one teaspoon of shredded or ground cramp bark and steep for half an hour. This provides a two-day supply. Take one third of a cup twice daily, and refrigerate the infusion between doses (it can be warmed before drinking).

HERBAL MEDICINE

Herbal medicine, also referred to as botanical medicine or phytomedicine (*phyto* is Greek for "plant"), has been used over the centuries in almost all cultures. Some herbs can be grown at home, and dried herbs are widely available and inexpensive. However, manufactured herbal preparations and concentrated herbal extracts available at health food stores may be quite expensive. Only a few herbal preparations are standardized; for many herbs, the active compounds have not been identified. The quality of herbal preparations sold in the United States is inconsistent. In an attempt to address this, the Food and Drug Administration (FDA) recently issued quality control guidelines to manufacturers.[3] However, the guidelines are voluntary, so it is important to purchase herbs from reputable sources. Herbalists in the United States are not certified or licensed to prescribe herbal medicines, but they may belong to the American Herbalists Guild.

The most common herbal medicines used in the United States are echinacea for cold and respiratory symptoms, St. John's wort for depression, ginkgo for dementia and garlic preparations for cardiovascular risk factors.[4] Many popular medicinal herbs are benign, but some are not, so it's a good idea to learn as much as you can about any herbs that you take. For example, St. John's wort can decrease levels of many conventional drugs such as digoxin, warfarin, protease inhibitors, and oral contraceptives[5] and, when combined with birth control pills, has resulted in accidental pregnancy.[6]

Much research is currently being conducted to evaluate the safety and efficacy of herbal medicines, since it is possible to evaluate them in much the same way as conventional drugs.[7]

ACUPUNCTURE

Acupuncture is one component of traditional Chinese medicine, which also includes a complex system of herbal medicine, diet, exercise, and *tuina*, a form of massage. In traditional Chinese medicine, symptoms are attributed to alterations in the flow of *qi* (energy) by trauma, stress, disease, or other factors. Acupuncture stimulates certain points along nonanatomic energy meridians to attract, disperse, or unblock the flow of *qi*.

A practitioner of traditional Chinese medicine uses several diagnostic techniques: questioning, observing, examining the tongue, listening (to breathing, voice, etc.), and reading the pulses. Acupuncturists take a person's pulses at twelve different places on the wrist. They believe that each position corresponds to an organ system, and that reading the pulse can detect subtle fluctuations in energy flow.

During treatments, disposable hair-thin stainless steel needles are inserted into acupuncture points. When the needle is inserted, the person receiving the treatment may feel a prick, tingling, numbness, pain, or nothing at all. Generally, from two to fifteen needles are used, and they are most commonly placed in the hands, forearms, lower legs, feet, back, abdomen, and ears. Needles may be placed far from the symptomatic area.

I was hit from behind by a drunk college student while backing out of a parking space. My head was twisted over my shoulder when it happened, and I suffered a very painful neck injury. After the accident, I could not move my neck at all. . . . That evening I saw my acupuncturist, who did an intensive treatment that included putting needles in a "neck spot" on my hand, and twisting the needles in, while I stretched my neck. I walked out of the office able to move my neck in both directions.

Acupuncture appears to be effective in postoperative nausea, morning sickness, recurrent headache, postoperative pain after dental treatment, and temporomandibular joint (TMJ) pain.[8] As more research is conducted, we may find out more about the efficacy of this method with other ailments.

Acupuncture is rarely associated with serious complications, but hepatitis and other infections have been linked to inadequately sterilized needles. Only disposable needles should be used.

Nonphysician acupuncturists are licensed or certified in more than forty states and the District of Columbia; even in states without licen-

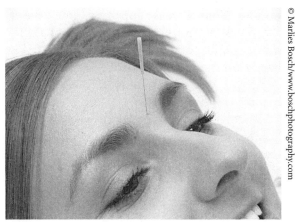

sure, an acupuncturist may choose to take the national exam administered by the National Certification Commission for Acupuncture and Oriental Medicine. This organization provides local referrals to certified acupuncturists. Many physicians have learned acupuncture, but nonphysician acupuncturists may be better trained. The amount of training required for physician acupuncturists (and, in some states, chiropractor acupuncturists) may be only two to three hundred hours; a typical education standard for a nonphysician acupuncturist is two to three thousand hours.[9] However, one advantage to a physician acupuncturist is that insurance may be more likely to pay for visits.

SPINAL ADJUSTMENT

Many women visit osteopaths or chiropractors for musculoskeletal problems or for preventive health care. The ways we habitually sleep, walk, or sit (for example, walking with our heads forward or standing with our knees locked) can cause misalignment. Trauma, physical strain from overexertion or holding one position too long, or muscle tension from mental and emotional stress, can cause pain or restrict motion. Both osteopaths and chiropractors use spinal adjustment to try to optimize the body's functioning. While there is controversy about the effectiveness of chiropractic techniques, one study found similar outcomes in patients with low back pain after six months of chiropractic care, compared with six months of medical treatment.[10]

Doctors of osteopathy (D.O.'s) are physicians licensed to do everything that M.D.'s do, but osteopaths also learn spinal manipulation (though some D.O.'s choose not to incorporate manipulation into their practice). Chiropractors are trained at chiropractic colleges and are not physicians. Some chiropractors restrict their practice to spinal adjustments, while others have expanded their practices to include other therapies. Chiropractors are licensed in every state of the U.S., and insurance generally covers chiropractic care.

BODYWORK

People turn to bodywork for a variety of reasons: to relax, to reduce tension, or to relieve pain.

Several forms of bodywork combine physical manipulation with movement education in an effort to help realign the body to create a more natural, comfortable posture, diminish tension, reduce chronic pain, and establish ease of movement. Rolfing involves deep manipulation of fascia, the connective tissue that covers muscles. The Alexander Technique, Feldenkrais, and Hellerwork make us more aware of our habitual movement patterns so that we can change or refine them. Some methods are practiced one-on-one with a practitioner; Feldenkrais and the Alexander Technique can be taught in a group setting.

Massage

Whether it's a simple hug or a complete body rub, touching is one of the most natural ways to communicate and offer comfort. It can also be an effective form of healing. We can do massage with our hands, thumbs, or feet, or with a massage ball or other instruments. We can massage our own bodies (at least the parts that we can reach), ask family or friends to massage us, or see a trained practitioner.

Foot rubs are my favorite kind of massage. They bring back childhood memories of my father rubbing my feet; they feel so good to give and to get. My children often ask me to hold and rub their feet when I go into their rooms to say good night. Some of my friends and I exchange them as a way of being close and helping each other relax.

In North America, Swedish massage is popular; this form uses long gliding strokes, friction, and kneading. Ayurvedic massage uses oil and gentle strokes. Chinese *tuina* massage utilizes deep and sometimes painful pressure. Shiatsu massage involves pressure at specific energy points. Some forms of massage are done while the person is clothed; others, which may use lubricating oils, are done with the person partially or fully nude.

Effective massage can relax the body, release muscle tension, improve joint flexibility, increase circulation and sensation, and generally enhance well-being. Practitioners often combine different massage techniques and may also use visualization and aromatherapy (use of essential oils made from flowers and herbs). A massage therapist says:

The way you touch someone is more important than the actual system you use. Whether you see yourself as channeling energy or are concerned with the muscle tone in your body and how you communicate it to someone else, you have to be rooted in your own body and pay attention to what is happening to you all the time you are giv-

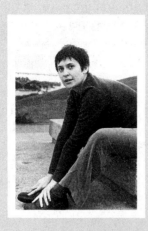

"THE CLASSES REMIND ME TO PAY ATTENTION"

AMY BOLLINGER

For the last two years, I've been periodically attending Feldenkrais Awareness Through Movement classes. One of the tenets of Feldenkrais is that you can't do what you want unless you know what you're doing—meaning that unless you pay attention to how you're moving or holding your body, you won't be able to change it. Through the classes, I realized I had changed and limited my movements to protect myself from an old back injury from a car accident. My self-image had adapted to the injury as well. I felt tighter, less confident physically.

The classes are at their core about problem solving. The teacher leads us through a series of movements. She describes them but rarely demonstrates, and she never touches or adjusts us at all. Through a combination of questions and suggestions, she helps us find approaches we may never have tried, to movements as simple as rolling over. Our goal is to find a comfortable place, not achieve an ideal pose. We're each trying to do the movement in a way that is most comfortable to our particular body. The movement itself is not important; it's how we approach it. When I'm feeling good, I can apply that same approach to problem solving in other parts of my life.

ing the massage. While I give everyone the same massage in the order of things I attend to, my touch feels different to different people.

Massage and other forms of bodywork can also release painful emotions.

When I arrived, she [the massage therapist] suggested to me that I might be storing old emotional wounds in my body, as indicated by my posture. I asked her what she meant, a bit defensively. . . .

She didn't give a mental explanation. Instead, she asked me to lie down, and she began to mas-

GIVING A MASSAGE

You don't need any special training to do general massage. Just get into a comfortable position and begin. Hold your friend's foot, head, hand, back, neck, or shoulders. Ask her where she wants pressure and whether you are applying too much or not enough. With your thumb or whole hand, find and rub tender areas or sore spots. Alternate gentle stroking with deep kneading. Avoid direct pressure on the spinal column; instead, press on either side. You don't need to massage the whole body—massaging just the feet or ears can be relaxing. Breathe regularly and deeply while giving the massage.

sage the vertebrae in my neck. . . . At first I felt only the degree of tension in my neck; gradually, I experienced a lump forming in my throat, my chest heaving, and a bunch of old sensations returning to mind. I began to cry, small jerky sobs at first, like the opening of a faucet that has been shut off for a long time. Then a burst of tears, and finally, several minutes of sobbing.

I was both terrified and relieved—terrified to think that there was so much deep emotion behind a stiff neck and relieved to know that it could be unlocked and soothed. . . .

Studies show that massage is helpful for back pain;[11] reduces lymphedema (swelling after lymph node removal) that some women have after breast cancer surgery,[12] and may benefit premature babies.[13] However, because massage may involve pressure and friction, you should not get a massage if you have phlebitis, skin infections, blood clots, inflammation, or skin that has become thin as a result of burn or injury.

Costs for massage vary, generally ranging from $50 to $85 for an hour-long massage. You may be able to find a massage school that offers less expensive massages, performed by supervised students. Some states prohibit male massage therapists from treating women and female massage therapists from treating men. If having a massage therapist of a particular sex matters to you, say so when you make an appointment. It's important to find someone with whom you feel comfortable and can communicate well. Massage therapists are licensed or certified in most states, and many are members of the American Massage Therapy Association.

MEDITATIVE PRACTICES

Meditative practices offer women ways to reduce stress and quiet the mind in order to rest from mental activity and be more present in our bodies. Many of these practices developed as part of spiritual traditions in Eastern cultures.

Meditation

A simple definition of meditation is "the intentional paying of attention from moment to moment." In the words of a woman who has taught meditation for fifteen years:

Meditation is different in its essence from every other human activity, but its essence is contained in every activity. Meditating, each one of us touches base with our deepest concerns, with the truth of our aliveness. . . . You could say it is acknowledging the radiant core of our being . . . our godliness, our Buddha nature, or whatever you like to call it.

People meditate for different reasons: to feel calm, to diminish stress or pain, to get through a crisis, or to engage in a spiritual practice. We might approach meditation for specific reasons, then discover that we want to attain a different level of consciousness or a deeper, more gratifying state of relaxation. In practicing meditation, we may feel more alert and resourceful in our daily lives.

My early-morning meditation is part silence, part chanting. Sometimes I actively pray while I sit looking out the window at the rising sun. It's important for me to meditate every morning, if only for ten minutes, to touch base with myself. I am continually surprised at how I get upset more easily on the days I don't meditate. Sometimes during the day, when I'm silent or alone, I find myself automatically feeling the tranquility I experience during meditation. This calmness helps me. Though usually my meditations are rather ordinary, on some days they are profound.

There are many ways to learn meditation: reading books, listening to tapes, or studying with a teacher. Meditation can take place indoors or outdoors, at home or in class, alone or with family, friends, self-help groups, or spiritual communities. Meditation doesn't have to be done in a cross-legged position, or even sitting down. Walking, swimming, dancing, listening to music, or rocking in a rocking chair can all be meditative activities. Any time that we focus on awareness may be meditative. (For information on another practice that focuses on awareness, see "Mindfulness Without Meditation" [W11] on the companion website, www.ourbodiesour selves.org.)

Yoga

Yoga includes *asanas* (physical poses) and *pranayama* (breathing exercises). Many types of yoga are practiced in the United States, and different teachers emphasize different aspects: Some teach yoga as a form of exercise, while others emphasize breathing. Some practices are entirely secular, while others incorporate a religious and spiritual aspect.

When doing yoga postures, I was asked to move slowly into the posture, to hold it still for some time, and then to gradually release. This way of exercising has dramatic effects on my mind. I often begin in some turmoil, filled with the concerns of my day. As I focus my attention on my movements and my breathing, I experience my mind slowing down and relaxing. The practice gives me some distance from my problems. Doing the postures releases new energy, relaxes me, and allows for another perspective to emerge.

We can learn some yoga on our own by using books, CDs, and videos, but beginners often find it helpful to learn from an instructor. Classes range widely in cost, with less expensive classes taught at local Y's, community centers, adult education programs, dance studios, and fitness centers. Once we learn the poses, yoga asanas are easy to practice on our own and don't require extensive equipment or much space.

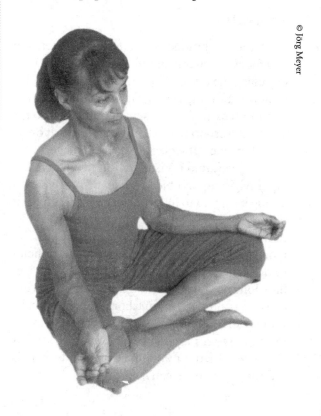

© Jörg Meyer

People with back pain often find yoga helpful, and studies have shown that yoga can benefit those with osteoarthritis[14] and carpal tunnel syndrome.[15] As with any exercise, it's important to pay attention to the fine line between exerting yourself and pushing beyond your individual limits. Benefits come from the effort rather than from reaching a specific goal.

T'ai Chi

T'ai chi, one form of Chinese martial arts, is moving meditation intended to balance the flow of energy, known as *chi* or *qi*. T'ai chi uses gentle, flowing body movements. The person practicing t'ai chi learns how to move the head and each leg, foot, hand, and arm in graceful and coordinated movements, while centering the mind. T'ai chi instruction is often available through Y's or community health centers.

Relaxation

Relaxation techniques allow us to release tension and focus the energy of our mind and body. One popular relaxation technique is progressive relaxation training (PRT), in which people first learn to tense and relax separate muscle groups and then learn to relax all muscle groups at once.

Relaxation practices that use imagery are called *visualization*. Visualization involves relaxing, imagining an object, scene, or process, and letting it expand to fill your consciousness until it becomes the only thing in your awareness. Meditative visualization is a learned skill; some achieve it quickly, others slowly, and some find it difficult to do at all. A teacher may be helpful. Midwives have long used positive images and relaxation exercises to calm women in labor. Whether visualization can be employed successfuly to rev up the immune system against cancer or other serious disease is a matter of intense debate, but there is little question that it can help us relax.

In the words of a scientist who underwent several operations for cancer:

The two years since I had the last operation have been the most productive of my life. I've had the opportunity to investigate healing in a way that I never did before. At first, when I felt the pain, I kept looking for an outside figure, a god figure, to help me, to care for me, to make it better. Then I said to myself, "Who's the most caring, best mother you know?" And I said, "I am." So I pictured myself cuddling myself. When the pain came, I went to it as a mother would to a child. I said, "How can I help it? How can I go to it?" Now when it comes, I say, "Poor baby." I tried to treat myself in a loving way. The more loving I was to myself, the more healed I felt. Now the pain is mostly gone.

TRY THIS HEALING VISUALIZATION

Relax and let your attention go to the particular body part that's causing discomfort or pain or isn't functioning as it should. Focus your attention on this place, and let yourself experience what it feels like right now. After a while, allow a positive image related to that area to come to your mind. It may be specific or abstract. Keep your mind focused until you are content with your image. Change it whenever you want. Now begin to visualize something happening within that part of your body to make it work better or start to heal. You might imagine energy, light, or color flowing into it; you might imagine it becoming warm or cool. Notice how this image affects how that part of your body feels.

DANCE AND MOVEMENT THERAPIES

Throughout the ages, women have danced and used movement for pleasure and relaxation. In many cultures, dance is a vital cultural and spiritual component of community. Some of us are learning the dances of our ancestors and of other peoples' traditions—Hawaiian, African, Native American, and other indigenous forms of dance—to develop both spiritual and physical well-being.

Movement also can be a more formal mode of healing. Dance therapy uses movement rather than words to address our physical body, emotions, mental attitude, and relationship with the world. A dance therapist observes us and moves rhythmically with us, mirroring not only our physical movements but also the feelings behind those movements. As we learn to identify certain details of our physical and emotional states while we move, we can begin to alter our movements so that we feel more comfortable with ourselves.

As part of an exercise, the group was physically lifting up a very large woman. This woman strongly believed that she always had to be supporting other people, but other people could not support her, especially because of her size. So the experience of being lifted up was a turning point for her. After this experience, she could believe that people would support her in other ways as well.

Spiritual Healing

The word "spirit" includes a wide range of concepts, including nonmaterial beings such as ghosts or ancestors, the soul, emotions, or one's true inner core or most fundamental self. For some of us, spirituality is associated with our deities or God; it is the "spirit" part of our being, along with our mind and body, that is addressed through spiritual healing practices. What constitutes spirit or spirituality depends on our religious and cultural orientations and upon the healing orientations of the practitioners we consult.

Spiritual healing is a way of life for many people. Venues for spiritual healing range widely and include home altars, shrines of *vodoun* practitioners, Protestant and Roman Catholic churches, synagogues, and prayer chains on the Internet. People may attribute healing to a nonphysical entity (spirit or deity or God or Jesus Christ), a group (prayer group, healing circle, church group), an individual (minister, shaman, psychic), or attendance at a "miraculous" place such as Lourdes. Techniques and rituals used in spiritual healing may include meditation and prayer, touching with healing intent, communication with the spirit realm, and connecting with sacred deities or ancestors.

In many communities of color, spiritual healing has a strong religious base, with roots in West Africa or in indigenous communities of the Caribbean and the Americas. Many religious healing practices are used not only to assist in curing an illness but for general cleansing, safety, and spiritual guidance. *Espiritismo,* a synthesis of Yoruban (West African) and Afro-Cuban spiritual traditions, is extremely popular in Puerto Rican, African-American, and Caribbean communities, where individuals will go to an *espiritista* to find comfort, guidance, and help with health problems.[16] An *espiritista* may also assist in removing negative influences from the individual's person or home. Often people will go to a *centro espiritista* or to a *botanica* to seek individuals with the gift of "sight" who can offer a reading and suggest ways of returning to a state of balance. Other forms of spiritual healing include *curanderismo* and Santeria.

ENERGY HEALING

Therapeutic Touch is a secular form of energy healing in which a practitioner channels energy to help the healing process in another person. Despite its name, the practice may not involve touching; the practitioner's hands are usually moved over the patient's body at a distance of several inches, in an effort to affect energy fields. Therapeutic Touch is practiced widely by nurses.

I went into the nurse's office as a migraine was just beginning. While I had heard about Therapeutic Touch, I had never tried it before. When the nurse offered me a choice of decongestants, pain relievers, Therapeutic Touch, or some combination, I decided to try Therapeutic Touch. (After all, I knew what the drugs could and couldn't do for me.) After the session, my head felt lighter and less congested.

Other energy therapies include Reiki and polarity therapy. All involve a healing intent on the part of the practitioner who seeks to affect a person's energy field.

HOMEOPATHY

Homeopathy is a system of medicine that uses highly dilute preparations made from plants, minerals, or animals in efforts to stimulate healing. Samuel Hahnemann, a German physician, developed homeopathy in the late 1700s. He articulated the Law of Similars, which holds that tiny doses of a substance that causes certain symptoms can be used to treat the same symptoms. For example, a homeopath would give a patient with a fever a dilute dose of a substance that, in larger doses, would cause fever.[17]

An initial visit with a homeopath generally takes an hour to an hour and a half and includes detailed discussion about a person's eating and sleeping habits, psychological and emotional state, fears, cravings, and family history as well as the specific ailments that are causing discomfort. After a homeopathic remedy is used, symptoms often worsen before they improve; homeopaths consider that a good sign. Oral homeopathic remedies usually come as liquid remedies or as tiny pills that are placed under the tongue.

The Council for Homeopathic Education accredits homeopathic training programs. Some practitioners are licensed in another health care practice, such as naturopathy or chiropractic. A few states in the U.S. license medical doctors specifically for homeopathy.

CHOOSING THERAPIES, SELF-HELP GROUPS, AND PROVIDERS

To determine which practices might work for us, we can read books, do research online, take classes, or talk with other people about their experiences. Many local libraries, community health clinics, and women's centers offer information about complementary health practices.

We can form support groups to help one another in our efforts to be healthy, to heal the wounds created by living in an oppressive and often violent world, and to research and share information about different methods of healing. Support groups that address concerns such as chronic illness, stress reduction, addiction, or eating disorders are low- or no-cost options frequently based out of hospitals, university health centers, or community centers.

Complementary health practitioners work in a range of settings, including clinics, private offices, health spas, and homes. To find a practitioner, ask for referrals from a health care provider, friends, or family, or seek local referrals from national organizations. Below are some tips to consider as you choose a provider:

- Seek practitioners who listen carefully and are willing to try different approaches and teach you skills to improve your health. Ask for personal referrals, interview several practitioners, and trust your intuition. If you are not comfortable with a practitioner for any reason, go to someone else.
- Look for practitioners who are willing to be part of a team of providers rather than someone who discourages you from getting other care. Avoid those who insist that any other therapy will undermine treatment.
- Avoid practitioners who seem to blame you for your health problems.
- If a treatment isn't helping after a month or two, or after three or four treatments, try something else. Be wary of those who try to get you to keep returning to them for additional services without improvement in your health or quality of life. Don't trust practitioners who try to commit you to a long series of treatments before you can expect to see any benefit. Avoid practitioners who ask you to purchase expensive equipment or expensive remedies, especially if they sell them from their office.
- Beware of practitioners and marketers of alternative approaches who offer miraculous results. Don't trust sweeping claims about curing cancer, AIDS, or other serious diseases.
- Be aware that good practitioners generally see themselves as facilitators of the healing process, rather than as conquerors of disease.
- Ask about the cost of the treatment. If you have health insurance, check to see whether the treatment is covered. If you are unable to pay the full rate, look for practitioners who have sliding-scale fees or who are willing to barter services. Massage schools and other training programs often offer affordable treatments for those who are willing to be treated by supervised students.
- Apart from traditional diagnostic techniques (such as pulse and tongue diagnosis in traditional Chinese medicine), beware of alternative diagnostics, including iridology (which claims to diagnose disease through examination of the iris), muscle testing, machines that purport to detect energy fields, etc. Alternative laboratory tests are almost always a waste of money. These include stool tests for candida; blood tests that detect food allergies; saliva testing for estrogen, progesterone, and testosterone levels; hair analysis; and any test that claims to measure aging or tells you what vitamins you should take.
- Competence matters. National certification exams exist for some complementary therapies; however, no piece of paper guarantees a person's ability to heal (nor does the lack of a recognized credential mean that a person isn't skillful or knowledgeable). Expect practitioners to be able to describe their training and experience in relation to the treatment they provide and ask about their experience in cases similar to yours. Be wary of practitioners who have no indicators of their qualifications.
- Explore the politics of the method you want to use. Ask yourself: Who profits from this mode of healing? Complementary and alternative healers can also be profiteers or use shamanic, Native American, and other traditional practices in exploitive ways, for example, to add a veneer of mysticism to what they do.

(For more information on finding the best care, see "How to Evaluate Health Care Information," p. 704 in Chapter 30, "Navigating the Health Care System.")

SOCIAL AND POLITICAL AWARENESS

Alternative modes of healing seem to promise a richer way of practicing health care than the standard drugs and surgery used in conventional Western medicine. However, holistic practices and practitioners can have some of the same weaknesses as conventional Western medicine and M.D.s, as well as additional problems of their own.

In complementary medicine, as in any system where practitioners or experts are the more powerful members of society, racism and elitism can affect the care of people of color. Some institutions devoted to holistic health deal with the broader issues of the people they serve, including racism. For example, La Clínica de La Raza in California is one model where complementary health care is offered in the context of community-based education and service.

When I first sought holistic health care practitioners, I was a little nervous, because many of the practitioners and clients didn't look like me, nor did they seem to have a broad cultural understanding. I remember walking into offices where people looked at me as though I were an intruder. But when other folks walked in the office, they were welcomed and greeted graciously. Nonetheless, after many attempts with practitioners who were afraid to touch me because of the color of my skin, I found people who looked like me, felt like me, and were eager to assist me in my struggle to keep healthy in a very unhealthy society.

When complementary approaches identify the locus of healing only in the individual, as conventional Western medical practice often does, they disregard political factors such as poverty, racism, and environmental degradation as major sources of ill health. For instance, a conventional practitioner might prescribe antidepressants or sedatives, while a traditional practitioner might prescribe herbs or a change in diet; neither may realize that health problems might be caused by domestic violence, a dangerous job situation, the rigors of parenting, or the grind of poverty.

Trusting our capacity for self-healing is not the same thing as blaming ourselves for illness. Some alternative practitioners imply—or state—that if we get sick or don't get well, it's our fault. They may suggest that wrong thinking, lack of will, a driven or meek personality, or insufficient faith in the practitioner is the real root of illness. This "blame the victim" attitude is both cruel and inappropriate.

ACCESS TO CARE

Many complementary therapies remain inaccessible to low-income people. Traditional methods may be affordable within specific ethnic communities but can be expensive when provided to, or by, outsiders to those communities. Complementary therapies are not always covered by insurance, though some insurance companies cover a limited number of complementary treatments or offer discounts on treatments with selected providers.

While insurance companies should cover complementary medicine, insurance is not a panacea. Many women are uninsured or have limited access to health care facilities. Also, insurance is designed to pay for treatment when we are ill, while complementary care emphasizes staying healthy.

Conventional Western medicine will have to change before complementary and alternative medicine can be fully integrated. This may not happen until the profit motive is removed from health care services. For example, herbs and dietary supplements are not patentable and cannot be as profitable as drugs. Effective botanical treatments and mind-body therapies won't be prescribed as long as most of doctors' continuing education is sponsored by pharmaceutical companies. Complementary therapies may best be utilized within a single-payer health care system, which could emphasize preventive care and a broad range of cost-effective therapies. We can promote such changes by writing to our legislators, joining organizations, and educating others and ourselves. As more research better defines which holistic practices are effective, we will be better able to advocate for their more widespread availability.

NOTES

1. National Center for Complementary and Alternative Medicine budget FY 2004, accessed at http://nccam.nih.gov/about/appropriations.

2. P. M. Wolsko et al., "Insurance Coverage, Medical Conditions, and Visits to Alternative Medicine Providers: Results of a National Survey," *Archives of Internal Medicine* 3, no. 162 (February 11, 2002): 281–87.

3. Guidance for Industry Botanical Drug Products, accessed at www.fda.gov/cder/guidance/index.htm.

4. K. Linde, G. ter Riet, M. Hondras, A. Vickers, R. Saller, D. Melchart, "Systematic Reviews of Complementary Therapies—An Annotated Bibliography, Part 2: Herbal Medicine," *BioMed Central Complementary and Alternative Medicine* 1, no. 2 (2001): 5.

5. A. Fugh-Berman, E. Ernst, "Herb-Drug Interactions: Review and Assessment of Report Reliability," *British Journal of Clinical Pharmacology* 58 (January 2001): 587–95.

6. U. I. Schwarz, B. Buschel, and W. Kirch, "Unwanted Pregnancy on Self-Medication with St. John's Wort Despite Hormonal Contraception," *British Journal of Clinical Pharmacology* 55, no. 1 (January 2003): 112–13.

7. E. Ernst, "Are Herbal Medicines Effective?," *International Journal of Clinical Pharmacology and Therapeutics* 3, no. 42 (March 2004): 157–69.

8. K. Linde, A. Vickers, M. Hondras, G. ter Riet, J. Thormahlen, B. Berman, D. Melchart, "Systematic Reviews of Complementary Therapies—An Annotated Bibliography, Part 1: Acupuncture," *BioMed Central Complementary and Alternative Medicine* 1, no. 1 (2001): 3.

9. T. J. Kaptchuk, "Acupuncture: Theory, Efficacy, and Practice," *Annals of Internal Medicine*, 5, no. 136 (March 5, 2002): 374–83.

10. E. L. Hurwitz, H. Morgenstern, P. Harber, G. F. Kominski, T. R. Belin, F. Yu, A. H. Adams, "A Randomized Trial of Medical Care with and Without Physical Therapy and Chiropractic Care with and Without Physical Modalities for Patients with Low Back Pain: 6-Month Follow-up Outcomes from the UCLA Low Back Pain Study," *Spine* 20, no. 27 (October 15, 2002): 2193–204.

11. A. D. Furlan et al., "Massage for Low Back Pain," *Cochrane Database of Systematic Reviews*, 2 (2002): CD001929.

12. A. F. Williams et al., "A Randomized Controlled Crossover Study of Manual Lymphatic Drainage Therapy in Women with Breast Cancer–Related Lymphoedema," *European Journal of Cancer Care* (Engl.) 4, no. 11 (December 2002): 254–61.

13. A. Vickers et al., "Massage for Promoting Growth and Development of Preterm and/or Low Birth-Weight Infants," *Cochrane Database of Systematic Reviews* 2 (2004): CD000390.

14. M. S. Garfinkel et al., "Evaluation of a Yoga-Based Regimen for Treatment of Osteoarthritis of the Hands," *Journal of Rheumatology* 12 (December 21, 1994): 2341–42.

15. M. S. Garfinkel et al., "Yoga-Based Intervention for Carpal Tunnel Syndrome: A Randomized Trial," *Journal of the American Medical Association* 18, no. 280 (November 11, 1998): 1601–603.

16. M. Singer and R. Garcia, "Becoming a Puerto Rican Espiritista: Life History of a Female Healer," in Carol Shepherd McClain, ed., *Women as Healers: Cross-Cultural Perspectives* (New Brunswick, NJ: Rutgers University Press, 1989).

17. For a review on the efficacy of homeopathy, see K. Linde, M. Hondras, A. Vickers, G. ter Riet, D. Melchart, "Systematic Reviews of Complementary Therapies—An Annotated Bibliography, Part 3: Homeopathy," *BioMed Central Complementary and Alternative Medicine* 1, no. 1 (2001): 4.

CHAPTER 6 ■ ■ ■ ■ ■ ■ ■ ■ ■ ■ ■ ■ ■ ■ ■ ■ ■ ■ ■

Sustaining our emotional well-being* is often challenging. Most of us feel sad, angry, frightened, or confused at various periods in our lives, and it often helps when family and friends give us emotional and practical support. But when we can't get through difficult periods even with their help, it can be useful and even life-saving to turn to other sources. These may include activities that help us feel better, specialized self-help groups, clergy or pastoral counselors, and mental health professionals.†

* This chapter includes practical guidelines and information about emotional well-being. For more information about emotional problems, including severe conditions and crisis situations, see "Resources" on the companion website, www.ourbodiesourselves.org, as well as *Treatment and Rehabilitation of Severe Mental Illness* by William Spaulding, Mary Sullivan, and Jeffrey Poland (New York: Guilford Press, 2003).

† A term commonly used to refer collectively to psychiatrists, psychologists, social workers, and other individuals who are trained to help people with psychological and emotional problems.

Figuring out what to do and where to turn can take some trial and error. You often have more resources available, both within yourself and within your family and community, than you might at first imagine. You can rely on your own intuition as well as the advice of people you trust.

You may be upset over work, money, relationships, illness, or other concerns. Discrimination (because of sex, race, class, age, looks, sexual orientation, gender identity or expression, religion, disability, or other factors) may have affected you in ways that are hard to handle. Life-altering events such as sexual abuse or the loss of a loved one may feel difficult if not impossible to deal with alone. You may have recently moved to a different area, lost your home, or migrated from one country to another. Regional or military conflicts may have turned your life upside down. Or you may simply feel bad and not know why.

During difficult times, doing positive things for ourselves—such as eating well, exercising, and enjoying simple pleasures (hot baths, time alone, or special time with friends) can bring some relief and comfort. These activities may also help prevent or manage the physical problems that can result from periods of excessive demands and pressures. These include headaches; neck, back, and shoulder pains; insomnia; skin rashes; jaw pains; cold sores; stomachaches; severely increased or decreased appetite; and diarrhea or constipation.

At times it is enough to talk, cry, ask friends for encouragement (or a foot rub), or find ways to laugh and play. Here are some other things you can try:

- **Wellness strategies** such as eating well, getting enough rest and exercise, meditating, and participating in relaxing activities. A healthy body and a calm mind can help you become more resilient.

- **Spiritual work,** including meditation, prayer, and involvement in a religious community.
- **Creative activities,** alone or with others: dancing, singing, arts and crafts, reading for fun, or learning about the kinds of dilemmas or problems you are confronting, through novels, biographies, or magazine articles.
- **Support, self-help, or common-interest groups.** Many groups exist that address various problems and challenges—becoming a new mother, recovering from addiction, growing older, choosing parenthood as a lesbian, understanding self-injury, living with a particular illness or disability, or separating from a long-term relationship. At their best, these groups help people to feel less alone and to see individual concerns within a larger societal context.
- **Friendships and community.** Find and reach out to a community of family, friends, neighbors, and spiritual advisers with whom you can celebrate and grieve life transitions. Sometimes a good listener is what we need most.
- **Working for social/political change.** Working to change social and economic factors that make life difficult, from expensive day care to racial discrimination on the job, can be meaningful, especially when the things you are trying to change are the things that cause you pain.

THERAPY AS AN OPTION

Sometimes those closest to you are unable or unwilling to talk about what's wrong, offer unhelpful advice, or are too much a part of your problem to assist you. Even when you have good support from people who care for you, you may still want additional help or a fresh perspective. If so, it can be useful to explore the option of therapy.

Choosing therapy is not a sign of weakness, as some people believe; nor is it "putting your business out where everyone can see." Therapists are supposed to keep confidential all that goes on in therapy as part of their legal obligation to a client. Moreover, you don't have to be concerned about protecting a therapist's feelings (as you might with a close friend or family member) and thus may feel free to talk more openly.

Many mental health professionals tend to assume that emotional distress, especially in a woman, requires medication, psychotherapy, or both. It helps to find a therapist who focuses not only on your problems but also on your strengths and resources, which are your essential raw materials for coping. Good caregivers recognize that even women who experience such traumas as child sexual abuse or rape have the capacity for resiliency. They also recognize the importance of holding abusers responsible, so that women are less likely to feel guilty or blame ourselves for these traumas. (See box: "Emotional Trauma and Psychiatric Diagnosis," p. 93.)

Therapy sessions facilitated by a mental health professional may occur one-on-one or in a couple, family, or group setting. Therapy involves an exchange between the client and the therapist. Through these discussions, you can seek to experience and express your feelings, understand your emotional life more fully, tell your story and possibly rethink it to come to a new understanding of your history. You can learn about your inner strengths, think about your concerns in various contexts (personal, interpersonal, societal), explore possible solutions for current life problems, and learn better ways to communicate your needs.

For the past five years, my husband and I have been struggling with a life-threatening illness. I felt out of control, and I looked for a therapist who could help me with overwhelming feelings of helplessness, fear, and rage. While I have a large network of supportive friends, talking with them did not stop my spiral into depression. I found a friendly, direct woman with forty years of experience. She helped me affirm and sort out my feelings and pointed me in a direction that enabled me to take action. My situation hasn't changed, and yet I feel more control over my life. Therapy is not a panacea, but it has been an instrument of enormous help in this very difficult life situation.*

Therapy can be useful for exploring in greater depth such painful and debilitating issues as a severe eating problem, an addiction, difficult childhood and family situations, or past or present trauma caused by emotional, physical, or sexual violence and abuse. Sometimes therapy helps people to deal better with anger and with unwarranted shame or self-blame about discrimination, abuse, and violence based on race, sex, sexual orientation, physical ability, or age. It can, for example, encourage you to confront and change discriminatory practices.

After my episode [two weeks in a mental hospital], I benefited a great deal from weekly individual meetings with a male psychiatrist. Sometimes it was frustrating because he wanted to avoid conflict or discussing my sexual abuse memories, but meeting with a male authority figure who treated me with caring and respect was also deeply healing. Participation in a support group . . . was wonderful for me. Our meetings were sometimes the only place I felt sane all week. "Oh, you feel that way, too!" could be more soothing than any pill. Currently, I see a therapist once a month . . . [take medication] and practice daily meditation. This combination allows me to be an attorney with a full caseload.

Sometimes therapists suggest drugs as a means of coping. Because long-term use of psychotropic drugs may produce significant negative effects, it is good to explore alternatives to drugs. Research has demonstrated that regular exercise, daily meditation and conscious breathing, and self-help groups can have positive helpful effects. In some cases, you may need to take drugs on a long-term basis, but there may be ways to lessen their negative effects.

When my partner of 12 years left me, I was so sad I didn't want to get out of bed. I saw a psychiatrist twice a week. . . . After seven months, I felt no better and ran out of money to pay her. Around that time, a friend urged me to join a hiking club, and that helped a lot—the exercise and the companionship!

DIFFERENT KINDS OF THERAPISTS

The categories of therapists include marriage and family therapists, mental health counselors, nurses, social workers, psychiatrists, and psychologists. The specifics about different specialists may be useful to know, especially since they affect insurance coverage. The type of therapy can have a significant impact on whether or not it will help you. For example, it may be useful to turn to a cognitive or behavioral therapist to deal with a particular phobia (like fear of crowded places). While psychiatrists (trained medical doctors) used to be the only therapists permitted to hospitalize people and to prescribe medications, many social workers and psychologists now also have hospital-admitting privileges, and some states allow psychologists, nurses, and other professionals to prescribe medications. In addition, some therapists routinely collaborate with psychiatrists or others who can prescribe medications.

Historically, *social workers'* training has included substantial focus on an individual in the context of family and community (social welfare issues). *Psychologists* are trained to administer and interpret standardized psychological tests and to practice psychotherapy or other types of clinical interventions. *Psychiatrists* are medical doctors with more training about physical diseases and psychopharmacology (the science of drugs that affect the mind). *Marriage and family therapists* and *licensed mental health counselors* tend to handle such problems as divorce and parenting.

Therapists of all kinds may use various approaches and usually have a particular style and approach that you can ask them to describe. (For more information, see "Approaches to Therapy" [W12] on the companion website, www.our bodiesourselves.org.)

While all these therapists may be licensed in your state, they may not all be reimbursed by insurance. Check with the professional organizations or licensing boards for each specialty in your state to find out whether they can accept third-party reimbursement. Be sure to ask about fees and insurance before you make a first appointment. Many of us do not have *any* insurance coverage for such professional help, and free care options are frequently not available (yet another reason we need major health and medical care reforms in this country). Some therapists offer sliding-scale fees.

If you are in a managed care plan with limited options, you may be able to see a provider outside your network. If going outside the network is not a standard option, ask if there is an appeal process. A practitioner outside the network does not have to accept only what the insurance company is willing to pay. Many practitioners actually prefer to avoid direct payments from insurers and instead ask that clients get reimbursed on their own. Find out how much your insurance pays for out-of-network providers, so you can know what you will be compensated for and have the flexibility to see the therapist of your choice.

FINDING A COMPETENT, CARING THERAPIST

To find a therapist whose training, style, and personality are suited to your needs, ask people whom you trust: friends, family, colleagues, neighbors, religious or spiritual advisers, current health care practitioners. You can also contact local mental health centers or places where therapists teach, such as colleges, therapy training centers, or hospitals. Culturally and linguistically appropriate mental health care is not yet recognized as a right in many institutions, so you may need help from others to help you address your particular needs.

After finding a possible therapist, here are some questions you may want to ask, either on the phone or at the initial meeting:

- Do you charge for the initial meeting? If so, how much? How much do you charge for ongoing sessions? Do you have sliding-scale fees?
- What are your training and theoretical orientation/approach?
- Can we discuss various options that you think might be useful for me?
- How do you prefer to work with people: individually, as part of a couple or family, or in a group?
- What are your specialties?
- Are you experienced in working with my specific concerns?
- Do you consult with other colleagues to discuss your therapy work when you have difficulties or concerns?
- Are you comfortable working with my particular race, ethnic or religious background, class, sexual orientation, or disability?
- How often would you suggest we meet, and would you have the time available?
- What are your policies about changing appointments? How much notice must I give?

- Can you be reimbursed by my insurance plan? What will happen if my insurance coverage runs out?
- If I have no insurance and no other way to pay, do you know of other resources I can turn to?
- What do you think about the use of psychotropic drugs?

As you speak to potential therapists, how do they sound to you? Do they answer your questions in a respectful manner? Do you feel comfortable with them? The quality of the relationship with any therapist is critical. Trust your own reactions to the initial interview. Think about whether the therapist's training and style might suit your needs. Don't hesitate to interview several people to find someone with whom you feel quite comfortable.

I've gone to a variety of therapists for shorter and longer periods of my adult life, by myself and with family members. The first time I went, I chose to see a woman, but men have helped me as well. The best of these therapists had these features in common:

They were gentle, friendly, and respectful.

They listened well and understood what I was saying.

They accepted the way I presented issues and didn't alter them to fit some theory.

Their own life problems didn't usually get mixed up with mine; when that happened, they were able to acknowledge it.

They helped me define my problems and see my way to making the changes I wanted to make.

They were open to my criticisms of them.

They cared that I succeeded without claiming responsibility for my success.

Working with the help of therapists who had these qualities, I felt stronger as a person and clearer about my life.

HOW TO KNOW IF A HELPER IS REALLY HELPING YOU

Finding your way through painful times and circumstances is not easy and often doesn't follow a straight line. Sometimes you will feel worse, as you realize that you misjudged someone you once trusted or you need to make changes in your life. If you think that your helper—whether a professional therapist, a friend or relative, a religious or spiritual leader, or anyone else—is consistently unsupportive, or if you feel increasingly worse about yourself over time, you should turn elsewhere or at least get a second opinion.

Good therapists are caring and supportive listeners. They may see *different* things in you than you see in yourself, and they are willing to challenge you in respectful ways that help you toward insight, or motivate you to make positive changes.

A professional title is no guarantee of the quality of therapy or the kind of person a therapist is. Each category of therapist includes individuals with various attitudes and beliefs about women and about healing and emotional health, as well as different degrees of awareness about the larger societal context in which you live. It may be important to you, for example, to find a therapist who is able to acknowledge power relations in your life as well as sexism, racism, homophobia, and other -isms that may make it hard for you to feel that you fit in with the world around you.

Some women mistakenly assume that male or female therapists who claim to be feminist therapists are inherently more likely to treat us with respect or to be somehow "better" than other therapists. Whether someone is a feminist

therapist, a behavior therapist, a psychoanalyst, or another type of professional may be less important than how you relate to that person.

You can stop seeing a therapist at any time, either because she or he is not right for you or because you no longer feel the need for that particular kind of help. But it may not be wise to stop therapy simply because it stirs up painful feelings, especially if you have a good relationship with your therapist.

Sometimes we encounter therapists who have limited skills or who are just not right for us. For example, women who seek counseling from clergy or other pastoral counselors may find that they impose traditional ideas of women's roles in unhelpful and limiting ways.

It is inappropriate for a therapist to try to create a social relationship with you, to discuss other clients by name or by other clearly identifying data, or to reveal inappropriate personal information. If a therapist suggests or initiates any sexual contact, it is crucial to leave immediately and make a report to the therapist's regulatory association. Encouraging a client to become a friend, lover, or business partner is wrong, as is other unprofessional behavior that may interfere with your therapy.

THE LIMITS OF THERAPY

Given that we live in an increasingly psychologized and psychiatrized climate, you might be inclined toward interpreting uncomfortable or upsetting feelings as a sign that something is wrong with you. You might assume mistakenly that friends would not be helpful because they are not trained therapists. It is sometimes hard to figure out what to do and where to turn.

Who is emotionally healthy? Who is normal? Who is mentally ill? Asking these questions is like asking "What is love?" or "What is art?" There are many answers. Mental health professionals have different definitions of emotional health and mental illness, and these definitions influence how they assess our problems. They also work in a field where intuition and sensitivity are as important as knowing the wide range of effects that antidepressants and other drugs may have on us.

Sometimes people may assume that you are mentally ill and may fail to consider that you are emotionally healthy but coping with difficult situations. Research has shown that therapists and laypeople—even women—often interpret as problematic in women the same behavior that they interpret as neutral or even positive in men.

It is important not to jump to the conclusion that you are sick simply because you are seeking help. Responsible therapists recognize that people are often the best experts on themselves and will work with you to interpret and understand behavior.

I was sent to Iraq in 2003 with my Army reserve unit. It was crazy-making, because we'd been told the Iraqi people would kiss our feet for liberating them, but most of them wanted us out of their country. And you never knew who was a friend and who might try to blow you up. After 10 months, I came home, and I couldn't sleep, couldn't say a civil word to anyone, just felt angry all the time. Nobody wanted to hear what it was like over there. They kept telling me I should "let go" of the past and get back to my nice, safe life here. Never thought I'd go to a therapist, but finally I saw a psychologist, and talking to her helped some. But it was rough, feeling the only person I could talk to got paid for listening, and I pulled away from my folks and my friends.

One day, my best friend, Sophia, asked if she had offended me because I never returned her calls. I told her straight out, and she was great. She said she'd listen to whatever I needed to say and would let me know if it got to be too much for her. That

was the turning point for me. She didn't make me feel weird or nuts for feeling like I did.

THE PROBLEMS WITH LABELS

The most influential diagnostic categories among mental health professionals are in the diagnostic bible, called the *Diagnostic and Statistical Manual of Mental Disorders (DSM)*. Although written and published by a committee of the American Psychiatric Association comprising mostly white American male psychiatrists, it is being used increasingly in other countries. Because it includes some blatantly sexist categories and other kinds of bias among its almost four hundred diagnostic labels,[1] it has been used in ways that hurt women.

Unfortunately, Medicaid, Medicare, and insurance company officials refuse to pay for psychological or psychiatric care unless the professional first labels the patient with a diagnosis of some sort. Even with such a label, insurance coverage may be quite limited, despite the fact that it may take time to establish the rapport and trust necessary to achieve a reasonable understanding of the problem.

Many emotional states or kinds of behavior *could* be classified as abnormal, but labeling a person mentally ill is problematic in itself when it creates feelings of fear and shame. Furthermore, labels can make it seem as if the problem is purely an individual one when it may stem from social, political, and cultural influences.

The matter of who gets what label is highly subjective. Furthermore, two people diagnosed with the same label can be substantially different and respond differently to the same treatments. At the same time, two people with similar problems might be diagnosed in totally different ways, or one of them might not be diagnosed at all.

Sometimes you may be aware that a doctor or other professional has placed a psychiatric label into your medical records. Since this can put you at risk for hurtful consequences or forms of discrimination,* it is important to know what these labels are and to discuss their implications with your caregivers. Often, "neediness" or "hysteria" in response to neglect is labeled in a negative way that results in a woman either feeling bad about having a legitimate human need or denying that she has this need at all.

IS IT ALL IN OUR BRAIN CHEMISTRY?

Historically, theories have varied about whether depression and other upsetting emotional states are biologically based or primarily caused by external events. In any case, how we respond to traumatic events in our lives is understandably influenced by past experiences, both good and bad.

The vast expansion of the mental health system, the rise of neuroscience, the profit motive of pharmaceutical companies, and health insurers who would prefer the quick fixes of drugs over longer-term talk therapy all intensify the push to identify most emotional distress as primarily brain-based. Even if this should prove true, it does not follow that every brain-based problem will have a simple, mechanical, or pharmaceutical cure.

Some authorities focus only on biological bases of emotional distress, often overlooking the critical roles of social, political, or interpersonal factors, as well as earlier traumatic experiences. Although chemical and other changes in the brain can alter emotions and moods, *changes in feelings can also alter the brain.* So if a woman who is distressed is found to have some below- or above-average level of a chemical in her body, it can be hard, even impossible, to know what was the cause and what was the effect. The interplay between biological and other factors is complex and still not well understood.

It is difficult to do good research about emotional distress, because the multitude of factors that might exacerbate or reduce it cannot be experimentally controlled. Scientists still have much to learn about how the brain, or any other bodily organs or systems, might create or aggravate emotional anguish.

CONCERNS ABOUT PSYCHOTROPIC MEDICATION

The two most common treatments professionals use for emotional distress are psychotherapy and psychotropic medications, drugs that affect the central nervous system and can change emotions or moods. Antidepressants are now commonly used, often recommended by family and friends, and prescribed frequently by health care providers. While these drugs help some people, their promotion and use are not without problems.

Prozac, Zoloft, Paxil, and Celexa are the brand names of some widely used drugs called *selective serotonin reuptake inhibitors,* or SSRIs. Like many drugs submitted for FDA approval, SSRIs have often been studied only for relatively short periods of time before they are approved, and their negative effects, such as sleep, digestive, and sexual problems, as well as a possible increased risk of suicide, tend to be downplayed or even concealed by the companies that sell them. Thus, it is not widely enough recognized that for some people who react well initially to SSRIs, the beneficial effects may wear off

---

* For example, losing custody of children; losing or being denied employment, even if illegal; being charged substantial increases in health insurance premiums or being denied health insurance altogether; being denied coverage for a pre-existing condition; losing the right to make decisions about one's medical and mental health care; and losing the right to make certain decisions about financial and legal affairs.

after a few months. For women who choose to take SSRIs or other mood-altering drugs in order to blunt disturbing feelings enough to get through a crisis, that might not be a problem. But women who hope that a drug will make us feel better over the longer term should know that good effects sometimes wear off or diminish, and in some cases the drug that originally made us feel better can begin to make us feel worse.[2]

Indications that you *may* be suffering from depression include prolonged periods of fatigue; loss of pleasure in activities; feelings of worthlessness, sadness, or hopelessness; decreased or increased appetite; indecisiveness; tearfulness; and suicidal thoughts. But those symptoms may not signify that a person is depressed, since many are common among the general popula-tion. Professionals differ in where they draw the line between the kind of depression that is sometimes just part of life and the kind that is serious and can include the risk of suicide. Furthermore, many symptoms may be effects of physical illnesses: For example, prolonged fatigue may be a symptom of the neurologically based condition chronic fatigue immunodeficiency syndrome,[3] a hormonal imbalance, or some other physical condition. If you believe that you are depressed, you may want to read more to help you make decisions about treatment options (see "Resources").

It is best to work with a medical provider who is knowledgeable about both drug and nondrug approaches. Some psychotropic medications can take several weeks before they have an effect, and often you have to try several before you find out whether one of them works for you. If you are seeing someone only for talk therapy, make sure that person knows which medication(s) you are taking.

If a doctor suggests medication, make sure that

- he or she informs you fully about all the possible benefits and adverse effects of this drug (the Internet also provides useful information).
- you find out about the wide variety of nondrug approaches that others have found helpful (see suggestions above and discuss these with your doctor).

Although some drugs have negative effects for a short period of time but positive effects that last longer, you should inform your doctor if a drug is making you feel more frightened, despondent, suicidal, or violent. Stopping a psychiatric drug abruptly can be physically dangerous, and there is high individual variability in the speed with which it is safe to stop, so it is important to learn about stopping drugs[4] and be mon-

FACING A CRISIS

If you are in danger of committing suicide or harming another person and do not know where to turn, you may need to go to the local hospital emergency room. If possible, ask someone you trust to go with you. Hospital staff may want to keep you for twenty-four to seventy-two hours, depending on state law, if they believe that you are a danger to yourself or others. (In some cases, people face involuntary commitment beyond that period. For more information, see "Inpatient and Outpatient Commitment" [W13] on the companion website, www.our bodiesourselves.org.) Once a crisis passes and you leave a hospital, try to learn about crisis hotlines and groups in your area that could be helpful in the future. There is still a tremendous unmet need for voluntary, non-coercive crisis programs (only a few exist).

Drug companies spend about $16 billion annually marketing their medications, $1 billion on antidepressants alone.[5] The advertisements usually minimize or omit mention of negative drug effects, so it is important to read package inserts and find knowledgeable pharmacists or others with more complete information. The example of Sarafem demonstrates well the growing problem of misleading prescription drug advertising:

THE TRUTH ABOUT SARAFEM*

Some television commercials, websites, and magazine advertisements have conveyed the message that women go crazy and act like shrews once a month. According to them, we don't just get bloated and experience chocolate cravings, breast tenderness, and irritability; rather, we have a medical problem that requires treatment with drugs. In the early 1980s, influential psychiatrists created a special disorder called *premenstrual dysphoric disorder* (PMDD)—to be distinguished from the PMS (premenstrual syndrome) that some women experience. To be labeled with this "disorder," a woman needed to have only one common, upsetting emotion such as irritability or anxiety, plus several physical symptoms such as bloating and food cravings. Some women were understandably so relieved to have our very real physical discomforts and distressing feelings recognized that we did not question the appropriateness of this psychiatric diagnosis.

There are hundreds of research studies about premenstrual days, but there is no proof that a psychiatric premenstrual disorder exists. In an important 1992 study, Sheryle Gallant and her colleagues[6] took the symptoms listed for "PMDD"—then called late luteal phase dysphoric disorder (LLPDD)—and asked three groups of people to document every day for two months the symptoms they experienced. The groups consisted of women who reported severe premenstrual problems, women who reported no such problems, and men. There were virtually no differences in the answers from the three groups. In addition, authors of the *DSM* themselves read hundreds of studies and concluded that (1) little research supported the existence of such a thing as a premenstrual mental illness (in contrast to PMS); and (2) the relevant research was preliminary and poorly done. In spite of this, "PMDD" continues to appear in the *DSM*.

From the beginning, the only recommended *psychiatric* therapy for "PMDD" has been antidepressants, usually Prozac. Although dietary and exercise changes and participation in self-help groups have been shown to help, these are proposed far less often than drugs.

In 1999, with its patent on Prozac about to expire, Eli Lilly (the drug company marketing Prozac) asked the U.S. Food and Drug Administration to approve Prozac to treat "PMDD." When the FDA's Psychopharmacological Drugs Advisory Committee met to consider that application, representatives of Eli Lilly attended and brought along a *DSM* "PMDD" subcommittee member to support their request. The Society for Women's

* Adapted from Paula J. Caplan, " 'Premenstrual Mental Illness': The Truth About Sarafem," *The Network News*, Women's Health Network, Washington, D.C. (May/June 2001), 1, 5, 7.

Health Research, a group heavily supported by drug companies, convened a roundtable discussion financed by Lilly and helped to produce a journal article that presented "PMDD" as a legitimate illness category. After the FDA approved Prozac to treat "PMDD," Eli Lilly packaged the drug as a pink and purple capsule, renaming it the feminine-sounding Sarafem. An early Sarafem commercial, which showed a woman frantic because she couldn't extract a shopping cart from a row of carts, featured a voiceover warning women that we might think we have PMS when we "really have" "PMDD."

The creation of Sarafem added untold millions to Lilly's bottom line, with questionable benefits for women now using this drug for "PMDD." Ironically, some women prescribed Sarafem won't know that it is a mind-altering drug; if we knew, we might choose not to take it. The negative effects, such as depression, digestive and sleep disorders, and/or sexual dysfunction, could be worse than our original symptoms.

The questionable promotion of Prozac for "PMDD" has been challenged in Europe. In December 2003, the European Committee for Proprietary Medicinal Products found that "PMDD is not a well-established disease entity across Europe" and criticized the industry-sponsored research purporting to show that Prozac was effective for the symptoms noted.[7] In response, Lilly sent a letter to health professionals there stating that it had removed "PMDD" as a reason to prescribe Prozac.

Sarafem is just one example of a drug whose benefits have been exaggerated and whose risks have been minimized. It underscores the importance of getting information from unbiased sources before taking a drug of any sort.

itored by a psychopharmacologist or psychiatrist as you go off the medication.

Taking medications may be an effective way to cope, particularly on a temporary basis. They can enable us to make the changes in our lives that will minimize external stress. But they can also be used inappropriately to muffle our true feelings.

I was married and had two kids. I had a job I loved, but the salary was low. My husband was CEO of a huge corporation, but he demanded I take a better-paying job doing work that bored me to tears. I didn't want to put my children through a divorce until they were grown up, but I felt trapped and depressed. I went on Zoloft, and it didn't get rid of my problems, but it allowed me to experience them as if from a distance.

CHALLENGES FOR CONSUMERS

Changes in the health care system are creating serious challenges for women who want access to therapy. Many of us do not have health insurance coverage, and even those of us who are fully insured may have limited mental health benefits that do not cover long-term care. You may be able to find therapists who have sliding-scale fees. You can also seek out self-help groups, which are usually free.

Managed care can have a particularly devastating impact on mental health services. One problem is that we often have to choose our providers from an approved list. Another is that insurers expect practitioners to identify problems quickly and to find fast solutions. Insurers vary (from state to state and from company to

EMOTIONAL TRAUMA AND PSYCHIATRIC DIAGNOSIS

The incidence of sexual and nonsexual physical assault of women, as well as of physical and sexual abuse of children, is disturbingly high, leaving many women and children emotionally traumatized. Two psychiatric diagnoses commonly applied to trauma victims are *post-traumatic stress disorder* (PTSD) and *borderline personality disorder* (BPD). Many feminist therapists were pleased by the description of post-traumatic stress disorder in the 1987 *DSM*[8] because the disorder was described as the result of an experience that would be traumatic for anyone. The focus of PTSD was on the traumatic events and their effects rather than on problems originating within the person.[9] It was indeed helpful in normalizing the flashbacks, hypervigilance, difficulties in concentrating, and other problems that so many victims of violence experience. Unfortunately, the authors of the *DSM*[10] revised the criteria for PTSD to exclude (1) people who have experienced even the most severe verbal and emotional abuse and (2) sexual abuse victims whose "physical integrity" was not threatened. (A definition of "physical integrity" is not included in this *DSM*, so the second category is open to interpretation.)

Borderline Personality Disorder is a label commonly applied to women who have endured extreme, usually ongoing, physical or emotional abuse or neglect.[11] It is rarely used as a diagnosis for men.[12] This diagnosis is often used to describe women who have intense needs for help and support, whom many mental health workers consider to be bothersome and untreatable. Rather than applying the stigmatizing BPD label,[13] it is usually more helpful to focus on healing from the effects of abuse and neglect and to try to understand how that mistreatment affects fears, longings, and the ability to monitor and control feelings.

When a person has been a victim of violence, labeling her "sick" can imply that the problem comes from within her, and it shifts the focus away from the perpetrator of the violence and the society that has failed so miserably to reduce such violence.[14]

company) in how many sessions they will pay for, depending on what diagnosis the therapist assigns.

Many of the values and guiding principles of good mental health care are in danger of being annihilated under the guise of efficiency and cost-effectiveness. Managed care companies often devalue psychotherapy and instead encourage practitioners to prescribe medication alone, which is cheaper and usually requires shorter visits than psychotherapy but may be less effective, ineffective, or even harmful. Ultimately, drugs cannot replace the human interactions and relationships that are at the core of good mental health care.

We may have to fight to get adequate care, to get the right kind of care, and to find a way to ensure that the confidentiality of our relationships is protected by insurance companies, HMOs, and therapists. There continue to be instances in which some families and state authorities lock away assertive women by labeling us "crazy." Yet for many other women, the problem is lack of access. Many of us are not getting enough or the

SELF-INJURY

Some women deliberately self-injure, possibly in response to trauma as a child or an adult. You may cut, hit, or burn yourself or pull out hair in an effort to cope with overwhelming feelings. The self-injury is not about suicide, but rather is an attempt to cope (although you might have suicidal feelings apart from the self-injury). Some mental health professionals find self-injury difficult to deal with and sometimes react with unhelpful frustration and blaming language (for example, "You are doing this just to get attention"). It is important to find someone experienced with this problem who can be sympathetic and supportive, and who understands how self-injury can serve as a soothing mechanism when difficult feelings become overwhelming. Some women have found it helpful to start or join a support group. Because there is a lot of shame involved in self-injury, it is often kept a secret that women bear alone.

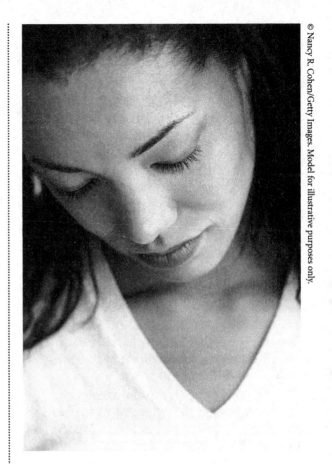

right kind of care, either because we don't have the money or because our insurance carriers won't cover it.

Prescribing psychotropic drugs to millions of women is not an adequate response to the pain that many women experience as a result of the complex social and economic realities that we face. Many of us have suffered physical or emotional abuse at some point during our lives, and recovery is a long process. We must continue to take action—individually and collectively—to get the care we want and need.

SOCIAL OR POLITICAL ACTION: AN OFTEN OVERLOOKED SOURCE OF HELP

Connecting with a group that is involved in working for social and political change can be an empowering and helpful step for many women. It has two advantages: It keeps in plain sight the external causes of our suffering, and it reduces the sense of powerlessness and isolation by providing a way to try to reduce these troubles.* It may also help us feel less ashamed or unusual.

* The documentary *Strong at the Broken Places* follows four individuals who offer powerful evidence of how working for social change can heal deep traumas.

Women who have experienced bad treatment in the mental health system or who have found the kinds of help we need unavailable or unaffordable may be particularly interested in helping to design caring and accessible forms of help and campaigning to make them a reality. Women who have had our rights violated by practices such as involuntary commitment and forced drugging may want to work for the social and political changes necessary to eliminate coercion from the mental health system. Especially for women who feel victimized or neglected by the system, working to reform mental health care can be empowering.

NOTES

1. Paula J. Caplan and Lisa Cosgrove, *Bias in Psychiatric Diagnosis* (Livingston, NJ: Jason Aronson/Rowman Littlefield, 2004).
2. Joseph Glenmullen, *Prozac Backlash: Overcoming the Dangers of Prozac, Zoloft, Paxil, and Other Antidepressants with Safe, Effective Alternatives* (New York: Simon & Schuster, 2001).
3. Jay Goldstein, *Tuning the Brain* (New York: Haworth Press, 2004).
4. Peter Breggin and David Cohen, *Your Drug May Be Your Problem: How and Why to Stop Taking Psychiatric Drugs* (New York: Perseus Publishing, 1999).
5. Dan Shapiro, "Drug Companies Get Too Close for Med School's Comfort," *The New York Times,* January 20, 2004.
6. Sheryle Gallant, Debra Popiel, Denise Hoffman, Prabir Chakraborty, and Jean Hamilton, "Using Daily Ratings to Confirm Premenstrual Syndrome/Late Luteal Phase Dysphoric Disorder. Part II. What Makes a 'Real' Difference?" *Psychosomatic Medicine* 54 (1992): 167–81.
7. Ray Moynihan, "Controversial Disease Dropped from Prozac Product Information," *British Medical Journal* 328 (February 2004): 365.
8. American Psychiatric Association, *Diagnostic and Statistical Manual of Mental Disorders-III-R.* Washington D.C. APA, 1987.
9. Laura S. Brown, *Subversive Dialogues: Theory in Feminist Therapy* (New York: Basic Books, 1994). E. H. Carmen, P. R. Rieker, and T. Mills, "Victims of Violence and Psychiatric Illness," *American Journal of Psychiatry* 141 (1984): 378–83. C. H. Cole and E. E. Barney, "Safeguards and the Therapeutic Window: A Group Treatment Strategy for Adult Incest Survivors," *American Journal of Orthopsychiatry* 57 (1987): 601–609. C. A. Courtois, *Recollections of Sexual Abuse: Treatment Principles and Guidelines* (New York: Norton, 1999).
10. American Psychiatric Association, *Diagnostic and Statistical Manual of Mental Disorders-IV* (Washington, D.C.: APA, 1994).
11. Dana Becker, *Through the Looking Glass: Women and Borderline Personality Disorder* (Boulder, CO: Westview, 1997). Dana Becker, "When She was Bad: Borderline Personality Disorder in a Posttraumatic Age," *American Journal of Orthopsychiatry* 70, no. 4 (2000): 422–32. J. M. Goodwin, K. Cheeves, and V. Connell, "Borderline and Other Severe Symptoms in Adult Survivors of Incestuous Abuse," *Psychiatric Annals* 20, no. 1 (1990): 22–31. J. L. Herman, J. C. Perry, and B. A. van der Kolk. "Childhood Trauma in Borderline Personality Disorder," *American Journal of Psychiatry* 146, no. 4 (1989): 460–65. S. N. Ogata, K. R. Silk, S. Goodrich, N. E. Lohr, D. Westen, and E. M. Hill, "Childhood Sexual and Physical Abuse in Adult Patients with Borderline Personality Disorder," *American Journal of Psychiatry* 147, no. 8 (1990): 1008–1013. J. Surrey, C. Swett, A. Michaels, and S. Levin, "Reported History of Physical and Sexual Abuse and Severity of Symptomatology in Women Psychiatric Outpatients," *American Journal of Orthopsychiatry* 60, no. 3, (1990): 412–17. T. L. Weaver, and G. A. Clum, "Early Family Environments and Traumatic Experiences Associated with Borderline Personality Disorder," *Journal of Consulting and Clinical Psychology* 61 no. 6 (1993): 1068–1075. M. C. Zanarini, J. G. Gunderson, M. F. Marino, E. O. Schwartz, F. R. Frankenburg, "Childhood Experiences of Borderline Patients," *Comprehensive Psychiatry* 30 no. 1 (1989): 18–25.
12. Vincent Fish, "Some Gender Biases in Diagnosing Traumatized Women," in Caplan and Cosgrove, 2004, 213–20.
13. Stefan, 1998.
14. Louise Armstrong, *Rocking the Cradle of Sexual Politics: What Happened When Women Said Incest* (Reading, MA: Addison-Wesley, 1994).

CHAPTER 7 ■ ■ ■ ■ ■ ■ ■ ■ ■ ■ ■ ■ ■ ■ ■ ■ ■

Where and how we live and work affects our health all the time. Increasing evidence suggests that hazards in our environment contribute to many human cancers and other diseases as well as reproductive problems, birth defects, and even behavioral disorders. ("Environment" here includes our diet and living habits as well as our surroundings.) Our bodies contain measurable amounts of industrial chemicals, pesticides, and other toxic wastes from the air, soil, food, and water. Chemicals in household products, biological hazards such as *E. coli*, and physical stresses at work and at home may also contribute to illness or injury.

Katsi Cook, a midwife of the Akwesasne Mohawk Nation, understands that the environment and the body are directly linked. "We know from our traditional teachings that the waters of the earth and the waters of our bodies are the same water," she says.[1] When a new mother on the reservation asked if her breast milk might be unsafe for her infant to drink, Cook saw the traditional teaching in a fresh light. The nearby General Motors facility had contaminated the area with PCBs (chemicals that may cause liver disorders and cancer). Cook recalls: "We quickly realized that Akwesasne is a veritable sink of the Great Lakes Basin, downstream and down-gradient from some of the world's most persistent and problematic pollution."[2] That pollution was affecting the community, just as it affected the water and the land.

Some environmental health hazards—such as the ones Cook describes—are caused by industrial practices and pollution. Others are caused by the way we live our lives. It is easier for private corporations and government at all levels to blame individuals for making unhealthy "lifestyle choices" than to spend the money needed to clean up our communities, purify our food and water supply, and make our workplaces safe. Our personal "choices" are in fact limited by economic resources, family obligations, and the available alternatives. Still, we may want to take what precautions we can in and around our homes to avoid creating environmental health hazards. For example, we may choose to buy mercury-free thermometers or check our homes for radon, the second leading cause of lung cancer. We may also press for more research on health risks that are poorly understood and for enforcement of regulations to keep our environment safe.

Learning that our home, workplace, or neighborhood may be hazardous to our health can be a catalyst to public action. As a twenty-eight-year-old community organizer from Maine says,

Toxic threats are like critical disruptions in people's lives; they can never continue on as before, and instead are driven to go door-to-door in their neighborhoods, stand up in front of strangers at town meetings, talk to reporters, and challenge traditional authority in a whole myriad of ways. When everything we thought was comfortable and normal is suddenly treacherous, our homes, our backyards, the air we breathe, we find that we can do whatever it takes to make things right again.

CONNECTING OCCUPATIONAL AND ENVIRONMENTAL HAZARDS

Occupational health and environmental health are sometimes considered to be separate fields of study, and different government agencies deal with them. The Occupational Safety and Health Administration (OSHA) focuses on workplace health and safety, while the Environmental Protection Agency (EPA) focuses on the larger environment. Yet many of the poisons and problems are similar. We and our families may be exposed to the same toxic substances or conditions in the workplace, at home, in schools, and in our neighborhoods.

Workers, community members, and even local health professionals may not be aware of the particular chemicals being used in an area or of their harmful effects. In rural communities, for example, pesticides may affect both farmworkers and everyone else who lives, works, and studies nearby. The connection to environmental conditions is strong in other occupations as well. Activists, researchers, and public health practitioners are now assessing the problems and developing responses. "Labor-neighbor" coalitions and their alliances with environmental justice organizations can help us see the larger context of shared, continuous risk. Our communities need not make dead-end "choices" between safe jobs and a healthy environment.

MYTH OR REALITY?

- *Women are more biologically vulnerable to environmental toxins than men.*

Reality. Research indicates that women, with as much as 10 percent more body fat than men on average, are able to store more fat-soluble toxic materials. These toxins have been tentatively linked to breast cancer and endometriosis.

- *Since harmful chemicals are regulated in the United States, I don't need to worry about being exposed to these chemicals.*

Myth. Every woman in the world now has some persistent pesticides and chemicals in her body, regardless of where she lives. For example, although DDT (a pesticide that can cause cancer) has been banned in the United States for many years, most American women have some DDT stored in our bodies.

PUBLIC HEALTH AND RESPONSIBILITY

Environmental and occupational hazards affect entire populations, not just individuals. They are public health issues. The National Institute for Occupational Safety and Health (NIOSH) sometimes emphasizes individual responsibility for prevention in its workplace safety and health programs, especially when eliminating the cause of the problem is claimed to be "economically infeasible." Too often, for example, employees are instructed to wear personal protective equipment (which may be ill-fitting and cumbersome), instead of the employer being required to change a practice or to substitute a less hazardous substance. This approach raises serious questions about who profits from exposing us to dangers at work or in our general environment. It also shifts responsibility for the dangers from public institutions and private corporations to us as individuals: We are told that our "lifestyle" or behavior is what makes us get sick or stay well. But we cannot avoid being exposed to toxic substances or dangerous conditions that we cannot control.

SHARED RISKS, UNEQUAL BURDENS

Today environmental hazards are so widespread that none of us can avoid them entirely. Chemicals called *polychlorinated biphenyls* (PCBs), once widely used in adhesives, paints, lubricants, electric insulators, and printing inks, can cause skin discoloration, liver disorders, cancer, and developmental delays in children. DDT, a pesticide now banned in the United States but still used widely in developing countries, can cause cancer and endanger wildlife. Lead, once used in plumbing, paint, and gasoline, damages the nervous system. These substances remain in the environment for decades. Even snow in Antarctica still carries residues of PCBs, DDT, and lead.[3] Human breast milk contains high levels of some toxins, and human sperm samples contain PCBs.

Economic and social power often determine how much we can protect ourselves from environmental health hazards. Some people can afford to buy bottled water or food without additives, to get better health care, or even to move away from a chemical dump or nuclear power plant. Others cannot. People of color are more likely than whites in the United States to work in more dangerous workplaces, to live closer to environmental hazards, and to dwell in substandard housing. Women of color thus bear a higher body burden (total accumulation) of pollutants than white women.

Communities of color and some low-income white communities face not only higher risks of hazardous exposure but also greater negligence by government agencies. The Commission for Racial Justice (United Church of Christ) found that three of the five largest commercial hazardous-waste landfills in the United States are located in mostly black or Latino communities; three of five blacks and Latinos live in communities with uncontrolled toxic-waste sites; and about half of all Asians/Pacific Islanders and Native Americans live near uncontrolled waste sites.[4]

Environmental health hazards are not only an urban problem. Rural people face heavy exposure to pesticides and herbicides, especially since agribusiness has taken over food production. Of the three million farmworkers in the United States, most are migrants, usually Latinos, and 25 percent are women. Female farmworkers' health issues are often neglected. Even without working in the fields, rural women and children who live nearby are exposed to similar conditions.

I lived where there was a lot of crop dusting. Every winter I got a sore throat as a reaction to this cotton defoliant they were spraying about the middle of December. When I remembered, I would always ask my doctor, and he was reassuring, even when I was pregnant and due to deliver in January.

Many Native Americans live with persistent low-level radiation from the uranium mining that has taken over much reservation land. Some companies have targeted reservations for toxic-waste dump sites, including sites for radioactive waste from military uses and nuclear power plants.[5]

Conditions that foster disease transmission are still common in many regions of the world: no garbage pickup, indoor plumbing, or sewer facilities; no access to clean water; and no awareness of how bacteria and viruses are spread. Pesticides, drugs, industrial chemicals, and processes banned as too dangerous in the United States are exported for use in developing countries where regulations are nonexistent or not enforced. How much prevention, protection, and enforcement of laws we can count on in each country varies by workplace and by the strength of labor unions.

Gender, racial, ethnic, and class discrimination intersects with workplace and environmental conditions so that health hazards are borne unequally by people with low incomes and people of color. The movement to right such wrongs is called the *environmental justice movement*.

WORKING CONDITIONS OF WOMEN

Women work in all sectors of the U.S. economy. A growing number of us face the same, often dangerous conditions that men face. We also may do work that involves sustained, repetitive effort or standing or sitting in a static position. When we speak up about health and safety concerns, we may not always find a receptive audience. Yet women's vocal presence in the workplace is changing the way people think about health and safety issues.

I had worked at the hospital for four years as a housekeeper when I got sick with hepatitis. I found out that a patient on my floor had hepatitis and nobody had bothered to tell me what precautions to take. I filed a claim for worker's compensation and the hospital fought my claim! I never thought that a thing like that could hap-

pen. I was working in a place that was supposed to care about people's health, and they never told me anything about protecting my health.

Many women work in low-paying and stressful occupations. Many of us have both paid work and responsibilities at home, so it's harder to get involved in after-work meetings about working conditions. We often have low seniority, or jobs that place us in caregiving roles or require us to support our bosses, so we hesitate to complain about hazards. Fewer women than men belong to labor unions, and many sectors where women work are not unionized, so organizing is more difficult.

Women living in poverty, rural women, and women of color are prime candidates for high-risk jobs. Approximately 85 percent of migrant farmworkers are people of color, mostly Latino,

many young, who rarely have access to worker's compensation, occupational rehabilitation, or disability compensation. While many are eligible for Medicaid and food stamps, not all can get these benefits, due to language barriers. For those of us who are undocumented immigrants, our children may be citizens who are eligible for benefits, but we may fear being deported if we come to the attention of the authorities. Many of us have no health insurance.

An immigrant in Chicago describes her days as a garment worker:

The work at the factory was hard. They had me going back and forth between cold and hot environments, which is how I got sick. . . . After five years I was still only making $6.25 an hour. And I had to pay $25 a week for my ride back and forth to work every day. I worked there for a year and a

THE PRECAUTIONARY PRINCIPLE OF PUBLIC HEALTH

Many people believe that environmental and public health regulations do not adequately protect either the environment or human health. One environmental organization, the Alliance for a Healthy Tomorrow,[6] delineates the fundamental flaws in our health and environmental regulations in the following way:

- Potential toxins are not usually tested for safety before use.
- The government generally takes action only after harm is proven and widespread.
- Certain levels of harm are accepted and allowed by government authorities.
- Powerful special interests obstruct government action to protect our health.

Some environmental health activists, concerned about the impact of toxins in our air, land, food, and water, are undertaking a global campaign to create new public policies based on an approach called the Precautionary Principle. According to the Precautionary Principle, "when an activity raises threats of harm to human health or the environment, precautionary measures should be taken even if some cause and effect relationships are not fully established scientifically."[7] The Precautionary Principle requires taking action in the face of uncertainty, shifting burdens of proof to those who create risks, and analyzing alternatives to potentially harmful activities.

(For more information, see "The Precautionary Principle of Public Health" [W14] on the companion website, www.ourbodiesour selves.org.)

half before I had any benefits. . . . I do not have health insurance because I cannot make the payments every month. When I started getting sick I was afraid that if I told them that work was making me sick, I would get fired.[8]

TYPES OF HAZARDS

CHEMICALS

Tens of thousands of chemical substances are in common commercial use in the United States, and new ones are introduced each year. The vast majority have not been tested over time for their potential ill effects, especially in combination—yet they are in our food, water, air, clothing, homes, and workplaces. Persistent and potentially harmful chemicals are globally distributed, contaminating both industrialized and developing countries as well as the earth's polar regions.[9] Many common chemicals threaten our health.

The total amount of toxic chemicals present in a human body at a given time, or sometimes the amount of a particular chemical, is called the *body burden.*[10] Our bodies respond to the total load of environmental influences from various sources, not just to each one separately.

WHERE	WHAT	RESULT
Air	Car exhaust; factory smoke, dust, ash; chemical and nuclear emissions; pesticides	Respiratory diseases
Atmosphere	Carbon dioxide, chlorofluorocarbons	Ozone depletion, global warming
Water	Industrial chemicals, agricultural pesticides, forestry herbicides, leaking dump sites	Disease, pollution
Food	Pesticides, fertilizers, preservatives, additives	Diseases, growth problems
Buildings	Lead-based paint (illegal since 1978);	Harms child development;
	household cleaners, personal-care products, dry-cleaning chemicals;	toxic fumes and residues cause disease;
	formaldehyde in carpet, pressboard, insulation;	disease, injury;
	radon gas; chemicals, carbon monoxide, air pollution	mood problems, harm to brain function

RADIATION

Low-level radiation from normally functioning nuclear power plants, weapons facilities, and testing sites contaminates our environment and our bodies in slow stages. Uranium mining and disposal of milling wastes (called tailings) and spent fuel create even more hazards. Waste from a nuclear reactor or a weapons plant remains radioactive for as long as 250 centuries. The U.S. government has downplayed the impact of nuclear testing on women's reproductive health, but research findings point to a pattern of difficult pregnancies, miscarriages, stillbirths, birth defects, and breast cancer near nuclear facilities.[11] If there were a meltdown at a nuclear power plant, thousands could die immediately, tens of thousands could suffer from acute radiation sickness within two or three weeks, and cancers might develop five to thirty years afterward. Nuclear war is the ultimate environmental hazard.

ELECTROMAGNETIC FIELDS

Electromagnetic fields (EMFs) are invisible lines of force created around power lines, electric wiring, and electrical equipment and appliances whenever electricity is generated or used. Women's neighborhood groups have taken the lead in calling attention to the potential dangers of exposure to EMFs. Some studies have shown increased leukemia and cancer rates among workers exposed to high magnetic fields, as well as leukemia among affected children. Much of the research in the United States on EMFs has been funded by the electric power industry. Scientists disagree about the harmful effects of EMFs, while admitting that more investigation is needed. Because of scientists' uncertainty, the federal government has not recommended any limits for worker exposure to EMFs. In the meantime, some simple and inexpensive mea-

sures can be taken to reduce the duration and range of EMF exposure. Magnetic fields often drop off about three feet beyond the source, so workstations can be moved and layouts for power lines can be redesigned to maintain at least that distance.

HEALTH EFFECTS OF ENVIRONMENTAL AND OCCUPATIONAL HAZARDS

To understand environmental health, we must understand that everything is connected—our body systems and organs, life habits, work, and the wider environment. Environmental hazards

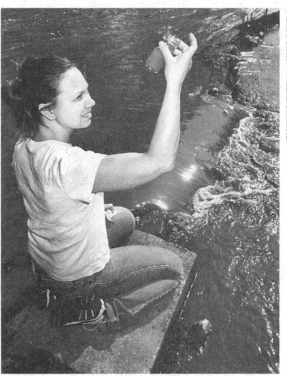

A local college student takes a water sample from Tar Creek in northeastern Oklahoma, a hazardous waste site targeted by the Environmental Protection Agency for Superfund cleanup.

can affect a particular organ or body system, directly damaging it and/or leading to further complications. While scientists generally test substances in labs one at a time, in real life our bodies always deal with more than one hazard at once. The combined interaction of two or more hazards may produce an effect greater than that of either one alone. The amount of exposure, the route of exposure, and the toxic substance(s) we are exposed to determine whether we will have health effects and whether they will be acute or chronic.

We can absorb toxic substances through the skin, the digestive system (eating or drinking), or the lungs. Often toxins cause damage on first contact: burns, rashes, or stomach pain. Once in the body, they can damage many internal organs and systems and build up in the bones and tissues. Both dosage and timing may influence the development and degree of damage; we might be more vulnerable at different stages of life.

In general, toxins affect women and men in similar ways: Anyone can have an allergic reaction or liver damage, chronic headaches or respiratory problems, mental retardation or lung cancer, or damage to reproductive organs. Environmental hazards put extra stress on our bodies and compound any other health problems that we might have.

SKIN DISEASES

Skin is our body's largest organ. Being porous, it is extremely vulnerable to chemicals and other contaminants. Skin diseases are the second most common type of occupational disease. Contact dermatitis—irritation from something that touches the skin—is caused by a wide variety of substances, including solvents, latex, and some pesticides, which may also trigger allergic dermatitis. Women often use rubber gloves as a barrier against toxic chemicals, bacteria, or infected body fluids, but the latex in the gloves can be a health hazard. Latex-free gloves have been developed as an alternative.

RESPIRATORY AILMENTS

Chronic bronchitis, emphysema, and adult asthma cases may result from exposure on the job to substances that can damage the airways, as well as from air pollution and smoking. Closed buildings and air-conditioning systems that recirculate air, as well as chemicals used in synthetic building materials and furnishings, may contribute to breathing problems. Preexisting asthma may be made worse by exposure to pollutants. Dust may be an irritant, particularly for workers with other respiratory problems. Cigarette and cigar smoking interacts with other pollutants, making people sicker than when we are exposed to each separately. The dust of coal, grain, and cotton cause respiratory ailments. Flour in commercial bakeries' air is a hazard for employees.

MULTIPLE CHEMICAL SENSITIVITIES

People with multiple chemical sensitivities (MCS), also called environmental or ecological illness, have a chronic reaction to chemicals and irritants at levels regarded as safe for most people. MCS can be triggered by ingredients in cosmetics and perfumes, newsprint, diesel fuel, solvent vapors, mattresses or other fabrics treated with flame retardant, pressboard, pesticides, molds, and permanent-press finishes. Symptoms can include lack of coordination, abnormal reflexes, vision and hearing disorders, memory loss, convulsions, and other problems (see p. 687 for details).

If you have MCS, the Labor Institute can help you demand "reasonable accommodation" in the workplace under the Americans with Disabilities Act. The National Center for Environmental Health Strategies, which monitors medical, policy, and legal issues, also provides practical advice about improving indoor air quality, reducing exposure to chemicals, getting diagnosis and treatment, and defending patients' rights.

INFECTIOUS DISEASES

Tuberculosis, hepatitis B and C viruses, and human immunodeficiency virus (HIV) pose a risk for health care and social service workers, prison staff, sex workers, and people in other occupations who handle body fluids or hazardous waste. Laboratory technicians can also contract contagious diseases from working with infected material. These hazards are particularly worrisome when they are transferred from patient to worker, or from worker to worker, through blood or through the air.

Bacterial contamination of food, especially salmonella and *E. coli*, can lead to sickness and death. For this reason, it is important to wash our hands well when handling food at home and to avoid using the same utensils for poultry and other food. Women in food-processing jobs may be working with contaminated products without knowing it, and may eat the unsafe food as well. A more reliable and efficient food-inspection system would be a boon for everyone.

REPRODUCTIVE HEALTH HAZARDS

A reproductive hazard is anything that has harmful effects on the male or female reproductive system and/or the development of a fetus. These hazards can be chemicals (such as pesticides), physical agents (such as X rays), or work practices (such as heavy lifting).

Because women bear children, reproductive hazards are too often considered a woman's problem, involving pregnancy alone. But reproductive health means more than having healthy babies, and men also experience reproductive disorders (such as impotence, decreased sperm count, and defective sperm). Infertility in either sex, a miscarriage early in pregnancy, and a baby with disabilities at birth can all be signs of a toxic environment.

Reproductive disorders affecting women also include menstrual problems and, in the babies we bear, low birth weight, premature births, developmental disorders, and birth defects. When toxic substances disrupt the reproductive hormones, they can cause menstrual disorders or loss of sex drive, or they can damage the ovaries directly. Substances in the environment can harm the genetic material in a woman's eggs.

Numerous occupational hazards (such as lead, solvents, and some pesticides) are known to affect reproductive functions. Chemicals used in the workplace have been shown to affect reproduction in animals, though most have not been studied in humans. Activities that upset the normal hormonal balance of the reproductive system (such as shift work) and substances that change estrogen levels or mimic the effects of estrogen (such as pesticides) need further study, too. Not enough attention has been paid to the effect on fertility and pregnancy of physical factors such as prolonged standing, reaching, or lifting, or to the interactive effects of workplace stressors and toxic exposures.

BREAST MILK CONTAMINATION

I learned about toxic flame retardants firsthand by finding out how much of them is in my breast milk. . . . When I got the information about toxic chemicals in my milk, I felt even more strongly that no mother should have to make a choice, to weigh the benefits of breast-feeding against the potential harm caused by contaminants in breast milk.[12]

Women around the world have toxic chemicals in our body fat and, when nursing, have

PRECAUTIONS FOR PREGNANT WOMEN

If you are pregnant, avoiding possible hazards becomes more urgent. Some toxins affect the embryo during the first three months of pregnancy, so early that a woman may not know she is pregnant. A fetus is usually exposed to toxins in the environment or workplace through the mother's direct exposure. However, toxins also can be brought home by other people who work with toxic dusts. (Changing clothes before returning home may reduce this problem.)

Possible risks to our reproductive organs should not be used as excuses to limit our advancement at work in the name of "protection." It is illegal to exclude women from working in an area because of concern about harm to future children. All areas must be healthy and safe enough for everyone, including women during pregnancy.

If you are pregnant, you may have certain rights to job transfer or to paid or unpaid leave. Under an amendment to the federal Civil Rights Act, women "disabled by pregnancy" must be treated the same as other temporarily disabled workers, like those who have had heart attacks or accidents. (*Disabled* is a legal term meaning unable to work.) Some states also have pregnancy disability acts.

Before taking a job, ask whether the company has a specific reproductive health policy, what it is, and whether it applies to both men and women. Some companies ask employees to sign waivers stating that they are aware of the job's possible reproductive hazards and will not hold the employer liable. Some lawyers think these waivers can be challenged in court. If your employer has a policy that seems unclear or unfair on fertility, pregnancy, childbirth, or any other issue related to reproductive health, contact a committee on occupational safety and health (COSH) or other workplace health advocacy group for support (see "Resources").

toxic chemicals in our breast milk. The level of toxic contaminants in many American women's breast milk is often reported to exceed the FDA's "acceptable daily intake" levels for other foods.[13] Some women and babies are at especially high risk because of diet or environmental exposures; among indigenous people in the high Arctic, babies take in seven times more PCBs than the typical infant in Canada or the United States.[14]

Still, breast-feeding is overwhelmingly preferable to infant formula feeding, unless a breast-feeding mother has high-level occupational exposure, extreme dietary exposure, or unusual residential exposure to hazardous or toxic chemicals. Breast milk offers tremendous protective qualities and benefits that outweigh the risks of low levels of chemicals in most cases. Providing uncontaminated air, water, and food is the best choice to protect mothers and infants from unwanted chemical exposures and risks. For more about breast-feeding, see Chapter 23, "The First Year of Parenting."

ENDOCRINE DISRUPTION

The endocrine system is the body's complex array of hormonal messages that affect almost every bodily function, including our reproductive health, thyroid gland, nerves, and immune system. Many industrial and pharmaceutical chemicals distort how our endocrine system functions. Research on endocrine-disrupting contaminants (EDCs), also called ecoestrogens or exogenous estrogens, is revealing environmental threats to women's health.

Breast cancer and other cancers in women, breast milk contamination, and other reproductive problems (such as endometriosis, miscarriage, and tubal pregnancy) may be related to EDCs in our food supply, air, and water; in industrial waste discharges; and in many synthetic household and personal-care products. These substances mimic, block, or alter the body's normal estrogen functioning, thereby putting us at risk for disease. Most scientists agree that breast cancer risk is affected by how much estrogen we have in our bodies and for how long over our lifetime. If the body's own "natural" estrogen levels are increased or changed in some way by chemicals that act like estrogens, our risk of breast cancer, endometriosis, and other diseases may go up.

BREAST CANCER

Women in the United States have a one-in-seven chance of developing breast cancer at some point in our lives. An extensive movement is pressing for more research on the causes of breast cancer, particularly the effect of the environment, so that preventive measures and better treatment can be developed (see p. 597). Certain chemicals are associated with cancer in lab animals and/or humans. Diets high in animal fat may increase the amount of fat-soluble toxins such as dioxin and some pesticides in your body. Over time, these compounds may trigger breast cancer by disrupting normal cell-regulation processes in sensitive breast tissue. Although women workers with high exposure to dioxin have significantly high rates of breast cancer, recent studies of endocrine disruptors and breast cancer were inconclusive.

The National Cancer Institute and other research institutions usually emphasize prevention—an approach that shifts responsibility for cancer onto individuals by advising us to change our lifestyles. This ignores the difficulties most women face in assuring our safety at work or in avoiding hazardous chemicals that we may not even know are present in our environment. It is more important than ever for us to insist that government and industrial interests take responsibility for their contribution to environmental and workplace hazards that may cause cancer.

HEARING LOSS

The most common occupational disease in the United States, hearing loss can reduce alertness to safety warnings and severely impair the quality of a worker's life. While hearing loss can occur from an acute injury, it is more likely to develop gradually over time, as a result of exposure to noise, solvents, metals, asphyxiants, or heat. Loss of hearing doesn't often hurt, so it may take a while to notice. Once it starts, it is usually irreversible. Most workers are unaware that exposure to certain kinds of chemicals can cause hearing loss.

BACK PAIN

Back disorders account for about a third of all recorded nonfatal occupational injuries and illness involving days away from the job. About 30 percent of workers perform tasks that increase the chance of developing back problems. Many of these workers are women, especially women of color. Lifting over a barrier, lifting too much weight, or lifting in an awkward position can strain the muscles.

Mechanical lifting devices, training, reorganizing tasks, and using a buddy system and a back belt may reduce risks. Redesigning materials, loads, and equipment can help those in occupations that involve lifting. Call the NIOSH hotline (see "Resources") for new recommendations on lifting.

FOOT AND LEG PAIN

Standing all day bothers many women, especially waitstaff, salesclerks, nurses, nurses' aides, and household and office cleaners. Sometimes these jobs combine stooping, kneeling, and lifting as well. Blood tends to pool in your legs, and varicose veins may develop. These jobs are particularly hard on pregnant workers. In addition, many of the jobs are stressful.

When possible, ask for a chair or stool to sit on, or a cushioned floor to stand on. If that is refused, ask to be rotated for part of the day so that you can alternate sitting and standing. For cleaning, request long-handled equipment that you can use standing or sitting instead of kneeling or bending over.

NECK, SHOULDER, AND HAND STRAIN OR INJURIES

These injuries are caused by repetitive movements or awkward positions. Musculoskeletal disorders—including stiff neck and carpal tunnel syndrome—occur in food processing, automobile and electronics assembling, carpentry, computerized data entry, store checkouts, garment sewing, and many other occupations where repetitive, forceful work affects the soft tissues of the neck, shoulder, elbow, hand, wrist, and fingers. According to the Bureau of Labor Statistics, such injuries represent almost 65 percent of all reported illness at work.

Unlike strains or sprains, which result from a single incident, repetitive motion disorders develop over time, and they can recur when we return to the task that produced the injury. The daily aches and pains that we ignore for all kinds of reasons—not least because we have to "get on with the job," paid or unpaid—may

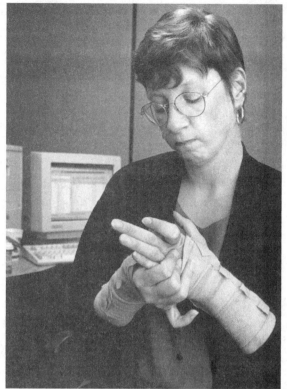

© Earl Dotter/www.EarlDotter.com

A data-entry clerk massages her hands, injured over a period of eight years at a computer keyboard.

add up to long-term problems. Forceful movements, vibration, working in cold temperatures, and insufficient recovery time can make injuries worse.

Ergonomics—the science of efficient work—can greatly reduce these problems. In practice, that means specially designed equipment, properly sized furniture, motion study, good lighting, sufficient rest, alternation of tasks, and reduced stress.

EFFECTS OF INDOOR AIR QUALITY

Many office and factory workers experience headaches, unusual fatigue, itching or burning eyes, skin irritation, nasal congestion, a dry or irritated throat, and nausea because of the air quality.

I take reservations for an airline. We have 800 people in the building, but only six or eight bathrooms. The windows don't open, so the air is never fresh. My section is supposed to be perfume-free, but people still use hair spray and aftershave. We take 90 to 120 calls a day, working eight and a half hours with only half an hour for lunch. All the calls are timed. If you get up and walk around, the supervisor yells at you. Also, we don't have designated workstations, so you're always sitting at a different keyboard, picking up everyone else's germs.

STRESS

Stress can result from physical factors, such as repetitive hand motions, poor seating conditions, excessive noise, heat or cold, eyestrain, lack of control, or general work overload. Other causes of stress range from relations with the boss and coworkers to lack of control over day-to-day tasks, sexual harassment, and concern about safety and health hazards. Many women are stressed out by low pay and no chance of promotion or retraining, sexual and racial discrimination, and limited educational opportunities. Women who have children or want to have them may worry about maternity leave, child care, and loss of seniority.

In the garment shop where I work, a lot of us who've been sewing there for a while have been having pains in our hands or our legs. The union is collecting information to find out whether there are any changes that would help, like changing the height of the tables or the angle of the machines. Anything that would make the job more comfortable would help my general level of tension! Between the noise from the steam presses, working fast enough to make a good rate, and bending over

the machine all day without enough light, I'm lucky if I get out of there without my shoulders all bunched up and a splitting headache at the end of the day.

Research shows that jobs characterized by high demand and low control, like those filled by millions of women, are the most stressful and most likely to be harmful to health. Though some companies today have stress management programs for employees, these programs usually define stress as an individual problem and allow the company to avoid changing the conditions that cause stress on the job.

EFFECTS OF SHIFT WORK

Shift work may cause physical and psychological hardship or make existing health problems worse. Digestion, the immune system, sleep, alertness, motor reflexes, motivation, and powers of concentration are all affected. Shift workers tend to smoke more, eat less nutritious food, have more risk factors for heart disease, and participate in fewer leisure activities and social networks than workers with a fixed eight-hour day. Frequent rotation continually upsets the body's eating and sleeping cycles; it's like having permanent jet lag.

Women who work shifts show high levels of job stress and emotional problems, and use sleeping pills, tranquilizers, and alcohol more frequently than women with regular hours. Shift work is hard on family life and friendships, especially if there is nobody at home to help or if we can't afford paid child care. We may become more isolated, losing valuable support networks and increasing our level of stress.

If you are on a rotating shift, try to avoid daily or weekly rotation; if you can, stick to one shift for at least three weeks so your body can adjust for a longer period of time. Try to get other workers to join you in demanding a less exhausting schedule. Unless you assert yourselves in a group, employers may resist making changes.

HARASSMENT AND VIOLENCE

Industries that employ many women—such as bars, restaurants, hospitals, and grocery stores—report a large number of serious nonfatal injuries. Homicide is a leading cause of occupational death for women. While robbery is often the motive, homicides are also committed by disgruntled workers, former employees, clients, or partners or ex-partners of women workers. A worker's risk for violence is increased if she exchanges money with the public, works alone or with few coworkers, works late-night or early-morning hours, or works in community settings.

For information in Spanish and English about workplace hazards, call the NIOSH information line (1-800-35-NIOSH).

REDUCING OUR EXPOSURE

Our homes, our workplaces, and indoor or outdoor community settings, including our children's schools, all may contain hazards that threaten our health. Sometimes we can reduce our exposure to these risks by changing our lifestyles, purchases, and other individual choices. In other cases, we need to take collective action with neighbors and coworkers to make these areas safer for ourselves, our families, and our communities.

HOME

The first environment to consider is your home. What are you buying, using, and storing, and how are you disposing of these things? What is in your furniture and carpets? Is there lead in your paint or asbestos wrapping on your hot water

HAZARDS AT HOME

HAZARD AND HEALTH THREATS	WHAT TO DO
Food Wide variety of problems over time	Read labels. If possible, buy organic produce without pesticides, fresh meat and poultry without hormones, and foods without preservatives. Check origin of fish; limit intake of tuna, swordfish, tilefish, and farmed salmon because of mercury exposure (see Chapter 2, "Eating Well").
Lead-based paint, lead dust, and paint chips Brain damage Kidney damage Anemia Reproductive problems Nerve damage	Have your home inspected for lead in the paint and lead dust or paint chips on floors and windowsills if built before 1977. Cover lead paint with lead-free paint. Never dry-scrape paint unless you are sure there's no lead in it. If you rent, call the local health department to find out how to get the owner to remove lead-based paint. Get children tested for lead by their health care provider. Wash children's hands before they eat; wash bottles, pacifiers, and toys often. Don't let children put paint chips in their mouth.
Carbon monoxide (CO) *Low levels:* Headaches Nausea	Install carbon monoxide monitors in your home (required in Canada and several areas in the United States). Have fuel-burning appliances, furnace flues, and chimneys checked and cleaned once a year. Do not use gas stoves or ovens to heat your home.

HAZARD AND HEALTH THREATS	WHAT TO DO
Carbon monoxide (CO) *(cont.)* *Higher levels:* Life-threatening	Don't sleep in rooms with unvented gas or kerosene space heaters. If possible, don't use portable stoves or heaters in the home at all. Do not use gas-powered equipment indoors. Never leave a car or lawn mower running in a closed or attached garage.
Mold Allergies Headaches Respiratory problems	Fix leaky plumbing. Insulate windows. Improve inside air circulation (if outside air is cold and dry). Dehumidify air (if outdoor air is warm and humid). Have heating and cooling systems cleaned for mold. Vent moisture-generating appliances (like dryers) to the outside.
Drinking Water Heavy metals such as lead, volatile organic compounds (VOCs), pesticides, and chlorine compounds Wide range of symptoms and illnesses	Check safety of your drinking water source. If you get drinking water from a public supply (city, town), the supplier must provide testing results every year, without being asked. If you have concerns about water quality between reports, call your supplier and ask for recent test results. Test private wells every year for contaminants—chemical, biological, and radioactive (radon or radium). Have your tap water tested for lead if you live in an older city and/or in an older house. Filter tap water. (However, not all filters will eliminate all contaminants.)
Radon gas Lung cancer	Install a radon monitor in your basement. Keep basements aired.
Chemicals in household products, home furnishings, and decoration Wide range of symptoms and illnesses	Use products with natural ingredients instead of chemicals. Buy natural fibers instead of synthetics. Air new carpets and furniture before installing. Open windows and wear a mask when using paint, glue, cleaners. Don't buy cosmetics or personal-care products with phthalates in them. Reduce or eliminate pesticide use; try integrated pest management.

pipes? Are there toxins in your water, and who is responsible for the local water supply? Is the food you eat safe? What's in the cosmetics and personal-care products, pesticides, and cleaning supplies that you use? How can you make your home a safe environment for children? How can you get your landlord to clean up your building?

WORK

Our workplace environment, where we spend most of our time during the day, is often where toxic hazards are first identified. The work we do affects our health, not only while we are working but throughout the rest of the day, on weekends and vacations, and even after we have left the

HAZARDS AT WORK

HAZARD AND HEALTH THREATS	WHAT TO DO
Chemicals Health effects depend on specific chemical	Find out what's in the materials you work with. Wear protective gear (gloves, dust masks, respirators, goggles) whenever needed. Urge union and coworkers to promote the use of safer materials. Report dangerous exposures to local health authorities.
Repetitive motion, uncomfortable workstation Repetitive stress injuries, backache, headache	Try to rearrange your workstation to limit or eliminate repetitive movements. Ask for furniture that fits your body (desk higher or lower, chair with support). Take breaks—walk around, stretch, get a breath of fresh air, do chair exercises.
Noise pollution Hearing loss, headache	In noisy workplaces, insist that your employer follow the written hearing-protection plan, as required by OSHA. Ask to see the plan; report violations. Wear earplugs or headphones. Make sure they fit properly.
Harassment and violence Stress, injury, death	Ask employer to separate workers from the public, install bulletproof barriers and alarm systems, add staff, and not force women to work alone. File class action lawsuits. Alert unions and the press.

job. Tens of thousands of workers die each year from known job-related diseases, and more suffer from other diseases not yet recognized as resulting from conditions at work. Poor working conditions should not have to be accepted as "just part of the job."

COMMUNITY

Women are learning to be both more aware of environmentally caused problems and more confident about the power of such awareness. Instead of accepting that "this is normal," we're investigating. And when we do, we often find that the problems are environmentally connected. Environmental damage can be hard to prove. Persist. Schools and public buildings are a good place to start.

ACTION STRATEGIES

IN THE ENVIRONMENT

Environmental health is basically a community issue, one we cannot fight alone. Luckily, we don't have to. Thousands of grassroots groups across the country are increasingly concerned about environmental conditions—from polluted water to toxic landfills—and many people are willing to make sacrifices (like paying higher taxes) to ensure a safer environment. Experienced activists agree on some basic ways to take effective action.

1. *Be a careful consumer.* Read labels. Demand full disclosure of all ingredients in your food, including the use of growth hormones in dairy, ge-

HAZARDS IN THE COMMUNITY

HAZARD AND HEALTH THREATS	WHAT TO DO
Pesticides Headaches Nerve damage Reproductive risks Learning problems	Find out what pest control policies exist for schools, public buildings, parks, and playgrounds in your town. Insist that staff, teachers, and parents be notified when pesticides will be applied anywhere on school or building grounds. Find out what's in the pesticides. Campaign for an integrated pest management (IPM) policy of non-toxic and least toxic approaches.
Supplies Headaches Respiratory problems	Insist on proper ventilation of rooms and safe use, storage, and disposal of paints, glues, glazes, and photographic development chemicals. Call manufacturers for clear instructions regarding safe use, storage, and disposal.
Carpeting/Furnishings Ear, nose, and throat irritation Headaches	Make sure the carpets in schools or other public buildings are vacuumed and steam-cleaned thoroughly, according to manufacturers' guidelines. Chemical cleaners and treatments for stains or mold/bacteria resistance may be irritating and otherwise harmful to people's health.

netically engineered organisms in fruits and vegetables, and pesticide use on produce and feed given to livestock. Learn about and join boycotts of unhealthy products.

2. *Investigate* environmental conditions where you live and work. Get information under worker and community right-to-know legislation, and use the Toxic Release Inventory (www.scorecard.org). Contact groups listed in the "Resources" section to learn about workplace and community monitoring and campaigning for preventive measures.

3. *Talk to your neighbors.* Develop labor-neighbor alliances between neighbors and unions around toxic exposure from factories, landfills, and waste shipment. Monitor health concerns, symptoms, and suspected exposure in the community. Conduct a community and workplace health survey. Watch for odd smells; bubbles or ooze; sick and dying wildlife, pets, and plants; abandoned oil drums; or illegal dumping. Find out whether local industries emit radiation. Pay attention to reproductive patterns in your area.

4. *Document your health* and that of your family. Keep a log of exposures, symptoms, and diagnoses. The health care providers you see should (but may not) be keeping an accurate medical and occupational/environmental history.

5. *Find out who paid* for the study when you or your group obtain information, statistics, or data. The answer should help you evaluate the data. Ask that information be presented in terms you can understand, not in the jargon of "experts."

6. *Use the consumer boycott.* Find out where pollutants come from and what products they're used in, and refuse to buy them. Boycotts are especially effective when networks of people participate.

7. *Work in coalition* with other organizations and movements. Don't limit your protest to "not in my backyard." Your efforts will be more effective, just, and inspiring if they don't develop at the expense of others whose resources and power are more limited than yours. Organizations such as the Center for Health, Environment and Justice; the Environmental Health Network; the Labor Institute; and the COSH groups can advise U.S. grassroots groups about filing legal challenges, conducting surveys, building relationships with sympathetic scientists, getting a company to accept a "neighbors' inspection," and using national data systems and community right-to-know provisions. The Center for Health, Environment and Justice also provides workshops for women leaders. Coalitions of environmental, labor, and other social justice groups are pushing beyond right-to-know* (the basic right of access to certain information about on-site toxins) and promoting right-to-act (the right to refuse work, change production activity, or enforce an emergency shutdown). (For more information, see Chapter 32, "Organizing for Change," and the "Resources" section.)

ORGANIZING FOR CHANGE

IN THE ENVIRONMENT

Taking action is often complicated—bureaucracies to fight, chemistry and biology to learn, the power of polluters to deal with—but it is not impossible. You can gain the skills necessary and follow in the footsteps of other women who have exposed environmental health hazards and worked to eliminate them.

* For more information on these regulations, see "Current Environmental and Occupational Health Right-to-Know Statutes" (W15) on the companion website, www.ourbodiesourselves.org.

ACTION STRATEGIES IN THE WORKPLACE

1. *Substitute.* Can a safer substance or equipment (chemical or process) be used? Use water-based products instead of those with solvents. Use natural, biodegradable cleaning products.
2. *Change the process.* Can the job be done in a different and safer way? If you can, rotate sitting and standing to reduce strain. Try to arrange materials or machines to reduce how many movements you need to make and how hard they are on your body.
3. *Mechanize the process.* Can parts of the task be automated? Can it be shared? Can some of it be done mechanically? Lifting devices can prevent back strain.
4. *Isolate or enclose the process.* Can the hazardous job be moved to a different time or area where fewer people or even none will be exposed to danger? Can the worker be isolated from the operation, or can the process be completely enclosed? Ventilating hoods or fans can keep workers from breathing fumes.
5. *Improve housekeeping.* Keep toxic materials from being reintroduced into the air by cleaning up. Keep dust levels down to protect the lungs. Move obstacles out of work areas and exits to prevent accidents. Wear masks and gloves, and use safety equipment.
6. *Improve maintenance.* Is equipment regularly serviced and repaired?

- Rachel Carson's book *Silent Spring* (1962) exposed the widespread use and dangers of pesticides in our environment. Her work brought this problem to public attention, led to the

ORGANIZING FOR WORKPLACE SAFETY

Efforts to improve conditions on the job may include the following elements:

- *Committees* can gather information, educate coworkers, help set priorities, and provide leadership and persistence to get things changed. A health and safety committee is most effective as part of a union. A unionized company is obliged by law to negotiate health and safety issues with the union.

- *Class action lawsuits* challenge sex discrimination and sexual harassment at work, as well as other health issues. They are difficult to win and are usually filed only against large companies that can afford to pay damages, rather than small companies, where many women of color and low-income white women work. Unions, COSH groups, the Labor Institute, and other advocacy groups (see "Resources") can help you decide whether class action is a good strategy for your situation.

- *Strike action* is the classic work stoppage organized by a labor union. *Contract negotiations* offer the opportunity to address hours, wages, and working conditions. If you belong to a union, discuss mobilizing around health issues with your union representative or organizer.

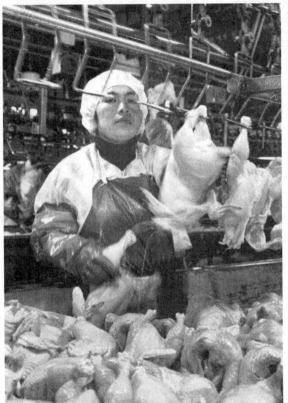

A "guest worker" from Central America handles chickens that are about to be processed.

ban on DDT in the United States, and helped launch the American environmental movement.
- Lois Gibbs organized the Love Canal Homeowners' Association in 1978, forcing New York State to recognize that toxic waste had contaminated their community and caused health problems. The members did health surveys, signed petitions, confronted officials, picketed, blocked buses, and testified in Washington until the government evacuated a thousand families, bought their homes, and established a safety plan and a health fund to cover future problems. Lois now leads the Center for Health, Environment and Justice, and in 2003 she launched the Be Safe Network.
- Peggy Shepard cofounded West Harlem Environmental Action (WE ACT), a coalition of young feminists and older neighborhood women, in 1988 to challenge the location of a

sewage treatment plant, winning a sizable settlement and the right to oversee the remedy. This legal victory also established a community's right to seek redress of a grievance.[15] Peggy and WE ACT are still doing community-based action, research, and public education linking health care to environmental justice.

- Erin Brockovich, who was made famous by a 2000 film starring Julia Roberts, investigated how contaminated water caused illness among residents of Hinkley, California. In 1996 her work led to the largest toxic tort injury settlement in U.S. history. Now director of research at a California law firm, she continues to challenge polluters.

- Patty Martin was mayor of a small town in Washington State in 1992 when she, along with farmers and neighbors, discovered that hazardous waste was being blended into fertilizers, causing crop failure, environmental damage, and health risks. In 2000, after being targeted by agribusiness and losing her campaign for reelection, Patty founded Safe Food and Fertilizer; in the fall of 2003, she took the fight to the federal courts.

- Hazel Johnson, the "mother" of the environmental justice movement, founded People for Community Recovery in 1982, when she learned about Southeast Chicago's high cancer rate. She documented health problems by going door-to-door; testified in Congress; and helped to educate and empower her community. She continues to lead "toxic tours" of Chicago neighborhoods.

- Rosalinda Guillen works with La Union del Pueblo Entero (LUPE), linked to the United Farm Workers, to fight for a healthy community as part of workers' rights. Rosalinda is at the forefront of the current struggle to connect pesticide exposure and environmental health to immigrants' rights, labor politics, daily working conditions, and consumer practices.

IN THE WORKPLACE

I was working in a supermarket as a meat wrapper. We take the cut-up meat and wrap it in plastic. The plastic comes off a big roll that we cut to size by pulling it against a hot wire. A bunch of us were having asthma attacks and getting acne real bad. The health and safety committee met and decided that it was from the fumes of the plastic when it melted. We talked to our supervisor, and he basically said, "Don't worry, ladies, it's all in your head." So we got mad and decided to try a new approach. We planned it so on one busy Saturday, we all came to work with respirators on. After about an hour behind the meat counter with the customers staring at us in shock, the manager decided we were serious and agreed to meet with us and discuss what could be done.

Women have a long history of collective action for health at work. The millworkers of Lowell, Massachusetts, struggled against hazardous conditions in the 1840s. In 1909 thousands of women in New York City's garment industry went on strike to protest sweatshop working conditions and low wages. In 1943 two hundred African-American women "sat down" at their machines in a North Carolina tobacco plant when a coworker died on the job after years of exposure to excessive heat, dust, and noise. In 1979 women led a strike to improve health and safety conditions and end sexual harassment at a poultry farm in Mississippi. In recent years, nurses have spoken out about the hazards of understaffing and mandatory overtime that affect both nurses and patients. With plenty of experience behind us, we continue to take action.

If you are thinking about taking action in your workplace, consider the possible results. Although the law says that you cannot be fired for raising health and safety issues, the reality may be different. If you work in the United States, you have the right to call an OSHA inspector to check health and safety conditions in your workplace. You can remain anonymous when you file an OSHA complaint. However, this does not ensure that your employer will not figure out who submitted the request, especially in small workplaces or when you have already been vocal about a potential problem.

Action on a particular health and safety problem often starts informally. When you organize at work, be sure to understand the difference between risk factors (hazards in the environment or workplace that may endanger health) and health outcomes (actual injury or sickness), and the consequences of focusing on one or the other. Try to show the connections. Show how a problem affects everyone. These are not individual issues, even if only a few individuals suffer at any given moment.

Whenever possible, try to form an ongoing workers' health and safety committee. Instead of responding just to emergencies, a committee can work preventively, uncovering potential problems before anyone gets hurt and approaching management about them. Members of a group may be less likely to be singled out as "troublemakers" and subjected to special harassment or even fired, than individuals working alone.

Know your group's strengths, weaknesses, barriers, and opportunities. You may find support in unexpected places. Ask what other workers in your shop or community can contribute to your questions and concerns. For example, female workers battling unhealthy indoor environmental conditions might enlist male maintenance or security workers who can help with ventilation, furniture, machines, or safety issues. Small acts of solidarity on the part of many women from all racial and socioeconomic classes can lead to substantial gains in a campaign. As the women's health movement has shown, we can work together to create healthier communities for everyone.

One of the best periods in my life was when we were on strike. We were all like one big family. Once I took a stand on what I knew to be right, I never felt freer in my life. Any average man or woman can do what we did. You can write press releases, push government, get things done. . . . You don't need a college education—just determination.

NOTES

1. Katsi Cook, "Women Are the First Environment," *Indian Country,* December 23, 2003, 1.
2. Ibid.
3. Carol Sue Davidson, "Antarctic Lore," in *The Cousteau Almanac: An Inventory of Life on Our Water Planet* (New York: Doubleday, 1981). Tom Conry, "Chemical of the Month: Lead," *Exposure* no. 13 (December 1981): 6.
4. Commission for Racial Justice, United Church of Christ, *Toxic Waste and Race in the United States* (New York: Public Data Access, 1987).
5. Robert Bullard et al., *We Speak for Ourselves: Social Justice, Race and Environment* (Washington, D.C.: Panos Institute, 1990).
6. Alliance for a Healthy Tomorrow, accessed at www.healthytomorrow.org/index.html in September 2004.
7. Wingspread Statement on the Precautionary Principle, Greenpeace. Accessed at archive.greenpeace.org/toxics/reports/gopher_reports/precaut.txt in September 2004.
8. Northwest Federation of Community Organizations, *Faces and Stories of U.S. Immigrants,* accessed at http://66.36.240.156/publications/immigration_storybook.pdf in July 2004.
9. Staci Simonich and Ronald Hites, "Global Distributions of Persistent Organochlorine Compounds," *Science* 269 (September 29, 1995): 1851–854.
10. "What Is Body Burden?" Coming Clean Network. Accessed at www.chemicalbodyburden.org/whatisbb.htm in September 2004.
11. "Marshall Islands Stand at a New 'Crossroads,' " *Health Research Bulletin* (Physicians for Social Responsibility publication) 3, nos. 1–2 (Winter 1996): 1–5, 19–20.
12. Erika Schreder, Washington Toxics Coalition, testifying before the Washington State Legislature, February 2004.
13. See www.nrdc.org/breastmilk and www.ewg.org/reports/mothersmilk.

14. Theo Colburn, Dianne Dumanoski, and John P. Meyers, *Our Stolen Future: Are We Threatening Our Fertility, Intelligence, and Survival?* (New York: Dutton, 1996), 106.

15. Vernice Miller, Moya Hallstein, and Susan Quass, "Feminist Politics and Environmental Justice: Women's Community Activism in West Harlem, N.Y.," in Dianne Rocheleau, Barbara Thomas-Slayter, and Esther Wangari, eds., *Feminist Political Ecology: Global Issues and Local Experiences* (New York: Routledge, 1996), 62–85.

CHAPTER 8 ▪ ▪ ▪ ▪ ▪ ▪ ▪ ▪ ▪ ▪ ▪ ▪ ▪ ▪ ▪ ▪

Violence against women is pervasive in the United States and around the world. Often the attacks come from those closest to us, further undermining our sense of safety. Almost one in every four women in the United States has been raped and/or physically assaulted by a current or former spouse, live-in partner, boyfriend, or date.[1] The attacks don't stop there. On average, more than three women are murdered by husbands or boyfriends every day in the United States.[2] Women are much more likely than men to be killed by an intimate partner; in 2000 intimate-partner homicides accounted for 33.5 percent of the murders of women in the United States and under 4 percent of the murders of men.[3]

The World Health Organization recognizes sexual violence,

intimate-partner violence, and the abuse of women and children as public health problems of epidemic proportions.[4] The United Nations has repeatedly called for the "elimination of all forms of violence against women." While the vast majority of violence against both men and women is inflicted by men,[5] women are also perpetrators of violence.

Violence against women is so woven into the fabric of acceptable behavior that many of us who are victimized feel that we are at fault or have no right to complain about violent treatment. Many of those who perpetrate violence feel justified by strong societal messages that say rape, battering, sexual harassment, child abuse, and other forms of violence are acceptable, or at least understandable. Every day we see images of male violence against women in the news, on TV, in the movies, in advertising, and in our homes and workplaces. The prevalence of these images makes it appear that violence against women is simply a fact of life.

In the broadest sense, violence against women is any assault on a woman's body, physical integrity, or freedom of movement through individual acts and societal oppression. It includes battering, rape, sexual and physical abuse of young girls, verbal and emotional abuse, murder by a partner or husband, "honor" killings by a family member (murder for perceived sexual activity that "dishonors" the family), forced sterilization, female genital cutting, stalking, sexual coercion in the workplace, getting women and girls "ready" for prostitution through rape and psychological manipulation, pornography that sexualizes violence and promotes violent sex, and trafficking of women and girls.

Every form of violence threatens all people and limits our ability to make choices about our lives. Sexual violence is particularly insidious because sexual acts are ordinarily and rightly a source of pleasure and loving human contact. Unfortunately, in the past three decades, persist-

ent cultural images linking sex with violence have caused violence itself to be seen as sexual or erotic.

Traditionally, most forms of violence against women and children have been hidden under a cloak of silence and tolerance. Today the general public is far more aware of this violence. The health care and justice professions have been forced to acknowledge the problem and provide better services, but still have a long way to go. During fiscal crises, these services are often some of the first to be eliminated. We must continue to be outspoken about the ongoing need to address the violence in women's lives.

UNDERSTANDING VIOLENCE AGAINST WOMEN

A man's act of violence against a woman may seem to result from his individual psychological

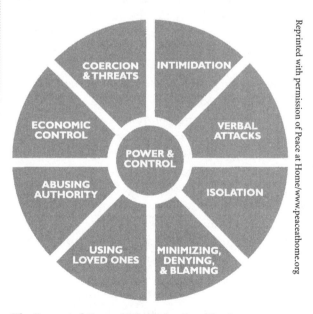

Reprinted with permission of Peace at Home/www.peaceathome.org

The Power and Control Wheel, developed by the Domestic Abuse Intervention Project of Duluth, Minnesota, is one model for understanding the dynamics of violence and abuse.

problems, or from sexual frustration, childhood abuse, unbearable life pressures, drug or alcohol abuse, or an innate urge toward aggression. All of these factors may contribute to the dynamic of violence. But these "reasons," often given to explain or even justify violent actions, oversimplify a complex reality.

Violence against women is about power and control. It is rooted in the power imbalances that exist between men and women. Our culture—like most other cultures in the world—assigns a superior position to men and an inferior or dependent position to women. Most people have been taught to relate to the world in terms of dominance and control, and many of us, particularly men, have been taught that violence is an acceptable method of maintaining control, resolving conflicts, and expressing anger. When a batterer uses beatings to confine a partner to the home and prevent her from seeing friends and family or from pursuing outside work, the batterer is exerting dominance and control. When rapists select victims or bosses sexually harass employees, they act out of a wish to dominate and control or to punish those who resist.

Little by little, he isolated me from my friends, he convinced me to quit working, he complained about how I kept the house, he kept track of the mileage on the car to make sure that I wasn't going anywhere. Eventually, when the beatings were regular and severe, I had no one to turn to, and I felt completely alone.

On the surface, it seems that men benefit from male dominance, control, and violence. On a deeper level, we know that men's violence against women harms men because it harms the women and girls in their lives and keeps men from having positive and loving relationships with women. Growing numbers of men are recognizing this, working to stop the violence, and becoming aware that violence against women is

MYTH OR REALITY?

• *Most women who are raped are attacked by a stranger.*

Myth. Two thirds of women who are raped are raped by an intimate or an acquaintance.[6]

• *A woman who is being battered should always take her case to court.*

Myth. There is no single right way to handle intimate-partner abuse. Some batterers are intimidated enough by the legal system to be stopped by a court order. However, other batterers may become violently enraged by the "betrayal" of legal intervention. In these instances, going to court may actually make a woman and her children less safe. An advocate at a local domestic violence organization may be able to help a woman decide whether to get a restraining order.

• *If I go to the hospital after being raped, I will have to be examined for evidence and I will have to file charges.*

Myth. If you have been raped, it is very important to receive medical attention as soon as possible regardless of whether you intend to press charges. You may refuse to be examined for evidence if you are sure that you will not want to prosecute the rapist. Bear in mind that even if you don't want to press charges right now, you might change your mind later. If you have evidence collected now, you don't have to use it.

a massive violation of human rights. The International Criminal Tribunal in The Hague has recognized rape as a war crime. Its ruling acknowledges that rape is not a private interpersonal matter but a weapon that is used to demoralize the enemy, as well as an institutionalized form of plunder.

RACE, CLASS, PREJUDICE, AND VIOLENCE AGAINST WOMEN

Violence against women and racism are profoundly connected. Rape has been used as a means of dominating other races and a tool of cultural genocide in wars, military and colonial occupations, and throughout the history of slavery. We can see this on a large institutional level and in individual cases.

While violence is often targeted toward us simply because we are women, factors such as race, class, sexual orientation, and age put particular women at greater risk and limit our access to resources. Women of color, older women, young women, immigrant women, refugees, lesbians, poor women, transgender individuals, and women with disabilities are especially vulnerable to violence. Violence against women may occur simultaneously with other hate-based violence aimed at a particular race, nationality, or religion.

Too often, organizations that aim to serve victims of violence are not aware of or do not have sufficient resources to serve the widest range of women. For example, hotlines in the United States may be available only in English, and courts may be inaccessible to women who have no telephone, transportation, or child care. These institutions can reflect society's race, class, and other ingrained prejudices.

Immigrant women with limited English-language proficiency are frequently in situations where the perpetrator speaks English better than the woman does and, because he knows her, is able as interpreter to have undue influence with the police. In these circumstances, the woman rarely gets the help she needs.

When women of color call the police to protect ourselves and our families against violence, we confront a range of issues. We may wonder, "Will we be treated fairly by a police officer of another race or culture?" or "Will we be accused of betraying our 'people'?"

The man who raped me was white, and the cops here are all white. I didn't report it. I just told a few people I trusted. It helped, but I still feel scared knowing he's out there and that nobody would do anything about it.

COMMON REACTIONS TO EXPERIENCING VIOLENCE

We usually experience violence as a private crisis. Many survivors feel isolated because of a lack of support or because sexuality and victimization are surrounded by shame in our culture. This creates a difficult set of reactions that may be experienced by women who have been raped, battered, sexually harassed, abused as children, robbed violently, or hurt by other forms of violence. Many of these reactions are common to all people who have experienced trauma, including soldiers in wartime, robbery victims, and friends and families of murdered loved ones.

It helps some of us to recognize the commonality in our experiences. The mental health professions have classified some of the common reactions listed below as post-traumatic stress disorder (PTSD). PTSD is a term used to describe the reexperiencing of trauma and the recurrent, intrusive, and distressing recollection of the event in images, thoughts, or perceptions. It can include flashbacks, hallucinations, nightmares, dissociation (feeling of detachment from one's body or surroundings), an intense negative response to things that remind you of the trauma, troubled sleep, irritability or outbursts of anger, difficulty concentrating, and hypervigilance.

Some common reactions to trauma:

- Self-blame and feelings of shame and guilt
- Fear, terror, and feeling unsafe
- Anger and rage
- Anger turned inward, depression, and suicidal feelings
- Substance abuse
- Eating disorders
- Physical symptoms
- Self-harm
- Grief and loss
- Loss of control, powerlessness
- Isolation
- Flashbacks and nightmares
- Sensory triggers
- Dissociation
- Changes in sexuality and intimacy
- Spiritual crisis

(For a detailed description of the above reactions, see "Common Reactions to Experiencing Violence" [W16] on the companion website, www.ourbodiesourselves.org.)

Although there are common reactions, the reactions of one person may vary greatly from those of another. And as we move through the healing process, different reactions may increase or decrease in intensity.

REGAINING OUR LIVES

Recovery is a gradual process of healing and empowerment. Since violence causes us to feel a loss of control, healing can occur when we begin to regain a sense of power. Reflecting on the following points can help us move through the healing process:

1. The violence was not our fault. Myths about violence against women get expressed in destructive ways: "It must have been her behavior, she must have provoked him somehow, it must have been what she was wearing, where she was. . . ." These things have nothing to do with the responsibility for the assault. We did not ask to be hurt and violated, and we do not deserve it.
2. We made the best choices we were able to. We may have been forced to make life-or-death decisions before, during, and after the assault.
3. There is no right way to feel or heal. Our reactions and healing process are connected to who we are as individuals. Our culture and economic background can influence our healing process in both positive and negative ways. We all take different paths to healing, and we must respect the choices each survivor makes.
4. We deserve support. We need to reach out to people who will believe us, provide support, and help us find the strength and capacity to heal. Rape crisis centers and domestic violence hotlines are available and often will help without regard to immigration status. A family member, friend, clergy member, or counselor may also be an option. We may decide to find a support group or try other kinds of healing support based on art, music, writing, physical activity, or meditation.
5. We need to give ourselves time to heal.

INTIMATE-PARTNER VIOLENCE

Intimate-partner violence and battering, also known as domestic violence, are among the most common yet least reported crimes in the world. While all couples at times disagree or

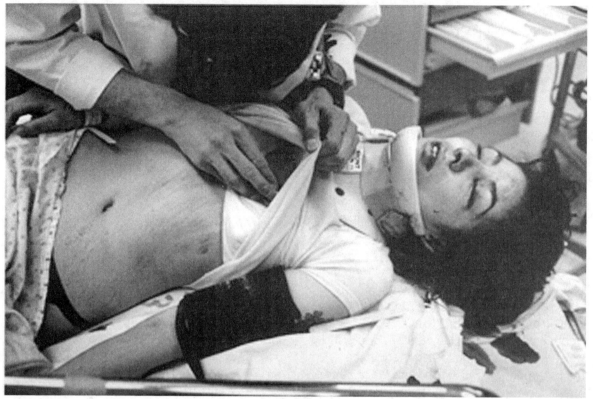

When Diana was rushed to a Minneapolis emergency room, her chest was covered with black tire marks. Her boyfriend had driven over her with his truck. Courtesy of Domestic Abuse Awareness, Inc.

argue or even have feelings of rage, not all aggressive behavior between intimates constitutes domestic violence. Domestic violence involves a *pattern* of behavior that causes fear and intimidation.

I was living with my then girlfriend, and everything was okay for a while. Then she started to . . . force me into doing things that I didn't want to do. She wouldn't take no for an answer to anything. If she wanted it, she would get it.

Domestic violence can be expressed in an array of threatening and harmful behaviors intended to assert power and control. It may include slapping, punching, choking, kicking, hit-

ting with objects, threatening with weapons, sexual assault, verbal and emotional abuse, control of finances or physical freedom, destruction of objects, and harm to children or pets. It may occur frequently or only occasionally.

I have been threatened when he's had a bad day and when he's had a good day.

Stalking may occur when the battered partner attempts to leave or does leave the relationship. In such cases, an abuser may feel loss of power and control; stalking may be an attempt to regain that control.

While some injuries experienced from certain acts may not appear life-threatening initially, this can be deceptive. For example, if a batterer resorts to choking, it may require just a little more force to crush your windpipe so that you suffocate and die.

If domestic violence is not adequately addressed in its early stages, it can escalate in magnitude and severity and ultimately end in murder. The easy accessibility of firearms makes domestic violence particularly deadly. Under federal law, people subject to protection orders are not supposed to own or purchase firearms, and in some states, abusers who are subject to an order of protection may not legally own, buy, or possess any firearm. But these laws have rarely been enforced, and few battered women are informed about our rights. We need to strengthen these laws, state by state, to protect women and families from lethal violence.

WHY DO WOMEN STAY?

A common question asked about women who are battered is "Why do they stay?" This question takes the focus off the real issue: "Why does the partner beat her?" There are many reasons why someone stays with an abusive partner. We may feel trapped and unable to leave, either because we still feel love for our partner and hope the battering will end, or because we are physically prevented from leaving. Battering often escalates at the point of separation, and we may feel safer staying. If we have children, we may think that we will not be able to support them and ourselves if we leave. People to whom we turn for support—clergy, police, friends, family—may not take the situation seriously or may not know how to intervene or provide help. We may know about the existence of shelters for battered women but feel that moving to a shelter in a new neighborhood or city will cause too much upheaval for us and/or our children. We may be afraid to leave if we believe our immigration status is dependent on the "goodwill" of the batterer. If we have been living with abuse for a long time, we may be so worn down physically and emotionally that we cannot see a way out or imagine a future without pain and fear.

THE IMPACT OF INTIMATE-PARTNER VIOLENCE ON CHILDREN

The effects of growing up in an atmosphere of domestic violence can be devastating to children. Children of battered women are more likely to be battered themselves. They often live in constant fear and can be torn physically and emotionally between their adult caretakers. They may develop severe physical and emotional responses to the violence, including symptoms of post-traumatic stress disorder. Children who grow up with intimate-partner violence may believe that violence is an appropriate way to resolve conflicts, and some of us live out our childhood experiences of violence in our adult relationships and our relationships with our own children.

Many batterers grew up witnessing abuse or experiencing physical or sexual abuse as children. They often came of age in families where male dominance was never questioned and where physical punishment "in the name of love" was accepted. When our families teach us to accept male dominance and violence as a way to relate to one another, this "education" is difficult to defy.

I was raped and beaten by my father. By the time I . . . started dating, I had lost my voice. I didn't think that I had the right to say, "No, you can't do this to me."

WOMEN WITH DISABILITIES AND IMMIGRANT WOMEN

Women and girls with disabilities experience a high rate of violence. We face many of the same struggles as other women who are abused, as well as some unique problems: We may be physically dependent on the batterer for daily care; the local shelter for battered women may not be set up to accommodate our disabilities. Finding appropriate help and alternative living arrangements that respect our right to privacy can be exceedingly difficult. Similarly, those of us who are immigrants or refugees in the United States may encounter systemic barriers that impede our ability to seek help. Fears of deportation, language barriers, and lack of information can make our problems worse. The Violence Against Women Act (1994) and its successors expanded access to legal relief and other services for immigrant women experiencing domestic violence and other crimes.

(For more information, see "Abuse of Women with Disabilities" [W17] and "Abuse of Immigrant Women" [W18] on the companion website, www.ourbodiesourselves.org.)

Efforts are beginning in many communities to break the intergenerational cycle of violence that exists in so many families. Often, they begin with community-based programs. Recently, programs like the Family Justice Center in San Diego have started providing comprehensive services under one roof, including social services for women, children, and batterers; law enforcement; a family court; prosecutors; and legal services. The aim of this model is to shift the emphasis from criminal justice to help for the whole family.[7]

Innovative programs that teach nonviolence and conflict resolution skills to preschoolers are being implemented in some child care centers. Workshops on dating violence are being offered to teenagers. These efforts aim to teach girls and young women that we have a right to be free from violence and terror, and to teach boys and young men a better way to relate to girls, women, and the world.

WHAT YOU CAN DO IF YOU ARE BEING BATTERED

If you are in a violent relationship right now, there are things you can do that may help you to be safer; assure the safety of your children, if you have any; and work toward ending the relationship, if that is what you want to do. No answer is right for all battered women. Overall, your safety can increase as you become more aware, inform others, find support, and implement a safety plan.

Here are some things you can do to take care of yourself during an attack:

- Stay as calm as possible.
- Try to shield yourself, especially your head and stomach.
- If you are able, and if it will not put you at greater risk, call 911 and get emergency assistance.
- Do the best you can to end the attack with the least amount of injury.

SAFETY PLANNING

Even if you are still in the situation and see no immediate way out, you can do the following to plan for your safety:

- Call the National Domestic Violence Hotline at 1-800-799-SAFE. Memorize this number. Ask if your area has a local domestic violence hotline.

WARNING SIGNS

This list identifies a continuum of abusive behaviors that come from the batterer's desire for power and control. The more behaviors that apply to the relationship, the more dangerous the situation may be.

Emotional and Economic Abuse

- Destructive criticism/verbal attacks
- Intimidation/pressure tactics
- Dominating you
- Disrespect/putting you down
- Overly jealous/possessive
- Lying
- Blaming you for everything
- Minimizing/denying his or her own behavior
- Abusing drugs or alcohol
- Threatening suicide or self-harm
- Isolating you from friends and family
- Controlling all the money
- Preventing you from getting or keeping a job

Acts of Violence

These may be done against you, your children, other people, or pets.

- Making angry gestures
- Destroying objects
- Threatening to hurt you or others
- Sexual violence
- Physical violence
- Use of weapons

All battering is dangerous. However, certain factors, such as the batterer's possession of weapons, extreme possessiveness or controlling behavior, or use of drugs and alcohol, can mean that you are at serious risk. (For more information on understanding how dangerous your situation is, see "Risk Assessment" [W19] on the companion website, www.ourbodiesourselves.org.)

- Become familiar with your state's laws and legal policies on domestic violence. Find out about protection (restraining) orders, including how to get them and where to get an advocate if needed. To find out how to get this information, contact your local domestic violence hotline or shelter.
- Build a support network. Get connected with your local battered women's service, join a support group, and develop a network of friends.
- Learn and watch for warning signs of your partner's abusive behavior/attitude.
- Teach your children how to call for emergency assistance.

- Prepare a safety plan. Write it down, if you can keep it in a place the abuser cannot find. Let others you trust know your plans when appropriate.
- If your abuser is using alcohol or drugs and you can get to Al-Anon meetings (see Chapter 3, "Alcohol, Tobacco, and Other Mood-Altering Drugs"), you may gain support and strength from the meetings to make a change.

If you are not a U.S. citizen, you may still qualify for benefits as a victim of domestic violence. To locate an advocate or a lawyer in your community with expertise in immigrant victims' is-

Increasing Safety While in the Relationship

- Carry important phone numbers for yourself and your children: for example, police, hospital, friends, battered women's shelter. Keep these numbers in a place that the batterer cannot find. Do not use your computer to store this information unless you are sure it cannot be accessed. Try to have a cellular phone or beeper, but make sure your phone does not have any tracking software.
- Find someone to tell about the abuse, and develop a signal for distress. Ask neighbors to call the police if they hear sounds indicating that violence is occurring.
- Think of four places where you can go and not be tracked down by your abuser if you leave in a hurry.
- Get specific items ready to take if you leave.
- Keep change for phone calls, and open your own bank account.
- Rehearse an escape route.
- Periodically review and update your safety plan.

What to Take with You if You Decide to Leave

Money, checkbook, bank cards, credit cards; identification, driver's license, keys, and car registration; important phone numbers; birth certificates, Social Security and health insurance cards, welfare identification; passport, immigration card, work permit; divorce or other court papers; school and medical records; house deed, mortgage; insurance papers and policies; information on past abuse, such as photos and police reports; medications and refill instructions; change of clothes.

Increasing Safety After You Leave

- If you have joint bank accounts, withdraw as much money as you can, and deposit it into a personal account.
- Use different routes as you go home, to work, or about your daily tasks.
- Avoid the stores, services, and banks that you know your batterer goes to often.
- Tell your child care provider who has permission to pick up your kids. Warn them if you think the batterer may attempt to kidnap your children. Tell them to call the police if the batterer appears for any reason.
- If it is right for you, get a protection order. Know what it orders and what will happen if your batterer violates it. Keep it with you at all times.
- At work, tell someone about the abuse, and have that person screen your calls. If possible, show other people a picture of your batterer and instruct them to call the police if he or she arrives at work. If you have a protection order, people at work should have a copy of it and a picture of your batterer.

sues, contact the Immigrant Women Program of Legal Momentum at 1-212-925-6635.

Making a safety plan while you are dealing with a violent partner can help in two ways. It can give you hope in what so often feels like a hopeless situation. It can also bring you closer to leaving a dangerous situation in a well-planned way. In many communities, battered women's service organizations can help you develop a plan to increase your safety and that of your children.

There are alternatives to enduring domestic violence. More and more women are leaving violent partners and making new lives free of violence. Women everywhere have been organizing to help battered women leave abusive situations, provide shelter, and demand a more responsive legal system.

LEGAL AND MEDICAL CONSIDERATIONS

There is no single right way to handle intimate-partner abuse. Each woman must decide what is best for herself and her family. However, if you decide to seek legal protection, know that batterers can be prosecuted for crimes such as assault and battery. In addition, special laws protect battered women in all fifty states. These laws are very consistent from one state to another.

All hospitals are mandated to train their staff about violence against women. The staff should be aware of the safety needs of battered women, especially if you are accompanied by the person who abused you. Hospital staff should also be able to assist you in getting help from the social services department.

The laws that protect battered women enable you to go to a local court and obtain an immediate protection order against the batterer. Orders of protection—often called restraining orders or protection-from-abuse orders—can provide different kinds of protection. They can order the batterer to stay away from you and your children and give you legal custody of your children. They can order the batterer to pay support. You can obtain protection orders even when you continue living with your abuser. Laws affecting women in lesbian relationships vary from state to state.

In addition to abuse prevention orders, all states have anti-stalking laws. Recognizing that women are often at greater risk right after leaving the batterer, these laws impose criminal sanctions against a batterer who continues to harass you or stalks you.

Some batterers are intimidated enough by the legal system to be stopped by a court order. If this is the case for your batterer, a restraining order may bring you some safety. However, the tendency toward violence is so deep-seated in some batterers that no court order will stop them. They may become violently enraged by what they see as a betrayal. In these instances, going to court may actually make you and your children less safe. An advocate at your local domestic violence organization may be able to help you decide whether to get a restraining order.

If you have had to defend yourself against a violent perpetrator and have injured or killed him or her, seek legal representation with an attorney who has experience defending battered women and who understands the dynamics of violence against women. Contact the Battered Women's Justice Project at 1-800-903-0111 or your statewide domestic violence or rape crisis coalition to find out about legal resources familiar with how your state's self-defense laws affect battered women.

RAPE

Rape, also called sexual assault, is any kind of sexual activity committed against someone's will. Whether the rapist uses force or threats of force is irrelevant. Rape, as a legal term, is defined slightly differently in each state. Most state laws define rape in terms of penetration with the use of force and without the person's consent. Penetration can be with the penis, fingers, or instruments like bottles or sticks. It can be perpetrated in the vagina, anus, or mouth.

The National Violence Against Women Survey reports that almost 18 percent of women said they have been the victim of a completed or attempted rape at some point in their lifetime, and most women were raped by someone they knew rather than a stranger.[8] Rape can happen

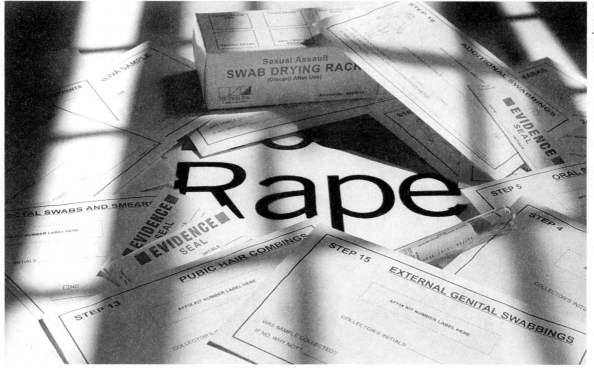

Rape kit, courtesy of the Boston Area Rape Crisis Center.

to us at any age, but girls and young women are at particular risk. In this same survey, which interviewed only women over eighteen, almost 22 percent reported that they were younger than age twelve when they were raped, and over half were under age eighteen.[9]

When we are raped, survival is our primary instinct, and we protect ourselves as best we can. Some women choose to fight back; others do not. Choosing not to fight back is also a survival strategy.

Although most rapes are perpetrated by men, women can and do rape other women. Women who are raped by women may feel isolated and confused, because we may have thought that only men can commit rape. (For information and resources, see "Woman–Woman Rape" [W20] on the companion website, www.our bodiesourselves.com.)

MEDICAL CONSIDERATIONS IF YOU HAVE BEEN RAPED

If you have been raped, it is critical for your physical and emotional health to receive medical attention as soon as possible, even if you have no obvious injuries. Your first reaction might be to take a shower and try to forget what happened. That is understandable, but you may wash away evidence that could be crucial if you want to prosecute the rapist. Even if you do not think you want to press charges right now, you could change your mind in a few months or years. If you have evidence collected, you can always use it later. Collecting evidence involves going to a hospital and asking to have a *rape kit* done. A rape kit is designed specifically for collecting evidence of sexual assault, including semen and blood.

If you go to the hospital:

- Try to have a friend, relative, or rape crisis counselor go with you as an advocate.
- Be aware that most states have passed legislation to assure that rape exams are free of charge.
- Bring a list of medications you are taking; a change of clothing if you are still in the same clothes; or the clothing that you were wearing during the assault, if you have changed your clothes.

Ideally, when you go to the hospital, an advocate from your local rape crisis center should meet you there. You should also ask to see a trained sexual assault nurse examiner in the emergency room.[11] Some hospitals have specialized programs staffed by nurses or doctors who have received extensive training in the medical, legal, and emotional issues associated with sexual assault. The programs are designed to provide sensitive medical exams and the best evidence possible for prosecution.

Rape can cause physical injuries to any part of the body. Therefore, you should request a thorough examination that includes and/or results in the following:

- **A verbal history of the sexual assault and related medical concerns.** You will be asked to give a detailed description of the assault, which will be written down. Although it may be difficult to talk about these details, they are important so that the medical provider will know where to check for injuries and what evidence to document, such as bruises, scrapes, or other injuries. Do not answer irrelevant questions about your sexual history or any past therapy, since the perpetrator's defense might try to gain access to your records later.
- **A pelvic exam.** In collecting evidence, the practitioner will look for the presence of semen if you were raped by a man. However, semen may not be present after a vaginal or anal rape. The practitioner will also comb your pubic hair for the possible presence of the perpetrator's pubic hair. This medical evidence will be made available to police or others only with your written permission. You or the person with you at the hospital should check the record for accuracy and objectivity as soon as possible after the exam. Try to do this while the doctor is still present. If you were raped vaginally, see p. 589 for more information about a pelvic exam. You will receive a rectal exam if you were raped anally.

CAMPUS RAPE

Colleges and universities are required by federal law to have a policy to deal with rape and sexual assault on campus. The sexual assault policy must include a disciplinary procedure against the perpetrator that is separate from what happens if you report the crime to the police.[10] Keep in mind that although your school might have sexual assault counselors, if they are administrators rather than service providers for sexual assault survivors, their priority may be the interests of the school and not your access to justice.

Most of the rape that happens on campuses occurs between people who know each other. This means that you will probably see the rapist in classes, the student center, or even the dormitories. You are legally entitled to get a stay-away order from your school, allowing you to change dormitories and preventing the rapist from coming near you.

(For more information on what to do if you have been raped, see "Campus Rape" [W21] on the companion website, www.ourbodiesourselves.org.)

- **Examination and treatment of any external injuries.** The practitioner will examine you for any external injuries and may photograph bruises or other marks to document the assault. If bruises emerge after the exam, take pictures of them and call the examiner so the information can be added to your record.
- **Treatment for prevention of sexually transmitted infections (STIs).** The practitioner will recommend giving you two shots of an antibiotic in your buttocks. Some STIs are not detectable until six weeks have passed, so it is a good idea to return for a six-week checkup (see Chapter 15, "Sexually Transmitted Infections").
- **Treatment for prevention of pregnancy.** If it is possible that you will become pregnant as a result of the rape, the doctor or nurse may offer you emergency contraception (sometimes called "the morning-after pill"). In some states, emergency contraception is available in pharmacies without a prescription (see Chapter 18, "Birth Control"). A pregnancy resulting from rape cannot be detected until several weeks later. If you become pregnant, see Chapters 19, "Unexpected Pregnancy," and 20, "Abortion."
- **Information about AIDS/HIV.** It is possible to be infected by HIV through a sexual assault. To treat potential HIV infection, you need medication immediately. Although not available everywhere, there are promising new treatments that help prevent HIV infection if taken right away. However, these drugs are controversial and should be taken only after they are fully explained to you. If you are offered testing for HIV, be aware that immediately after the assault is too soon for HIV antibodies to show up. Also, the test results could become part of your medical and legal record. (For more information, see Chapter 16, "HIV and AIDS.")
- **A follow-up exam.** Although you may feel physically recovered shortly after the rape, a follow-up visit that includes tests and treatment for STIs and a pregnancy test, if indicated, is an important part of taking care of yourself.

LEGAL CONSIDERATIONS IF YOU HAVE BEEN RAPED

Although improvements have been made in the legal system, prosecution of a rapist can still be a drawn-out and painful process. Most communities have rape crisis centers that provide advocates to help you move through the legal system. Many local district attorney offices offer victim/witness advocates who can provide information and support. In some states, you can report a rape anonymously or without prosecuting. Whether you report it or not, write down everything you can remember so if you decide to file a criminal complaint later, your statement will be accurate. (For more information about deciding whether or not to report a rape, see "Legal Considerations if You Have Been Raped" [W22] on the companion website, www.ourbodiesour selves.org.)

WHAT TO DO IF SOMEONE YOU CARE ABOUT HAS BEEN RAPED

If you are a friend or family member of someone who has been raped, you might not know what to say. Just being there and listening is helpful. The rape may bring up strong feelings for you, but avoid expressing opinions that are critical of her behavior. (For more ideas on how you can be supportive, see "What to Do If Someone You Care About Has Been Raped" [W23] on the companion website, www.ourbodiesour selves.org.)

PROTECTING OURSELVES AND EACH OTHER FROM RAPE

Most sexual assaults are committed by someone we know rather than a stranger. In either case, we can take steps to protect ourselves.

- **Safety in social situations.** Pay attention to how you feel. If you want to end a date or leave a party, say so, even if you are afraid or embarrassed. If you drink alcohol, keep an eye on your drink. Drugs are available that can be slipped into drinks to tranquilize a person and induce a blackout.
- **Safety in intimate relationships.** Learn to recognize potentially abusive relationships. An abusive or unhealthy relationship involves disrespect, fear, jealousy, possessiveness, and controlling behavior.
- **Safety at home.** Make sure entrances are well lit and windows and doors are securely locked. Use only your last name on your mailbox. Find out who is at your door before opening it for anyone.
- **Safety in your neighborhood.** Arrange to walk home with people you trust. Get to know the people who live in your apartment building or on your street.
- **Safety on the street.** Be aware of what is going on around you. Walk at a steady pace, and look as if you know where you are going. Dress so you can move and run easily. If possible, walk in the middle of the street, avoiding dark places and groups of men. Carry a whistle around your wrist. Always check the backseat of your car before getting in, and keep the car doors locked while driving. Avoid groups of men on public transportation. Avoid hitchhiking.
- **Calling for help on the highway.** Usually, 911 will connect you to emergency services, but there are still many places in the U.S. that do not have 911 systems. In some places, #77 or

*77 will get the state police. If you are pulled over by an unmarked vehicle, especially at night or in a secluded area, you do not have to stop immediately. Slow down, turn on your emergency flashers, and drive to a well-lit, populated place before stopping. Keep your doors locked, and roll down the window only an inch. Ask to see a badge and photo ID. If you have a cell phone, use it to contact a police dispatcher to check the person's authenticity.

These tactics can help you, but they are not foolproof. Practice tactics for dealing with situations that make you feel most at risk and least powerful. Try to remain calm and act as confident and strong as possible.

INCEST AND SEXUAL ABUSE OF CHILDREN

One common form of violence against children is incest, which is defined as sexual contact that occurs between family members. Incest can be perpetrated by adult male or female relatives against male or female children. Sexual abuse can be perpetrated by friends, coaches, teachers, babysitters, or clergy. Unfortunately, people in such positions can use the child's trust and dependence to initiate sexual contact and often to ensure that the relationship continues and remains secret.

The extent of incest and childhood sexual abuse is hard to measure because of lack of reporting and uniform definitions and the limits of memory. A conservative estimate is that one in five girls and one in thirteen boys have been sexually abused as children.[12,13]

Incest and sexual abuse of children take many forms and may include sexually suggestive language; prolonged kissing, looking, and petting; vaginal and/or anal intercourse; and oral sex. Because sexual contact is often achieved without overt physical force, there may be no obvious signs of physical harm.

Whether or not the signs of abuse are physical and obvious, sexual abuse in childhood can have lifelong consequences. We often blame ourselves long after the abuse has ended—for not saying no, not fighting back, telling or not telling, having been seductive, or having trusted the abuser.

As victims of incest and abuse, we may have lots of sex with many partners in order to feel accepted, or to erase or overpower the memories of abusive sex. We may run away from home to escape the abuse; we may experience depression; and we may use drugs and alcohol to dull the pain.

To heal from the trauma of incest or early sexual abuse, we need to tell our stories to people who can understand and empathize. Talking with others in counseling or in support groups may break the silence, help us gain perspective, and end the isolation. Some women find it necessary to confront the family member who perpetrated the abuse. This is a frightening task, but it can also be rewarding.

SEXUAL HARASSMENT

Sexual harassment is unwanted sexual attention. It includes leering, pinching, patting, repeated comments, subtle suggestions of a sexual nature, pornography in the workplace, and pressure for dates. Sexual harassment is not limited to the workplace or school. It can include doctors with patients, welfare workers with clients, and police officers with the public. Sexual harassment involves the abuse of power. In addition to men harassing women, women can harass other women, and men can be harassed by other men or by women. Because sexual harassment can escalate, people who are being sexually harassed are at risk of being physically abused or raped.

In the workplace, we may experience a direct or implied threat, such as "Have sex with me or you will be fired" (called *quid pro quo*). A hostile work environment can interfere with the ability to do our job, whether the harasser is an employer, a supervisor, a coworker, a client, or a customer.

Socializing at work often includes flirting or joking about sex. Although it may be a pleasant relief from routine or a way to communicate with someone we are interested in, this banter can turn insulting or demeaning. It becomes sexual harassment when it creates a hostile, intimidating, or uncomfortable working environment. Refusal to comply with the harasser's demands may lead to reprisals, which can include escalation of harassment; poor work assignments; sabotaging of projects; denial of raises, benefits, or promotion; and sometimes the loss of a job with only a poor reference. Harassment can drive women out of a job or the workplace altogether. Poor women, immigrant women, older women, and teenagers are especially vulnerable to sexual harassment because of difficulties in finding other employment.

When sexual harassment happens in a school setting, it can have devastating effects on the course of a young person's life. One sixteen-year-old girl describes her experience:

It came to the point where I was skipping almost all of my classes, therefore getting me kicked out of the honors program. I dreaded school each morning, I started to wear clothes that wouldn't flatter my figure, and I kept to myself. I'd cry every night when I got home, and I thought I was a loser. . . . Sometimes the teachers were right there when it was going on. They did nothing.[14]

Because there is such a taboo against identifying sexual harassment, when we first experience it, we may be aware only of feeling stressed. We may develop headaches, anxieties, or resistance to going to work in the morning. It may take us a while to realize that these symptoms come from being sexually harassed. We may blame ourselves and wonder if we did something to provoke the harassment. We may also be afraid to say no or to speak out because of possible retaliation. But when we take the risk and talk with other women, we find others who are being or have been harassed and have responses similar to ours.

(For more information, see "What You Can Do if You Are Being Sexually Harassed" [W24] on the companion website, www.ourbodiesourselves.org.)

PROSTITUTION AND SEX TRAFFICKING

Prostitution is sometimes portrayed as a way to make vast amounts of money, live the "good" life, or meet a rich man who will become your boyfriend. In reality, even though billions of dollars are made annually in the sex industry, the rich Hollywood prostitute is extremely rare.

The prostitution industry attempts to glamorize prostitution as a choice for a sexually liberated woman. Some middle-class women do choose to enter prostitution out of curiosity or a sense of adventure. But poverty is the major force that drives people, especially women of color and runaway teenagers, into prostitution. One of the few groups funded to study prostitutes found that the average age of entry into prostitution in the United States is fourteen, and many of these girls are running away from abusive homes.[15] Girls who enter prostitution are not consenting adults and do not exercise free choice. Prostitution is a means of survival when other work is not available.

I ran away from home, and I met a woman who brought me to her boyfriend, who I later found out was a pimp, and that guy raped me, over

and over. . . . He then brought me to his friend, another pimp, and sold me to him, and from the age of 12 years old until I was 35 and too drugged out to work, I was a prostitute.

Prostitutes are particularly at risk for violence from pimps and customers. Women who are prostitutes suffer a higher rate of sexually transmitted infections, including HIV/AIDS and hepatitis, but most of the health studies have focused on prostitutes as vectors of disease rather than as disease victims.[16] Female and transgender prostitutes have little or no protection from police harassment and lack police protection when victimized by crimes such as robbery, battery, and rape. The criminal justice system prosecutes prostitutes, while the johns routinely go free.

Prostitutes have organized in the U.S. and Europe to demand decriminalization (the abolition of all laws against prostitution). Decriminalization is not the same as legalization, which would put prostitution under state regulation and legitimize the sex industry. Decriminalization organizations advocate abolishing laws that punish the prostitute, and seek laws that would make it illegal to be a customer of a prostitute or to engage in sex trafficking, pimping, or owning brothels. Such laws would put the johns, rather than the prostitutes, at risk of being arrested and fined.

Prostitutes need resources and services that will provide medical testing and treatment, condoms, and help with negotiating safer sex. Prostitutes should be able to keep and control any money earned through prostitution, and social services need to provide all people with economic alternatives to prostitution.

Because the demand for prostitutes exceeds the supply, a criminal trade in women and girls has developed throughout the world. Traffickers use force, coercion, and lies to recruit, transport, and exploit people as forced labor or slaves. The CIA estimates that between 700,000 and 2 million women and children are trafficked internationally into prostitution, sex entertainment, and forced labor and that about 50,000 women and children are trafficked into the United States every year.[17] The growth of sites on the Internet promoting sex tourism fuels the rapid growth of the trafficking industry.

A twenty-two-year-old prostitute in Calcutta recalls how she was trafficked from her native Bangladesh at age seventeen:

I didn't come of my own wish; I was sold. They picked me up from the street over there and brought me . . . There were no police. There was one, whom they had bribed . . . For the first two or three days, I was very stubborn about not joining this line [of work]. They starved me for those two or three days and never even gave me water to drink.

Traffickers often provide fake passports and visas for the women they recruit. They commonly charge large fees for documents, airline tickets, and room and board, and then require the women to pay them back. The women are often indebted for years and are moved from city to city and brothel to brothel. Women who are trafficked are also routinely criminalized by immigration services, do not have access to health care, and are isolated. Traffickers and pimps use the technique of "seasoning" by repeated rapes so that new recruits will accept being prostitutes. Trafficked women and children are also extremely vulnerable to battering, injury, and sexually transmitted infections, but this violence is frequently defined as acceptable "rough sex" or "an occupational hazard."

DEFENDING OURSELVES

The most important step in ending violence against women is to stop people from using violence to get their way. At the same time, we must learn to protect ourselves as best we can. Learn-ing self-defense boosts our physical and emotional self-confidence and can increase our options in a situation where we are at risk of violence. The actual use of these skills when we are in danger is a choice made at a particular moment. Each of us makes the best decision we can based on our resources and knowledge at the time. If you decide to learn self-defense, also prepare yourself for the real possibility that the person you may defend yourself against may be your date, friend, partner, parent, teacher, or coworker.

The study of self-defense includes many activities: assertiveness training, exercise, and boxing and other sports that promote self-confidence, self-knowledge, and self-reliance. Self-defense is not simply responding to violence with violence. While there are increasing numbers of girls and women willing to act violently, responding this way does not necessarily

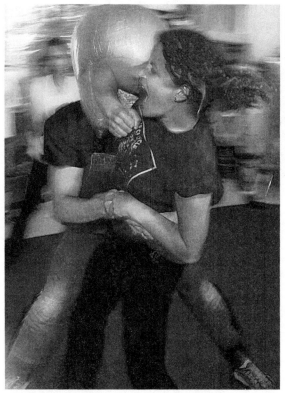

increase women's safety. Self-defense classes may help us think clearly if we are under attack, so that we can mobilize our thoughts, assess the situation, make a judgment about the level of danger, and then carry out the response we have chosen. We can also use this self-awareness in other uncomfortable life situations.

I have experienced such profound changes in my self-image and in the way that I see the world and relate to people that I really can't separate my study of self-defense from the rest of my life.

Several myths can prevent us from defending ourselves effectively against a physical assault. They include that we do not know how to defend ourselves; that the assailant is invulnerable; and that greater physical strength determines who prevails. Yet women have defended ourselves against attacks through both resourcefulness and force. For example, one woman frightened off three adolescent males who were following her along a city street: She turned quickly and let out a bloodcurdling yell. Another woman stopped a would-be assailant with a kick in the midsection.

Street techniques, which depend upon surprise and causing damage, do not work as well against repeated assault by men we live with. Other skills developed in the practice of self-defense may be useful. As we begin to feel more self-confident, we will be able to consider how we might resist the battering or how we might eventually leave the batterer and the violence behind us.

ENDING VIOLENCE AGAINST WOMEN

Over the past thirty-five years, women have focused much effort on the problem of violence against women and made great progress.

Women have started talking about our experiences, built rape crisis centers and shelters, advocated for changes in laws, been joined in our efforts by men, become recognized as part of the international public health and human rights movements, and influenced other survivor movements, such as the one working on abuse by clergy. (For more information about the history of work on the issue of violence against women, see "Ending Violence Against Women: A Brief History" [W25] on the companion website, www.ourbodiesourselves.org.)

There is still much to be done. We need to:

- Speak out against the messages in our society that glorify and encourage violence, domination, and exploitation
- Teach and model nonviolence
- Intervene whenever we see the seeds or expression of violence against women, realizing that our silence helps perpetuate it
- Strengthen family, community, and neighborhood sanctions against violence as opposed to relying exclusively on the criminal justice system
- Work to maintain a strong network of services for all of us who are at risk of and who have survived violence
- Demand that our government officials take violence against women seriously and make it a key part of their agendas if they want our votes

For the future, we must pursue our vision of a violence-free world loudly and clearly. Noeleen Heyzer, the executive director of UNIFEM (a United Nations fund that promotes gender equality), describes that vision:

Imagine a world free from gender-based violence: where homes are not broken into fragments; where tears are no longer shed for daughters raped in war, and in peace; where shame and silences break into new melodies; where women and men gain power and courage to live to their full potential. Into such a world, I pray, let the twenty-first century awake.[18]

NOTES

1. U.S. Department of Justice and the Centers for Disease Control, National Violence Against Women Survey.
2. Bureau of Justice Statistics Crime Data Brief, *Intimate Partner Violence, 1993–2001,* February 2003.
3. Ibid.
4. World Health Organization, "Report on Violence and Health," October 2002, www.who.int/gender/violence/en/.
5. Patricia Tjaden and Nancy Thoennes, "Full Report of the Prevalence, Incidence, and Consequences of Violence Against Women," National Institute of Justice, November 2000. Accessed at www.ncjrs.org/pdffiles1/nij/183781.pdf on September 30, 2004.
6. U.S. Department of Justice, Office of Justice Programs, *Bureau of Justice Statistics National Crime Victimization Survey,* June 2001, www.rainn.org/Linked%20files/NCVS%202000.pdf.
7. Family Justice Center, www.familyjusticecenter.org; 707 Broadway, Suite 700, San Diego, CA, 92101, 1-866-933-HOPE (4673).
8. Tjaden and Thoennes, "Full Report."
9. Ibid.
10. Jodi Gold and Susan Villari, eds., *Just Sex: Students Rewrite the Rules on Sex, Violence, Activism and Equality* (Maryland: Rowan G. Littlefield Publishing, 2000).
11. Sexual Assault Resources Service and Sexual Assault Nurse Examiners Program, www.sane-sart.com.
12. D. Finkelhor, "Current Information on the Scope and Nature of Sexual Abuse," *The Future of Children* 4 (1994): 31–53.
13. D. Finkelhor, "The International Epidemiology of Child Sexual Abuse," *Child Abuse and Neglect* 18 (1994): 409–417.
14. Nan Stein, "No Laughing Matter: Sexual Harassment in K–12 Schools," in Emile Buchwald, ed., *Transforming a Rape Culture* (Minneapolis: Milkweed Editions, 1993).
15. E. Giobbe, "Juvenile Prostitution: Profile of Recruitment" in *Child Trauma I: Issues & Research* (New York: Garland Publishing, 1992): 117.
16. Sachi Sri Kanta, *Prostitutes in Medical Literature* (Westport, CT: Greenwood Press, 1991).
17. Amy O'Neill Richard, "International Trafficking in Women to the United States: A Contemporary Manifestation of Slavery and Organized Crime" (Washington D.C.: Central Intelligence Agency, 1999).
18. In her address to the forty-third session of the U.N. Commission on the Status of Women, March 1, 1999.

Relationships and Sexuality

CHAPTER 9

Our attractions and identities are powerful and intimate parts of who we are. More and more, people are understanding gender identity and sexual orientation as aspects of life that don't fit neatly into boxes. This chapter addresses these separate yet intertwined topics that affect our relationships with ourselves, each other, and the world.

CHALLENGING SEX AND GENDER

Moving beyond the concept of two fixed gender identities is a new challenge for some of us and a very personal story for others.

"Sex" and "gender" are two separate yet connected concepts. Sex is commonly understood to be based on a person's biological features: the penis, testicles, vagina, uterus, etc., that anatomically define a person as male or female. "Gender" is used in several ways. It may refer to gender roles or expression: the behavioral characteristics considered "masculine" or "feminine" in a particular culture at a particular time. These can range from hair and clothing styles to the way people speak or express emotions. "Gender" may also refer to gender identity: our internal sense of ourselves as man, woman, or transgender (not fitting conventional norms). In mainstream U.S. culture, gender is believed to follow directly from one's sex. In other words, a baby born with a vagina is considered female, called a girl, and expected to grow up to be a woman who acts, dresses, and talks in a "feminine" manner, who dates boys, marries a man, and has children.

Many people challenge the expectation that the genitals we are born with should dictate almost all of our physical, emotional, and psychological attributes. Feminists and others have long objected to strict gender roles that require women to be "feminine" and men to be "masculine." And some people are contesting the idea that our gender identity is inextricably tied to our biological sex and that there are only two genders. What if being a woman isn't about having a vagina? What if people don't have to fit neatly into "masculine" or "feminine" boxes? For some of us, how we see ourselves and how others perceive us in the galaxy of masculinity, femininity, and the million points swirling between them cannot be constrained within the two simple categories of man and woman.[1]

Recently, I have been in the process of informing others of my true gender identity. What I am is androgynous—both man and woman. What my birth sex is, is irrelevant. I'm finding . . . that more and more people are saying things like "What sex is . . . he? . . . she?," though always to

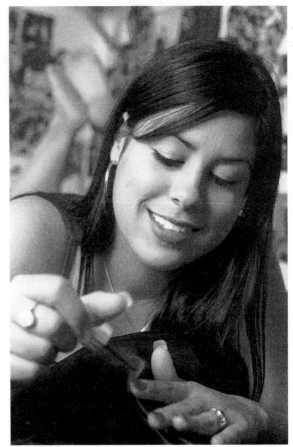

© Jörg Meyer

friends, never to my face. I'm finding this very pleasing, although I wish people would say it to me. I do take it as a compliment!

Some of us grapple with and analyze our gender; others take our gender for granted. Where does gender come from? Its source may not be the same for all of us. Our race, class, geographical, physical, and sexual identities affect and shape our gender, and it may change over time; some people maintain that gender is not necessarily an identity that remains the same from birth to death.

Some women believe that gender norms should be expanded or eliminated altogether, so that the full range of human behavior is accepted in all people. We may not fit traditional stereotypes of how women should act, yet we still consider ourselves women and question why a particular feeling or experience cannot be a woman's experience. Other people born with female sexual anatomy want our adoption of a masculine gender identity to be accepted. We, too, may not fit traditional stereotypes of how women should look or act, but we call ourselves transgender. Others of us were born with male sexual anatomy but identify as and want to be recognized as women.

The idea that gender is separate from sex has opened doors for many of us to express ourselves in ways that may conflict with how society dictates we should look and act.

GENDER IDENTITY: WHAT WE CALL OURSELVES

Each of us has a gender identity, whether we choose to label it or not. A new vocabulary is evolving to describe identities that fall outside the two gender categories our society has traditionally recognized: man and woman. Most of these new terms originate in medical, academic, or activist settings that are often middle-class and white, and many of them have entirely different meanings, or are not used at all, in communities of color, immigrant communities, or working-class and other communities. The terms below are some of the most widely used.

Transgender: A broad umbrella term referring to people whose gender identity and/or presentation do not fit traditional norms. Often abbreviated to "trans."

Transsexual: A person who lives as the opposite gender. The process of changing gender can involve any or all of the following: changing use of pronouns; changing names; changing clothing;

THE ABCS OF COMMUNITY

The language of the early gay liberation movement has expanded to include people who identify as bisexual, transgender, transsexual, questioning, queer, and intersex. As queer communities have become more inclusive, the acronyms we use to describe ourselves have shifted from L&G to LGBTQI. The changes are more than semantic; they are political. They acknowledge the variety of identities and experiences within queer and trans communities. (For definitions of the words listed above, see "Gender Identity," on this page, and "Sexual Orientation," p. 146. For a discussion of intersex issues, see p. 232.)

taking hormones; and undergoing sex reassignment surgery.

Female to Male Transsexual (FTM): Someone who was born biologically female and identifies as male. FTMs are also sometimes referred to as transmen. Some of us have undergone sex reassignment surgery.

Male to Female Transsexual (MTF): Someone who was born biologically male and identifies as female. MTFs are also sometimes referred to as transwomen. Some of us have undergone sex reassignment surgery.

Genderqueer: Someone who blurs, rejects, or otherwise transgresses gender norms. Also used as a term for someone who rejects the two-gender system.

Gender identity labels used in different communities also include "tranny boys," "two-spirit," "femme queen," and on and on. While some people who fit the criteria of these definitions use these terms, others do not. Regardless of gender identity or sexual orientation, we have a right to use the term with which we feel most comfortable, or to use no label at all.

Gender-related labels are not used to describe only those of us who are trans. Within queer communities, "butch," "femme," and "androgynous" are a few of the terms we may use to describe our place on a spectrum of masculinity and femininity. Within straight communities, we may use terms like "girly-girl" and "tomboy" to label gender characteristics or expressions.

We all hope that others respect our identities. It can be painful and awkward when people assume that we identify a certain way based on appearances alone. If you're not sure how a person identifies or what pronoun to use, try asking politely. In addition to "he," "she," "her," and "him," some of us in the trans community use "ze" and "hir" to describe ourselves. It's not easy for transgender or transsexual people to educate others on a daily basis, so try to connect to transgender allies.

TRANSGENDER

Those of us who are transgender defy conventional gender definitions, though others may ridicule or attack us for doing so. We express our gender identities in a range of ways. Some of us who have been raised as women may present

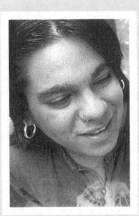

© R. A. McBride

"I CLAIM THE RIGHT TO CHOOSE MY ULTIMATE GENDER"

SUNEEL(A) MUBAYI

I identify as a male-to-female (or male-to-feminine androgynous) transgender or genderqueer person in a male body. I was born and raised as a straight male but started questioning both my gender and sexuality around the age of 16 for many complex reasons. . . . When I was little, kids in school would make fun of me by calling me "Suneela" to characterize a perceived weak and effeminate nature. I decided to reclaim this, but in a way that would make people think and not assume my gender when they look at my name (Suneel is a boy's name in Hindi). It gives me an androgynous quality, which I like.

Often I'm plagued by self-doubt—am I doing this just to attract attention? I answered it myself when I expressed these doubts to my friend Erica (thank god for her) and she asked me the most fundamental question of all: What does being a woman mean to you? To me, being a woman means having an identity that is feminine, but without any preconceived notions, ideas, or mind-sets about what a woman is or what a woman should be—in any sense, be it in terms of looks, actions, habits, social roles, or anything else. Everybody feels like there is some kind of "ideal" man and "ideal" woman. Well, I reject that. I am a woman with no conditions and no strings attached. And no presumptions, either. You may find me rather androgynous, deviant, and gender-bending. I like to dress up, be pierced, and be "effeminate" or "girly."

Yes, I am all those things, or rather, I possess all those qualities. But I claim the right to choose my ultimate gender beyond my traits, looks, qualities, and features, even if it is different from the sexual organs I possess. And whether that's feminine or hermaphrodite or my desired blend of masculine and feminine is my choice. You can love it, be okay with it, be uncomfortable with it, be revolted by it, or leave it. But it's my choice. Being a woman means being a woman.

ourselves in ways that men customarily do. We may buy our clothes in the men's department. We may cut our hair very short. We may let our facial and other body hair grow, bind our breasts, or take male hormones. Some of us were born and raised as men but now identify as women. We might take estrogen, get breast implants, or wear wigs. Some of us live our public lives as women and our private lives as men, or vice versa.

TRANSSEXUAL

Many transsexuals feel that the sex assigned to us at birth does not accurately reflect who we are.

There is no doubt that from very early on I knew something was wrong. I was a girl, yet my parents named me John Joseph and insisted that I was a boy.

According to medical science, transsexuals have a "gender identity disorder," with the word "disorder" implying that something is wrong with us. Some transsexuals prefer the term "gender dysphoria" because we feel we were born in a body that doesn't match who we are inside. Others feel that both of these terms are stigmatizing. Many transsexuals take hormones; undergo sex reassignment (plastic reconstructive) surgery, breast reduction, or mastectomy; and/or go through intensive retraining on how to walk and talk and present ourselves as the gender that we feel inside. Medical science has developed ways of creating a vagina out of male genitals (called *vaginoplasty*) and creating a penis and scrotum out of female genitals and skin grafts (called *phalloplasty*). Surgery and hormones may help some transsexual women and men achieve a better fit between our bodies and our identities, but these medical interventions also carry significant health risks and may impair sexual functioning.

From the moment I realized I was transsexual, EVERYTHING changed. Although I'm now legally and "aesthetically" male, I was raised and socialized female, and no amount of hormones or surgery can ever erase that. Nor should it. I have no interest in denying my past, for the years I lived as a woman make me a better man today. . . . I am a strong, proud, transsexual man; I love my life and my body (and am now more inclined to take good care of it); I have a wonderful wife and family; and I am working hard to make the world a better place for those who share my experience.

Some transsexuals do not undergo surgery. Some of us cannot afford it or are unable to have it due to preexisting medical conditions such as HIV or hepatitis. Some avoid medical providers because of transphobia in the health care system or concerns about complications from surgery. Others aren't interested in surgically altering our bodies but may take hormones and live in a gender identity different from our assigned sex. Some of us believe that surgery is an individual, medicalized "solution" when what really needs to change are social attitudes about gender.

I always loathed being considered male, but it took years to get up the courage to identify myself as a woman. I have always felt this way, though, even as I have continually butted up against

society's dictates about what it means to be a woman. I don't think having this mixed body, including breasts, hips, and a penis, disqualifies me.

SEXUAL ORIENTATION: WHAT WE CALL OURSELVES

Many of us confuse gender identity and sexual orientation. The distinction between the two is simple: Our gender identity is about who *we* are; our sexual orientation is about whom we find attractive. Of course, how we identify our gender influences how we name our sexuality, and whom we are attracted to may change throughout our lives. Following are a few common terms used to describe various sexual orientations. The terms "women" and "men" are used below for simplicity; however, these are meant to include anyone who identifies with them, including MTFs and FTMs.

Straight/Heterosexual: Refers to women who are sexually attracted to men and men who are sexually attracted to women.

Gay/Homosexual: Describes women who are sexually attracted to women and men who are sexually attracted to men. Often used to refer to men exclusively.

Lesbian: Refers to a woman who is sexually attracted to women.

Bisexual: Describes people who are sexually attracted to men and women.

Queer: Still a powerful derogatory term for gays in some communities, this word is now used positively by many lesbian, gay, bisexual, and transgender people to refer to ourselves. It is sometimes used to describe an open, fluid sexual orientation.

Asexual: Describes someone who is not experiencing or is not acting on sexual attraction at a given time.

Pansexual: Describes someone who is attracted to people across the range of genders. Often used by those who identify as transgender or genderqueer or who are attracted to people who are transgender or genderqueer.

Some of us have reclaimed historically negative terms, such as "queer," "fag," and "dyke," and use them affirmatively to describe ourselves. This is a political act that attempts to take the power out of these slurs. Some of us choose not to label our sexuality at all. It's important not to assume that we know another person's sexual orientation or identity.

CONFUSING SEXUAL ORIENTATION AND GENDER IDENTITY

All lesbians look like men, right? Since we sometimes confuse gender identity and sexual orientation, we may end up forming stereotypes. For example, when we picture a lesbian, we may picture a woman with short hair, broad shoulders, and a motorcycle jacket. We are assuming that because a woman is a lesbian, she must be masculine. Likewise, we might assume that because a woman is masculine, she must be a lesbian. But some straight women appear masculine, and some lesbians appear feminine. Being lesbian or bisexual doesn't mean our gender looks or feels a certain way.

The fact that I am femme (that is, traditionally feminine in appearance, with mannerisms perceived as feminine) throws people off; I'm often told I don't "look gay."

In the same vein, identifying as transgender does not automatically make a person lesbian or gay. Some transgender people identify as straight, and others identify as lesbian, bisexual, pansexual, or queer.

BISEXUALITY

Bisexuality has historically been misunderstood and maligned. Labeled as confused, sex addicts, or not queer enough, people who identify as bisexual have often been stigmatized in both gay and straight communities.

I have always known I am a bisexual woman. For as long as I can remember, that is how I identified myself. I've had fondness for both men and women. And . . . those who acknowledged homosexuality as legit . . . often tell me that bisexuality is just "greedy," wanting sex wherever it can be found.

In the last few decades, bisexual activists have helped increase acceptance for our orientation. Bisexuality can take many forms, including being single, being married, being in a monogamous relationship, or having several lovers. Some of us choose to have sexual relationships with men at one point in our lives and with women at another point. We may become lovers with men only or with women only, without acting on our other attractions. For some, being bisexual means dating both men and women at the same time. Sometimes thinking of ourselves as bisexual is a stopping place in a transition from one identity to another. Yet for many of us, bisexuality is not transitional at all. We are comfortable with our desires and accept that we don't have to be *either* straight or gay.

I'm a woman who has primarily dated men but has had two short-term relationships with women. I'm in a committed relationship with a man. He is a wonderful, articulate, sensitive feminist whom I hope to marry; and yes, he knows of my past experiences and is open to me having continued relationships with women. . . . My desire for women isn't based on the inadequacies of my current lover but rather a need for some other, some different, some similar thing—all of which I find in women.

The concept of bisexuality, and sexual orientation in general, can become more complicated if we are transgender or if we are dating someone who is transgender. For example, some women identify as lesbian and date transmen, while other women identify as lesbian and date transwomen. Questions arise: How should we identify? Are we lesbian? Straight? Bisexual? Some of us use the word "pansexual" to describe being attracted to people across genders. This term gives more room to those who are attracted to or identify as transgender or genderqueer and feel limited by defining attraction to men and/or women.

When I first became involved with my partner, I had just begun identifying as a lesbian. It was important to me that I only be with females from that point on. I really didn't know a lot about transgender issues at the time but shortly after getting involved, my partner told me that she had in fact always felt like a "he" and wanted to begin taking testosterone. We have been together for five months, and he has just begun to actively transition.

For a detailed discussion of lesbian identity and relationships, see Chapter 11, "Relationships with Women"; for a similar discussion of straight relationships, see Chapter 10, "Relationships with Men."

COMING OUT TO OURSELVES

Coming out is the process of accepting and affirming our sexual orientation or gender identity and deciding how open we will be about it. Before we come out to others, we usually come out to ourselves. We admit to ourselves that we are attracted to people of the same sex, or that we don't identify with gender traits considered appropriate for our sex. Because we grow up in a culture that assumes everyone is heterosexual and that everyone's gender matches their sex, becoming aware of our identity and accepting it is often a gradual process. Coming out to ourselves can happen at any age or stage in our life.

Coming out of the closet as a lesbian was the hardest thing I ever did. I tried everything to "avoid" being gay. . . . I tried to stay away from women I was attracted to, but finally, after many years, I began to feel much more comfortable with the idea.

Some of us come out to ourselves more than once in our lives. For instance, we may come out as lesbian or bisexual, then later as transgender or transsexual. The process of questioning our sexual orientation or gender identity may be extremely challenging, but accepting ourselves for who we are can also be an affirming experience.

After my last suicide attempt, I found my soul. . . . At the age of 45 I declared myself female and, in a sane and sober state, worked on matching my body, soul, and spirit into one complete female. It took me five years. Today my body is mine. . . . My birth certificate reads "female."

COMING OUT TO FAMILY, FRIENDS, AND THE WORLD

Letting other people know that we identify as lesbian, bisexual, queer, or trans can be one of the most challenging and life-changing decisions we face. Each of us must decide for ourselves to what extent we want our family, friends, and acquaintances to know about our sexuality and gender identity. Some of us, depending on our job, family, age, geographical location, or culture of origin, can come out in relative ease. Increasingly, our families and friends may embrace us, and our coworkers may accept us.

I'd only realized that there were female-to-males out there about two months before (all my life, I figured that a lot of girls wanted to be boys, and that male-to-females had so much attention, because who would want to give up being male?). But that day my mother was cooking sauce. We're one of those Italian families, I guess, and I offer to stir . . . hypnotically, stirring, I start talking, and the next thing I know, I've told her. She wasn't

thrilled, and almost four years later, she's still not, but she's my strongest ally in my family. She's just a great mom.

For many lesbian, bisexual, and transgender people, coming out is a long and difficult process. We may have to make the decision to come out over and over as we encounter new people and situations. Some transsexuals have no choice but to come out, due to physical changes we are going through.

Though coming out may mean that we risk losing friends or family, our jobs or our homes, it can also be a liberating experience to be open with others about our identity.

It took me until I was 27 to decide that I am a lesbian and very proud of it. The coming-out process meant that I gained friends and lost friends. Family made choices to continue their relationships with me or not. Either way, I grew as a woman who loved women. I'm now 40 years young and am enjoying being with the woman of my dreams. I cannot fathom what took me so long. . . . Then again, you can't change what was, only what is and what will be.

The decision whether or not to come out, and what coming out is like for us, is influenced by our circumstances. The experience varies greatly based on class, gender, race, religion, ability, and other aspects of our lives.

I was the only openly queer African-American person at my college. When I came out sophomore year, my black friends were supportive yet oftentimes more reserved around me. Many were very religious, and very socially conservative. Others had never met a queer person before. There was always something unspoken between us—was I still as black as they were? Was my white girlfriend a sign that I had betrayed my race, black men, my friends? Who were these new white queer people that I was now spending time with? Many of my black friends became my closest allies as they learned and grew with me. Those who didn't I lost touch with quickly. But my race will never be separated from my sexual orientation, and vice versa.

Many people of color are faced with difficult choices around sexuality, gender, and coming out. We risk alienation from our communities by coming out. We also experience racial discrimination within queer communities, which creates division and conflict.

Some white lesbians are unaware of the pervasiveness of racism or unwilling to confront our own racism. When white lesbians assume that our experience parallels that of people of color in the U.S., we ignore both our own privilege as white-skinned women in a racist society and the complex layers of discrimination that affect the daily lives of lesbians of color.

Women of color may find ways to live openly in both worlds, and we may learn to come out in our communities in ways that are culturally appropriate. Some of us may be able to seek out queer communities of color.

Some people think that queer and trans are Western concepts and that femme equals looking like Barbie, but that's not how I see it all. As a South Asian queer femme woman, my models for my gender are my grandmother and great-aunties who organized for independence from Britain and [for] labour and women's rights—in short skirts and bobbed hair—in Sri Lanka and Malaysia in the twenties. . . . When I hold my hot-pink "Desi divas against war and racism" sign at the antiwar rally, I am continuing that tradition.

Our jobs and our workplaces may affect how out we can be. Some of us work in faith-based organizations, where being queer may be unacceptable. We might work in jobs that are not very secure, and coming out could jeopardize our employment. In most places in the United States, it is legal to fire employees because they are trans, lesbian, or bisexual, though some states and municipalities have enacted civil rights protections based on sexual orientation.

Those of us in traditionally religious families or conservative communities might face additional challenges around coming out.

Being brought up in an Irish Catholic family meant getting married to a man, having babies, and living life as one was "supposed" to. However, since the second grade, I knew something was very "different" about me.

Lesbian, bisexual, and transgender people with disabilities face additional trials around coming out and being queer. We may face homophobia or transphobia within the disabled community, and we may have to struggle to find places and events in able-bodied communities that are wheelchair-accessible, smoke- and scent-free, or sign-language-interpreted.

Fat lesbians face size discrimination within both the queer and the straight worlds. People may assume that we're queer because we can't find a man, or that we're asexual. Some queer spaces are more accepting of fat women.

I'm a queer fat femme of Italian-American and middle-class background. How I experience my sense of self in regard to gender and sexual orientation shifts depending on the context. In straight spaces I'm likely seen as a straight, fat girl. Being fat, my sexuality is not celebrated or recognized in mainstream society, because fat people are not supposed to be sexual . . . in queer contexts, however (when other queers perceive my femmeness as queer), I feel quite different. My fat femmeness is celebrated as hot and sexy. I feel motivated to wear clothes that show off my curves, large ass, hips and breasts.

Some of us, because of our race, gender, class, and ability, receive unjust benefits.

I experience privilege within the queer community: I am a dyke and I am masculinely gendered; I am white, I am upper-middle-class, and graduated from an elite college. My white privilege means that I see myself reflected in many representations of queer people, and I do not experience racism within queer communities in the ways that queer people of color experience. My class and education privilege mean that I have access to a specific language for talking about my own identity.

HOMOPHOBIA, HETEROSEXISM, AND TRANSPHOBIA

In many of our families, schools, and workplaces, people either don't mention lesbians, gay men, bisexuals, or transgender and intersex people at all, or they joke cruelly about these groups. Our culture teaches us to fear and hate homosexuality and gender transgression in others and in ourselves. This hatred hurts all of us, no matter our sexual orientation or gender identity. It turns us against friends and family members, depriving us of important relationships. It causes us to deny attractions or identities that may be natural to us, and it may prevent us from choosing the partners or claiming the identities that are right for us. It prevents us from publicly acknowledging our friendships with queer or transgender people. It divides us from one another.

I am now a freshman in college and still haven't come out to my parents. A couple of years ago, my father asked me if I was a lesbian. With much hesitation, I answered, "No," because I was scared. . . . He said, "Good, because I don't want a fucking faggot for a kid." This statement tore me apart and has delayed my decision to come out to my

LGBTQI YOUTH

Many teenagers of all orientations and identities question our sexuality and gender. Some of us first realize that we are queer or trans when we are in junior high or high school. We debate whether or not to tell our friends. The process can be frightening, exciting, or both. It can be difficult to find friends who will listen to us without judging us or freaking out. We risk our families not accepting us. We may be told that we're "going through a phase" or aren't old enough to make any decisions about our identity. Queer and trans youth are at high risk for depression, suicide, and homelessness.

But there are queer and trans teens across the country—we just need to find each other! Look for local queer or trans groups, or get online. Many cities have a center that offers free or sliding-scale counseling, support groups, and social services. Some larger cities have centers specifically for queer or trans youth. It's totally normal to feel confused, depressed, or angry about being different, and it's important to find people who will understand and relate to us. (For more information on teens coming out, see Chapter 11, "Relationships with Women," and "Resources.")

parents. Most everyone who knows me (including my siblings) knows my orientation. I am currently waiting to tell my parents, for fear that they will kick me out or stop paying for my college.

Homophobia—the fear and hatred of homosexuality or gay, lesbian, or bisexual people—affects the lives of queer people in many ways. It put us at risk of discrimination, harassment, rejection, or violence in our everyday interactions with family, friends, and strangers, and it can affect our ability to accept who we are. Internalized homophobia occurs when we take on, often unconsciously, our society's prejudice and stereotypes regarding gay, lesbian, or bisexual people. Internalized homophobia may lead to self-hatred, denial of our identities, or attempts to live a heterosexual life.

The internalized homophobia—the nagging fears of incompetence, being too different, being unlovable—are still hanging around in my head. But getting up each day . . . each time I do something positive, the homophobia inside me has less power. And each time we do something positive for each other, the homophobia in society has less power.

Heterosexism—the assumption that heterosexuality is the only normal orientation—denies us legal, religious, and social privileges. We are prevented from getting married (for more information on changing civil marriage laws, see Chapter 11, "Relationships with Women"), filing joint tax returns, and being covered under a partner's health insurance (except in companies and cities that allow coverage for domestic partners). We face job and housing discrimination and stereotypical, homogenous, or nonexistent representation in the media. Lifesaving safer-sex material, when presented in schools, sometimes omits homosexual relationships.

Heterosexism can also occur on an interpersonal level. Our "queer-friendly" friends and family may ostensibly support our choice of partners and our queer identities but still make heterosexist assumptions or unwittingly offer more emotional or financial support to straight couples in the family than to us and our partners.

Much of what we refer to as "gay bashing" or "homophobia" is actually based on gender. We

FINDING OUR COMMUNITIES

For many of us, finding communities of people who are similar to us can be life-affirming. We not only find friends, we find family. In most major U.S. metropolitan areas, there are an increasing number of venues or groups where we can find other queer or trans people who share our interests and backgrounds. There are groups for older women, women with disabilities, women of color, youth, mothers, and fat dykes, to name just a few. There are groups organized around politics, around gender identity, around performance, around religion. The list is endless. Rural women who have fewer local options but have access to the Internet may want to check out numerous online resources (see "Resources").

are targeted because our gender expression does not fit within society's expectations for conventional masculine and feminine behavior. The system of two rigid genders gives rise to the prejudices and practices that endanger the lives of lesbian, bisexual, gay, transgender, and intersex people.

Transphobia is the fear and hatred of transgender or transexual people. It involves much more than a slanderous term being uttered on a street corner late at night. Because the two-gender system is so prevalent in society, people who don't fit this norm find it difficult to attend school, hold jobs, or even go to public restrooms without fear of rejection, harassment, violence, or even arrest.

As a female-bodied genderqueer, I choose to use the women's restroom, but often find myself dealing with unpleasant comments or looks and, on a few occasions, verbal or physical threats/assaults.

As a result, I have avoided using public restrooms, as much as possible, for 17 years and have now developed urinary tract problems.

Gender-based discrimination is a serious human rights problem that plagues United States society today. Violence, homelessness, police brutality, chronic underemployment, and poverty disproportionately affect transgender people. It is exceedingly difficult for trans people to access many services such as rape crisis centers, emergency medical care, homeless shelters, group homes, and domestic violence shelters because these spaces are sex-segregated.[2] Trans people often avoid getting needed medical care because of the discrimination and harassment we face in the health care system. Trans people of color and low-income trans people also are affected by racism and class discrimination.

Transgender and transsexual people also sometimes face discrimination within the queer community. Transwomen are sometimes denied entrance to all-women's spaces because we are not perceived to be "real" women, and transwomen who have intimate relationships with women are sometimes not welcomed into lesbian spaces.

Everybody talks about surgery, about feminization . . . about electrolysis. No one talks about the mental difficulties faced before—and especially after—the transition. Like, for instance, being a (trans) dyke. Like being referred to as "he" in lesbian groups. Like being banned from places, like Mountain Moving Coffeehouse in Chicago and the Michigan Womyn's Music Festival.

Those of us who are heterosexual can use our privileged status to challenge heterosexist laws and practices. Those of us who do not identify as transgender can fight for education on trans issues, safe and inclusive facilities and programs for trans people, and a greater understanding of gender outside of a binary system. For those of us who are queer or trans, it's important to fight discrimination, work for equal rights, take care of ourselves, stay healthy and safe, and find communities that accept and support us.

NOTES

1. "Transgender Introduction," www.srlp.org/TLC%20new%20trans%20101.htm. The idea of a galaxy of gender was previously published by Gordene O. MacKenzie, "Fifty Billion Galaxies of Gender: Transgendering the Millennium," in Kate More and Stephen Whittle, eds., *Reclaiming Genders: Transsexual Grammars at the Fin de Siècle* (New York: Cassell, 1999).
2. See the Sylvia Rivera Law Project (www.srlp.org) for information and resources on discrimination.

CHAPTER 10 ▪ ▪ ▪ ▪ ▪ ▪ ▪ ▪ ▪ ▪ ▪ ▪ ▪ ▪ ▪ ▪

Those of us who look to men for love, friendship, support, sex, or some combination of the above face unique satisfactions, comforts, and joys. We also face unique challenges and questions to which there are no easy answers. How do we negotiate safer sex with our male partners? How do we protect ourselves from violence as we try to get to know potential lovers? How do we build long-term relationships that are satisfying and equitable? How do we continue to develop our individuality and personal power while fostering mutual interdependence? How do we balance romance with educational and/or career goals? How do we approach being single—its potential for loneliness as well as its promise of satisfaction—as we navigate multiple possibilities for companionship?

In a world where people are so divided by gender, the connections we make with men sometimes feel especially precious. This chapter focuses on how, as heterosexual and bisexual women, we relate to the men with whom we flirt, make love, and build lives—and on how we relate to ourselves in the process.

"THE PERSONAL IS POLITICAL" AND FEMINISM'S THIRD WAVE

"The personal is political," a phrase the women's movement made famous, expresses the belief that individual problems are symptoms of larger social problems. The second wave of feminism in the United States both coincided with and was greatly shaped by the so-called sexual revolution of the late 1960s and 1970s, in which it became more acceptable to be sexually active outside marriage. As many feminists pointed out, although this sexual revolution could often be a raw deal for women—adding yet another societal expectation for us to fulfill—it also ushered in positive changes for women's sexual health, including wider availability and choices of birth control, the legalization of abortion, and the gradual lifting of moral sanctions against premarital or nonmarital sex.

Today, in what is often called feminism's third wave, women and girls are again being encouraged to explore sexuality and express it in ways that generally weren't allowed previously, at least not with such gusto. But feminism's third wave also coincides with a powerful mainstream popular culture in which messages about sex are often superficial and rarely examine sex in the context of real relationships. What about intimacy and vulnerability? What about the demands of balancing family and/or career? How does any *one* woman navigate this new landscape—with all her unique characteristics of race, ethnicity, age, sexual orientation, socio-economic background, political stance, religious beliefs, etc.—without losing her integrity, her "self"? Or is the self, at least somewhat, meant to be lost when in love?

In keeping with the mantra that the personal is political, it's important to remember that individual men and women enter into relationships not just with our own background or "baggage" but also with the weight of generations of cultural and familial expectations. Although real people are much more complex than stereotypes, few of us are immune to their influence. Fortunately, many of us—men as well as women—are struggling to unlearn and rebel against these expectations. It is challenging work, but it can also be exciting, especially as we strive together with the men in our lives to create new ways of relating to and loving each other.

BEING SINGLE

Whether as a temporary interlude or as a life choice, being single can be a deeply rich and satisfying experience, despite negative messages from family and/or popular culture to the contrary. Depending on how we choose to define it for ourselves, being single may mean having one or many lovers, an occasional casual sexual encounter, a committed relationship without marriage, or no sexual or romantic relationships at all.

I like the independence of being single, which for me means that I date men occasionally but don't sleep with them . . . Not being responsible for half the maintenance of a relationship means that I can spend time with more friends, and a lot more time thinking for myself about my own ideas and questions. In relationships, I tend to let myself get wrapped up in my partner's issues, problems, and ideas, and don't think for myself as much.

I plan not to get involved in another exclusive long-term relationship. I am enjoying the lifestyle I am living now (I currently have about five men that I keep in contact with casually). I am always straight up with the men I date. In other words, I let them know right from the start that I have no intention of getting involved in a committed relationship. I do not want to mislead or hurt anyone. Most men are not used to that type of attitude from women, but most deal with it just fine. I do know that this will get old at some point, and there are definitely lonely times involved. So what will my ultimate solution be? Time will have to answer that.

And yet being single can also be difficult, especially if we feel we haven't *chosen* singlehood, but rather that it has chosen us, particularly through some trauma, illness, or loss.

I was raped about three years ago, right after college, and I'm still dealing with it. I have a good support network of friends and a therapist who is helping me through recovery. It was an acquaintance rape. It really hurt my ability to trust men. I know that for a while I won't be sexually involved with any man. . . . I need time to feel better about myself, work through some pretty heavy feelings that still haunt me, and get love from people I know won't hurt me. That includes male as well as female friends. Someday I'll date again. But for now, I'm happy being single and celibate. Except, of course, for those times when I get super-down and blame some of that loneliness on the rape. Generally, though, I'm discovering personal inner resources I never knew I had.

Some single women who want biological children but see no father in sight also speak about the pain of loneliness as we get older, despite the fact that more and more women are choosing to have children on our own. One thirty-four-year-old single woman relates:

A few years ago, after a painful breakup, I went through a spate of calculations: What would it cost, monetarily and in terms of life sacrifice, to raise a child on my own? To adopt? To try in vitro? I spoke to my parents about it. . . . I got a lot of emotional support. In the end, though, I decided the timing wasn't right. I need more financial and professional stability to give a child a good home. Just thinking it through, though, helped me feel less sad and more proactive. I was able to move through the question. I know now there may be more options ahead than I had originally imagined. Being single isn't so scary anymore.

Those of us who are single mothers—whether by choice or by circumstance—face a unique set of challenges and rewards. A forty-seven-year-old psychotherapist and divorced mother of two boys says that when it comes to raising children alone, "what is most important is a strong support system." She continues:

I read recently about single mothers who share a house together with their kids; that seems like an idea with great potential. I guess I still believe that when it comes to raising children, "it takes a village."

Although many communities admire independent single women, most of us are told from childhood that our lives will be incomplete until we find a man. The hardest thing about being single, women sometimes say, is not loneliness but the negative stereotypes we must confront from others and, to the extent we have internalized such stereotypes, in ourselves.

I'm 30, and I'm not married. I get hints from people that they think I'm irresponsible, or that I must be a slut. When my parents and people at work ask me again and again if I've "met someone," I turn it into a joke, but inside I think,

"I'm as happy as I can be right now, and you can't understand that."

Many of us were taught from a very young age—either explicitly or implicitly, through familial or cultural forces—to find a man with potentially supportive qualities and attach ourselves to him. In this way, we could become complete. Many girls begin to face this pressure in middle school, if not before, and notice it increasing through high school.

When I was growing up, especially in high school and college, there was this overwhelming cultural and social pressure to pair off and become some guy's "girl." In college, all my best friends eventually wound up with boyfriends, and they spent all their time trying to please him and find out all about him instead of find out about themselves. I often felt the push of everyone around me to find someone to "belong" with, but I wanted simply to become my own person, without the weight of someone else. I'm 27 and still a single woman, with an ambitious career, and very happy that I didn't pair off when everyone else did. There's nothing wrong with getting married and having kids, but it shouldn't be a fallback when you're lonely or don't know what else to do. I wouldn't have done half the things I've accomplished, or seen what I've witnessed, or written or even thought about my own ideas if I hadn't chosen to be single. And there are lots of single women like me out there, single and loving it just fine.

Many single women also stress the importance of being strong enough to know how and when, if at all, to move on—either to deeper intimacy or to a new relationship.

When I broke up with my lover, I luckily had a circle of warm, affectionate friends who would give me a hug or a pat on the back. Yet, I feel the lack of that very intimate whole-body contact. I

Increasingly, women are meeting men through dating services and the Internet. (For more information, see "Online and Speed Dating" [W26] on the companion website, www.ourbodiesourselves.org.)

didn't want to rush precipitously into a new relationship just because I felt so hungry to be touched. One answer was to get a massage every other week for several months.

When we are happy and strong on our own, we are better able to choose freely and carefully the men we do become close to. Creating a safe and equal relationship with a man can then become a challenge we seek and enjoy out of mutual attraction, admiration, and love.

PERSONAL POWER AND RELATIONSHIPS

To me, personal power vis-à-vis relationships with men means being in touch with what I want and need and communicating those needs to my partner in a direct way. In practice, this can be a very challenging process—to get in touch with what one wants is in itself a lifelong exercise. Communicating that in real time to one's partner is no easy feat. I think women are so focused on what others need and want that we easily lose touch with our Id [our instinctual needs and desires]! Men, on the other hand, have overdeveloped Ids (if you ask me) and less developed awareness of serving others.

Personal power means different things to different people: self-esteem, sense of identity (group and/or individual), positive body image, self-confidence, enjoyment in what one does, a sense of contributing to the community, financial stability/earning power, self-reliance, ability to communicate . . . the list goes on. For many of us, finding personal power means finding inner strength—a sense of ourselves and who we are, what we need, and what we want.

For me, body image is a factor in how I feel about myself; it is a part of self-respect. Physical activity (in my case, running regularly) helps me to feel physically and mentally strong, which affects my willingness and ability to be intimate. . . . I believe that having a strong sense of oneself makes it much easier to be in a relationship with someone else. This means feeling committed and positive about myself as a communicator, feeling strong in how I move through life (physically and emotionally), feeling supported by people around me, and feeling invested in things that I do outside the relationship (work, friends, etc.).

Social and cultural factors can make a big difference in how one understands oneself in the context of relationships. Every woman faces a unique set of choices and challenges that both limit and enable her life.

A thirty-five-year-old woman who grew up in Japan and who now lives in the U.S. says:

I often find myself fighting off this image of Asian women who are passive, submissive, reserved . . . and as a result, I behave overly opposite just to show I am not a stereotypical Asian woman. I am very cautious of men who are too familiar with Asian culture, especially those who have been spoiled because they are white (or American). . . . For me, self-esteem is always an issue. Being a minority . . . and fighting off a stereotype (which I may only have in my head) makes it hard to be myself. Although I love the way my boyfriend respects my decisions, I often find myself expecting him to behave more paternally or protectively.

Folded within the personal, then, are external social, cultural, economic, and historical factors

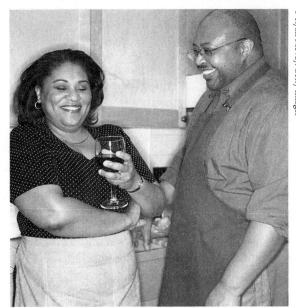

that contribute to the formation of that person. Feminists have long pointed out that earning power and actions in the public sphere are intimately connected to personal power and self-esteem—and therefore to intimacy—in the private sphere.

Women who face discrimination due to physical disability, for example, grapple with a host of public and private issues that women without those challenges do not. A woman in her forties who was born with severe muscular dystrophy because of problems her rural Native American mother faced during delivery now cycles to work every day on a bicycle made especially for her. Though she lived at home longer than many other women do, once she started to live independently and to hold a rewarding job (as director of an independent living program tailored for Native Americans), she was able to pursue more adult relationships with men:

I've always known a lot of people through family and tribal connections, and I've always been a pretty outgoing person. Hey, I'm good at making people laugh. Until I knew I could make it on my own, though, I often felt frustrated and suffocated. I lived with my parents. I didn't work. I blamed the world. Sometimes I blamed myself. As a member of the Omaha nation, I'd always been a strong person connected to a strongly spiritual worldview: respect for life, the interconnectedness of all living beings, views like that. They helped me a lot. Also, once I started living alone and gaining more confidence to do so . . . once I started meeting so many more people through work and travel, and started gaining their respect—I started to respect myself more too. I started developing deeper, more intimate connections with people— including men—outside my family and my tribe. Something really changed. . . . I started to feel like I had something very special to offer. Of course I always had; I just didn't always know it.

Racism and classism can likewise affect women's power in the public and private spheres. At the other extreme, pressures on women to "have it all" can debilitate a sense of personal power by creating internal confusion, if not utter exhaustion. A young lawyer says:

I think that the myth of the "superwoman" is damaging to women. I have a lot of professional female friends, and most of us still want marriage and children. We expect to continue our careers and have equal household/child care responsibilities with our partners. I honestly don't know how this can happen, though. Our workplaces are still modeled with the idea that the workers (men) have spouses (women) at home to take care of all the details of life and leave the workers to concentrate on their job. . . . This lifestyle is not good for men, women, or families. Instead of creating the ideal that women can "have it all," it would be more sensible to improve the workplace so both men and women can enjoy a better quality of life with their families and friends.

The demands of economics bear a very real weight on us. As our bodies can be exhausted by work or poverty or illness, so, too, can they be buoyed, through work or activities outside of work, to access more power, health, and strength. Some of us who have weighed our physical power against that of men and have found ourselves lacking have tried to cultivate compatible levels of physical power and/or assertiveness.

One of the things I plunged myself into at age 54 was to take tae kwon do [a Korean martial art]. I had always been fascinated by martial arts but never had enough nerve to try it. I was stirring up long years of status quo; one more unorthodoxy didn't matter, I reasoned. All through our marriage, I was never able to stand up to my husband, and I felt that taking a martial art might perhaps help me to become more assertive. My husband was totally put off by such a "masculine" activity. But I have persisted.

Some of us find that cultivating centering practices—such as prayer, meditation, walking, writing, playing or listening to music—likewise provides us with a source of inner strength we can tap into when trying to sustain relationships.

On the other hand, some women who have a well-developed sense of personal power— whether or not it's accompanied by financial success or physical strength—find that men are threatened by our confidence and successes.

I have had many more men be intimidated by my career, financial stability, and poise, than not. I work on my own car, fix my own lamps, travel alone. I have been told I don't let men feel needed enough. I feel this has severely limited my dating options. I choose being single over compromising.

INTIMACY: UNDERSTANDING SOME OF THE BARRIERS

My idea of the perfect man would be a woman trapped in a hot man's body. That way I could get the sensitivity and attentiveness I am after, along with tight buns and broad shoulders.

When we say "intimacy," what do we mean? Why do we all crave it so, and what *is* it, exactly, that we crave? Physical contact? A best friend with whom we share everything? Total, unconditional acceptance? Clear conditions within which we can explore? All of the above? Can any *one* person give it all? Does it last? How do we find it? How, if at all, can we help it along?

For me, intimacy is a precious state of relationship in which we feel safe enough to expose our whole selves and know that we will still be loved. The great challenge with intimacy is that, in order to achieve it, we must risk the possibility of rejection. Intimacy affords us the safety to be more loving toward ourselves and toward our partners. . . . The barriers I have experienced around intimacy with men include my own fears about being inadequate, a partner's lack of communicativeness (and my feeling like I can't "get inside his head"), and partners' breaches of trust that have made me feel unsafe or unloved.

Intimacy requires honesty. That means having the courage to share difficult feelings, needs, or problems, even if we are afraid they will scare our partner away. Holding back on honesty for fear that we will hurt the other almost always backfires: We cheat ourselves out of feeling connected with our partner, and we likewise cheat our partner out of the opportunity to truly know us, and to respond out of love.

Just as fear breeds more fear, insecurity breeds more insecurity. Feeling safe, then, can also come from a sense that our partners feel secure about who they are—secure enough not to be threatened by our own strengths or needs, nor by their, our, or others' sexuality.

For me, one of the main barriers to intimacy with straight men is their frequent homophobia. A straight boy with a nasty attitude towards two guys in an intimate relationship together has always seemed to translate into a straight boy with problems with women as equals, as well. Since intimacy is about trust, and since I think you need a strong sense of self to be able to trust someone else, guys who feel threatened in their own sexuality over gay coupling are, in my book, incapable of intimacy with anybody, and are to be avoided by straight women.

Cultural differences, furthermore, can present challenges to intimacy. A twenty-two-year-old Argentinean immigrant to the U.S. says that the most difficult challenge to pursuing intimate relationships with men has been integrating American guys into her family:

It was very hard for them to understand the close relationship I had with my mother. Telling her some of my secrets and sharing things with her were not things that these guys understood or even liked much. It was hard for me to accept a boy without my parents' consent or opinion. Another issue was sex. I was not willing to have sex with someone I didn't love. . . . Most boys wanted to make out or have sex on our second date—many times the first date. Lots got scared that I was a virgin at age 19. It took someone with an open mind and interest in understanding my relationship with my family to overcome the fear of my parents' powerful influence on me and to respect my virginity. . . . Nevertheless, having been raised in a more conservative culture, I had to play around with the rules and norms from this coun-

try in order to have a healthy relationship with my partner.

Our conceptions of intimacy—and what we want from an intimate partner—may also change over the years as we grow into both ourselves and our relationships. After fourteen years of marriage to a Chinese-American man, a thirty-six-year-old Catholic, half-Mexican graduate student and mother of two small boys now defines intimacy as "a meeting of the minds":

Or is that because that's about all that meets these days with the kids in our bed, on our couch, at the table, in the car? Intimacy has become something snatched from the margins of our kid-centered life. Before, it used to consist of snuggling on the couch. The couch used to be our touchstone. Now it is the place we collapse upon in exhaustion at the end of the night, maybe watch a movie. Can I tell you, though, what at this stage of our relationship I crave most? Taking a long walk on a beautiful beach . . . alone. I crave intimacy with MYSELF! . . . I think also that intimacy is something created in a space of total trust. I know I can be myself—the good, bad, and the ugly—and, within limits of sanity, [my husband] will still love me. I spend so much time in my life trying to prove myself to other people: my dissertation committee, the random folks at workshops, job

STAYING SAFE

Single women confront particular risks as we start new relationships with men. Below are some ideas to help you stay safe.

- If you are dating, take a man's number rather than giving him yours. Meet in a public, well-populated place. Tell a friend where you will be and that you will call her the next morning to let her know you got in all right. Avoid excessive alcohol or drugs on a first date.

- If you pick up a stranger, play close attention to your surroundings and keep an eye on your drink; sexual predators have been known to slip in drugs that cause short-term memory loss. Know that you are taking big risks if you bring home a person you've only just met.

- Be prepared to discuss and practice safer sex with a male partner. Learn about precautions against STIs, including HIV (see Chapter 14, "Safer Sex"), and about birth control (see Chapter 18, "Birth Control"). If you think you might have intercourse, have condoms ready. Don't assume that if your partner goes inside you unsheathed, it means he cares enough about you to have been tested already. Many an HIV/STI-free woman has mistakenly so assumed and has been heartbroken—if not infected—upon finding out otherwise.

- Learn beforehand about all the fun and satisfying sex you can have while protecting your health (see Chapter 12, "Sexuality"). That way the conversation doesn't have to be just about things you *can't* do.

- Know your own rules. Every woman who is sexually active makes choices about which risks she is willing to take and which she isn't. Know *your* limits and requirements for protection before you get into a sexual situation, when your decision-making abilities may not be at their best.

interviews, my parents *still! Even people on the streets: Am I behaving in public like a "good" mother, an attractive woman, a decent human being? [My husband] is probably the one person in my life that I am not "performing" for.*

A woman in her thirties who describes herself as bisexual says of her first relationship:

My first lover and I were both total beginners, but best friends, too, so we shared an honesty and an intimacy—a willingness to learn, experiment, joke, and basically not take ourselves too seriously. So even though we've grown up and are very different people now, we still share some almost tangible something.

It's more of a struggle as I get older to have that kind of carefree openness in a love affair. People seem to get both tougher and more fragile with age, but the lovers I've found who could do that— joke and be direct—are the ones I still know and rely on and, frankly, the ones I still love.

FEARING INTIMACY

Crossing over into spaces of new physical and/or emotional intimacy comes with risks. We may fear that we will not be met halfway, or that if we try to go the distance, we will lose ourselves in the crossing—physically, emotionally, or psychologically. Or we may fear that we will be rejected because we are not "enough."

And yet fear is a natural instinct, a healthy reaction to dangerous or potentially dangerous conditions. The first trick to understanding fear is to notice it. Only then can we discern where and when it is legitimate, and only then can we try to work through it. A writer in her fifties says:

I believe fear of intimacy is a rationalization— an adaptive defense that keeps you from getting entangled with the wrong person. With luck, it dissolves when you meet the right person. At that

point, you stop worrying about your sagging breasts and ruffled thighs, your need to be in control, and your fear that he will start farting in bed if you get too familiar. The energy that's freed up in this process can now be diverted to asking for what you need, fantasizing about what you want, and making concrete plans to realize your dreams.

Many of us who have experienced some sort of sexual and/or emotional trauma in our lives may feel fear even in safe situations. Difficult, confusing feelings can arise around sexual intimacy as a result of earlier trauma, sometimes for a lifetime (see Chapter 8, "Violence and Abuse"). Discussing such trauma with an intimate partner can be difficult; it can also be part of the healing process. A partner's response can be a clue to his sensitivity, and to his ability to deal with significant issues, communicate, and relate to strong feelings. Heightened sensitivity on both sides to past sexual trauma can create new barriers as well as, with good communication, more intimacy.

It has been said that loving takes two whole people. No one, of course, is perfectly whole. Still, we can reach toward wholeness as we relate to loved ones. Indeed, wholeness can be sought even after something has been taken away, injured, broken, or left undone. Past hurts, while they can create fear and barriers to intimacy, can also teach courage and allow us to approach relationships with greater wisdom and compassion. Whether pursuing new relationships or strengthening old ones, we can integrate our past experiences with the "now" of each moment as we negotiate tensions between interdependency and self-sufficiency, intimacy and the need to remain separate.

One thing that's clear about my second marriage is that because I'm older and because of who Rob is, I am much closer to him than I was to my first husband. I am able to care for him much more deeply. And there are moments when he's away, even overnight, that are very painful for me. It's not "Oh my God, I can't take care of myself," because I have and I can—but it's deeply, passionately missing somebody. And it's ironic, because I had so strongly identified with the women's movement's "superwoman agenda" of being self-sufficient. Yet it's come home to me just how painful it would be if something were to happen to Rob, how empty life would be. Not because my life isn't full in addition to him, but because I risked having a certain depth of commitment and feeling.

COMMITMENT, MONOGAMY, AND MARRIAGE

Many of us forging monogamous, long-term commitments with male partners decide to get married. We do so for a wide variety of reasons: because we want our love and connection with our partner to be celebrated and supported; because we believe marriage offers spiritual and material stability; because we want health benefits, property rights, residency privileges; because we want children and we want them to grow up in a legally recognized family.

I married because I wanted a sense of permanence; I wanted a legal binding relationship like marriage can usually afford.

I feared that marriage would disable my ability to fulfill my passion—a career. I married at age 28 because I met a man who made me feel as if my self-actualization was the most important thing to him. I wanted to marry my best friend, and he is and has been my best friend.

The institution of marriage has a long history of oppressing women, by denying us our rights to own property and to defend ourselves against

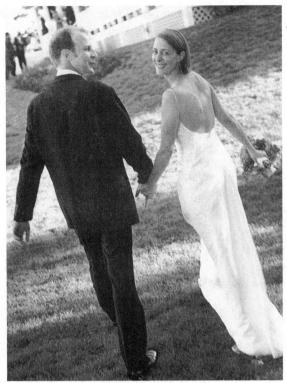

© Jörg Meyer

abusers, and by reinforcing traditional gender roles. Half of all marriages in the United States end in divorce. Yet whether we see marriage as a flawed, even discriminatory, institution, an ideal foundation of a family, or a circumstance that is hard to imagine, many of us still want to get married.

Call it cognitive dissonance, but I have decided that I can live within the bounds of legal marriage and enjoy it. I can "choose the path of least resistance" while at the same time helping to ingrain new ideas of what marriage is. And in little, seemingly insignificant ways, I can chip away at some of the baggage that marriage—and weddings in particular—carry with them. I can walk down the aisle without the escort of my father; I can decline an engagement ring; I can keep my name; I can prefer "partner" to "fiancée" or "wife" or "spouse." My partner and I can express our exist-

ing and lasting commitment in a way that society and our parents understand, and enjoy a great party and health insurance to boot.

Many women feel that, "traditional" or not, a marriage ceremony is a deeply symbolic act that can bind the couple more deeply to each other as well as to the community.

By enacting the ritual of marriage, I demonstrate that I too think this is a sacred contract; it is above the daily routine while at the same time it enacts the sacredness of daily life with another. Commitment without community reinforcement is bound to crack easily. Ritual gives the couple the opportunity to open up its private discourse to communal support.

Some women find that marriage brings both social recognition and a more personal sense of stability and peace. This may allow a relationship to flourish further.

I swear, my mother referred to Colin quite often as "that guy" (as in her oft-repeated "When is that guy ever going to marry you?"). As soon as the engagement ring was on my finger, he became "Colin"—a full-fledged person, not the guy who was "getting the milk for free." Colin, such a great guy, so happy to have him in the family, etc. Of course I wanted to get married. The big wedding and the gift registry—how long had I looked forward to that?! But seriously . . . until Colin made that commitment—saying: "I want to marry you"—I was always a little insecure, and the trust was not complete.

And yet it is important to try to put aside familial or social pressure when making the decision to marry. In the long run, it's our life and our partner's, side by side, that will matter most. When it comes to longevity, a fifty-something woman with two grown children says there is not enough space or time to describe the intimacy of a marriage and "where it takes you."

Not in the sexual sense but in the helpless place of vulnerability. When I was between my second and third spinal surgery, not only could I not walk but I could not pull my panties up. I remember trying my best to scoot down the hall to the bathroom when my husband entered the room to assist me. His tender touch, his look, his acknowledgment that I was in pain that he would have carried if he could. . . . There is an exchange that you have with no other. Outside marriage, there is always an open door ready to cross through if things don't go your way. Inside marriage, there is a recognition that our bodies connect in ways beyond the physical. . . . It is as if we are constructing our own sense of space and time, our own language of being.

Many women marry with the consciousness that marriage remains an unjust social arrangement in most religions and states, because only heterosexual relationships get such recognition.

I think we didn't marry for the first four years of our relationship as a protest, more or less. . . . It's always bothered us that this right is conferred on nice straight people like ourselves, while our queer sisters and brothers get laws made against their ever being able to legally have a union. So it didn't seem fair to us that we could share in the benefits and a whole other group of people—whether they wanted to take advantage of the system or not— were denied them.

A growing number of couples who disagree with the institution of marriage prefer to live happily together in commitments of their own making, which may or may not involve children. Communities also look to such couples for coherence, support, and continuity.

I can't imagine life without my partner—he anchors me, supports me, and continually delights me. We are absolutely committed to one another, and have been so for eleven years. But marriage seems completely irrelevant to the life that we share—quite simply, it's got nothing to do with our love or commitment. For the most part, our families and friends have been understanding and extremely supportive of our choice not to marry. Last year, we used our tenth anniversary as an excuse to throw a fabulous party for our family and friends, so they could celebrate our commitment with us.

While most of us hope our partnerships will last a lifetime, the stark reality is that a good number of them will end in divorce or separation. A thirty-one-year-old publisher describes her unexpected marriage—and even more unexpected divorce:

I never expected to get married at all. In fact, I consciously avoided seeing marriage as a goal in and of itself. When I met the man I did end up marrying, I was very much taken by surprise by my desire to live with and marry him. It was an intense relationship that got serious fast, and we wanted to make a public statement of commitment (partly to get the message across to friends and family that it was serious, whirlwind nature notwithstanding) and, I admit, take advantage of the straight shot to relationship "legitimacy" that marriage (and heterosexual privilege) offers. To make a long and complicated story short and simple, four years later he had an affair, and it soon became clear that the partnership was unsalvageable (and, in fact, had been deeply flawed in ways I had refused to acknowledge).

While the ending of a relationship, especially one that was pledged to be a lifelong commitment, may be very painful, it can also lead to new awareness of one's self and ideals. The thirty-one-year-old publisher continues:

The period of separation and divorce was intensely painful. More than a year later, I am still feeling its effects, but after coming through it

(with the help of my friends and family and a really good therapist), I have a much more well-developed sense of what I want and need from a partner, a renewed resolve never to be blinded to those ideals again, and a confirmation of what I always knew: that I am very, very happy as a single person.

While some look to lifelong monogamous relationships as the ideal, others seek open relationships—having two or more romantic and sexual relationships at the same time—either for a short term (say, during a period of dating) or for a lifetime (as in an open marriage). Other women practice *polyamory,* in which we maintain committed relationships to more than one person at a time.

For me, polyamory is about having a range of intimate relationships that aren't polarized into "sexual" and "nonsexual." Occasionally, I might have sex with a friend; at other times, I might have a deeply committed, long-term relationship with someone where sex isn't involved. Right now I have three wonderful partners, all of whom I love very deeply. I've been with two of them for about four years, and the other relationship is just a few months old. They are different enough that I find each of them is able to fulfill me in a way the others can't. That's what I love about polyamory! I can watch cheesy TV shows with one partner, and geek out about computers with another one. Love is not a finite resource—I believe the more you share it, the better it gets.

For some of us, monogamy is not a given but something that we grow into as a way of expressing our commitment to a partner.

Monogamy was never really a big deal to me, to be honest. I think this is due mainly to Nancy Reagan! I was a young teen during the Reagan years, just trying out my sexuality (among other things), and the mantra back then was "Just Say

No." A lot of us responded with "Let's Try It." So, there was a lot of experimenting going on for me and my peers that I think was very healthy, very liberating. I'm in a monogamous relationship for 11 years now, because my husband requires this of me in order to be in a relationship with him— that's just the way he's wired. It was difficult at first, but at this point, no problem.

If you are thinking about marriage or commitment and wondering if it is for you, talking to your partner is of course a good idea. Beyond that, friends or peers who have considered marriage and other kinds of partnership can offer new perspectives. If you're in a committed relationship and discussing marriage, premarital counseling can be helpful (and is actually required by some religious organizations). There are also organizations that provide legal tips, advice, and political advocacy for couples who do not wish to marry but are concerned about having a partnership legally and socially validated.

MAKING IT WORK: SHARED POWER

In any relationship, problems arise regardless of how "right" we are for each other, of how hard we have worked to build the relationship, and even of how solid and stable we feel together. It can be frightening to look squarely at what is difficult and hurtful. We want to believe that we have chosen a good partner and that we have made wise decisions. To become aware of aspects we have been afraid to face, or to admit deep conflicts, may mean that we have made a major error, that it will take a lot of time to address this issue, or that it is time to move on.

While a whole and healthy sense of personal power is the necessary foundation for a good relationship, a balance of power is a simultaneous goal. Sharing power in a good relationship both

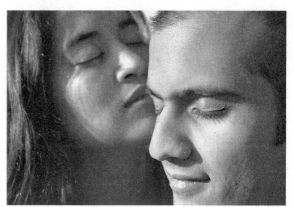

requires and cultivates continual personal growth—and has the potential to reinvigorate the relationship endlessly. Confronting problems and taking steps to change can be frightening, but with self-confidence and the support of our communities, and with the trust that comes from sharing deeply, men and women can find new ways of being together that feel more free.

Making relationships work requires skills. Luckily, these can be cultivated. Below are some basic skills many women and men have tried to cultivate to help make things work.

DEVELOPING GOOD COMMUNICATION

Avoiding confrontation is more likely to result in stagnation and resentment than in keeping the peace or making things better. *Conflict can be part of a creative process of working things out.* We can start by identifying the aspects of our conflicts that we have inherited from society or our families, and avoid the common pitfall of blaming each other (or ourselves) for everything that goes wrong.

QUESTIONING EXPECTATIONS

Taking a step back and trying to see through our partner's eyes—developing a sense of empathy—may help shift the discussion in a creative way. Trying to set aside old roles, particularly those that stem from social conventions, and trying to engage without assumptions or expectations may also help us to see our own patterns of relating to men. The earlier we are able to do this, the better off the relationship will be. We all come to relationships with expectations. The question is, to what extent are we willing to shift them in order to be with our partner?

PAYING ATTENTION TO EACH OTHER

So many things vie for our attention: work, friends, children, our various activities and chores. A new love eclipses everything else, but before long, it can get squeezed in between our family's needs, our work commitments, our friends. Intimate relationships form the background and sustenance for the rest of our lives, but at times they require our full attention. That may mean having a special date once a week, or setting aside time to talk about the day and the details of what happened at work or at home; it may mean, on occasion, staying up until the wee hours trying to work out a crisis and/or making passionate love. For many of us, it means trying to be watchful, responsive, and fully present with our partner.

ENJOYING SEPARATENESS

It may feel natural for many of us to go on separate vacations or to see separate friends. Others may take it as a sign that something is wrong. Sometimes one member of a couple may be threatened when a partner's life excludes him or her in some way. And yet keeping some distinct turf for ourselves—whether it's separate checkbooks, separate vacations, separate friends, separate rooms, or not rushing into living together—doesn't have to threaten our relationship. It can contribute to the vitality and growth of what goes on between us.

DEVELOPING OTHER FRIENDSHIPS AND COMMUNITY

Sometimes couples close in on themselves. We may come to attach less importance to other friendships and let them drop. But it is unrealistic to expect that one person can meet all our needs. Our friendships and communities—religious, artistic, political, neighborhood, etc.—are crucial to our emotional well-being, happiness, and growth. Furthermore, by expanding our intimate circles, we relieve some of the pressure on our main relationships, and when times are hard, other people can then give us support. This includes having male as well as female friends.

KNOWING WHEN TO LEAVE

If you wind up accommodating your partner just to prevent fights, rather than having some hope that it's worth trying to work things out; if your relationship is based on evasiveness, deception, and withholding; if it is characterized by lack of room for change and growth; or if it just doesn't seem that your life is better in the relationship than it would be out of it, then it is time to consider ending it. You don't need to do this alone. Friends can be an excellent source of support and insight. Individual or group therapy can help, too. There are also good books on the subject (see "Resources"). As important as it is to work very hard on building a relationship, it is also important to leave before we are damaged by it. (If you are concerned that your relationship may be abusive, see Chapter 8, "Violence and Abuse.")

GETTING HELP

If we do not want to leave, or if we are struggling to discern whether it is time to do so, we may need help. Sometimes problems are resistant to change, and it seems as if talking to our partner and to friends and family gets us nowhere. When we feel that we've gone around and around on the same issues with no improvement, we may become completely overwhelmed and feel stuck in patterns we can't change on our own. That's when we might seek therapy, either as individuals or together.

My boyfriend and I both grew up in abusive households. As a result, we had no models of fair fighting. Our arguments would get completely out of control—by the end of each we had exploited each . . . other's weakest points, and hurt each other so badly that civilized discourse was nearly impossible. . . . Coming from South Asian families, my boyfriend and I decided to seek out a South Asian counselor—perhaps then we would find someone whom we didn't have to explain cultural issues to, and who could approach our problems, which extended to family, with a South Asian vantage point. [Our counselor] was wonderful. She encouraged us to draw up "boundaries" and pledge never to overstep them. When we noticed the other hedging near a personal boundary, we gave our partner notice, asking them not to go there. We also learned to "replay" our arguments afterward, creatively pondering how the other would have reacted had one partner done something differently. These dispassionate reenactments have allowed us to better understand where the other person is coming from.

While we can use therapy to help improve communication about painful issues, choosing the right therapist is crucial. It is important to find a therapist whose definitions of health and normalcy are based on a worldview that sees women as having a full range of options, not on narrow beliefs, such as the idea that women's only role is to "service" men and take care of children. (For more information, see Chapter 6, "Emotional Well-Being.")

CREATIVE TENSION

Though it may seem contradictory to advocate seeking intimacy with our partners while at the same time pursuing personal power and other friendships, these multiple aspects of our lives can and do enrich one another. They can also provide a balance that stimulates growth and promotes mental, physical, and spiritual well-being.

One sixty-four-year-old, herself long married and glad to be so, avoids the term "marriage" while stating that she believes "wholeheartedly in lifelong commitment as the context in which intimacy can really grow." She adds:

Of course, physical intimacy can happen quickly and can be a harbinger for intimacy on all levels. True intimacy (i.e., intimacy that reaches into the core of your soul) takes time and, for me and my husband of going on 40 years, a heck of a lot of work, not to mention forgiveness. Balancing individuality and togetherness is always a high-wire act, but with commitment to the relationship, the tension can be—and, to last, must be—creative tension.

We are perhaps the typical couple in that my husband has had to fight a reluctance to "open up" and become vulnerable, and I have had to persevere in encouraging such mutual openness while respecting where he's coming from in the moment. It is our desire for an evolving relationship that has kept us trying (sometimes two steps forward, one step back). Ironically, neither feels diminished in the bigger picture of things, but enriched. With each breakthrough in understanding each other, the intimacy goes deeper.

CHAPTER 11

The new millennium is a promising time for women who have intimate and/or sexual relationships with women. With issues important to the lesbian, gay, bisexual, and transgender communities increasingly in the news, more people all over the country and around the world are recognizing who we are and supporting how we live our lives. The debate over the legal recognition of gay marriage, domestic partnerships, and civil unions has engaged the nation. More and more television shows and movies attempt to portray our lives (albeit not always in the most accurate or satisfying ways). Many people in positions of power and authority—politicians, business owners, and celebrities—are out and proud. There have never been more resources and support available to members of the queer community who have been traditionally neglected, including youth, women in rural areas, transgendered people, women with disabilities, and women of color. Thanks largely to activism from within the queer community and an increasing emphasis on coming out, many women who love women are living more freely and openly than in generations past.

As women who have, want, or are considering sexual relationships with women, many of us identify our sexual orientation as lesbian, bisexual, queer, gay, pansexual, questioning, or bicurious. For personal and political reasons, though, plenty of us prefer not to be labeled, or we use another label that feels more encompassing of our unique personal identity. This chapter uses the acronym "LBTQ," as well as the word "queer," in an attempt to include as many people as possible. "LGBT" is also used to refer to the larger queer community, including gay men. (For definitions of the terms used in this chapter, see Chapter 9, "Gender Identity and Sexual Orientation".)* In addition, this chapter uses the word "partner" to refer to people in different types of relationships, from casual sexual partners to monogamously or nonmonogamously committed partners.

Despite the fact that we have increased visibility and acceptance in the mainstream, homophobia and heterosexism continue to have a strong hold in our society. As LBTQ people, we risk losing connections with homophobic friends and family and endanger our access to equal civil rights when we come out about our sexual and/or gender identity.

---

* The inclusion of transgender/transsexual women in this chapter isn't meant to imply that all transgendered/transsexual people are gay or lesbian, or that all the social and legal progress for lesbian, bisexual, and gay people has been extended to transgendered and transsexual people. Instead, it's meant to address and acknowledge those of us who are transwomen, transmen, and other genderqueers—who have self-identified as women for at least part of our lives—and are currently involved in or interested in having romantic or sexual relationships with women.

All LBTQ women are affected by the social and legal obstacles currently depriving us of the rights and protections we deserve. These difficulties are exacerbated when we have low incomes or are imprisoned, or when we are women of color, immigrants, or noncitizens of the United States. While the laws affecting us are constantly changing, sometimes in our favor, many legislators, judges, and lawyers in the U.S. judicial system still perpetuate our society's bias against the queer community and other communities with which they don't identify.

In recent decades, we have won recognition of our individual rights in some contexts and have seen new laws passed to expand our rights toward full equality in other contexts. In 2003 the Supreme Court struck down "homosexual conduct" laws that criminalized oral and anal sex between same-sex couples. This landmark case, *Lawrence* v. *Texas,* reinforced our right to privacy, which means that law enforcers can no longer enter our homes and arrest us for engaging in private, consensual sex acts. Rescinding this anti-queer legislation paved the way for increased legal recognition of the civil rights of LBTQ individuals and families.

This chapter offers information and support to all queer women. It is a limited space to cover such an infinitely diverse topic as women's relationships with women; because of this, every attempt has been made to ensure that the other chapters in this book are relevant to and inclusive of the LBTQ community and the issues that directly and indirectly affect our relationships. Readers may find the other chapters in this "Relationships and Sexuality" section particularly useful in navigating relationships.

FINDING LOVE

When we're looking for potential life partners, casual dates, or sexual experiences, we must start

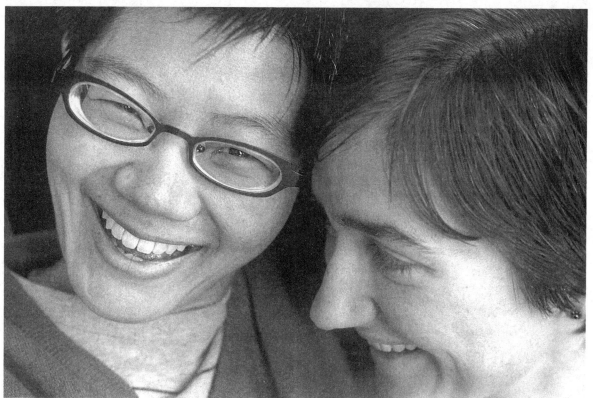

by taking risks, which often means moving out of our comfort zones and confronting our fears. We each have a unique array of challenges around relationships, but some common ones are fears around rejection, intimacy, commitment, sex, abandonment, or enmeshment. In some cases, we worry about how people will react when we come out. But our reward for overcoming our fears is meeting other queer women with whom we can connect emotionally, sexually, spiritually, and/or intellectually.

With the advent of the Internet and increased visibility and acceptance of LBTQ women, this is an exciting time to be connecting with and dating other queer women. But that doesn't mean dating women is painless. Because so many of us have been socialized by heterosexual society to wait until we're asked out, we often find ourselves wondering (okay, obsessing) over whether an attraction is mutual. Perhaps the title of Mo Brownsey's comedic book about dating women best sums up this quandary: *Is It a Date or Just Coffee?*

Especially if we haven't met someone in an obviously queer setting, we may find ourselves wondering "Is she queer, too?" Sometimes it's easier to be direct and ask; if we're not in a queer-friendly environment, we may want to get to know someone slowly, perhaps gauging how she responds to general queer topics before we decide to come out or to ask her out. It's important to protect ourselves and avoid situations that seem like they will be unsafe for us emotionally or physically.

When we first start dating women, many of us have a lot of questions. We may wonder how the experience compares to traditional gender roles in straight relationships. Who asks out whom? Who pays? Who makes the first sexual move? One forty-two-year-old who has been out for five years says of her experiences dating women:

I've always dated men, so my dating experience with women has also been a kind of cultural shock. Where men usually "make the first move," I've had to relearn my dating "techniques" and sometimes feel as if I'm going through puberty again or for the first time.

Sometimes queer relationships may allow more space to negotiate our own rules with our partners than do relationships with men. Communication is the key. We will likely find that with each new partner, certain things will fall right into place, and others will be more awkward at first. That's just the nature of dating. The important thing is to have fun with it, and to leave the space to create a unique relationship that best fits the preferences of everyone involved.

But first things first: We have to meet women before we can date them! Those of us having trouble finding potential partners don't have to feel like our only options are getting back together with our exes or giving up altogether. We just have to keep putting ourselves into situations where we meet new women.

Many of us find love in our own backyard, dating longtime friends, friends of friends, or coworkers. One woman met her partner at the factory where they work.

I asked her to go for a cup of coffee with me after work where we were at the time, after being at work with her for about two weeks. . . . I couldn't stand it anymore. . . . She looked so wonderfully sexy, butch, beautiful . . . everything . . . and she said yes, she'd go have coffee with me. . . . And now the rest is history.

I was introduced to my first girlfriend at a party. I dated a couple of my current, lifelong friends (who still remain my friends to this day), and I met my current girlfriend at work.

Many of us spend a tremendous amount of our time and energy at work, and we are likely to meet people there with whom we have shared interests. Of course, dating coworkers is a path that should be walked with caution. Before proceeding, refer to your company's dating policies and consider how it could affect your work life if you are turned down or have a messy breakup with a coworker down the line.

There are also plenty of ways to meet completely new people. For those of us who enjoy the nightlife, numerous bars and nightclubs exclusively serve a queer clientele or have a regular girls' night for women to meet each other. Many bars and feminist or queer bookstores offer poetry readings and open mikes for those of us who enjoy a creative bent. And for something more formal, we might try lesbian-focused dating services or speed dating, in which women have several short "dates" in one night to increase our odds of meeting someone who is queer and available.

The Internet has dramatically enhanced our ability to connect with other women, especially for those of us who live in rural areas or who are computer-savvy teens seeking a community of peers. Online chats and dating services can bring women to us from all over the world, although many of us use these methods to find the queer girl next door. Most online dating services include a section for women who want to meet women, and there are also many sites dedicated specifically to the queer community.

I met my first long-term girlfriend through the newspaper personals. When we broke up, Internet personals had become popular, so I tried those, as well as speed dating. I think I've been pretty successful meeting women this way; it's a lot less painful than going out to bars.

Trying online dating or chats necessitates safety precautions. People are not always who they seem to be (for example, men can pose as women, or adults can pose as teenagers). It's important to keep your identifying information—such as home phone, home address, school, or workplace—private and to trust yourself if you feel uncomfortable with where the conversation is headed. If you decide to meet in person, do so in a public place, and tell trusted friends or family where you will be and with whom.

Becoming a part of an ongoing queer group or organization is an excellent way to get to know women while simultaneously expanding your community of friends and acquaintances. For those of us who live in an area that has an LGBT community center, it is a great place to find events and groups. Others may enjoy meeting people with similar priorities and passions while pouring energy into volunteer work for a political or social organization. A forty-two-year-old polyamorous woman met her partners through various community activities.

I met A via a Usenet newsgroup. I met N at a pagan ritual. I met M at a polyamory support group that A and I were organizing. I met J at a fat-acceptance support group for women that J organized.

A sixty-year-old woman who is exploring her attraction to women began by volunteering for a local feminist bookstore.

I went over and bought a few books and asked to be a volunteer. . . . No, I haven't found anyone I want to get closer to, but at least it is nice to find people of similar interests who also like to read.

There are queer-specific community activities for practically any interest we can come up with, including athletic teams, book groups, religious or spiritual organizations, and support or discussion groups. Many of these groups advertise in local queer newspapers or free alternative weeklies, when available. In addition, some cafés and restaurants are owned by or cater to queer clientele; look for telltale signs like pink triangles, the rainbow stripes of the pride flag, and Human Rights Campaign logos (which look like a blue box with a yellow equal sign inside).

If none of the offerings in your area meet your interests, consider starting something new, such as a gay-straight alliance in your school, or a group where women enjoy or discuss books, movies, favorite TV shows, or other cultural events. If you are seeking to meet or date other queer women of color, transpeople, or people who share your political ideals, you may want to start social or discussion groups specifically for those populations. It's okay to build whatever kind of community you need in order to feel fulfilled and find the women you are attracted to. When you create something, you often bring others to you.

BUILDING HEALTHY RELATIONSHIPS

Some of us choose to be single or to have casual lovers. Some of us aim to foster long-term connections with a partner, whether we stay together for a few months, a few years, or a lifetime. Being in a relationship generally involves planning our lives with our partner, helping each other through personal changes and difficulties, working through conflicts, and sometimes having children.

I like being with someone who follows all the threads of my life, even the most mundane.

FLYING SOLO

Being single can be a legitimate, healthy destination; a time to tend to ourselves and get our bearings after a breakup; or a challenging time in which we must face our deepest fears about seeking the love we long for.

As people who are identified based on whom we are intimate with, have sex with, and share our lives with, some of us may find it challenging to feel confident and accepted as a single queer woman. We may worry that others doubt our sexual orientation. If we have never been in a same-sex or same-gender relationship, we may not feel that we have "earned" our queer identity. This can cause self-doubt, or fears that we'll be rejected by the queer community or by potential partners due to our inexperience—even though we all have a first time sometime.

Of course, sometimes we aren't single because it's our ideal. Some of us may not be ready to come out to others or ourselves. Perhaps our desires have been silenced or overpowered by homophobia, or we have distanced ourselves from our sexual desire. Others of us may be uncomfortable dating, or feel hopeless about finding the right partners, and thus find it difficult to confront the painful feelings that dating can raise. In these instances, seeking queer-positive counseling or support groups may help us sort through the issues that are keeping us from what we want. (For more information on counseling, see Chapter 6, "Emotional Well-Being.")

When our gender identity doesn't correspond with our physical body, we may want to abstain from sex or partnership until either our bodies are transformed, our circumstances change, or our painful emotions about our experiences are healed. A fifty-two-year-old postoperative transsexual woman is exploring her sexual orientation following her transition, which she pursued for decades before she had access to hormones and surgeries:

I could not relate sexually with a partner in the wrong body. . . . The denial of transition also denied me the possibility of forming a sexual orientation—of any sort. That was all burned out of me in the pain of those decades of hopelessness. Perhaps I shall be able to recover some of it now that I am post-op, I do not know. Since my transition, I have begun to form friendships with women, but I feel no sexual attraction to women. My childhood experiences with males were violent and abusive, and overcoming the deep fears this gave me will not be easy.

In our society, we experience a lot of pressure to be in a relationship—especially to have a straight partnership. It's important that we look inward to discover what relationship status we really want for our lives, then take action to make our desires a reality. Singlehood can be a marvelous time for us to explore ourselves, live our lives without compromise, and build close friendships and a strong community.

I love the freedom, spontaneity, and calmness of living alone. Love the creativity of celibacy: all the energy and passion that once went into coupling now released to move in surprising new directions.

I like being poly because it seems to me that being able to express the romantic/sexual aspects of relationships binds people more closely together, so my social structure feels more like an "extended family" or "network" than a group of friends.

When I hear another lesbian talking about being involved as lovers and friends with lots of women, it excites me. I know that by choosing to be with one woman, I am missing out on a certain kind of emotional adventure. But for my lover and me, there is a kind of adventure I prefer at this point.

After we meet someone with whom there's a mutual attraction, we begin the process of getting to know each other. We learn about the other person's likes, dislikes, work life, family, and hopes and dreams. We tell her about our own interests and passions. At some point during this process, we may begin a sexual relationship. Many of us begin to consider whether the relationship has the potential to become long-term. Dating isn't a precise science: Some relationships begin with sex or with a friendship that has grown over time. Some move fast, some almost achingly slow, and others have fits and starts. However it looks, this is the groundwork of building a relationship.

Sharing information about ourselves causes us to be more vulnerable. This risk can be both exciting and terrifying. Many of us feel exposed on a number of levels as we seek to achieve intimacy in our relationship. These challenges, faced in all kinds of romantic partnerships, can be complicated further if we encounter or sense a homophobic reaction to our choice of partners.

I didn't realize I was "passing" as an "ungay" woman until I felt an attraction to and pursued a relationship with a butch woman. When we are together, there is no question what our relationship is. The smiles that I would encounter alone are absent when I am with her. I have decided to

be brave and meet the challenge of a generally uncelebrated relationship. Celebrating being gay in the closet is no longer enough.

Internally, we may also find that particular issues around intimate relationships can be challenging. Sometimes we have well-meaning but unrealistic expectations about how easy a relationship with another woman is going to be. While our connections with each other can certainly be thrilling, they aren't free of the work required of any relationship.

The only thing that we have in our heads is: You meet a woman, you feel for her, you enter into a relationship, you relate only to her. It's been the downfall of many intimacies.

Although there are endless differences between any two women, a particular closeness often results from our connections. We have similar bodies, similar socialization, and many of the same challenges as women in an often homophobic and sexist world. This intimacy can be incredibly fulfilling, though it also has the potential to feel suffocating. We can help prevent our relationships from becoming enmeshed by achieving a healthy balance between closeness and distance, defining our individual selves assertively, and encouraging each other to grow as individuals. While the importance of such boundaries is not unique to women's relationships with each other, it may be that our similarities sometimes make appropriate boundaries more difficult to ascertain. If possible, it can help to establish and communicate boundaries from the beginning of the relationship, changing them over time as we each feel comfortable.

It's critical that my lover and I really understand our boundaries, where we want to say no and where we want to say yes. If I don't build my own privacy right away into a relationship, then the

TEEN DATING

More and more queer teens are out to family and friends, which allows us to date and be more fully ourselves in all areas of our lives.

My mom could not be greater in accepting me for who I am. All she wants is for me to be happy. And, when I decided to take a girl to the prom with me, she was overjoyed because she saw how happy it made me.

I realized I was bisexual when I was about 13 and started to be attracted to other girls. When I came out at school, at the beginning of freshman year, I was amazed at how accepting and supportive everyone around me was.

Others of us find it more challenging to meet and identify other queer and questioning teens, understand or define our sexual orientation, or find guidance and support in order to come out to family, friends, and the world around us. QueerAmerica.com is a good source for organizations serving youth. Local queer and feminist newspapers and bookstores can also point you in the right direction.

When we experience unsupportive, abusive, or homophobic family or friends, we can feel isolated, depressed, even suicidal. We may want to run away and leave our parent's or guardian's home. Our difficulties are not due to our sexual orientation or gender expression; they are due to not getting the support, love, and acceptance we need and deserve. If your parent threatens to throw you out of your home, connect with an adult you can trust, such as a therapist, a guidance counselor, or a counselor at a queer or queer-friendly organization. These resources can be found in the phone book or on the Internet. (For more information, see "LBTQ Teen Dating" [W27] on the companion website, www.ourbodiesourselves.org.)

---

next thing I know I'm either spacing out or leaving.

When we have poor boundaries, our relationships may be emotionally painful. We may avoid intimacy out of fear of being "swallowed up." Or we may become so close to our partner that we don't know where her needs, desires, and personhood end and where we begin. As trust deepens in a relationship over time, we must let down our guard and take the risk of communicating openly and honestly with our partner.

If a relationship is strong and healthy, it can better withstand conflict and change. It will encourage personal and interpersonal growth. The ability to communicate with our partner allows us to establish a strong foundation for intimacy, which can last a lifetime if that's the commitment we choose to make.

For those of us who keep our sexual orientation a secret, open communication can be a particular challenge. We may edit out important information about our lives with those we care about, including family, friends, or coworkers—using words like "friend" or "roommate" to disguise whom we love instead of using "girlfriend," "partner," or a clear equivalent. Although we may feel that being in the closet is necessary for our safety or well-being, it invariably diminishes our access to expressing our full truths—sometimes with our partners or ourselves.

SEEKING EQUALITY
WITH OUR PARTNERS

As women, we tend to invest a lot in the idea of equality in our partnerships. But just believing in the idea of shared power and control isn't enough to make it so. The reality is that discrepancies in power exist in our partnerships just as they do in straight ones, and they undermine us when left unchecked.

As D. Merilee Clunis and G. Dorsey Green write in *Lesbian Couples: A Guide to Creating Healthy Relationships,* "Shared intimacy also requires attention to the balance of power in the relationship. If one partner makes all the decisions, controls such important aspects of the relationship as money, conversation or sex, or is looked up to by the other but does not look up to her partner, the balance of power is not equitable. There are real-world power differences such as skin color, gender, ability, education, financial resources, physical size and age. There are also interpersonal power differences such as ability to express feelings, comfort with oneself and verbal quickness. It is vital that couples become aware of and discuss the impact all of these differences have on each of them and their relationship."

It's important that we don't take advantage of a power imbalance, especially once we recognize it. Instead, we can strive to bring fair communication, respect, and love to the situation.

HONORING OUR DIFFERENCES

By acknowledging and celebrating our differences with our partners, we honor each other and gain the opportunity to learn more about our partners and ourselves. This can help to ease the pain that may arise when our differences get in the way of understanding each other's values, decisions, and behaviors.

Because racism is still so prevalent in our society, racial or ethnic differences can prove challenging.

Within the black community, we are still facing an incredible amount of homophobia, and then there is the racial prejudice in the world that we also face. . . . White people cannot understand what we are faced with. So, when I met my partner, [who is a white woman,] it was a little surprising that I was really attracted to her and her soul and we had a lot of things in common— we still have our differences, and I help her to understand my race, and she helps me to understand hers.

Age is also a difference that can create tension or a power imbalance in our relationships. One woman who is many years younger than her partner says they "grew up in different worlds":

What she wants for her life is not what I ever wanted or expected for mine. As long as both of us notice, respect, and understand these differences, we do well together. In a way, the age span is good—it makes us see that we can't be everything for each other, that we need friends our own age.

Differences in class and nationality can be challenging as well. One Korean-American woman who is the daughter of immigrants is partnered with a woman of mixed ethnicity who immigrated to the United States with her mother from Vietnam when she was five years old.

She grew up working-class, with the idea that the ability to go to school and to choose her type and place of work were privileges probably out of her reach. I grew up poor also, but with parents who had the dream and the resources to achieve eventual economic stability, and the certainty that I was meant for education and . . . a profession, not a trade. . . . The different expectations . . . are, in many ways, a result of class differences caused by our countries' different respective histories of immigration. . . . Understanding our differences, our privileges, our burdens, and our histories [is a way to] build bridges between and within our communities.

It is also important for our partners to acknowledge our health issues or disabilities.

As a woman with fibromyalgia, I often appear to be healthier than I am. My disability is hidden so much so that many people, including my wife, often forget that it exists. She has learned over the past five years how to help me manage my time and energy to maximize my energy.

There are numerous other differences we may have from our partner, including but certainly not limited to our gender identity, sexual orientation, health and physical ability, religious or spiritual beliefs, political values, and unique methods of self-expression. With a willingness to fully see and be seen, and to communicate openly, we can develop a deeper relationship and an opportunity for greater intimacy.

CREATING SUPPORTIVE COMMUNITIES

Most straight couples can hold hands in public, be safe going out together, feel welcomed by their families and at religious services, and celebrate their relationships openly. Though some straight couples who date across lines of race, ethnicity, class, and religion may not share all of these freedoms, they still are able to marry legally and access the rights to make decisions for each other in times of sickness and provide for each other's material well-being in case of death, among hundreds of other essential civil rights. Women in intimate relationships with women can take none of this for granted.

I think that every woman who comes out to her family wants them to be accepting of her life and her relationships. It's very hard to have a close, loving relationship with a parent who . . . [has] difficulty with their own homophobia. After ten years, I would like to think that my mother could tell her friends that I'm a lesbian in casual conversation, instead of staying silent when the issue of homosexuality comes up.

Many of us have family members or other people in our social network who are either hostile, unsupportive, or ignorant about our relationships with our partners. Even if our straight family members and friends mean to be supportive, they may still be prone to making heterosexist assumptions about our relationships, such as that we're attracted to every woman we encounter, that we won't or shouldn't have children, or that our weddings are less significant or not as important to attend as a straight ceremony. Because of this, many of us find strength in developing a community of supportive friends that includes other queer people.

Finding a network of queer people who share similar experiences, feelings, and questions can be particularly helpful when we are coming out or first exploring our sexual orientation. The queer community is incredibly diverse, and with diversity comes difference. Because of this, it can sometimes be difficult to find our place in the community, where all of the aspects of our identity can be acknowledged and appreciated. One Latina longs for a space where she's not approached by men or hit on by women who exoticize her ethnicity:

In the majority of "straight" bars, we're vulnerable to men asking one of us out and the awkwardness of one of us having to watch the other getting picked up. . . . In "lesbian" bars, the looks are more about how we look: GAY WOMEN OF COLOR! It's sooo great that you're here! . . . There's got to be a place, somewhere, for us.

Another woman who is in a relationship with "a woman who is now a man" says this about their partnership:

He is still the woman I fell in love with, the strong, brilliant, tender person I fell in love with, but in a shiny new skin. He is now stronger, just as our love is stronger, because he is finally wholly himself.

The same woman speaks of the couple's challenging search for community:

We do not know where we fit now, except among the tiny group of transmen and their partners. We are an anonymous, straight couple to strangers, queer and straight alike, and a strange couple to our queer friends. . . . Where do we fit? When do we come out? What are we? How do we explain? And will people accept us?

A bisexual woman speaks to how people respond to her sexuality within the queer community:

I feel bisexuals are invisible in the queer community. I'm particularly shocked that some folks continue to argue that we don't even exist. . . . Thankfully, I don't experience as much outright hostility as when I first came out 15 years ago. At the same time, I never feel fully at home in lesbian space. I've been in a relationship with a woman for over six years, and part of me still feels "less than" among queers—like I'm crashing the party. My wife and I met at a social event for bi folks, and I thought, "What a relief! At least I don't have to worry about whether she's biphobic."

Finding people who can fully support us and rejoice in who we are is incredibly affirming and life-enhancing. At different periods in our lives, we may focus on building support around particular circumstances. Whether we're coming out, having children, moving to a new city, finding ourselves single, or going through any of life's transitions, we can find solace in and support from others who are at the same point in their lives.

There are many ways to build a supportive and diverse community of people around us. Outside of our immediate network of family and friends, there are support groups, individual or group therapy, and LGBT centers. There are also thousands of local and national listservs, or online e-mail communities, that allow people with similar interests to share resources and stories, and many of these are specifically for the queer community.* If a religious or spiritual practice is part of our lives, we can find a place to join together with others who share our beliefs and who accept us for who we are. Some queer-friendly spiritual centers use the phrase "open and inclusive" to indicate that we are welcome. Queer newspapers or local e-mail communities can help you locate these places more quickly.

As LBTQ women, we are often faced with discrimination because of whom we love. It's essential that we take care of one another. We can ask one another about our relationships and give our queer friends a loving place to discuss all of life's ups and downs. We can offer our time or money to organizations that support the rights and well-being of queer people. And we can do this by being out and proud.

---

* QueerNet (http://groups.queernet.org) and Yahoo! (http://groups.yahoo.com) are two great resources for those interested in listservs, with thousands of groups to join. PlanetOut (www.planetout.com) hosts chats specifically for queer folks.

NAVIGATING HOMOPHOBIA AND HETEROSEXISM

We grow up in a society that largely condones negative messages about queer people. It's almost impossible not to internalize, to some extent, the homophobia around us. Sometimes this means that we reject our desires for women, consciously or unconsciously, and sometimes it can lead us to self-hating or self-punishing behaviors. We may feel uncomfortable seeing other queer couples together, or we may have trouble thinking of ourselves as queer. These issues can prevent us from achieving intimacy and connection, which can be incredibly painful. Some of us are caught between our cultural upbringing and the desire to find love.

I come from a Caribbean/Latin background, which aggressively frowns upon homosexuality. My mother has said that she would literally disown me if I choose such a lifestyle. People in parts of the Caribbean are actually stoned and terrorized if they dare be flamboyant with their homosexuality. . . . I am in a mental and spiritual tug-of-war on this issue.

It was the first same-gender relationship for both of us, and with the yin of beauty came the yang of terror. I didn't sleep well or eat well the entire time we were dating. My family was scared . . . and I had to be careful about who I told and how we acted in certain public places. This also made my girlfriend very nervous and seemed to inhibit her from considering a long-term relationship with me. When our relationship ended, I grieved deeply. Who knows what would have happened if we didn't feel constricted in any way by family or cultural opinions.

Sometimes our society's negative views are so insidious that they cause us to hurt ourselves and our partners. If you are closeted or passing as a gender that mainstream society might not acknowledge as your own and your partner threatens to expose you to anyone you don't want to tell, that is emotionally abusive. If your partner seems to blame all problems on your internalized homophobia or transphobia, or if she uses your bisexuality against you, it's important to get outside perspectives and make sure you aren't being manipulated.

The homophobic and heterosexist attitudes in our society are not our fault. They are bred by ignorance and intolerance, and we don't deserve to have these negative messages inflicted upon us. While cultural attitudes toward our relationships are improving, we will still invariably be affected by prejudice. We can't force people to accept us, but we can build a supportive community, face our fears, and work through our internalized homophobia over time, which will give us greater access to intimacy and love.

GETTING SUPPORT RAISING OUR CHILDREN

More and more queer women are deciding to have children. For queer parents, creating a supportive community can be particularly necessary to help our families thrive in a largely unsupportive society.

If we have children from previous relationships, our ex-partners can be a great source of support, provided they are accepting of who we are and they don't try to undermine our relationships with our children.

Our biggest support has been our kids' other parents. We had a "family meeting" every other week to transition the boys, as they lived two weeks with us and two weeks with them. We also celebrated major holidays and birthdays together. We parented by committee. It worked.

There are also groups where we can talk about our feelings and experiences as mothers. It can be a huge relief to know that other LBTQ mothers live with problems similar to ours, to realize the problems aren't our fault; to discuss new approaches; and to share the daily surprises and delights we experience with our kids.

What I've always wanted for my children is a wider network of caring adults, and we're making one in [a support] group. It's not enough just to come in and talk about being lesbian mothers; we include our kids, having parties for us all, going to the beach together. . . . The kids at some point look around the room and say to themselves, "All these kids have lesbian mothers," and feel less isolated.

We may find that we can also get support from straight parents who are queer-friendly. Still, for many women, it helps to have others to talk with about the particular experiences associated with being a queer parent. For instance, having children can make it more difficult to be closeted, and we might need to out ourselves to protect our children's well-being.

When shopping around for day care, I was forced to come out to complete strangers constantly. I obviously needed to explain our family situation and get a sense of acceptance among staff and administration before deciding whether or not to send our kids there. . . . I am not completely out at work and not to my immediate supervisor, so when sharing stories and photos, I find myself concocting evasive stories to explain the "adoption," "the complicated situation," the "friend" staying with the sick child. There was discomfort at first in lining up teenage babysitters. It is uncomfortable being outed in public places to total strangers every time your kid refers to two people as "Mommy."

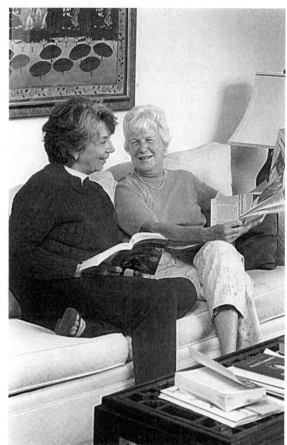

© Jörg Meyer

There are many organizations that support LBTQ parents. For more information on parenting, adoption, conception, and fertility issues, please see "Resources"; Chapter 17, "Considering Parenting"; and the section on donor insemination in Chapter 25, "Infertility and Assisted Reproduction."

MAKING A COMMITMENT

By the time we embark on making a commitment to our partners, we have ideally built a strong foundation of love, mutual respect, and open communication. Our pledges to each other may be emotional, spiritual, and/or legal. They may be private, just between us, or public, inviting our communities to celebrate and support our unions. They may or may not include monogamy as one of their tenets. Regardless of the specifics, when we commit to a shared life, we make a promise to grow together and to turn toward each other in difficult times.

LIVING TOGETHER

Many of us choose to live with our partner at some point in our relationship. Some of us move quickly from the getting-to-know-you stage to living together, and others do it after years of knowing each other. Many of us make this move because we want to come home to our partner at the end of a long day and have someone with whom to share the daily aspects of our life.

Living with one partner works better for me than living alone. Although I'm an introvert and sometimes don't get enough alone time, when I have lived alone, I have gotten somewhat too detached for my own good.

Living together can offer more opportunities for emotional and sexual intimacy and fulfill our desire to share our lives fully with another woman. At the same time, moving in raises the need for much more negotiation and responsibility to each other. We must decide how we will split up household chores, how integrated our finances will be, and how we will negotiate time together and time apart. Over time, we may need to go out of our way to keep things fresh, making sure sex and romance aren't buried under daily responsibilities. Living together transforms a relationship on many levels and heightens the need for good communication.

GETTING HITCHED

Many of us have public ceremonies to honor our relationships and celebrate our commitment with our friends and family. We come together to affirm our identities, honor our commitments, and celebrate the new family that our relationship has created.

We had a commitment ceremony after having been together five years (we celebrate ten years in September). It was very solidifying. It was in our yard with my ex-husband on the video camera and his wife as our officiant. Our kids participated by reading poetry and escorting us. My daughter carried the rings. There wasn't a dry eye in the house.

It can be incredibly fulfilling to get support around our relationships. At the same time, not all of us are supported by those we love. Sometimes members of our family refuse or don't bother to attend our ceremonies or weddings. This can happen because they are homophobic, disapproving outright of our union, or because they are heterosexist, assuming that our rituals are less important because they aren't legally or socially sanctioned. Regardless of the reasons, those absences can be painful.

We are waiting, for financial reasons, to have a wedding. Things cost money—rehearsal dinner, officiator, dresses, shoes, gifts for wedding party, location, dinner and drinks, DJ and/or band—the whole nine yards. Why should we not have that? . . . It's exciting and thrilling and such a big fuss.

We each get to choose whether we make a private commitment, have a small ceremony or a big traditional ceremony, or forge partnerships that look completely different. What's important is that we choose based on what best honors our relationships and feels most fulfilling.

WHEN A RELATIONSHIP ENDS

When a relationship ends, we may grieve the loss of our partner or our idea of what might have been. We also may grieve over the things we wish we had done differently in the relationship.

In my first long-term relationship with a woman . . . I spent an enormous amount of time focusing on my partner and how to make our relationship work . . . After we broke up, I was very angry for all the time that I felt like I had lost—time that I could have spent in a more healthy relationship.

Sometimes our partners say or do the most hurtful things at the end of a relationship. One woman's partner of seventeen years undermined the fundamental understanding of their relationship when she left:

When my life partner dumped me, she announced that because we had never been married, I should not have expected commitment; fidelity was my own personal illusion.

Breaking up can be one of life's most difficult experiences. Yet it can be a relief when a relationship that isn't working ends. As queer women, we may experience the additional pain of not getting the support we need, especially if we didn't have enough support around our relationship in the first place. This can make us feel even more isolated when a relationship is over.

Since I've left and returned back to my hometown, I rarely receive any acknowledgment of my relationship. Sometimes it makes me feel like a shadow or half a person to be grieving for an unrecognized relationship. . . . I was very happy recently when a woman who is a friend of the family . . . asked me how I was doing and said something like "Now weren't you out there with your partner for a long time?" It made me feel so whole to have it acknowledged.

Because our relationships face so much social scrutiny, we may feel pressure to hide the problems we had for fear that they will reflect badly on all queer partnerships. Ultimately, we must take care of ourselves after a breakup and get the support we need. It's not our responsibility to hide our pain because of the homophobia of others.

Many of us try to be friends with our ex-partner after a breakup. This isn't always possible, but it may be quite fulfilling if there is still a healthy bond and genuine caring. Going to couples therapy together to process a breakup, or having a divorce ritual or ceremony that acknowledges the change in relationship, can be particularly healing.

MAKING IT LEGAL

The United States does not offer federal recognition of same-sex marriage. In 1996, President Clinton signed the so-called Defense of Marriage Act, which defined marriage as a relationship between a man and a woman and allowed states to refuse to recognize same-sex marriages should they be legalized by other states. In 2004, President George W. Bush endorsed a federal marriage amendment, which would amend the U.S. Constitution to say essentially the same thing, and would also prohibit individual states from making their own decisions on the matter.

Civil marriage is a state-recognized institution providing 1,049 federal rights and responsibilities, as well as hundreds more state rights and responsibilities, including inheritance rights, hospital visitation rights, joint ownership and spousal support, joint tax returns, joint parenting and child support, joint insurance, joint pension and other benefits, and joint decision making and exemption from property transfer taxes. Most same-sex couples are currently being denied all of these essential civil rights.

Some states now recognize our relationships, to varying degrees. The Massachusetts Supreme Court ruled in 2003 that same-sex marriages were constitutional in that state; legal licenses were first handed out on May 17, 2004.

Like so many other couples planning a June wedding, we are excited, nervous, detail oriented, and just a little giddy. But the giddiness has a different spin for us—we never really thought we would see this day come. . . . Then, last week, we did the most ordinary thing that couples planning to marry check off on their to-do list—we got blood tests. . . . We cried with happiness all the way there in the car—there is nothing we take for granted these days. The attendant was kind and efficient, chatting, asking questions and filling in forms as if it were the most ordinary thing to have two brides arrive together for blood tests. But it is NOT ordinary—it is extraordinary!

Other states may follow suit, while some offer more limited rights for civil unions and domestic partnerships. On the other hand, many states have laws that explicitly discriminate against us. In addition, heterosexual transsexual people can also be denied the right to civil marriage, as the 11th District Ohio Court of Appeals demonstrated in 2004.

The country is currently engaged in a heated

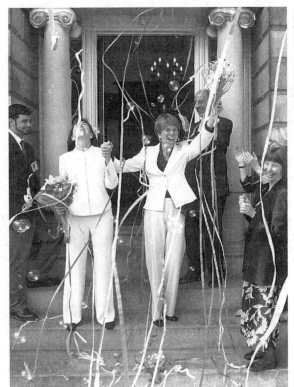

Hillary Goodridge, right, lets out a yell as she and her new spouse, Julie Goodridge, left, leave the Unitarian Universalist Church in Boston after being married on May 17, 2004. The Goodridges were the lead plaintiffs in the Massachusetts lawsuit that led to the legalization of same-sex marriage in that state.

debate about queer civil rights. In the past, U.S. laws discriminated against women and people of color, and interracial marriage was prohibited. Many citizens and public officials are standing up against the legal discrimination same-sex couples face, saying that our current laws are just as much in error as the legal race and sex discrimination of the past. When San Francisco mayor Gavin Newsom ordered that city's clerk to issue marriage licenses on February 12, 2004, hundreds of couples lined up to receive a license. Although the California Supreme Court later invalidated the licenses, the experience was life-changing for many. As one woman who had been with her partner for twenty-two years said,

I would never have expected it, but in some way we both feel different, more committed and more solidly connected. How could that simple process have such a profound effect after such a long time being together and all the other things we have done in our lives to assure we were recognized as a couple? I still don't know.

For some of us, the idea of marrying brings up questions about the institution of marriage and its patriarchal underpinnings. It focuses attention on how much the state regulates our sexualities and relationships, especially since we aren't allowed access to legal marriage throughout the United States. In addition, some of us question whether "couple" relationships, either gay or straight, should be legally sanctioned and receive special benefits. Some of us choose to forgo the institution of marriage altogether and to create new visions for our relationships, while others claim our right to celebrate our relationships any way we choose.

While we continue to fight for our equal rights as citizens of this country, we can take measures to protect ourselves in the meantime. Many couples who cannot marry opt for legal relationship contracts to specify what should happen in the event of a breakup or a partner's illness or death, including the protection of children and the dispersion of shared property.

The laws in regard to our rights as queer women are changing every day. For updated information, see the websites in "Resources" for Lambda Legal Defense and Educational Fund, the National Center for Lesbian Rights, Gay & Lesbian Advocates & Defenders (GLAD), and the Human Rights Campaign.

Legal and social recognition of our relationships is imperative to protect our individual rights, our relationships, and our families. But until we receive such recognition, we must continue striving to love ourselves as queer women, as well as rejoicing in our partners and the members of the supportive community we have built around us.

CHAPTER 12 ■ ■ ■ ■ ■ ■ ■ ■ ■ ■ ■ ■ ■ ■ ■

SOCIAL INFLUENCES

We are all sexual beings, from the moment we are born till the day we die. Whether or not we are in a sexual relationship with another person, we can feel good in our bodies, appreciate sensual pleasures, and learn what excites us sexually. Our sexuality has the potential to be a powerful and positive force in our lives, filling us with energy and deepening our most intimate connections.

The society we live in shapes and often limits our sexuality. Child-rearing practices, governmental policies, religion, images of girls and women in the media, male-centered medical views, powerful pharmaceutical companies, violence, and stereotypes based on aspects of ourselves, such as race, class, gender, age, disability, and sexual orientation—all these can affect how we experience our sexuality.

Even our sexual desires reflect social influences and contradictions. A particular sexual act may feel affirming in one situation but degrading in another. We might think that a man whistling at us on the street is crude, but also like the attention. We may think that pornographic magazines are harmful, but still find them enjoyable to look at. We may fantasize about sexual acts we would never wish to do.

It's important to talk with each other and work in our communities to redefine our sexuality according to our own pleasure and well-being.

GROWING UP

I watch my daughter. From morning to night, her body is her home. She lives in it and with it. When she runs around the kitchen, she uses all of herself. Every muscle in her body moves when she laughs, when she cries. When she rubs her vulva, there is no awkwardness, no feeling that what she is doing is wrong. She feels pleasure and expresses it without hesitation. She knows when she wants to be touched and when she wants to be left alone. It's so hard to get back that sense of body as home.

Childhood experiences shape our adult sexuality. Ideally, we grow up with adults who talk comfortably and openly about sex and respect our boundaries. If, as children or as teenage girls, we learn to think of sex as forbidden, dirty, and shameful, and if we experience sexual abuse, it may take years of positive experiences to heal our relationship with our bodies. (For more information on sexual abuse, see Chapter 8, "Violence and Abuse.")

BODY IMAGE*

We often see ourselves through the eyes of our families, lovers, coworkers, health care practitioners, athletic coaches, and others. Influenced by the images of girls and women in the media (magazines, music videos, TV, movies, advertisements, and the Internet), we may lose respect for our uniqueness, our own smells and shapes. We may judge ourselves. All this can affect our sexual lives.

For years I wouldn't make love in a position that exposed my backside to scrutiny, for I had been told it was "too jiggly." Needless to say, this prevented me from being sexually assertive and creative and limited my responses.

We have a good sex life with lots of variety, fantasies, games. The fact that my disability prevents me from bending my leg limits us in some positions, but we just try different ones. Yet I don't have orgasms with my husband, only in masturbation. I am still struggling with my body. When I am unclothed, I still feel like parts of me are really ugly. I think that when I can finish mourning and cry out my anguish over the disability, then sex will get better for me.

If we like the way we look and feel good about our bodies, we may feel better about making love.

One of the difficult things about being large is that more often than not, other people are the problem, not me. Many times I have felt that people I know wonder at my friendship with my lover. They wonder how a thin person can make love to a large one. The idea, I suppose, is that large women aren't attractive. Nonsense, of course. I enjoy my body immensely when I make love, either to my-

* See Chapter 1, "Body Image."

self or my boyfriend. I never think about my largeness. I simply am it and positively luxuriate in it. I love my body when I make love. It is beautiful to me and to my boyfriend. For six years, we have both exulted in good lovemaking.

STEREOTYPES

Media images perpetuate harmful stereotypes like the "Hot Tamale" Latina woman who is flirtatious and tough, the "Good Muslim Wife" who is repressed and subservient, or the African-American "Foxy Flygirl" who is sexy and seductive.[1] Such stereotypes often arise from contexts of racism and white dominance. During the enslavement of Africans in the U.S., for example, white owners and overseers raped the enslaved women freely, yet the stereotypes that developed at that time and continue to this day blamed the women rather than the white men who raped them. The image of the Asian woman as a "China Doll"—exotic, meek, and eager to please—grows out of and contributes to the sex tourism, sexual slavery, and forced prostitution that have developed in many Asian countries in response to U.S. militarism and global economic injustice. (For more on the international sexual exploitation of women, see p. 739.)

If we are lesbians, we may face stereotypes of being ugly, masculine, or aggressive. If we are bisexuals, we may be stereotyped as promiscuous for refusing to be boxed into an either/or definition of sexual attraction. Those of us who express sexuality openly may find ourselves called sluts. "Slut" is a slur that is also used against those of us who are "different" in ways that have nothing to do with sexuality at all.

These and other destructive stereotypes influence the ways we do or don't assert our desires and the ways that we judge ourselves and other women. They affect how others treat us, and when we internalize them and believe them, they affect how we treat ourselves. In reality, there are enormous differences in sexual experiences and attitudes among women within any racial, cultural, or sexual orientation identity. We can begin to free up the range of sexual values and expression available to *all* of us, by approaching one another with curiosity, to listen and learn.

POWER

Power differences often play out in sex, especially in our relationships with men, but also with women. Men as a group have more power in our society than women do; they may earn more than women for the same work, and they tend to hold more respected leadership positions in government, religion, and community. Even if we feel equal to a husband or male lover, the culture we live in often values men more. A female sexual partner may also have more "status" than we do due to her earning power, level of education, class, race, or other factors. This supposed superiority (though our partner may not feel superior at all) can surface in sex in the following ways:

- You should make love when s/he wants to, whether you're in the mood or not.
- You should make sure the kids don't interrupt while you are making love.
- You should have orgasms to show what a good lover s/he is.
- You shouldn't ask for what you want, especially if it's different from what your partner is doing.
- You shouldn't use a condom or a dental dam if it interferes with your partner's pleasure, even if this leaves you unprotected against sexually transmitted infections, including HIV.
- If you don't have intercourse with a man, you should help him have an orgasm to relieve him of his sexual tensions.
- You should take care of birth control if you're with a man, and you shouldn't use birth control at all if he doesn't want you to.

Becoming aware of such power dynamics is an important step toward developing respectful and mutually satisfying sexual relationships.

VIOLENCE AGAINST WOMEN*

It is a cruel fact of our lives that many women experience abuse—more often from men, but also from women. Childhood sexual abuse, rape by a date or partner or stranger, sexual harassment by a boss or coworker or teacher, battering in our homes: Any of these can affect our sexual lives. Even if we don't experience violence directly, the

* See Chapter 8, "Violence and Abuse."

possibility leers at us from pornography, news stories, movies, crude jokes, and so on.

Sometimes when I hear about a rape that's happened, I can't make love with my husband, even though I love him and usually enjoy sex. I know he is a gentle person, but for a moment I don't see him; I see all the men who use their penises as weapons to dominate and hurt women.

I went through several one-night stands and found that I did not have to love or really know the person to have sexual physical contact. In the past couple of years, I have wondered why this detachment exists. The therapy I went through clarified many things for me. I wondered how my sexual assault experiences had affected my sexuality. I find now that I am much more deliberate about my sexuality, about balancing pleasure and intimacy. I think I am still capable of detaching feelings from sex, but I choose not to anymore.

We must work for a just and nonviolent society in which sex is used not as an instrument of dominance but for consensual and mutual pleasure.

RELIGION AND SPIRITUALITY

Spirituality and religion can influence how we experience our sexuality. Many religions have teachings that prohibit certain sexual thoughts and behaviors, especially outside of monogamous heterosexual marriage. These can leave us with negative feelings about our bodies and sexuality. If we grew up in a religion in which spiritual "goodness" is associated with celibacy or the denial of sexual feelings, we may have come to believe that sexuality and spirituality are completely split.

I was taught to be ashamed of my body and that it is not all right for a single woman to desire sexual pleasure for any reason. I do not even masturbate, the way I've heard other women have, because I feel so guilty and ashamed if I bring myself pleasure. . . . I cannot seem to rid myself of that guilt/shame, and the "you aren't doing it right" voice.[2]

All through my teen years, [my] church leaders stressed sexual purity. . . . While I was busy staying sexually pure and modest, . . . I learned absolutely nothing about my body or how I felt sexually. The guilt and shame stopped me in my tracks, and this did not go away when I married. . . . [Recently] I spent a lot of time on a female-oriented sexuality website. . . . After immersing myself in all this female-friendly sexual literature, I finally got in touch with my sexuality and started enjoying sex.

I was raised in a strict Southern Baptist environment in a small town in southern Arkansas. I knew I was a lesbian at around 9 or 10 years old. Having repressed my sexuality until I was 28 was very hard. I had no role models to look to, growing up. In my mind, church and being a lesbian just did not go together. Now I know that sex can be a very spiritual, uplifting experience. I wish I experienced it more.

At the same time, some of us have found positive messages about our sexuality within organized religions.

I was raised in Roman Catholic schools forty to forty-five years ago. . . . I was taught that the body was the "temple of the Holy Spirit," and I thought then, as I think now, that having the spirit of God, however we each define God, dwelling within us is . . . beautiful.

Some of us leave our religions of origin because of the sexual prohibitions. Some seek out liberal congregations within our own denominations, and others seek denominations that are more sex-affirming. For example, Reconstructionist Jews, Unitarian Universalists, the United Church of Christ, Metropolitan Community Churches, and Quakers (Society of Friends) have a wider acceptance of women's roles and sexuality and may include female clergy and leaders, recognition of same-sex relationships, and comprehensive sexuality education.

Our sense of spirituality may exist within an organized religion or separate from it. Spirituality can include tapping into one's deepest self, creating a sacred bond with a friend or lover, developing a personal relationship with the divine or a higher power, feeling part of a community, and/or being connected to nature and all beings. Some of us are focusing on unifying sexuality and spirituality—finding the integration of body, mind, and spirit. Our bodies and sex can be sacred.

I have experienced sex as a gateway to the soul—my soul, the soul I am making love to and god and all that is—including spiritual guides. By experiencing sex as a spiritual tool, I have grown strong in intuitive and telepathic abilities, and grown closer and closer to god. More one-ness with All and more power to open doors to create what I choose.[3]

There is something extremely powerful in Spiritual Union, be it same-sex or opposite-sex union. Having experienced both, [I know that] each is an awe-inspiring experience in and of itself; both awaken you to new depths and levels of your body, spirit, love, and existence.

There are many paths to sacred sexuality. A recent survey found that the connection of sexuality and spirituality for women often occurs in relationships with some degree of commitment and is facilitated by self-esteem, intense sensuality, being in love, and sharing deep feelings.[4] Drawing upon ancient cultures in which women's bodies, sexuality, and fertility were honored as an integrated part of nature and life, some of us have found wisdom and strength in connecting sexually with a partner and a divine feminine energy. Others have turned to tantra, an Eastern spiritual philosophy, to explore sexual practices that focus on the interconnectedness of life. By investigating sensations of touch and breathing, creating rituals, and paying attention to subtle energies, we can create a sacred connection with our partner(s) and higher power(s). (For more on tantra, see "Anand" in "Resources.")

SEXUAL PLEASURE

Women experience sexual pleasure in many different ways: physically, emotionally, spiritually, and intellectually. We may enjoy a gentle caress, an erotic dance, or a sweaty orgasm. Traditionally, male researchers' descriptions of sexual pleasure have focused on genital sensations and stages of physical arousal. But pleasure and eroticism are much more than these. Sounds, tastes, sights, smells, emotions, and touch can arouse our sexual feelings, as can fantasies, an engaging conversation, a favorite song, writing a poem, or the sensation of wearing a slinky dress. The erotic can be a source of power and information for us as we access our deepest feelings and creative energies in all aspects of our lives.*

Sexual pleasure is a universal human right. For more information, see the Declaration of Sexual Rights at www.worldsexology.org.

DESIRE

Sexual desires can be a source of pleasure at any age. In our teen years, most of us learn that we are supposed to make ourselves beautiful and sexy in order to become objects of (boys')

desire—but not to enjoy our bodies, not to have desires ourselves. We may come to fear that if we have desires, they will automatically lead us into risky sexual behaviors that will, in turn, lead us into danger—unwanted pregnancy, forced sex, sexually transmitted infections.[5] Yet when we become aware of our desires, we can choose whether and how to act on them. Perhaps we will masturbate, fantasize, write erotic stories, dance, express them with a partner, or just simply notice them.

VARIATIONS IN DESIRE

We may have ideas about how much desire we think we "should" have. Many movies, television shows, and magazines portray women as highly sexual. Drug companies and the popular media capitalize on these images and bombard us with messages about how to increase our sexual appetites. While these portrayals are accurate for some of us, they represent only a narrow slice of the wide range of women's experiences. Paradoxically, while desire is supposed to be undetectable in *girls,* pharmaceutical companies (and medical researchers often hired by those companies) have begun to define low sexual desire in *women* as a medical disorder deserving of medical treatment. Yet what they label a disorder may in fact be a variation in sexual desire.

Thanks to feminist researchers such as Leonore Tiefer and other authors of *A New View of Women's Sexual Problems,*† we can resist the attempt to medicalize sexual desire. While affirming that certain medications can help some women with sexual problems caused by specific physiological conditions, *A New View* names a whole range of causes for women's sexual problems: sociocultural, political or economic, relationship-based, psychological, or medical.

---

* See Audre Lorde's "Uses of the Erotic" in "Resources."

† See "Resources," and the following website: www.fsd-alert.org/manifesto.html.

Moving beyond the strictly physical, the book defines women's sexual problems broadly as "discontent or dissatisfaction with any emotional, physical or relationship aspect of sexual experience."[6] (For more information, see "Female Sexual Dysfunction: A Feminist View" [W29] on the companion website, www.ourbodiesourselves.org.)

If we apply this broader view to the question of sexual desire, we see that in much of the world, women do not have full access to services crucial to our enjoyment of sex—sexuality education, protection from unwanted pregnancy and sexually transmitted infections, and legal abortion when we need it. We may have learned that sex is intended for reproduction only, not for pleasure. We may feel physically or emotionally unsafe. We may have been sexually abused and find that certain situations bring up frightening memories. We may work so hard, or be so engaged in some other creative pursuit, that we do not have much time or energy for sex. Or we just might not feel like having sex, period. Not feeling sexual is not necessarily pathological.*

In a relationship, there may be a "discrepancy" or difference in sexual desire, where one partner has a higher level of desire than the other, creating tension for the couple.

I want sex a lot more often than my husband does. I try not to take it personally when he says no, but sometimes it hurts. I feel rejected. The images on television and in the movies and the jokes that circulate on the Internet always show the man wanting sex more than the woman. Women who want more sex are "nymphomaniacs." It's insult-

ing. And sometimes I wonder if there is something wrong with me. However, when I check in with my friends, they're often experiencing the same thing. Being really horny at 30-something is normal, and it's also really hard. I wish more people would talk about it.

For some couples, a desire discrepancy may be simply the result of different preferences and bodily rhythms. We, along with our partners, can seek to bridge these differences by communicating clearly, learning about our own and each other's needs, and taking responsibility for finding the middle ground. For other couples, the discrepancy may be due to lack of attraction, or to problems in the relationship that need attending to.

A discrepancy of desire may exist in male/female relationships because men are "supposed" to know more about sex, to initiate it, to have a stronger sex drive. Women are "supposed" to be passive recipients. According to the Mars-Venus framework, men want sex, and we want love. Such generalizations are false and damaging. Perhaps what's at issue is not male sex drive but the fact that men are raised with different ways of expressing their emotions. Sexual intercourse is one of the few permissible ways for a man to be close to someone. For many men, it is the only acceptable place for their tender, loving feelings. It may be this limitation, rather than a greater sex drive, that prompts many men to initiate intercourse often, and leads to the stereotype that women are less sexual than men. The stereotype may also arise from deep cultural fears of women's sexual passion and power.

We may need to change how we think about desire. Traditionally, desire has been understood as a spontaneous motivation to have sex. More recent models point to an important component of a woman's desire as willingness or arousability. Particularly in long-term relationships, we may find that exploring intimacy with our part-

---

* For a few of us, conflicts about ourselves and sex are so deep that we are never interested in sex. We may feel an extreme, unpleasant sensitivity to touch, or we may feel so ticklish that we can't relax. Our bodies are reacting this way for a reason—they are protecting us from sexual experiences we can't handle at this point. This may well be a time to look for professional help (see "AASECT" in "Resources").

ner(s) can help us move toward physical arousal even if initially we do not crave sex.[7]

SEXUAL AROUSAL AND RESPONSE

When we act on our sexual desires, we may become sexually aroused and go through a series of physical and emotional changes, sometimes called *sexual response.*

When I'm feeling turned on, either alone or with someone I'm attracted to, my heart beats faster, my face gets red, my eyes are bright. My whole vulva feels wet and full. My breasts hum. When I'm standing up, I feel a rush of weakness in my thighs. When I'm lying down, I may feel like doing a big stretch, arching my back, feeling the sensations go out to my fingers and toes.

The most important part of sexual response is what feels good, what works, what makes us feel more alive in ourselves and connected with a partner. There is no one "right" pattern of sexual response. Our patterns will change at different points in our lives.

Despite the wide variations among women, sex researchers have tried to develop models to describe women's sexual responses.[8] In the 1960s, the researchers William Masters and Virginia Johnson observed and measured women and men engaging in sexual activities in a laboratory setting, and reported their research in *Human Sexual Response.* By choosing to focus their study on people who were very experienced with orgasm during masturbation and intercourse, Masters and Johnson missed the fact that women with different patterns could also be satisfied and happy. As a result, their work reinforced a belief that orgasm and intercourse are necessary to human sexual response. Thus, while the work was valuable for women in exploring

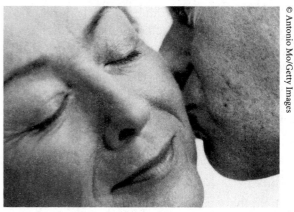

the role of the clitoris in sexual response, it had significant limits.[9] In the 1970s, for example, feminist researcher Shere Hite polled several hundred women and discovered that most of them did not reach orgasm through intercourse alone.[10] In the 1970s and 1980s, several researchers and clinicians such as Helen Singer Kaplan[11] and Bernie Zilbergeld and Carol Rinkleib Ellisons[12] expanded on the Masters and Johnson model. They included emotional aspects of sexual response, such as desire, arousal, and satisfaction.

Despite the limitations of the Masters and Johnson model even as it has been revised, psychiatric and medical clinicians, along with pharmaceutical companies, continue to use it to create definitions of sexual health and sexual problems. For a critical alternative, see *A New View of Women's Sexual Problems,* mentioned on p. 191, which includes the relational aspects of women's sexuality and allows for a wide range of differences among women's experiences.

TWO MODELS FOR WOMEN'S SEXUAL AROUSAL AND RESPONSE

It can be helpful to understand the Masters and Johnson model, not as a standard that we should try to follow, but because aspects of it may fit our experience, and because so many clinicians still use it. The model outlines four stages of physiological arousal: excitement, plateau, climax, and resolution. (For anatomy details, and drawings that may help you understand these stages, see Chapter 13, "Sexual Anatomy, Reproduction, and the Menstrual Cycle.") In sexual *excitement,* our whole pelvic area may feel full, as erectile tissue in the pelvis, vulva, and clitoris swells with blood, and nerves in that area become more sensitive to stimulation and pressure. In the vagina, this increased blood circulation produces the fluid that makes the vaginal walls and inner lips get wet—often an early sign that we are sexually excited. (In women who are past menopause, there may not be much lubrication.) Sexual tension rises throughout the body as muscles begin to contract. We may breathe more quickly, our nipples may become erect and hard, and a flush or rash may appear on our skin.

If stimulation continues, we move into what Masters and Johnson called the *plateau* stage. The responses may continue to intensify as the vagina becomes more sensitive and the clitoris retracts under its hood. With enough stimulation of or around the clitoris and (for some women) pressure on the cervix or other sensitive areas, we may build up to a peak, or *climax.* Orgasm is the point at which all the tension suddenly releases in a series of involuntary and pleasurable muscular contractions. We may feel contractions in the vagina, uterus, and rectum. Many women experience orgasm as a total-body release. If stimulation doesn't continue, we enter the *resolution* stage: During the half hour or more after climax, the muscles relax, and the clitoris, vagina, and uterus return to their usual positions (except in the rare disorder known as persistent sexual arousal syndrome).[13]

In her book *Women Who Love Sex,* sex therapist Gina Ogden offers a very different model.[14] Ogden visualizes sexual response as "three dancing spheres of energy": pleasure, orgasm, and ecstasy. We may experience pleasure without orgasm or orgasm without ecstasy, and so on. In some cases, we may experience all three. Our sexual responses are linked to intimacy, lust, fantasy, full-body stimulation, satisfaction, and more. In addition to explaining physical and emotional responses, Ogden explores the spiritual aspects of sex. She observes that ecstasy can be a transcendent experience that is also rooted deeply in the body, and suggests that it may be more easily described in poetic or mystical language than in physiological terms.

We do not have to rely exclusively on "experts" for accurate information about our sexuality. If the models proposed by sexologists and researchers (*or* feminists) don't fit our experiences, then we must trust ourselves and learn more from each other. We can obtain powerful data by discussing our experiences in settings of our own making. In some cases, this information can be enhanced by respectful research that attempts scientifically to record and measure our experiences.

ORGASM

For some of us, orgasm is a special source of sexual pleasure. It can be mild, like a hiccup, a sneeze, a ripple, or a peaceful sigh; it can be a sensuous experience, as the body glows with warmth; it can be intensely physical or even ecstatic, as we lose awareness of ourselves for a time. Orgasm can be primarily physical but usually has emotional aspects as well. Feelings of intimacy can enhance our orgasms with a partner, and orgasms can enhance intimacy. Orgasm may feel totally different at different times, even with the same person, and different when we masturbate or make love. It may feel different with a finger, fist, penis, or dildo in the vagina, or a vibrator on the clitoris.

Masters and Johnson asserted that all female orgasms are physiologically the same (brought about through stimulation of the clitoris, with contractions occurring primarily in the outer third of the vagina). Yet some women describe orgasms that don't fit this model. One such orgasm is brought on by penetration of the vagina and feels "deep" or "uterine." The buildup may involve a prolonged involuntary holding of breath, which is released explosively at orgasm, and there do not seem to be any contractions of the outer third of the vagina. Some women with spinal cord injuries, who have no feeling in the pelvic area, report experiencing orgasm and its sensations elsewhere in the body (see "Sex and Disability," p. 215). Women without physical disabilities may also experience such extragenital sensations.

Women have the potential to respond to sexual arousal throughout the entire body and especially the pelvic region. When the muscles around the outer third of the vagina (pubococcygeus muscles) are strong and well exercised, many women find it easier to reach orgasm (see "Kegel exercises," p. 235).

Farther up in the vagina are the *cervix* and *uterus*, which some women find crucial to orgasm. Women who have had a total hysterectomy, in which the cervix and the uterus have been removed, may have to learn to focus on different kinds of sexual stimulation and feelings.

For many women, the *clitoris* is the organ that is the most sensitive to stimulation and has a central role in elevating feelings of sexual tension. Although it's sometimes called "the joy button," the clitoris is actually much more than a single spot. (For a complete description of the clitoris, see Chapter 13, "Sexual Anatomy, Reproduction, and the Menstrual Cycle.")

Some of us may not have our full clitoris intact due to a clitoridectomy (see "Female Genital Cutting [Circumcision]" on p. 209), an accident, or sex reassignment surgery. Although certain types of touch or movement may be painful, we may still have the capacity to experience great pleasure and even orgasm. The removal of the outer portion of the clitoris does not reduce the expansive network of erectile tissues, glands, muscles, and nerves that allow us to feel sexual pleasure. And, of course, genital surgery does not prevent our ability to fantasize and get turned on by our thoughts and feelings.

You or your lover can stimulate your clitoris in many different ways—by rubbing, sucking, stroking, kissing, body pressure, or using a vibrator. Any rubbing or pressure in the pubic-hair-covered mons area or the vaginal lips (even on the lower abdomen and inner thighs) can move the clitoris and may also press it up against the pubic bone (see "Learning to Masturbate," p. 199).

Searching for the one and only "right" model of women's orgasm does not reflect the diversity of women's experiences.

The way I've heard about orgasms is there's supposed to be a big release, but that's not the way it works for me. I feel a really intense buildup that feels great, and then suddenly, my clitoris becomes too sensitive to keep stimulating, so I stop. I no longer have a desire to keep going, and I just feel relaxed and tired, in a good way. I always wonder, did I miss the climax? Or was that not really an orgasm?

If we become aroused at a time when we can't get enough stimulation to reach orgasm, sexual tension will subside eventually without orgasm, though it takes longer, and our genitals and/or uterus may ache for a while.

Some women reach orgasm once, some twice or more in quick succession. Knowing that multiple orgasms are possible has made some of us feel we ought to have them and that we are sexually inadequate if we don't. Men may expect it, too; yet one orgasm can be plenty, and sex without orgasm can be pleasurable. It's important that orgasm doesn't become one more performance pressure.

When I try too hard to have an orgasm, it usually doesn't work and I end up frustrated and bored. For me, it's best if I relax and let it happen if it's going to.

At the same time, we can learn how to have orgasms, how to increase our capacity for more and longer ones. We can think of orgasm as a skill we can learn, an ability that we can expand and enhance.

PROBLEMS WITH ORGASM*

Quite a number of women have never had an orgasm or have difficulty reaching one. Sometimes we just need more information. Sometimes shame about exploring and touching our bodies may keep us from learning to bring ourselves to orgasm through masturbation. Sexual, physical, or emotional abuse (past or present) may also impair our ability to have orgasms. If we have been sexually abused in the past, sexual arousal may restimulate mental and/or physical memories of the abuse, and we may experience fear, terror, flashbacks, even a loss of sensation sometimes called sexual anesthesia; physically, we may have an aching sensation, discomfort, or even pain (see Chapter 8, "Violence and Abuse").

If we want to explore how to have an orgasm, we can try it through masturbating (see p. 197), using a vibrator, reading books or watching a video about it (see "Resources"), asking a partner to help, or joining a therapy group focused on sexual issues.

With a partner, here are some problems that may get in the way of having an orgasm:

- We don't notice or we misunderstand what's happening in our body as we get aroused.
- We're too busy thinking about how to do it right, why it doesn't go well for us, what our

lover thinks of us, whether our lover is impatient, whether our lover can last.
- We are afraid of asking for too much and seeming too demanding.
- We are afraid that if our lover concentrates on our pleasure, we will feel such pressure to come that we won't be able to—and then we don't.
- We are trying to have simultaneous orgasms, which seldom occur for most of us.
- We are in conflict about, or angry with, our sexual partner.
- We feel guilty about having sex and so cannot let ourselves really enjoy it.
- We, or our partner, think that women should have orgasm through penetration of the vagina, and that isn't working for us.
- We have fallen into a pattern of "faking" orgasm to please a partner or to get it over with.

Not being able to reach orgasm with a partner may be a clue that the relationship itself has problems and needs to change in some way. It may also be that our partner(s) need to learn more about women's sexual arousal and response—or that we do! Or perhaps we and our partner(s) would benefit from learning how to communicate better about sex (see p. 213).

G-SPOT AND FEMALE EJACULATION†

A lesser known part of the clitoral system is the *G-spot*,[15] or the *urethral sponge*, which is the erectile tissue surrounding the urethra (the tube through which we urinate). Sometimes called the female prostate, the urethral sponge is filled with blood vessels and glands; it produces a fluid similar to that produced by the male prostate.

---

* See L. G. Barbach's *For Yourself: The Fulfillment of Female Sexuality*, in "Resources."

† For more on the G-spot and female ejaculation, see Deborah Sundahl's *Female Ejaculation and the G-spot* in "Resources."

The G-spot can often be felt by pressing on the interior front wall of the vagina, and it may produce pleasurable sensations when stimulated.

For some women, continuous stimulation of the G-spot may lead to *ejaculation:* the release of fluid from the urethra. Some people doubt the existence of female ejaculation, but from ancient Greek writings to the Hindu *Kama Sutra* to sixteenth-century Japanese artwork, female ejaculation has been described and honored.

Female ejaculation can bring a wonderful feeling of release and pleasure. It can occur with or without an orgasm. Ejaculation can also occur without stimulation of the G-spot, through other methods of arousal. Some of us may have ejaculated without realizing what it was, or we may have mistakenly thought that we peed. Although ejaculate is released through the urethra, the fluid is different from urine. It consists of prostatic fluid mixed with glucose and trace amounts of urine. It can be clear or creamy, and the smell and taste may vary during our menstrual cycle. (Note: If you are ejaculating with a partner, remember that HIV can be transmitted through vaginal secretions, including female ejaculate. If you are HIV-positive or think you could be, practice safer sex when ejaculating with a partner: Ejaculate away from your partner's body to avoid mixing your bodily fluids with your partner's; also, have a partner wear latex gloves for penetration and a male partner wear a condom during intercourse.)

MASTURBATION

Masturbation—touching ourselves sexually—is one way of exploring and enjoying sexual pleasure. When we were infants, touching and playing with our bodies, including our genitals, felt good. Then some of us learned from our parents, and later from our schools and religious institutions, that we were not to touch ourselves sexually. Some of us heeded their messages, and some did not. But by the time we became teenagers, many of us thought masturbation was bad, whether we did it or not. Others never discovered masturbation at all.

I never even knew about masturbation. When I was 21, a man friend touched me "down there," bringing me to orgasm (I didn't know that word, either). Then I had a brilliant thought—if he could do it to me, I could do it to me, too. So I did,

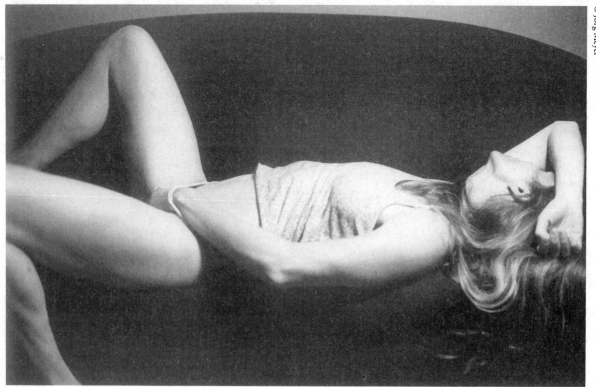

though it was a long time before I could feel a lot of pleasure and orgasm.

Masturbation allows us the time and space to explore and experiment with our own bodies. We can learn what fantasies turn us on, what kinds of touch arouse and please us, what tempo and where. We can learn our own patterns of sexual response without having to think about a partner's needs and opinions. Then, if and when we choose, we can tell our partners what we've learned or show them by guiding their hands to the places we want touched. We can achieve freedom by knowing how to give ourselves sexual pleasure. We become less dependent on our partners to satisfy us, which can give them freedom, too. Through learning to pleasure ourselves, we are more likely to be satisfied with our sex lives overall, and to reach orgasm more

easily alone or with a partner. Some women may even experience masturbation as a spiritual experience—a unification of mind, body, and spirit, or a connection with the divine.[16]

I used to think masturbating was okay only if I didn't have a lover and only for a quick release. Now I see it's part of my relationship with myself, giving myself pleasure. My rhythms change. Sometimes I masturbate more when I have a lover. Sometimes I'll go for weeks without doing it.

After menopause, especially if we aren't having partner sex, masturbating helps keep our vaginal tissues moist.

For me at 73, masturbation is better than a sexual relationship, as most of the time, I'm more interested in nonsexual pursuits. Sustaining a relationship with all the time and thought involved would be a nuisance.

LEARNING TO MASTURBATE*

If you have never masturbated and want to, you may feel awkward or self-conscious, even a bit scared at first. You may have to contend with voices within you that repeat "Nice girls don't" or "A happily married woman wouldn't want to." You may fear losing control of yourself, or you may feel shy or guilty about giving yourself sexual pleasure. Many of us have these feelings, but they can change in time.

Some suggestions: Find a quiet time when you can be by yourself without interruption. Make yourself as comfortable as possible: You are expecting a lover, and that lover is you! Take a relaxing bath or shower. Rub your body all over with cream, lotion, oil, or anything else that feels good. Slowly explore the shape of your body with your eyes and hands. Touch yourself in different ways. Put on music you like, keep the lights soft, light a candle if you want to. Think about people or situations you find sexually arousing. Read some erotica if you wish. Let your mind flow freely into fantasy. Let your body relax. Of course, such a relaxed and special atmosphere isn't always possible—or necessary! Desire can overtake us at the most unexpected moments. We can find ourselves sexually aroused and masturbate while cooking a meal, working at a desk, riding a horse or bicycle, or gardening.

Women have many ways of masturbating. We can moisten our fingers (with saliva, fluid from the vagina, or a lubricant) and rub them around and over the clitoris. We can gently rub or pull; we can rub the hood or a larger area around the clitoris. We can use one finger or several. We can rub up and down and around and around, and

try different kinds of pressure and timing. The clitoris is exquisitely sensitive, and for many of us, direct touching or rubbing of the glans (or tip) is painful; indirect or intermittent touching of the glans may be more pleasurable. As women grow older, the hood of skin covering the glans may pull back permanently, so if you are past menopause, you may need extra lubrication in order to tolerate having your clitoris rubbed.

Some of us masturbate by crossing our legs and exerting steady and rhythmic pressure on the whole genital area. We may use a vibrator. We may insert something into the vagina—a finger, a cucumber (room-temperature and peeled), or a dildo. A finger in the anus may stimulate some of us. (To avoid causing a bacterial infection, wash your finger before touching your vagina.) We may rub our breasts or other body parts and play with tension and relaxation.

At 16, I gave up masturbation for Lent. Since I defined masturbation only as touching my genitals in a sexual way, in those six weeks, I learned that I could have wonderful orgasms through a mixture of fantasy and quietly tensing up and relaxing the muscles around my vagina and vulva.

Still other ways of masturbating include using a pillow instead of your hands, a stream of water, or an electric vibrator. (Vibrators are sold at many drugstores, often as body or neck massagers. There are also many sex-positive companies that provide information as well as discreet service. For mail-order catalogs, see "Resources.")

I can direct our shower nozzle so the water hits my clitoris in a steady stream. I have a real relationship with that shower! I wouldn't give it up for anything. It's nice when I get up for work and don't have time for sex with my lover but do have a little time for the shower. Those few minutes are real important for me.

---

* See books and videos by Betty Dodson and L. G. Barbach in "Resources." Also see "G-spot and Female Ejaculation," p. 196.

Women experience a variety of sensations and feelings when masturbating. As you get sexually aroused, your vagina may become moist. Experiment with what you can do to feel even more: Open your mouth, breathe faster, make noise if you want to, or move your pelvis rhythmically to your breathing and voice. As you become more aroused, you may feel your muscles tighten, and your pelvic area may feel warm and full.

For me, the most pleasurable part is just before orgasm. I feel I am no longer consciously controlling my body. I know there is no way I will not reach orgasm now. I stop trying. I like to savor this rare moment of true letting go!

It's this letting go of control that enables us to have orgasms. If you do not reach orgasm when you first try masturbating, don't worry. Simply enjoy the sensations. Try again some other time.

Masturbating opens me to what is happening in my body and makes me feel good about myself. I like following the impulse of the moment. Sometimes I have many orgasms; sometimes I don't. The greatest source of pleasure is to be able to do whatever feels good to me at that particular time. I rarely have such complete freedom in other aspects of my life.

Not everyone enjoys masturbating.

I have tried masturbating because I read about it, not out of natural desire. Sometimes it seems like a chore. I feel like I should take the time to explore my body, but I quit after a few minutes because, quite frankly, I'm bored. It just doesn't seem to have the effect another person would.

If masturbating doesn't bring you pleasure, trust your own preferences and don't do it.

MEDICATIONS, HORMONES, AND SEXUALITY*

MEDICATIONS

Certain medications can play a role in sexual desire, as well as in the likelihood and intensity of orgasm. If you are taking a prescription drug or herbal supplement and notice a change in your sexual functioning, there may be a connection. Antidepressants, in particular, are known to affect sexual functioning sometimes.

When I got in a relationship, I found that some of the sexual side effects [of taking Prozac] are more subtle. I found that while I still experienced desire, it has become really difficult to have an orgasm. And when I do, the quality is different. In the old days, I felt a slow buildup that ended with intense, sudden contractions; now I most often feel a wave of excitement that ebbs and flows but never quite peaks in the same way.

Some SSRI antidepressants (selective serotonin reuptake inhibitors) such as Prozac, Paxil, and Zoloft may reduce sexual desire and the ability to orgasm. However, other antidepressants, such as Wellbutrin (bupropion), have been shown to cause less sexual dysfunction than SSRIs (some women even report an increase in sexual desire). Adjustments in drug dosage sometimes affect sexual side effects. (For more on antidepressants, see Chapter 6, "Emotional Well-Being.")

HORMONES

Estrogen, progesterone, and testosterone are hormones that affect a woman's sexual desire

---

* For more information, see Elizabeth Davis, *Women, Sex, and Desire: Understanding Your Sexuality at Every Stage of Life*, in "Resources" on the companion website, www.ourbodiesourselves.org.

and functioning. In terms of sexual desire, the most influential hormone is testosterone, sometimes called the "libido" or "male" hormone. In fact, testosterone, like estrogen, is present in both men *and* women, though the proportions differ between the sexes. In women, testosterone is produced through the operation of the adrenals (two small glands near the kidneys) and the ovaries.

Many factors affect our hormone levels at any given time, including the following:

1. *The menstrual cycle.* Hormone levels fluctuate throughout our cycle. Many women who menstruate have a peak of sexual desire (libido) before and around ovulation, with a second, less intense peak during menstruation. Many women's lowest level of libido is prior to menstruation, although there is much variation from this pattern. Postmenopausal women, and many women using hormonal birth control methods, have less variation in sexual desire. (For more on hormones in the menstrual cycle, see Chapter 13, "Sexual Anatomy, Reproduction, and the Menstrual Cycle.")

2. *The Pill and other hormonal birth control methods* such as the "patch" (e.g., Ortho Evra), injectable contraceptives (e.g., Depo-Provera), and the vaginal ring (NuvaRing). Some hormonal birth control methods suppress the usual cyclical nature of our hormones and may affect our desire and sexual functioning.[17] Some women may have less desire, reach orgasm less easily, and/or experience vaginal dryness. The specific effects of these methods vary greatly among individual women.

3. *Pregnancy.* Estrogen and progesterone levels are higher during pregnancy, and blood flow to the genitals increases. These changes, along with other physical and psychological effects of pregnancy, may lead to increased desire for some

women. For others, however, fatigue, nausea, pain, fears, or issues with changing body size and self-image may squelch desire. (See "Sandra Margot" in "Resources.")

4. *Nursing.* Breast-feeding can suppress ovulation for months after the birth of your baby, as a result of the high levels of the hormone prolactin and reduced levels of estrogen. Many women report a drop in sexual desire while nursing. Some have no libido at all and become nonorgasmic. This is normal during breast-feeding; libido will return when the baby is weaned or nursing much less. This normal postpartum variation in desire can be stressful to our intimate relationships.

5. *Menopause.* Estrogen and testosterone levels drop during and after menopause. We may experience less desire and increased vaginal dryness. For some of us, relief from the fear of pregnancy may allow newfound sexual freedom. (For more on menopause, see Chapter 26, "Midlife and Menopause.")

6. *Adrenal or ovary removal (oophorectomy).* These surgeries may result in a dramatic decrease in sexual interest and frequency of orgasm, in part due to a reduction of testosterone.[18] This is one of many reasons for avoiding unnecessary removal of the ovaries or adrenals.

Hormonal changes and their effects on sexual desire and functioning are not necessarily a problem. Menstrual and menopausal changes, for example, are a normal part of a woman's development. However, if a hormonal change leads to a drop in our desire or sexual pleasure, and we feel dissatisfied with this, we may want to explore our options. We may want to change or alter medications or a birth control method. Some women have turned to hormonal supplements, such as estrogen or estrogen/progestin pills and patches, or estrogen cream applied topically in the vagina. (For more about the risks and benefits of hormonal products, see Chapter 26, "Midlife and Menopause.")

There is some evidence that testosterone supplements may increase sexual arousal and desire in women who have had an oophorectomy (removal of ovary/ovaries) or hysterectomy (removal of uterus),[19] but there is a great need for more research on this hormone. Testosterone supplements, which may come in a pill, patch, or gel, were developed to help men and have not been approved by the Food and Drug Administration (FDA) for use by women. Though doctors can still legally prescribe such drugs to women (known as "off-label use"), the doctors must guess at the right dosage or use a special compounding pharmacy that will mix lower-dose products for women. Even for men, the efficacy and safety of testosterone supplements have been called into question.[20] Furthermore, the side effects of testosterone supplements can include hair growth, muscle mass increase, and deepening of the voice.

Pharmaceutical companies have rushed to develop other types of medical products to address women's problems with sexual desire and functioning.[21] For a while, they tested some drugs originally created for men, but the results have been disappointing so far. Examples of drugs now sold to men to address impotence problems include Viagra (sildenafil), Levitra (vardenafil), and Cialis (tadalafil); nonprescription remedies such as Zestra (which contains herbal oils) and ArginMax (an amino acid); and vibrating apparatuses such as Eros. These are all designed to increase blood flow to the genital areas. It is not clear how safe or effective these products are for women.

It's important to remember that variations in our sexual desire and pleasure may not be medical disorders at all; they may arise from many factors in our lives (see *A New View of Women's Sexual Problems* in "Resources"). Some women have had good results with hormonal or other pharmaceutical solutions, while others have experienced no improvement or even harmful side effects. Research continues to evolve in this area, and it is prudent to investigate the latest data available.

SEXUAL EXPRESSION

VIRGINITY

A virgin traditionally is someone who hasn't had sexual intercourse. Although both men and women are virgins before they have had sex, the main pressure to be a virgin has been on women. Today there are conflicting pressures about virginity.

My mother told me it's a gift I can give only once, so I'd better hold on to it.

Among my girlfriends during senior year of high school, I was the only virgin. This caused me embarrassment and teasing from my friends. I was branded as a nice girl, chicken, weird, etc., even though I did all the same things they did except have sex.

Whether virginity is revered or denigrated, judging girls and women solely on the basis of our sexual behavior limits who we are.

Young women experiencing pressure to be sexually active need accurate, comprehensive sex education to help us decide what we want. We may choose to abstain from intercourse or other sexual activities because we are not ready, we are not with the right partner, or we are concerned about sexually transmitted infections or pregnancy. We also may choose abstinence because of our religious beliefs or because we are focused on developing other aspects of our lives.

We must be free to have sex or not, as we think best. Having sex usually changes a relationship. It makes sense to think about this decision, talk it over with people we trust, choose a method of birth control if necessary, and learn how to protect ourselves from sexually transmitted infections. We have the right to say no to someone who is pushing us to have sex when we don't want to.

(For more on this topic, see *Changing Bodies, Changing Lives* in "Resources.")

CELIBACY

Traditionally, celibacy has meant choosing not to marry. Today many people use it to mean not having sex with a partner for a certain period of time, and sometimes no masturbation as well. Sometimes we choose celibacy in response to our culture's overemphasis on sex, as a break from feeling we must relate to others sexually all the time: "I was tired of having to say yes or no." It can be a personal adventure.

I'm exploring myself as a sexual person but in a different way. My sensitivity to my body is heightened. I am more aware of what arouses my sensual interests. I am free to be myself. I have more energy for work and friends. My spirituality feels more intense and clear.

I spend part of each day in yoga and meditation. Sometimes I go for days without thinking about my sexual identity at all. I masturbate only when inspired, which is seldom these days. Yet in meditation last week, I found myself having an orgasm. It was ecstasy!

In couple relationships, we may choose celibacy when we want some distance or solitude or when we just don't want to have sex for a while. This can require careful communication.

I say to my woman lover, "I don't feel like making love this month, and I may not next month."
Now, who does that? Is it okay? Am I allowed? The last thing we were ever taught was that it was okay to try what we want.

Some couples choose celibacy together. It can help us get out of old sexual patterns, expand our sensual/sexual focus beyond genital sex, and make us feel more self-sufficient and independent, which can strengthen the relationship.

Having a new baby may enforce a time of virtual celibacy. Sometimes we are faced with celibacy when we don't choose it—after a breakup or divorce; when a partner or lover dies or is separated from us; or during a dry spell. Though these circumstances may be painful, celibacy can surprise us with its own satisfactions.

LOVEMAKING*

Lovemaking or partner sex allows for endless possibilities: massaging, hugging, licking, kissing, caressing, biting, rimming (oral to anal stimulation), direct clitoral stimulation, oral sex, vaginal or anal penetration, intercourse, nipple stimulation, fisting, playing with power and roles, tribadism (rubbing a body part against your partner's genitals), erotic talk, or sleeping together without genital sex.

Sex with another person can be extremely pleasurable, but we also may bring certain experiences or assumptions with us into lovemaking that make it difficult to enjoy ourselves. For example, many of us have experienced the fear of being assaulted or have perceived our sexuality as dangerous, even if we have not experienced abuse. This fear may crop up in our intimate relationships. Even with a partner who would

* For more on sexual techniques, see *The Good Vibrations Guide to Sex* in "Resources."

never dream of harming us, a sudden touch or grabbing of the genitals may trigger what some call the "sexual alarm system"[22] and cause us to tense up. We may have to show our partner how to "disarm" the system, by warming up with nongenital touch, intimate conversation, or relaxation.

Whether we make love with a man or a woman, it is important to plan for safer sex. (For more information on enjoying sex and staying healthy, see Chapter 14, "Safer Sex.")

(For personal descriptions of how sex can change throughout the years and in long-term relationships, see "A Lifetime of Sexual Relationships" [W30] on the companion website, www .ourbodiesourselves.org.)

TOUCHING AND SENSUALITY

Massages, backrubs, stroking—these are wonderful at any time. As part of lovemaking, they can make sex slower and more sensual.

Eric likes me to nibble his feet and suck his toes. I think that gives him as much pleasure or more than anything else we do in sex.

Tender touching can be a way of making love.

We always sleep right up next to each other naked. There's always a lot of touching and feeling, so even though we don't have intercourse that often, I consider us having sex all the time.

I yearn to feel the crook of her arm under my neck as I sleep. I long to stroke her face and enjoy how good it feels to wake up with her arms around me in the morning. The heat and passion of sex is great, but I think that a gentle caress is more personal. That's what I crave most right now.

When a couple has problems in sex, it may turn out that they have been focusing on each other's genitals and not taking time or learning how to touch and stroke each other lovingly all over. Many men are more focused on genitals than women are and need to learn the pleasures of touching.

One lover told me with great puzzlement at first that I made love slower than any woman he knew, and he didn't just mean it took me a long time to come. Later, he got used to my "style" and said he liked it.

It took making love with women for me to see that all the other things—oral sex, having my breasts sucked, rolling around or just lying still and feeling the sensations, touching my lover and turning her on—all these are lovemaking for me. Now, when I make love with men, I do it more like making love with a woman—slower, more sensually and tenderly, sometimes without penetration at all.

The hour or so after active lovemaking can be a special time.

After sex we talk tenderly, laugh deeply, whisper, cry, sleep like babies in each other's arms. Some of the most important conversations in our relationship have come in those satisfied and intimate moments.

LOVEMAKING WITH A MAN

Most people learn to define sex between a woman and a man mainly in terms of intercourse.

I have orgasms easily during intercourse. Sometimes I love his thrusting deep inside me. Sometimes I don't want the penetration, I want something else. But he feels [that] if we haven't had intercourse, we haven't actually made love.

I feel shy to ask for more foreplay when I know what he's really waiting for is the fucking.

Intercourse is a form of lovemaking that is often well suited to men's orgasm and pleasure but not necessarily well suited to ours. Vagina-to-penis intercourse may give only indirect clitoral stimulation. To reach orgasm during vagina-to-penis intercourse, many of us need direct and sometimes prolonged clitoral stimulation both before and during intercourse. Many women with male partners who get infrequent erections find that sexual pleasure actually increases, partly because penetration by the penis is no longer the focus of lovemaking.

Standard male definitions call all the touching, licking, sucking, and caressing that turns us on "foreplay" to the big act—intercourse. But "outercourse," all the other stuff that we do in bed, can be as important as intercourse or more so.

I love rubbing his penis against my clitoris and vulva. It gives both of us great pleasure and always brings me to the verge of orgasm.

For many of us, the most satisfying aspects of lovemaking are not specific types of stimulation but feelings of closeness with our partners before and after sex.[23]

Men's increased use of drugs such as Viagra has affected the sexual lives of many women. Some of us welcome a male partner's firmer erection and more sustained thrusting; others, for whom penetration isn't necessarily desirable all the time, may find that the drugs contribute to an unwanted focus on intercourse and longer periods before a man reaches orgasm.*

* For a thoughtful discussion of these issues see Abraham Margentaler's *The Viagra Myth: The Surprising Impact on Love and Relationships* (San Francisco: Jossey-Bass, 2003).

LOVEMAKING WITH A WOMAN

There is no single way to be sexual with another woman. Our desires are as varied as we are.

The more women I sleep with, the more I realize you can't assume [that] what you like is what she likes. There are tremendous differences.

I felt weird because [as a woman with a disability,] I had to explain what my sexual needs were to anyone I wanted to sleep with, until I realized that everyone has to explain what their needs are in order to get them met. I don't have sensation in my pubic area, but since there is no set standard to what lesbian lovemaking is, it leaves a whole world of sexuality and sensuality open to explore.

I want my lover on her back, my first two fingers curling up, as if to say "Come here, baby," inside her, my thumb on her clit, her voluptuous body shuddering. I like the same thing, but lying on my stomach. My lover says she loves hands because their possibilities are endless.

When we make love with a woman, our own sexual impulses and preferences may make us uncomfortable if they seem to follow a male

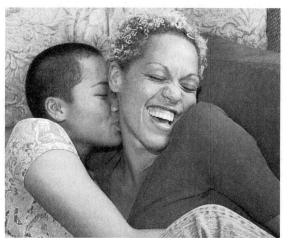

© Thinkstock

model. We may feel uncomfortable with lust, for instance, or with acting aggressively, having fantasies of dominance, or using erotic materials. Yet these may be aspects of sexuality that we would enjoy. A dildo, for instance, is not a "penis substitute"; it can give us pleasure if we enjoy penetrating or being penetrated in sex. We have a chance to move away from male-defined sexuality and to reclaim all the dimensions of sexuality that deepen our intimacy, pleasure, and love.

When I make love with a woman, the challenge is to be honest more often; to say what I am really feeling; to explore when I'm not feeling present instead of pretending that I am; if I am spacing out, to ask what's the fear.

In finding out what turns my lover on, exploring her body, tasting her, learning her odors and textures, I am growing to love myself more, too.

MASTURBATION WITH A PARTNER

Pleasuring ourselves while we are with a partner can be part of lovemaking.

My lover rubbed her breasts and clitoris while I made love to her yesterday. After I got over feeling a little inadequate (I should be able to do it all), I found it was like having another pair of hands to make love to her with. It was a turn-on to both of us.

When one person in a relationship wants sex or orgasm more than the other, masturbating is a possibility. Here are some different views.

It's typical for my husband to want to make love at night, but I'm too tired. Then by morning I'm very horny, and he wants to get up. I always tease him in the morning, ask whether he jerked off or not. Sometimes he did. Sometimes I'll be going off to sleep and feel the bed shaking.

I guess I'm old-fashioned enough to say that no husband of mine is going to have to masturbate because I wouldn't satisfy him.

Masturbation is such a private thing, and I want to keep it for when I'm alone with myself. Also, doing it with someone else would be the ultimate in showing that I'm a sexual person, and maybe I'm shy about that.

VAGINAL PENETRATION

Some of us experience tremendous pleasure in having a male or female lover enter our vagina with fingers, fist, dildo, or other object. (For penetration by a penis, see "Vaginal Intercourse," p. 207.) If we are with a female lover, we may enjoy entering her. Vaginal penetration can be gentle, playful, intimate, or passionate. Some women do not like penetration at all and prefer to stick with external stimulation. As with all sex, it is important to communicate and to respect both your partner's and your own desires.

Vaginal penetration can be thought of as reciprocal, with one of you enveloping the other's hand as it explores and penetrates. If you want your partner to enter you, make sure your vagina is wet with vaginal fluid or lubricants. The partner who is penetrating should keep his or her fingers free of rings and the nails well filed, and wear an unpowdered latex glove or finger cot (resembling a cutoff finger of a glove) to protect against the transmission of HIV/AIDS through any cuts on the fingers.

In penetrating a female partner, we can stroke, tap, circle, thrust, and experiment with different rhythms and speeds. Try stimulating her G-spot (see p. 197). Or you can put one or more fingers inside her and, if you both like, gradually put your whole hand inside (called *fisting*). Inside her vagina, it can feel warm, wet, and wonderful.

VAGINAL INTERCOURSE

If you make love with a man, you may want to have intercourse—to feel his penis in your vagina. Intercourse, too, can be reciprocal: You open up to enclose him warmly, you surround him powerfully, and he penetrates you. It can be infinitely slow and gentle, hard and thrusting, or both—at its best, an exceptional part of lovemaking.

I can so clearly remember moving in and around him, and him in me, till it seemed in the whole world there was only us dancing together as we moved together, as we loved together, as we came together. Sometimes at these times I laugh or cry, and they are the same strong emotions coming from a deep protected part of me that is freer now for loving him.

For intercourse to give you pleasure, you must feel sexually excited, your vagina wet and open. Often it takes women longer—sometimes much longer—than men to become aroused. Although you may feel open and ready for intercourse immediately, more often you will want your partner first to touch, rub, kiss, or lick your vulva and clitoris, using his hands, mouth, or penis. To add extra "juice," you or he can apply water-based lubricants or use a lubricated condom; some people use saliva. Do not use Vaseline or any oils. They destroy latex condoms and diaphragms.

If you are sexually inexperienced, frightened, not ready, not in the mood, or angry with your partner, or if you have a partner who practices only the "in and out" of intercourse and not the lovemaking that surrounds it, then penetration (especially when your vagina is dry) can be boring, unpleasant, even painful. If it doesn't feel good to have him inside you, stop. You can play more with external stimulation and wait until you're very aroused, then try again.

Certain positions at certain times will feel more exciting to you than others. The "man on top" is not a "naturally" better position at all. You can sit or lie upon him or lie side by side. Sit up with your legs over his and his penis in you. Or he can enter you from behind and reach around to caress your clitoris. (You can caress your clitoris, too, in this position.) Pressure of the penis at the back of the vagina can be the key to orgasm for some women. If you want deep penetration and pressure on your cervix, choose positions that make these more possible. We are all different shapes and need to find positions that suit us. If we have injuries or disabilities, being creative and using pillows for support may increase our comfort. Communicate with words, sounds, or movements what feels good to you (see "Communicating about Sex," p. 213).

Intercourse is about pleasure and connection, not necessarily orgasm. Many women don't experience orgasm during intercourse alone. Trying to have an orgasm may make you self-conscious and tighten you up. On the other hand, sometimes it's exciting to strive for orgasms.

If you are not ready for orgasm and the man is highly aroused when you begin intercourse, he might reach orgasm too soon for you if he moves back and forth inside you and you move your pelvis against his quickly. Both of you can slow your movements until you become more excited yourself. Experiment with holding your bodies still for a time when he enters you, then begin to move together slowly. Moving slowly can help men learn to delay ejaculation, which can make intercourse more pleasurable for both of you.

Over time you and your partner can learn your mutual rhythms of desire and arousal, and explore what gives each of you the most pleasure.

PAINFUL PENETRATION

We may experience discomfort, even pain, with vaginal intercourse or other forms of vaginal penetration. If penetration is at all painful, don't put up with the pain! Find out what is causing it, and do something about it. Get regular gynecological exams to find out whether there are physical causes. As an alternative to penetration, we can try masturbating with a partner, oral sex, and other ways of giving ourselves pleasure.

Local Infection

Some vaginal infections—like monilia (yeast) or trichomoniasis—can be present in a nonacute, visually unnoticeable form. The friction of a penis, dildo, or finger moving on the vulva or in the vagina might cause the infection to flare up, resulting in stinging and itchiness (see Chapter 28, "Unique to Women"). A herpes sore on the external genitals can make friction painful (see Chapter 15, "Sexually Transmitted Infections").

Local Irritation

The vagina might be irritated by a birth control foam, cream, or jelly you are using. If so, try a different brand; however, if the irritation persists, it may be in reaction to the spermicide nonoxynol-9. This spermicide can irritate the vaginal membranes and thereby increase the transmission of HIV. Alternative spermicides are extremely hard to find, so you may want to consider another birth control method. Some of us react to the rubber in a condom, diaphragm, or latex glove (though latex allergy is fairly rare). Alternatives include polyurethane condoms, including female condoms. Vaginal deodorant sprays and scented tampons and all so-called feminine hygiene products can irritate the vagina or vulva, as can body wash, soaps, bubble bath, and laundry detergents.

Insufficient Lubrication

In most women, the wall of the vagina usually responds to arousal by *sweating*—giving off a liquid that wets the vagina and the entrance to it, which makes penetration easier. Sometimes there isn't enough of this liquid. Some reasons: We may be nervous or tense about making love (for example, it's the first time, or we're worried about getting pregnant). We may be trying to let the penis, hand, or object in (or your lover might be putting/forcing it in) too soon, before there has been enough time and stimulation to excite you and set the sweating action going. Be sure to give the vagina time to get wet. Lowered levels of estrogen can affect the vaginal walls in such a way that less liquid is produced. This affects some women after childbirth (particularly if we are nursing) and some women after menopause. After menopause, we may need to look for signs other than vaginal wetness to signal that we are aroused (see Chapter 26, "Midlife and Menopause").

One way to address the problem of vaginal dryness is to use a lubricant. Saliva can be used as a natural lubricant, or we can purchase a "lube," now available in a wide variety of formulas, tastes, and textures. Preferences for lubes are personal—try out different kinds until you find one you like. If you are prone to yeast infections, try a glycerin-free lubricant like Liquid Silk or Slippery Stuff, since the sugary content of glycerin may feed yeast. If using condoms, you can also buy lubricated condoms. Avoid condoms or lubes that contain nonoxynol-9; this spermicide can irritate the vaginal membranes and increase the transmission of HIV. Never use Vaseline or other oil-based lubricant with a latex condom or diaphragm. It will deteriorate the rubber.

Tightness in the Vaginal Entrance

The first few times we have intercourse or any other form of vaginal penetration, an unstretched hymen can cause pain. Also, when we are tense and preoccupied, the vaginal entrance is not likely to loosen up enough, and getting the penis, finger, or dildo in might hurt. Even if we feel relaxed and sexy, timing is important. If we try penetration before we are fully aroused, we might still be too tight, though we are wet enough. So don't rush, and don't let yourself be rushed.

Pain Deep in the Pelvis

Sometimes the thrust of penetration hurts way inside. This pain can be caused by tears and scarring (known as *adhesions*) in the ligaments that support the uterus (caused by obstetrical mismanagement during childbirth, a botched abortion, pelvic surgery, or violent intercourse); infections of the cervix, uterus, and tubes (such as pelvic inflammatory disease—the end result of untreated sexually transmitted infection in many women); endometriosis; cysts or tumors on the ovaries; or a vagina that may have shortened with age. Intercourse in these cases is sometimes less painful when we are on top or lying beside a partner. Consult a health care practitioner if penetration consistently causes deep pelvic pain.

Vulvodynia and Vaginismus

Vulvodynia is a chronic burning or stinging sensation in and around the vagina, which makes any kind of penetration, including entrance by finger, tampon, speculum, or penis, acutely painful. In some cases, this condition may be related to *vaginismus,* a strong, involuntary tightening of the vaginal muscles, a spasm of the outer third of the vagina. (For more information, see Chapter 28, "Unique to Women.")

Female Genital Cutting (Circumcision)

Some of us from parts of Africa and Asia have had our genitalia cut as a cultural rite of passage that was intended to maintain virginity and ensure marriageability. Part or all of the clitoris and labia may have been cut or removed *(clitoridectomy),* and the vaginal opening sewn shut, thus preventing penetration or making it extremely painful. *Deinfibulation* (surgical repair) is possible to allow penetration and childbirth, although many doctors are not familiar with this procedure. (For more information, see p. 643.)

ORAL SEX

We can suck or lick our partner's genitals, which, when done to a woman, is called *cunnilingus* (slang: going down, eating, eating out) and, when done to a man, is called *fellatio* (slang: giving head, blow job, cock sucking). For some of us, oral sex brings orgasm more surely than other ways of making love.

We're really into oral sex, and he's always ready and willing. He'll say, "Do you want to have an orgasm?" And he'll go down on me. It's terrific.

To enjoy oral sex, it helps to like our partner's genitals and to feel good about our own. Yet we are often ashamed of our "private parts."

For ages I thought my lover was doing me a favor when he did oral sex on me. I couldn't imagine that I tasted good. Finally, he convinced me that he loves doing it. Also, I tasted my juices, and they're not bad!

At first I was repulsed by the idea of going down on a woman. I thought we smelled bad, that vaginas were nasty. It was a little pungent and intimidating in the beginning (though less so than a penis had been!). I soon learned to lose myself in the wonderful textures, tastes, and formations of a woman's genitals. I realized that lesbian sex is about loving myself, overcoming my hatred of my own body.

In oral sex with a man or woman, there is a risk of getting HIV/AIDS or another sexually transmitted infection, because both ejaculate and vaginal secretions can contain HIV and other organisms. We can have safer oral sex by using dental dams and/or condoms.

Like everything in sex, oral sex is good only if we want to be doing it.

Often a guy I'm dating will say, "If you won't have intercourse, just give me a blow job." But if I didn't want him in my vagina, I probably don't want him in my mouth. Oral sex can feel like rape to me if I'm not in the mood to be doing it.

Sometimes it's incredibly erotic for me to have his penis moving in my mouth. Since I don't enjoy swallowing his semen, I usually spit it out or let it flow out on the sheets, and that's fine. Sometimes, however, blowing him makes me gag—I don't want his penis filling up my mouth at all. Then we do something else. Or we get in a position where I have more control, like being on top of him with the base of his penis in my hand.

What feels good in oral sex may differ from time to time and from person to person.

I like tongue, lips, moisture, not too much sucking and pulling, and time for exploring—my lover's got to be willing to stay with it for a while.

It can be done rather crummily! I hate it when I feel like he's eating me up with his teeth, or when the pressure's too hard and it hurts, or when he moves around from place to place and doesn't keep the stimulation steady.

For me there's no right or wrong place, just the places I want concentrated on, on a particular day. I'm getting better at telling my lover where it feels best.

ANAL STIMULATION

The anus can be stimulated with fingers, tongue, penis, dildo, or any slender object (so long as it has a flared base and can be retrieved easily). For many of us, it is a highly sexually sensitive area. You can give or receive anal stimulation with a male or female partner.

I like having something small in my anus during lovemaking—no pressure or movement, just there.

Having the area around my anus licked during oral sex is a real turn-on. And anal intercourse when I'm in the mood is incredibly sexy. I love the sensations deep inside me and the thrill of doing something so unusual.

The anus is not as elastic as the vagina, so be gentle. If you have anal intercourse, go slowly, wait until you're relaxed, and use a lubricant—saliva or a water-based jelly such as K-Y, Astroglide, or Probe. Anal bacteria can cause serious vaginal infections and cystitis, so if you want your partner's finger(s) or penis or a dildo in your vagina after being in your anus, be sure they have been washed well first, and use a condom on a penis or dildo. If you or your partner want to use a tongue in the anus (sometimes called *rimming*), be sure to use a dental dam with lubrication to protect against getting a stomach infection or a sexually transmitted infection.

Anal sex is a very risky activity for HIV/AIDS transmission. The delicate tissue in the rectum is prone to small tears that make an entryway for the AIDS virus. Latex or polyurethane barriers (condom, gloves) must be used (see Chapter 16, "HIV and AIDS" and Chapter 14, "Safer Sex").

Anal intercourse isn't for everyone.

My husband wants to have anal sex a lot because he likes the tight fit and the exoticness of it. Once it happened and I almost didn't know it was happening. There was lubrication, and everything was right and it felt fine. At other times I've really not wanted it, and a few times it's been almost painful and I've stopped it. I wish I liked it better, because I'd love to give him that pleasure, but I have to be honest—I just don't enjoy it.

In our one great try at anal intercourse, I ended up jumping three feet in the air and squealing like a stuck pig. This so terrified him that he completely lost his erection, and we laughed and laughed. I don't think it ever really got in or anything—somehow we hadn't quite worked out the logistics of it.

FANTASIES

Today as I stretched out before my run, I closed my eyes and imagined my lover's naked body floating a few inches above me. I could feel her breasts on my face and in my mouth, our bodies reaching out, drawing close, and then wrapped together. The images and feelings sailed me through an hour of strong running.

I had the fantasy of making love with two men at once. I pictured myself sandwiched between them. I acted on this one with an old friend and a casual friend who both liked the idea. It was fun.

Nearly everyone has fantasies, in the form of fleeting images or detailed stories. They express depths within us to learn about and explore. The thoughts and images we carry in our minds can evoke strong physical responses. Some sex researchers assert that the *brain* is the most important organ of sexual pleasure, and some women report that they have orgasms from fantasy alone.[24] In fantasy, we can be whatever we imagine.

We may share our fantasies with a lover.

We've just started to talk about the fantasies we have during sex. At first it felt somehow disloyal that I've needed fantasies when the other person was such a good lover. Now, we figure, the more pleasure, the better.

Sometimes it can be difficult to accept sexual fantasies.

I imagined I was sitting in a room. The walls were all white. There was nothing in it, and I was naked. There was a large window at one end, and anyone who wanted to could look in and see me. There was no place to hide. There was something arousing about being so exposed. I masturbated while having this fantasy, and afterward I felt very sad. I thought I must be so sick, so distorted inside, if this image of myself could give me such intense sexual pleasure.

We might worry that we are bad or sick for imagining something different, or feel disloyal when we fantasize about someone other than the man or woman we are with. Yet our fantasies treat us to *all kinds* of erotic experiences, including situations that seem taboo. It takes a while to learn that this is okay and that we can enjoy these stories and images without having to act on them.

Some people say that if we fantasize about having sex forced on us, that means we want to be raped. This is untrue. Totally unlike actual rape, fantasizing about rape is voluntary and does not bring us physical pain or violation. For those of us who grew up learning that "good girls" don't want sex, a fantasy of being forced to have sex may free us of responsibility and can be highly erotic. It can allow us the feeling of being desired uncontrollably. There is a huge difference between having a fantasy and wanting to act on it.

In one of my juiciest fantasies, a woman and a man tie me up and make love to me and to each other. There is something extremely erotic in imagining being that powerless. In real life, my lover and I do at times feel totally vulnerable to what the other does or wants. This fantasy lets me play around with the power dynamics that are sometimes so intense between us.

We may distrust fantasies that seem to play into male pornographic images of women as submissive or masochistic, and we may imagine that in a less sexist future, fantasies of dominance would come to us less often. Yet this is difficult to predict. For now it seems important to accept that all kinds of fantasies may be erotic and free up our sexual energies. (If you repeatedly have fantasies that disturb or scare you, they may be a sign that you need help. You might want to talk about them with a trusted friend or a trained counselor.)

ROLE-PLAYING, SADOMASOCHISM (S/M), BONDAGE AND DISCIPLINE (B&D)

With our partners, we can playact situations and fantasies that excite us. We can dress up. We can be our child selves as well as our adult selves, our lusty and vigorous selves as well as our needy selves.

Sometimes when I'm feeling good, I'll create a strip scene for my husband—and for me, since our mirror is strategically placed—and we both get very excited. Now he does it, too, standing in front of the bed, moving his body rhythmically, slowly taking off and throwing down his clothes. I love it. His strength and vulnerability come through at the same time.

In sadomasochistic sex play (S/M) or bondage and domination (B&D), the playacting is based on fantasy situations of dominance and submission. Partners act out roles like master–servant, police–citizen, and monarch–subject. One will enforce her or his will on the other. Some of us may like light spanking or having our hands restrained, and some experiment with activities involving some physical pain, until the other gives a prearranged signal to stop. The practice of S/M is highly controversial among feminists and has caused debate and division among lesbians. Women who support S/M point out that between partners who both fully want to be doing it, S/M play can increase sexual pleasure and open up hidden issues of power that are present in most human intimacy. For some women, the appeal of S/M lies in the joy of experiencing intense physical sensation in an atmosphere of trust. Some key words in the B&D–S/M community are "safe, sane, and consensual."

S/M, like regular sex, allows people to share an intimate physical experience and an intimate emotional experience, but beyond that, S/M allows my partner and me to share a fantasy life, which is a deep kind of intimacy, very special and unique, that I would not trade for anything.

Others argue that dominance and pain infliction have no part in "healthy" sexuality. At times, S/M can camouflage truly oppressive behavior.

I was a battered wife. My husband, a professional with a good job, said he was into bondage. I bought in to it at first. Toward the end, he said that he could relate to me sexually only if he tied me up. At the end, he was threatening to kill me. For him, bondage had to do with low self-esteem and wasn't a healthy expression of sexuality.

It's important to say no to anything we don't want to do. If we are confused or upset by pressure from a sex partner, we may want to discuss the situation with a friend or counselor who can help us decide how to respond.

EROTICA

In recent years, women have begun to make inroads into the male-dominated industry of erotic entertainment. Much of traditional pornography has been based on men's fantasies and has depicted women's bodies as depersonalized objects. Today we can choose from a wider selection of sexually explicit videos, magazines, books, and sex toys created by and for women of all sexual orientations. Still, what some women consider erotic, other women may consider demeaning.

Sex toys and aids can spice up sexual encounters, make safer sex fun, and be an outlet for creativity. We can try edible body paints or flavored condoms, an egg-shaped electric vibrator or a double dildo, a strap-on harness or a G-spot stimulator, an anthology of erotic short stories or a hot and sexy video. There are also instructional videos and books available on masturbation, orgasms, sexual intimacy, female ejaculation, and much more.

Erotica can be bought in women's sexuality boutiques. These boutiques, the first of which opened in the 1970s, are often discreetly located and offer information and workshops for women and men. There continue to be attempts to censor and legislate against sexually explicit

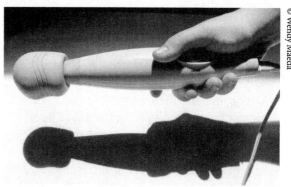

© Wendy Maeda

material. We may feel awkward or embarrassed entering a sex shop, and feel as if we are doing something bad. However, there is nothing wrong with seeking information or buying products to make sex fun. The store clerks are used to answering questions from customers—you're almost certainly not the first one to ask! For those of us who don't live near a store or don't feel comfortable going to one, many products are available by mail order and on the Internet. For information on obtaining catalogs, see "Mail Order" in "Resources."

We all have different ideas of what is erotic. We are not limited to what's available in a catalog. A cucumber dildo, a shower nozzle spray, or looking at our own love letters and photographs can be intensely arousing. We can use our imagination and resources to create our own erotic pleasures.

COMMUNICATING ABOUT SEX

We all face certain issues in a sexual situation, whether it's with a date, a longtime lover, or a spouse: How do I feel at the moment? Do I want to be sexually close with this person now? In what ways? What if I don't know—can I say I'm confused? Can I communicate clearly what I want and what I don't want?

Talking about sex can be challenging. We

LET'S TALK ABOUT SEX

- Invite a group of women friends over to watch and discuss a video on orgasms.
- Attend, get on video, or invite a bunch of friends to read aloud from the play *The Vagina Monologues* (see www.events .vday.org).
- Join or create a support group (see *The Self-Help Group Sourcebook* in "Resources").
- Seek out a sex therapist through the organization American Association of Sex Educators, Counselors and Therapists (AASECT) in "Resources."
- Host a sex-toys party (like a Tupperware party, but more fun!).

may prefer "proper" terms such as vagina, penis, fellatio, and intercourse or slang terms such as cunt, cock, and fucking. If we find slang terms degrading, we may need to be creative and come up with our own sexy and affirming language. Sometimes the vagueness of expressions like "hooking up" and "making love" can lead to miscommunication if both partners are not clear on the meaning. Finding a common language can help communication.

We may want to find a time to talk with our partners when we are *not* having sex and there's no pressure to respond right away. Talking about safer sex, birth control, sexual techniques, or specific preferences can temporarily "kill the mood" but can ultimately lead to heightened intimacy. We can practice saying what feels good while exchanging massages, for example, when the atmosphere is less intense.

Our body language and the sounds we make are just as important as the words we use. Making the sounds that let a partner know we are feeling good, speeding up or slowing down our hip movements, placing a firm hand on the shoulder meaning "Let's go slow" are all ways of communicating.

I've liked just saying "Watch" and showing.

We were both really excited. My lover began rubbing my clitoris hard, and it hurt. It took me a second to figure out what to do. I was afraid that if I said something about it, I would spoil the excitement for both of us. Then I realized I could just take my lover's hand and very gently move it up a little higher to my pubic hair.

We also need to be aware of the relationship between our words and our body language. We may be verbally saying yes to some sexual activity, but our body is pulling away or tensing up. Or we may be saying no to further sexual intimacy while continuing to stimulate ourselves or our partners. We can seek to make our words and movements consistent.

Communication about our sexual needs is a continuous process. A woman who had found the courage to talk with her lover about their sexual relationship said in angry frustration, "I told him what I like once, so why doesn't he know now? Did he forget? Doesn't he care?"

He would come almost instantly when we began to make love after marvelous kissing. A little while later, we'd make love again, when I'd be more aroused—aching for him, in fact. I never knew how to alter this pattern, never dared talk about it, and later on found out that he had resented "having" to make love twice.

We had a wildly passionate sex life for a year and a half. When we moved in together, sexuality suddenly became an issue. It turned out our patterns were very different. My lover needs to talk, to feel intimate in conversation, to relax completely before she can feel sexual. I need to touch and to make a physical connection first before I feel re-

laxed enough to talk intimately. I'd reach out for her as we went into the bedroom, and she'd freeze. We battled it out for months, both feeling terrible, before we figured out what was going on.

Even in the most loving relationships, asking for what we want may be hard.

- We feel that sex is supposed to come naturally, and having to talk about it must mean there's a problem.
- We are afraid that being honest about what we want will threaten the other person.
- We are embarrassed by the words themselves.
- We have been making love with the same person for years, and it feels risky to bring up new insights.
- We aren't communicating well with our partner in other areas of our relationship.
- Our partner seems defensive and might interpret our suggestion as a criticism or a demand.
- We don't know exactly what we want at a particular time, or we prefer to react to something our partner does.
- Even with a willing partner, we may feel inhibited about asserting our sexuality openly and proudly.

If we do ask for what we want, we may be relieved and gratified to get our desires met. However, if our partner has different preferences, we may have to do some negotiating or look below the surface and figure out the underlying needs. For example, let's say that you want to spend long hours in bed on a Sunday morning making love, but your partner wants to get up and go for a run. What are your needs that aren't being met? Do you want more intimacy? Do you need time to unwind? Do you want more sexual attention? What are your partner's needs? Instead of getting locked into positions over whether to cuddle in bed on Sundays, you and your partner can focus on how to get your needs fulfilled in

For information on communicating about safer sex and birth control, see Chapters 14 and 18.

other ways. Perhaps you can create special times throughout the week for relaxing together. Expanding the focus to include your underlying needs can open up a lot of possibilities.

SEX AND DISABILITY

Some of us were born with a chronic disease or disability, like cystic fibrosis or blindness, or developed one later in life, like multiple sclerosis or bipolar disorder. No matter when we become an individual with one or more disabilities, we are all women with unique feelings and attitudes about our sexuality and our disability.

We seek fulfillment of our sexual desires and want to feel good about how we express our sexuality. Yet we find that some people, including health care providers, assume we are childlike and sexless.

Recently, I told a doctor I wanted to be tested for HIV/AIDS. Without even asking me any other questions, he just said, "No, no, people with your disability never get AIDS."

Disability may trigger feelings of alienation or disconnection from our own bodies, causing us shame and embarrassment. Reclaiming our bodies for positive experiences of sexuality takes time and patience, as well as experimentation and support.

After my brain injury, I couldn't get spontaneous pictures of people masturbating in public out of my mind and even flirted with the idea of lifting my skirt and doing it myself. These new thoughts were disturbing, and I was afraid to tell my part-

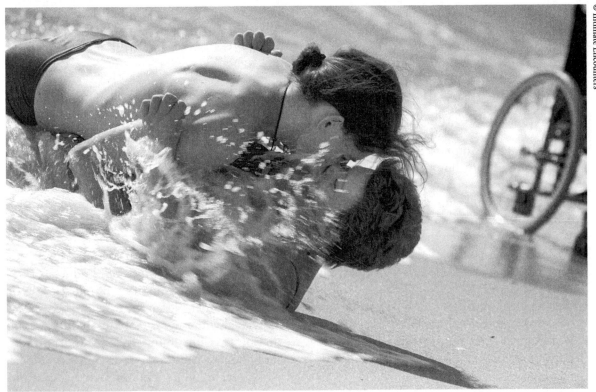

"We love each other passionately and often," says Samantha of her relationship with her husband, Michael. "While the disability does, in reality, affect how we do things and what we are able to do together, it does not define our relationship. Assumptions are always the problem. People can assume that because I am disabled, that my sexuality, and my ability to enjoy and participate in sex, has been taken away from me. It is fun to be part of an education process aimed at challenging this perception." Samantha has quadriplegia.

ner, because I worried it would damage our relationship. Then I learned in a support group how a brain injury can change our ability to maintain appropriate sexual boundaries. Eventually, my urges were less frequent, and I became more comfortable with my sexuality.

I have a lot of diagnoses, including bipolar disorder, and when I'm manic, I sleep with more women and have fewer barriers. But because of my PTSD diagnosis, I have a hard time receiving pleasure and only want to please the woman I'm with, so that way, no one can get close to me. It's different when I'm in a relationship, though— I have to love her before she can touch me.

When I'm not manic, sex doesn't appeal to me as much.

The first time I had sex with my boyfriend after I became paralyzed, it was awful. But then, over time, it got better with communication and experience. I was surprised that I could still orgasm after my injury, since no one at the hospital had discussed it with me.

From dating to the logistics of lovemaking, challenges may arise, especially with a major disability. Lack of knowledge, poorly designed spaces, and inaccessible transportation systems can turn simple issues into huge barriers. We must also decide when and how much to disclose if our disability is "hidden."

I have been surprised at how little most men I have had sex with are bothered by my urostomy [in which urine is collected from the bladder in a small bag attached to the abdomen]. I do tell them before we are in the buff, and it hasn't been too much of an issue. I think they must already accept my disability to some extent before becoming intimate, so perhaps they just see the urostomy as more of the same—part of the disability, which is how I see it. Also, I accept it and don't treat it as a big deal, so they feel more comfortable as well.

A great deal of sexual expression involves verbal and nonverbal communication. Being honest and frankly discussing whatever makes us feel good can be a model for all lovers, whether or not we have a disability.

I needed to find out if I could actually feel comfortable and communicate to someone who really didn't know me before my accident in order to have sex. At this party, I met a guy, and we eventually had sex. The morning after, I asked him what it was like to be with me, and he answered, "Honestly, at first I was afraid I might hurt you because you are so small, but you talked to me and told me what felt good, and what to do that was good for me, too, so it was great!" In more ways than one, it was great for me as well.

When one partner is deaf, hard of hearing, or has a speech disability, we may need to learn new ways of communicating, such as American Sign Language.

The cultural pressure for sex to be spontaneous is hurtful to those of us who need some accommodation to our disability. A personal-care assistant may be needed to help us prepare for sex, whether one or both partners have a disability. That way we can feel more independent in the relationship, and our sex partner has a choice about being involved in the preparation. Like anything else in our lives, sexual expression is better when we focus on what we can do rather than on what we can't.

Even when [you're] sexually aroused, the spontaneity can soon disappear when your partner has to help empty your bladder and carefully clean and position you. . . . My sexual fantasies relate to spontaneous sexual behavior—sex in an elevator, in any room of the house, and in numerous positions—on the floor, up against the wall, and so on.[25]

My husband and I are both disabled, so we need a lot of help. We decided that hiring a personal-care attendant was too much of an invasion of our privacy, though. It is very frustrating, but we just don't have intercourse anymore. We have our orgasms through oral sex now, and my husband says we are lucky and that other people would be jealous if they knew.

Certain chronic illnesses and disabilities such as fibromyalgia and some spinal cord injuries have associated pain, so there may be times when we want sex but can't bear to be touched. However, some of us have discovered that direct stimulation of our genitals can help block the pain[26] and take our minds someplace else.

We don't do much "hard-core sex" but find our greatest fulfillment in slow, deep touching and holding. We can't seem to get enough cuddling.

Members of the disability community have taught the medical establishment much about sexuality over the years. It has finally validated what we knew all along—that our orgasms are real and can result from stimulating our genitals or other highly eroticized places on our bodies.[27]

I have erratic, vague sensation in my vagina and clitoris. When I have an orgasm, I feel most of the pleasure in my knees—it's a nerve transfer thing, I guess. I'm probably the only woman in the world whose knees come.

Disability is part of who you are, as is your sex drive. When you have confidence in yourself, you can also be confident you are no different from anyone else sexually; maybe you express yourself sexually in a physically different way, but all in all, my instincts, desires, and expressions are the same as everyone else's. Sex knows no disability.

SEX AND DISABILITY*		
CHRONIC DISEASE OR DISABILITY	EFFECTS ON OUR SEXUALITY	HELPFUL HINTS AND SPECIAL IMPLICATIONS
Cerebral palsy (CP)	Muscle spasticity, rigidity, and/or weakness may make certain sex acts and self-pleasuring difficult to impossible for us. Contractures of our knees and hips may cause us pain under the pressure of a partner, and spasms may increase with arousal. Some of us experience a lack of vaginal lubrication. Menstruation, fertility, and pregnancy are not affected. During delivery, those of us with severe CP might need a cesarean section.	Nongenital lovemaking, using different positions, and propping our legs up on pillows may ease spasms. We can use a vibrator to make love alone or with another person if our arms and hands are involved. Because of an increased risk of clotting, the birth control pill is not advisable for those of us taking seizure medication (anticonvulsants) or if our mobility is greatly restricted by severe CP.[28] **A, B, D, E**
Brain and cognitive disabilities (including epilepsy, traumatic brain injury, and stroke)	Our sexual abilities may vary depending upon the location of injury. We may experience a changed level of interest in sex as well as difficulty with vaginal lubrication and having an orgasm, sometimes caused by our medications or associated depression.[29] Stroke and TBI may result in communication, cognitive, and visual-perceptive impairments, as well as loss of sensation, paralysis, and incontinence. Those of us with severe TBI may show sexual indiscretion and be impulsive. Some of us get confused about public versus private matters and act in ways others find socially inappropriate.[30] Many of us have irregular periods and may experience difficulty becoming pregnant. We may also go through menopause earlier than we expected.	If our balance, strength, or coordination is not good, it may help to engage in sexual activities in positions that support our bodies or that require little exertion. If we experience cognitive or behavior problems, social-skills retraining or help from a neuropsychologist may assist us in better understanding our disability and gaining greater self-control and confidence. An understanding friend or partner often provides the best help during the slow recovery process. Birth control pills should be used with extreme caution if we have paralysis or circulatory disorders, and they are not advisable for those of us taking seizure medication. There are complex interactions between the hormones (estrogen and progesterone) contained in birth control pills or devices and some of the medications used to control seizures. Some of these

*Some of the more prevalent disabilities have been included in this chart.

CHRONIC DISEASE OR DISABILITY	EFFECTS ON OUR SEXUALITY	HELPFUL HINTS AND SPECIAL IMPLICATIONS
Brain and cognitive disabilities (cont.)		medications increase the breakdown of contraceptive hormones in the body, making them less effective in preventing pregnancy.[31] **A, B, C, D, E**
Diabetes	Recently, several studies have examined the effects of diabetes on women's sexual response. Some diabetic women report that orgasms gradually become more rare and less intense. It is possible that the threshold for orgasm increases because of damage to the nerve fibers in the pelvic region. A lack of vaginal lubrication and recurrent infections may make some lovemaking unpleasant.[32] While most research indicates that sexual difficulties in women with diabetes have a physical cause, a recent study suggests there may be psychological causes as well.[33,34] Diabetes that is difficult to regulate may cause fertility problems and stop menstruation. Depending on how stable our blood glucose levels are, pregnancy may be complicated and should be closely monitored.	Using a vibrator allows some women to reach orgasm because the stimulation is more intense. Healthy women with diabetes can generally take birth control pills safely, but women who have complications such as hypertension should avoid taking the Pill.[35]
Renal failure	In chronic renal insufficiency, menstruation may stop or become extremely irregular. Many women become infertile and rarely carry pregnancies to term. We may have difficulties becoming sexually excited, and our orgasms may become more rare and less intense.[36] Sometimes we have a decrease in vaginal lubrication and breast tissue mass.	Maintenance hemodialysis often brings on excessive and sometimes painful menstruation but may improve our desire for sex, though not necessarily sexual responsivity. Kidney transplants usually improve both our desire for sex and sexual response, and fertility improves dramatically. Many of the drugs used to lower hypertension are likely to dampen our sex drive. The birth control pill is usually not advised.[37] **D, E**
Rheumatoid arthritis (RA)	Swollen, painful joints; muscular atrophy; and joint contractures may make it difficult for us to masturbate or make love in some positions. Pain, fatigue, and medications may decrease our sex drive, but genital sensations remain intact.[38] Menstruation, fertility, and pregnancy are not affected, but birthing may be complicated if our hips and spine are involved. However, symptoms may improve during pregnancy because of changes in our immune system.	To avoid pain and pressure on affected joints, we can be creative in sexual positioning. If our symptoms respond to heat, we can plan sexual play after a hot compress or a hot bath with our partner. Choose the best time, when you have the least pain and stiffness, for lovemaking. Try sex instead of corticosteroids—it is said to stimulate the adrenal glands and so increases the output of natural cortisone, which alleviates painful symptoms.[39] The birth control pill

CHRONIC DISEASE OR DISABILITY	EFFECTS ON OUR SEXUALITY	HELPFUL HINTS AND SPECIAL IMPLICATIONS
Rheumatoid arthritis (RA) (cont.)		may not be good for us if we have circulatory problems or greatly restricted mobility. However, if we do not have these problems, the birth control pill is safe for use and may even improve the symptoms of RA.[40] *A, B, C, D*
Systemic lupus erythematosus	Many difficulties are the same as in RA (above). However, because individuals may have quite different symptoms, often related to other disorders, one cannot generalize. Research on the female sexual effects of lupus is scarce, despite the fact that nine out of ten people with lupus are women. Sometimes we have sores in and around the mouth and vagina and a decrease in vaginal lubrication, so we may have pain during vaginal penetration.	For helpful hints, see RA (above). Choose birth control methods with extreme caution, especially if symptoms or complications other than RA exist. Estrogen-containing birth control pills are not advisable due to risk for blood clots.[41] *A, B, D, E*
Myocardial infarction (MI)	For those of us with very serious conditions, chest pain, palpitations, and shortness of breath may limit our sexual activities. However, many of us can resume regular lovemaking once we can climb two flights of stairs at a brisk pace without inducing symptoms.[42] Taking an exercise stress test is a good way to tell if you are physically ready to resume sexual activity.[43] (The cardiac responses during step climbing and lovemaking are similar, the average being 125 beats per minute.)	We should consult a physician to see when and if we can safely begin an exercise regimen. We can participate in lovemaking activities that require little or no exertion with our arms (for example, on our side or back). Go slow in the beginning to minimize stress and fear of stress, because the majority of sexual problems arise from anxiety and misinformation about this ailment. The American Heart Association suggests engaging in sex when we are rested, relaxed, and free from interruptions, waiting one to three hours after eating a full meal to allow time for digestion, and, if prescribed by your doctor, taking medications before sexual activity. Birth control pills should not be used, but an IUD may be used except in women with cardiac valvular disease.[44] *A, D*
Multiple sclerosis (MS)	Depending upon the stage and severity of MS, our symptoms will vary and may come and go. Some of us experience difficulty in having an orgasm, decreased genital sensitivity, dryness of the vagina, muscle weakness, extreme fatigue, pain, and bladder and bowel incontinence.[45] Our menstrual and fertility patterns may change.[46] The symptoms of MS often decrease during pregnancy but may increase slightly after pregnancy.	Because sexual difficulties may come and go with other MS symptoms, it helps to be creative. Some medication for spasms and topical anesthetics for pain may be helpful. If our balance is not good and we tire easily, we can use a vibrator or participate in lovemaking activities that require little exertion. Some women say that vaginal penetration is painful but having their clitoris stimulated feels good. The birth control pill is

CHRONIC DISEASE OR DISABILITY	EFFECTS ON OUR SEXUALITY	HELPFUL HINTS AND SPECIAL IMPLICATIONS
Multiple sclerosis (MS) (cont.)		not advisable if we have paralysis or restricted mobility, but recent studies have shown that it may help symptoms in early stages of MS.[47] **A, B, D, E**
Ostomy	More is known about the sexual functioning of men with ostomies than about women with ostomies, even today. Surgery should not impair our genital responsivity or fertility.[48] However, a few women report pain during vaginal penetration or a lack of vaginal sensations after ileostomy and colostomy surgery.	An ostomy is a hidden disability until our clothes are off; therefore, it may help to find a comfortable way to tell potential partners before sexual relations begin. The opening or appliance may be covered or secured before lovemaking, both for aesthetic reasons and for support, so it does not get in the way. We can use lovemaking positions in which we feel most secure that the bag will not get pulled out. If odors are a problem, we can bathe and empty the bag before making love. Consider alternatives to the birth control pill, and consult a physician if taking it, because sometimes it is not absorbed properly.
Spinal cord injury (SCI)	SCI may result in paralysis, spasticity, loss of sensation, incontinence, skin ulcers, pain, and a dry vagina, sometimes complicating making love. Changes in our ability to lubricate or feel genital sensations will depend on the level and severity of our injury.[49] We may continue to have orgasms, regardless of the level or degree of paralysis. They may be similar to those before injury or may be diffuse, either in general or to specific body parts, such as our breasts or lips. Exploration is the key to discovering these changes. Our neck and ears and the area above the injury may become more sexually exciting. Arousal, self-pleasuring, and lovemaking may increase spasms and the risk of incontinence. Although we may stop menstruating for several months after the injury, fertility is not permanently disrupted.[50]	It can help to make love in ways other than vaginal penetration, which may be difficult or painful because of increased bladder infections, spasms, and vaginal irritation and tearing. Taking our time and using a vibrator helps some women experience orgasm. Be aware that for some women with high-level paralysis, intense vaginal stimulation (as in childbirth, or in penetration/vibrator use that is especially prolonged and vigorous) can cause autonomic dysreflexia (AD). AD can lead to a life-threatening disruption of the nervous system. Its symptoms include elevated blood pressure, severe headache, increased spasms, and chills.[51] Routine bowel and bladder programs can decrease the risk of "accidents" during sex, and a towel will help if there is any leakage. We can also tape down the catheter or move it out of the way so it doesn't get pulled out. Some spasm medications may be of assistance. Pregnancy increases the risk of blood clot development and bladder infection, but many women have healthy and painless births. During labor and delivery, be on

CHRONIC DISEASE OR DISABILITY	EFFECTS ON OUR SEXUALITY	HELPFUL HINTS AND SPECIAL IMPLICATIONS
Spinal cord injury (SCI) (cont.)		guard for signs of autonomic dysreflexia and uterine prolapse.[52,53] Birth control pills are usually not advisable and should not be used if taking anti-hypertensive medication.[54] **A, B, C, D, E**

A: Many medications are directly responsible for the negative effects on our sexuality—often much more so than the disability itself! Examples of such drugs are antihypertensives (i.e., diuretics), antidepressants (i.e., selective serotonin reuptake inhibitors), tranquilizers (i.e., phenothiazines), spasticity medications (i.e., baclofen), and antiseizure medications (i.e., phenytoin), as well as medications such as lithium, digoxin, reserpine, and naproxen.[55]

B: The diaphragm may not be recommended if you have poor hand control, recurrent bladder or vaginal infections, or very weak pelvic muscles. If the use of your hands is limited, ask your partner or attendant to help insert the diaphragm. Also, devices are available that can make it easier to insert the coil-spring diaphragm, but some hand control is required.

C: The IUD is not a good birth control method for women with a loss of sensation in the pelvic area because of the risk that puncture or pelvic inflammatory disease may go unnoticed.[56] Also, some hand coordination is needed to check the strings every month and make sure the IUD is still in place.

D: Estrogen-containing birth control pills can increase the risk of clotting and cause serious medical problems such as embolism, deep vein thrombosis, and stroke. Progestin-only pills ("minipills") or progestin-containing injectable contraceptives such as Norplant may be a good alternative because they do not contain estrogen.[57,58] Newer contraceptive methods such as low-dose oral pills, contraceptive patches, and NuvaRing release less estrogen than earlier versions of the Pill.[59] However, the dangers of these methods are similar to those of estrogen-containing pills, so check with your health care provider before using any new method.

Because some birth control medications may interact poorly or be rendered less effective when taken in combination with other drugs, be sure to inform your health care providers about the medications and dosage you are taking when seeking contraceptive services.

E: A water-soluble lubricant can often help with a dry vagina.

NOTES

1. The Guerilla Girls, *Bitches, Bimbos and Ballbreakers: The Guerilla Girls' Illustrated Guide to Female Stereotypes* (New York: Penguin Books, 2003), 85–87.

2. Personal anecdote from Gina Ogden's study "Integrating Sexuality and Spirituality (ISIS)," conducted in 1999.

3. Ibid.

4. Gina Ogden, "Sexuality and Spirituality in Women's Relationships: Preliminary Results of an Exploratory Survey," in *Working Paper 405* (Wellesley College Center for Research on Women: Wellesley, MA, 2002).

5. Deborah L. Tolman, *Dilemmas of Desire: Teenage Girls Talk About Sexuality* (Cambridge, MA: Harvard University Press, 2002).

6. The Working Group on a New View of Women's Sexual Problems, "A New View of Women's Sexual Problems," in Ellyn Kaschak and Leonore Tiefer, eds., *A New View of Women's Sexual Problems* (Binghamton, NY: Haworth Press, 2001), 1–8.

7. R. Basson, "Women's Sexual Desire—Disordered or Misunderstood?", *Journal of Sex and Marital Therapy* 28, Supplement 1 (2002): 17–28. For practical suggestions, you might want to read "When I'm Hot and You're Not," in *Hot Monogamy* by Patricia Love and Jo Robinson (New York: Plume, 1994).

8. This section draws from the description of models of sexual response in *Exploring Our Sexuality* by Patricia Barthalow Koch (Dubuque, IA: Kendall/Hunt Publishing Company, 1995).

9. Leonore Tiefer, "Arriving at a 'New View' of Women's Sexual Problems: Background, Theory, and Activism" in Ellyn Kaschak and Leonore Tiefer, eds., *A New View of Women's Sexual Problems* (Binghamton, NY: Haworth Press, 2001), 77–78.

10. Shere Hite, *The Hite Report: A National Study of Female Sexuality* (New York: Seven Stories Press, 2004).

11. Helen Singer Kaplan, *Disorders of Sexual Desire* (New York: Brunner/Mazel, 1979).

12. B. Zilbergeld and C. R. Ellison, "Desire Discrepancies and Arousal Problems in Sex Therapy," in S. R. Leiblum and L. A. Pervin, eds., *Principles and Practice of Sex Therapy* (New York: Guilford, 1980), 65–104.

13. In a rare condition called "persistent sexual arousal syndrome," a woman sustains unwanted, persistent, and intense genital arousal, unaccompanied by sexual desire, which is only temporarily relieved by orgasm. The condition can be extremely distressing and may be caused by medications such as trazodone, or a combination of physical, psychological, or emotional factors. Boston Medical Institute for Sexual Medicine, accessed at www.bumc.bu.edu/departments/pagemain.asp?departmentid=371&page=8105 on November 12, 2003.

14. Gina Ogden, *Women Who Love Sex: An Inquiry into the Expanding Spirit of Women's Erotic Experience* (Cambridge, MA: Womanspirit Press, 1999), 45–71.

15. The G-spot was named by the sex researchers Dr. John Perry and Dr. Beverly Whipple, after Dr. Ernst Grafenberg, who wrote about it in 1950.

16. Martha Cornog, *The Big Book of Masturbation: From August to Zeal* (San Francisco: Down There Press, 2003), 183–86.

17. Lorraine Dennerstein, "Female Sexuality, the Menstrual Cycle, and the Pill," in S. Zeidenstein and A. Moore, eds., *Learning About Sexuality: A Practical Beginning* (New York: Population Council, 1996), 257.

18. Helen Singer Kaplan and Trude Owett, "The Female Androgen Deficiency Syndrome," *Journal of Sex and Marital Therapy* 19, no. 1 (Spring 1993): 3–24.

19. Ibid. and also Jan L. Shifren et al., "Transdermal Testosterone Treatment in Women with Impaired Sexual Function After Oophorectomy," *The New England Journal of Medicine* 343 (September 7, 2000): 682–88.

20. Catherine T. Liverman and Dan G. Blazer, eds., *Testosterone and Aging: Clinical Research Directions* (Washington, D.C.: National Academies Press, 2004).

21. Steve Dow, "The Pinking of Viagra," accessed at www.alternet.org/story.html?StoryID=15096 on February 4, 2003.

22. Thank you to psychologist Judy Leavitt for this concept.

23. Carol Rinkleib Ellison, *Women's Sexualities* (Oakland, CA: New Harbinger, 2000), 204.

24. Ogden, *Women Who Love Sex*, 128–48.

25. Jo Campling, ed., "Julie," in *Images of Ourselves: Women with Disabilities Talking* (London: Routledge and Kegan Paul, 1981), 17.

26. Barry R. Komisaruk and Beverly Whipple, "The Suppression of Pain by Genital Stimulation in Females," *Annual Review of Sex Research* 6 (1995): 151–86.

27. Marca L. Sipski, Craig J. Alexander, and Ray C. Rosen, "Orgasm in Women with Spinal Cord Injuries: A Laboratory-Based Assessment," *Archives of Physical Medicine and Rehabilitation* 76 (1995): 1097–102.

28. K. Best, "Epilepsy Drugs May Reduce Method Effectiveness," *Network* 2, no. 19 (Winter 1999): 12.

29. State Government Victoria Department of Human Services, Australia, Disability Online, "Traumatic Brain Injury and Sexual Issues," accessed at www.disability.vic.gov.au/dsonline/dsarticles.nsf/pages/Traumatic_brain_injury_and_sexual_issues?OpenDocument on September 29, 2004.

30. The Sexual Health Network, "Possible Effects of a Traumatic Brain Injury on a Person's Sexuality," accessed at www.sexualhealth.com/article.php?Action=read&article_id=336&channel=3&topic=12 on September 29, 2004.

31. Epilepsy Foundation, "Birth Control for Women with Epilepsy," accessed at www.epilepsyfoundation.org/answerplace/Life/adults/women/weibirthcontrol.cfm on September 29, 2004.

32. S. Morano, "Pathophysiology of Diabetic Sexual Dysfunction," *Journal of Endocrinological Investigation* 26, Supplement 3 (2003): 65–69.

33. P. Enzlin et al., "Prevalence and Predictors of Sexual Dysfunction in Patients with Type I Diabetes," *Diabetes Care* 26 (2003): 409–14.

34. Morano, "Pathophysiology of Diabetic Sexual Dysfunction."

35. J. Bringer et al., "Which Contraception to Choose for the Diabetic Woman?," *Diabetes & Metabolism* 27, no. 4 (2001): S35–41.

36. J. Guan et al., "Sexual Dysfunction in Patients with Chronic Renal Failure," *Zhonghua Nan Ke Xue* 9, no. 6 (September 2003): 454–56, 461.

37. S. Wysocki and S. Schnare, "Current Advances in Oral Contraceptives: OC Use in Patients with Common Medical Conditions," Excerpt from National Institute of Child Health and Human Development June 2001 meeting, *Preventing Unintended Pregnancy: Advances in Hormonal Contraception,* accessed at www.npwh.org/Oral-Contraception/.

38. J. Hill et al., "Effects of Rheumatoid Arthritis on Sexual Activity and Relationships," *Rheumatology* 2, no. 42 (February 2003): 280–86.

39. Florence Denmark, "Myths of Aging," *Eye on Psi Chi* (Fall 2002) 7, no. 1, 14–21, accessed on September 29, 2004 at www.psichi.org/pubs/articles/article_38.asp.

40. Sandra Welner, "A Provider's Guide for the Care of

Women with Physical Disabilities and Mental Conditions," North Carolina Office on Disability and Health, 1999, accessed on September 29, 2004 at www.fpg.unc.edu/~ncodh/Provider.pdf.

41. Ibid.

42. *Merck Manual of Geriatrics,* "Effects of Medical Disorders on Sexuality," accessed on September 29, 2004 at www.merck.com/mrkshared/mm_geriatrics/sec14/ch114.jsp.

43. Annette Owens, "Cardiovascular Disease: Sexual Problems and Their Management," Sexual Health Network, accessed on September 29, 2004 at www.sexualhealth.com/content/read.cfm?ID=64&theTopic=Disability%20or%20Illness&topicID=36&subtopicID=48.

44. Welner, "A Provider's Guide for the Care of Women with Physical Disabilities and Mental Conditions."

45. A. J. McDougall and J. G. McLeod, "Autonomic Nervous System Function in Multiple Sclerosis," *Journal of Neurological Science* 215, no. 1–2 (November 15, 2003): 79–85.

46. Welner, "A Provider's Guide for the Care of Women with Physical Disabilities and Mental Conditions."

47. S. Subramanian et al., "Oral Feeding with Ethinyl Estradiol Suppresses and Treats Experimental Autoimmune Encephalomyelitis in SJL Mice and Inhibits the Recruitment of Inflammatory Cells into the Central Nervous System," *Journal of Immunology* 170, no. 3 (February 1, 2003): 1548–55.

48. *Merck Manual of Geriatrics,* "Effects of Surgery on Sexuality."

49. The Sexual Health Network, "Possible Effects of SCI on Sexual Functioning," accessed on September 29, 2004 at www.sexualhealth.com/article.php?Action=read&article_id=248&channel=3&topic=11.

50. F. Biering-Sorensen, "Sexual Function in Patients with Spinal Cord Injuries," *VgesKrift for Laeger* 164, no. 41 (October 7, 2002): 4,764–68.

51. L. Pereira, "Obstetric Management of the Patient with Spinal Cord Injury," *Obstetrical and Gynecological Survey* 58, no. 10 (October 2003): 678–87.

52. W. M. Helkowski et al., "Autonomic Dysreflexia: Incidence in Persons with Neurologically Complete and Incomplete Tetraplegia," *Journal of Spinal Cord Medicine* 26, no. 3 (Fall 2003): 244–47.

53. G. P. Earl, "Autonomic Dysreflexia," *MCN: American Journal of Maternal Child Nursing* 27, no. 2 (March–April 2002): 93–97.

54. B. T. Benevento and M. L. Sipski, "Neurogenic Bladder, Neurogenic Bowel, and Sexual Dysfunction in People with Spinal Cord Injury," *Physical Therapy* 82, no. 6 (June 2002): 601–12.

55. EngenderHealth.org, Sexuality and Sexual Health Online Mini-Course, "Drugs That Affect Sexual Function," based in part on EngenderHealth's *Self-Instructional Module: STIs, HIV/AIDS, and Sexuality,* written by Dr. Mark Barone and Julie Becker and produced in 1999. Accessed on September 29, 2004 at www.engenderhealth.org/res/onc/sexuality/response/miw/pg7.html.

56. E. Hakim-elahi, "Contraception for the Disabled," *Female Patient* 16, no. 10 (October 1991): 19–20, 24, 27.

57. Welner, "A Provider's Guide for the Care of Women with Physical Disabilities and Mental Conditions."

58. International Planned Parenthood Federation, *IMAP Statement on Contraception for Women with Medical Disorders,* 1999, accessed on September 29, 2004 at www.ippf.org/medical/imap/statements/eng/pdf/199906a.pdf.

59. D. M. Plourd and W. F. Rayburn, "New Contraceptive Methods," *Journal of Reproductive Medicine* 9, no. 48 (September 2003): 665–71.

Sexual Health

Sexual Anatomy, Reproduction, and the Menstrual Cycle

This chapter offers a tour of female sexual anatomy, including parts both inside and outside the body.* The first part of the chapter talks about names of body parts, where to find them, and what they do. How are parts different, and how do they work together? What is "normal"? The second part of the chapter covers periods and fertility awareness. It explains how the menstrual cycle works, as well as the practical issues: choices about menstrual products, physical and emotional changes across the cycle, and the debate about voluntarily stopping periods.

* Note that this chapter describes female sexual anatomy, but some of us who identify as women do not have this anatomy. Others have parts of both male and female anatomy. Yet still others identify as men or as neither man nor woman but have female sex anatomy.

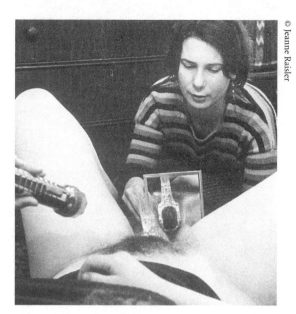
© Jeanne Raisler

SEXUAL ANATOMY:
THE SELF-GUIDED TOUR

One way to learn about your body is to take a self-guided tour. This is your road map. It describes the sexual and reproductive organs both outside and inside your body. Many of us find it empowering to learn about our bodies in this way. If you are not interested in or able to take the tour physically—looking at and touching your own body—you can still learn about female anatomy by reading the following descriptions. Find a comfortable place to sit, with good lighting, either to read the words or to see your body. If you are taking the tour yourself, you may want a speculum,* flashlight, and hand mirror. This is your tour, and you may take it as many times or in as many ways as you like; you may read and experience this alone or with another trusted person. (For more detailed information, see "Sexual Anatomy Tour" [W31] on the companion website, www.ourbodiesourselves.org.)

* You can buy a speculum at your local medical supply store or order online or via phone. The Feminist Women's Health Center is one resource, www.fwhc.org/sale3.htm#plainspec and 509-575-6473 x121.

STOPS ON THE TOUR

The tour has six parts:

1. **Exits, entrances,** which discusses the following openings to your body: introitus, urinary opening, and anus.
2. **On the outside (and just beneath)** discusses parts of the vulva and its neighbors: vulva, pubic hair, mons, pubis symphysis, labia majora, labia minora, perineum, and vestibule.
3. **The vagina and its neighbors,** including the following: vagina, hymen, urethral sponge, fornix (part of the vagina), cervix, os (part of the cervix), and pubococcygeus (PC) muscle.

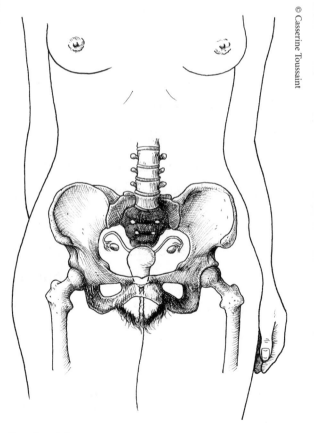
© Casserine Toussaint

Female pelvic organs

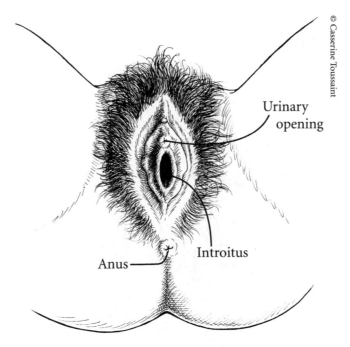

Urinary opening

Anus

Introitus

© Casserine Toussaint

Exits, Entrances

EXITS, ENTRANCES			
COMMON NAME	ANATOMICAL NAME	FUNCTION/ROLE	CAN YOU SEE IT?
Vaginal opening	Introitus	Opening to the vagina	Yes
Pee hole	Urinary opening (Meatus)	Opening to the urethra–the tube that leads to your bladder, where urine is stored before it exits your body	Yes
Butt hole	Anus	Opening of the rectum, the end of the large intestine	Yes

Notes

1. Opening 1, the introitus: This is the vaginal opening and leads to the vagina, where menstrual blood flows out. The vagina is the birth canal through which babies travel to the outside world (unless they're delivered by surgery). Some women may insert a tampon, finger, penis, dildo, or speculum here.

2. Opening 2, the urinary opening: This is where your urine (or pee) comes out.

3. Opening 3, the anus: This is where you defecate (or poop) from. Some women may insert a finger, penis, dildo, butt plug, or anal beads in the anus.

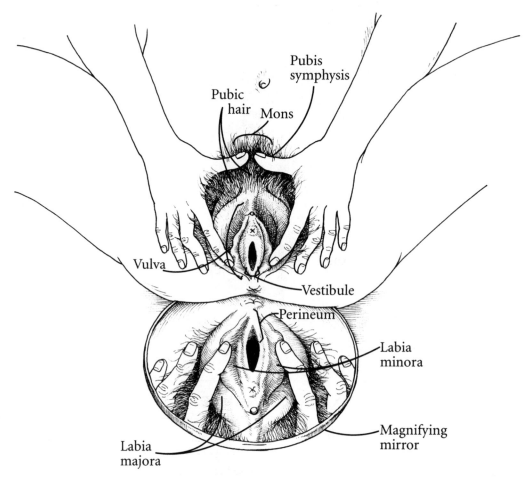

On the Outside (or Just Beneath)

ON THE OUTSIDE (OR JUST BENEATH)			
COMMON NAME	ANATOMICAL NAME	FUNCTION/ROLE	CAN YOU SEE IT?
Genitals, pussy, yoni, cunt	Vulva	An area consisting of many of the parts that follow. The vulva protects your sexual organs, which are the sites of sexual response.	Yes
Pubes	Pubic hair	Protects, cushions, and prevents irritation during sexual intercourse	Yes

COMMON NAME	ANATOMICAL NAME	FUNCTION/ROLE	CAN YOU SEE IT?
Mound	Mons, mons veneris, mons pubis	Skin and fat covering pubic bone; protects and cushions during sexual intercourse	Yes
Pubic bone	Pubis symphysis	Joint of the pubic bones. To feel it, try placing one hand on each hip and tracing your hip bones down in a V-shape toward your vulva.	No
Outer lips	Labia majora	Protect the inner lips	Yes
Inner lips	Labia minora	Swell during sexual stimulation	Yes
Taint (t'aint, derived from "it ain't either vagina or anus")	Perineum	Between vaginal opening and anus, stretches during childbirth	Yes
	Vestibule	Area between sides of labia minora, contains urethra and vagina	Yes

Notes

1. Be careful not to confuse "vulva" with "vagina." The vulva is the outside that you can see easily, and it includes many parts. The vagina is just one part on the inside of your body. People often incorrectly refer to the vulva as the vagina, but they are different.

2. The terms "yoni," "pussy," and "cunt" also describe the vulva. Sometimes these words are used in a derogatory way to disempower women, but some women have reclaimed the words' power by using them with pride.

3. Not only is looking at our vulva a way to learn about our bodies, but regularly examining the vulva is a good habit to develop. We can observe what is "normal" for us and detect anything out of the ordinary to discuss with our health care provider.[1,2]

4. **Find your orgasm here!** This section is all about the clitoris and its many wonderful parts: clitoris, hood of clitoris, glans of clitoris, shaft of clitoris, suspensory ligament, crura, bulbs of the vestibule, and vestibular glands.

5. **All the way in** focuses on the following parts of our internal sexual anatomy: uterus, fundus, fallopian tubes, and ovaries.

6. **Our breasts** details the parts of breast anatomy: areola, nipple, sebaceous glands, fat, connective tissue, and milk-producing glands.

INTERSEX

"Intersex" refers to a variety of conditions in which a person is born with sex chromosomes, external genitals, or an internal reproductive system that is not clearly male or female. The clitoris may be larger than usual, or the vagina may be small, lack an external opening, or be absent altogether. Intersex is not always evident from an external examination; for example, a person may be born with external female genitals and with XY chromosomes and internal testes (male reproductive glands) rather than ovaries.

The traditional model of medical management, developed in the 1950s, was based on the idea that intersex people could be helped to live a "normal" life only if their condition were hidden. Doctors concealed information and promoted early cosmetic genital surgery (frequently removing parts of the clitoris) and later hormone treatments. People treated this way often grew up with a sense of intense shame, depression, and compromised sexuality.

Most specialists continue to surgically alter intersex babies, although there is growing controversy over this practice. While some intersex conditions may involve health issues that require medical intervention, the primary rationale for most intersex surgeries is to make genitals look clearly male or female to prevent emotional trauma. Such surgeries can create health problems, impair sexual functioning later in life, and actually contribute to emotional trauma. For these reasons an increasing number of specialists agree with patient advocates that cosmetic genital surgery should be performed only when chosen by a well-informed patient, and never on infants.

Angela Moreno describes her experience of surgery:

"When I was twelve, I started to notice that my clitoris (that wonderful location of pleasure for which I had no name but to which I had grown quite attached) had grown more prominent. Exactly one month later, I was admitted to Children's Memorial Hospital in Chicago for surgery. They told me a little bit about the part where they were going to 're-move my ovaries' because they suspected cancer or something like that. They didn't mention the part where they were going to slice off my clitoris. All of it. I guess the doctors assumed I was as horrified by my outsized clit as they were, and there was no need to discuss it with me. After a week's recovery in the hospital, we all went home and barely ever spoke of it again. I'm now twenty-four. I've spent the last ten years in a haze of disordered eating and occasional depression. Four months ago, I finally got some of my medical records from Children's Memorial Hospital in Chicago. They are shocking. The surgeon who removed my clitoris summarized the outcome as 'tolerated well.'" [3]

Organizations such as the Intersex Society of North America (www.isna.org) are fighting to end the secrecy and shame around intersexuality and to develop better approaches to health care for intersex people.

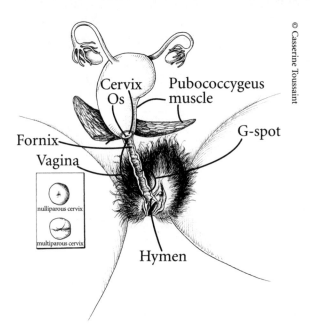

The Vagina and Its Neighbors

THE VAGINA AND ITS NEIGHBORS

COMMON NAME	ANATOMICAL NAME	FUNCTION/ROLE	CAN YOU SEE IT?
Vagina, birth canal	Vagina	Pathway for menstrual blood, and babies at birth; place where tampon, penis, dildo, fingers, or vibrator may be inserted	Yes
Cherry	Hymen	Thin membrane around vaginal opening	Maybe, if it's still there—sometimes you can see its remnants
G-spot	Urethral sponge/ perineal sponge	Erectile tissue against front wall of vagina; orgasm and pleasure site	No, but you can feel it with your fingers
	Fornix (part of vagina)	Back end of vagina, near cervix	Yes, with a speculum

(continued)

THE VAGINA AND ITS NEIGHBORS (*continued*)

Cervix	Cervix	Entrance to uterus from vagina; dilates during labor	Yes, with a speculum
	Os (part of cervix)	Opening to uterus; part of cervix	Yes, with a speculum
Pelvic floor muscle	Pubococcygeus (PC) muscle	Supports pelvic organs and other organs; see "Pump Up Your Pelvic Floor: Kegel Exercises" p. 235	No

Notes

1. If you try to put a finger or two inside your vagina, and it hurts or you have trouble, take a deep breath, relax, and use a lubricant such as Astroglide or K-Y jelly. You may be pushing at the wrong angle, or your vagina may be dry. Shifting positions, breathing deeply, and using lubricant should help.

2. You may or may not be able to see the remains of your hymen, which disappear for different reasons and at different times. Exercising, using a tampon, and sexual activity all can cause the hymen to disintegrate. Whether or not you have a visible hymen says *nothing* about whether or not you have had sex. It is *impossible* to tell simply by looking at a woman's hymen whether she has had sexual intercourse.

3. Wet and dry: If you move your fingers around (in small circles inside the vagina or gently in and out of it), you may notice that your finger slides around inside the vagina as you move it. The walls of the vagina range from almost dry to very wet. How wet your vagina is depends on you (some women naturally have wetter or drier vaginas), and your own wetness may change during different parts of your menstrual cycle or lifetime. Wetness often increases with sexual arousal.

4. G-spot: A particular area near the vagina is the urethral sponge (also called the perineal sponge), or G-spot. Some of us know exactly where our G-spot is; for others of us, locating the G-spot is more challenging. The G-spot (named for Dr. Ernest Grafenberg, who originally wrote about it) refers to an area inside our bodies. It surrounds the urethra, but we can feel it when we press up against the front wall of our vagina. Stimulation of this area may lead to orgasm and/or ejaculation (see "G-spot: Can You Spot It?" on p. 197). Some women find orgasms from stimulating the G-spot more pleasurable than orgasms from stimulating the clitoris; some women find them harder to achieve than orgasms from stimulating the clitoris. To feel your G-spot, try to touch the front wall of your vagina, below your belly button. You may feel it about one third to half the way up your vagina, not as high up as your cervix. This stop on the self-guided tour may be more difficult to find, but many women report that it's a hidden jewel.

5. A rosebud or a smile? The opening of the cervix is the os, the opening to the uterus. Women who have never had a vaginal birth have an os that feels like a rosebud. Women who have given birth vaginally have an os that feels like the curve of a smile. The cervix also feels like a cartilage spot, such as the tip of your nose; it's not as soft as other parts inside your vagina. The texture and position of the cervix change throughout the menstrual cycle.

6. It won't get lost! Except when the os opens wide to have a baby come out (and at that time, it expands enormously), the os has only a tiny opening that is normally closed with mucus for most of the cycle. No tampon, finger, or penis can go up through it. This is why you never need to worry that a tampon, dildo, or anything else can get "lost" inside your vagina. If you hear horror stories to the contrary, rest assured that they are not true.

PUMP UP YOUR PELVIC FLOOR: KEGEL EXERCISES

Did you know that exercise can lead to better orgasms and an easier time giving birth? Not just any exercise, but a particular set of exercises to strengthen the pelvic floor. In addition to the positive effects on orgasms and birth, these exercises can restore muscle tone after giving birth, improve bladder control, and possibly treat vulvar pain conditions. They are called Kegel exercises, after Dr. Arnold Kegel. You may also hear them called strengthening exercises, elevators, or PC exercises.

The pelvic floor muscles surround our three openings (bladder, vagina, and rectum) and are also called the *pubococcygeus (PC) muscle.* An easy way to find the pelvic floor muscles is to pretend that you're holding in pee (it's not a good idea to do this while you are peeing). Also, you may put your finger halfway inside your vagina and try to grip your finger with your vagina. Think of pulling muscles up and in, and try to relax your abdominal muscles and buttocks. It's easy to involve them in these exercises, but if you use your abdomen, you're not exercising the PC! Try squeezing up and in for ten seconds and then relaxing for ten seconds. Repeat for a few minutes. You also may experiment with quick flicks or squeezes in and out, to get the feel for the muscle. You can do these exercises anywhere and at any time. Try making a habit of doing them while waiting at red lights or standing at the sink doing dishes.

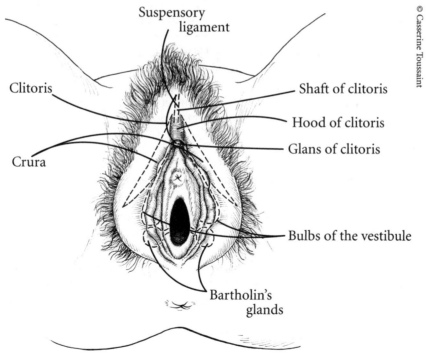

© Casserine Toussaint

Suspensory ligament

Clitoris

Crura

Shaft of clitoris

Hood of clitoris

Glans of clitoris

Bulbs of the vestibule

Bartholin's glands

Find Your Orgasm Here! (Dotted lines indicate areas inside the body.)

FIND YOUR ORGASM HERE!

	COMMON NAME	ANATOMICAL NAME	FUNCTION/ROLE	CAN YOU SEE IT?
NOW YOU SEE IT . . .	Clit	Clitoris; it has many parts, described below	Sexual arousal and orgasm	Parts of it
	Hood	Hood of clitoris	Protects and connects to the glans	Yes
		Glans of clitoris	Tip of the clitoris: most sensitive part; contains thousands of nerve endings that experience sensations of pleasure	Yes
. . . NOW YOU DON'T—FELT BUT NOT SEEN		Shaft of clitoris	Like a cord; has blood vessels that fill during arousal	No, but can feel it
		Suspensory ligament (part of clitoris)	Connects the shaft to the ovarian ligaments, passing over the pubic bone	No
	Legs	Crura	Tips of erectile tissue that attach shaft to the pelvic bones	No
		Bulbs of the vestibule	Fill with blood during arousal	No
		Vestibular glands, Bartholin's glands, or vulvovaginal glands	Produce a few drops of fluid during arousal; provide immune protection	No, but can feel them

Notes

1. The glans of the clitoris is the most sensitive spot in the entire genital area. It is made up of erectile tissue that swells during sexual arousal.

2. Remember how many people confuse "vulva" and "vagina"? Well, many people confuse the *glans*—only the tip of the clitoris—with the whole clitoris. The clitoris is a complex organ with many parts, and the glans is only one (very important) part of it.

3. Did you know that the whole clitoris and vestibular bulbs are the only organs in the human body that are designed solely for sexual sensation and arousal? (For more information, see Chapter 12, "Sexuality.")

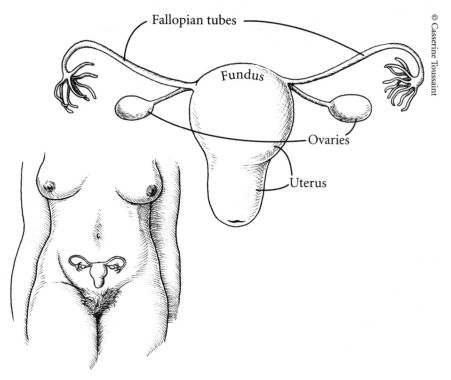

Fallopian tubes

Fundus

Ovaries

Uterus

© Casserine Toussaint

All the Way In . . .

ALL THE WAY IN . . .			
COMMON NAME	ANATOMICAL NAME	FUNCTION/ROLE	CAN YOU SEE IT?
Womb	Uterus	Where menstrual blood is developed; where fetus may grow	No
	Fundus (part of uterus)	Top of the uterus	No
Tubes	Fallopian tubes, oviducts	Pathway between ovaries and uterus; where egg may be fertilized	No

(continued)

	Ovaries	Where eggs are housed and matured; site of hormone production (such as estrogen, progesterone, and testosterone)	No

Notes

1. Often when we see drawings of the uterus, fallopian tubes, or ovaries, we don't have a good idea of where those parts are located inside our bodies. The base of the uterus starts at the cervix. You can see your cervix with a mirror and feel it as well; envision the uterus beginning just behind that.

2. The ovaries are organs about the size and shape of unshelled almonds or large grapes, located on either side of and somewhat below the uterus. They are about four or five inches below the waist.

3. The fallopian tubes start right next to the ovaries, circle down, and end in the uterus. The ovaries aren't actually connected to the fallopian tubes. There is a small gap between the ovary and the end of its neighboring fallopian tube. This gap allows the egg to float freely after it has been released from the ovary. The fingerlike ends (fimbria) of the fallopian tube sweep across the surface of the ovary and propel the egg into the tube after ovulation.

OUR BREASTS

In popular North American culture, women's breasts get an enormous amount of attention: How big are they? Are they real? Do bigger breasts make women sexier? Despite all this attention, or perhaps because of it, many of us do not take the time to get to know our own breasts and realize what they do or do not mean for us. Like fingerprints, no two breasts are alike, and there is no "perfect" pair.

If you never have looked at your breasts in the mirror, try it. Since their appearance or feel may change during your menstrual cycle or as you age, it is important to know for yourself what "normal" is for your breasts. Your breasts may have areas of hardness or softness, different textures, and varying areas of sensitivity. Examining your breasts regularly can help you learn your usual patterns as well as detect anything out of the ordinary. (For more information about examining your breasts, see Chapter 28, "Unique to Women," p. 597.)

When you look at your breasts in the mirror, you may notice that they are not the same size or shape. Sometimes the right one is smaller than the left, or vice versa. If you observe the shape of your breasts over time, you will also notice that they usually become droopier over the years as your skin becomes less elastic and your milk glands get smaller. This happens even faster after menopause, when the milk glands are no longer stimulated to grow. Because the breast reacts to sex hormones produced by the ovaries, you may notice pronounced changes during the menstrual cycle—your breasts may be bigger and fuller right before you menstruate. This fullness can produce tenderness in some women and can

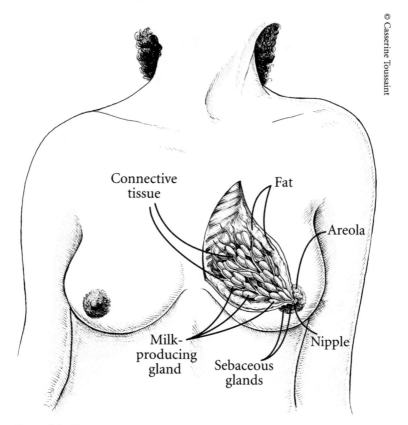

Connective
tissue

Fat

Areola

Milk-
producing
gland

Sebaceous
glands

Nipple

Parts of the Breast

© Casserine Toussaint

PARTS OF THE BREAST

NAME	LOCATION/APPEARANCE	FUNCTION/ROLE	CAN YOU SEE IT?
Areola	Circle of skin (may vary in color) in the middle of breast, surrounding the nipple; may be a different color from other parts of breast; may have bumps or hairs growing out. In many women, the areolae get darker during pregnancy.	Surrounds the nipple and contains muscle that makes the nipple stand out in response to cold, sexual stimulation, and breast-feeding (stimulation point for milk letdown). This is where an infant's mouth closes on the breast when nursing. Has a pleasure function as well.	Yes

(continued)

Sexual Anatomy, Reproduction, and the Menstrual Cycle ■ ■ ■ 239

PARTS OF THE BREAST (*continued*)

Nipple	Center of the breast; may lie flat, stick outward, go inward (be inverted)	Contains milk duct openings (many tiny openings for milk to pass through); with the areola, it may become harder or pointier (erect) in response to sexual arousal (a pleasure function), heat, or cold	Yes
Sebaceous glands, oil glands	Bumps on the areola	Secrete lubricant that protects the nipple during nursing	Yes
Fat	Throughout breast	Protects and surrounds glands and connective tissue	No
Connective tissue	Throughout breast	Provides support and structure for breast; holds the milk ducts, milk-producing glands, and other structures in place	No
Milk-producing gland (mammary gland)	Made up of milk-producing sacs and tubes (ducts)	Carry milk to the nipple for lactation; may produce clear fluid even when we are not lactating	No

be felt down into the armpit in the part of the breast called the *tail*. During pregnancy and nursing, breasts can enlarge considerably. They may also swell during sexual arousal.

With the great increase of sex hormones during adolescence, the milk-producing gland in each breast starts to develop and increase in size. All women have approximately the same amount of milk-producing tissue at the same points in our reproductive life cycles. Most of the breast consists of fat that surrounds the gland as well as connective tissue. The amount of fat in the breasts is determined partly by heredity. This fat causes breast size to vary, and it explains why breast size is not related to the sexual responsiveness of the breast or to the amount of milk produced after giving birth. (For more on breast-feeding, see Chapter 23, "The First Year of Parenting.")

MENSTRUATION AND REPRODUCTION

In addition to the growth of breasts and pubic and armpit hair, the onset of menstruation is a major marker in the transition from girl to woman. Women talk about periods in many different ways, but it's amazing how little we use the words "bleed" or "blood." There are a vast number of menstrual euphemisms that women may use to describe the cycle. English-language eu-

If you choose to shave, wax, or pierce your genital area, the important words are "clean" and "caution." Use only very clean tools and exercise caution, since this is a sensitive area of your body. Particularly if you pierce, make sure you go to a trained professional who uses sterile tools. Check out the Association of Professional Piercers' statement, "A Piercee's Bill of Rights" (www.safepiercing.org/rights.html or call 1-888-888-1APP).

phemisms include "my red friend," "the curse," "my period," "Aunt Flo," and "on the rag." Consider how you talk about and feel about menstruation. (For an online list of euphemisms, see www.mum.org/words.html.)

This section explores our bodies' differences and variations regarding the menstrual cycle. It also discusses fertility awareness, a method of observing and charting body signs that reflect fertility, which can be used for birth control or to increase the likelihood of conception and to learn about our health. As with our bodies, we can describe menstruation with a set of basic physical facts, but there is no one right way to experience menstruation. We embrace variety, difference, and unique experiences.

BROAD STROKES— MENARCHE TO MENOPAUSE

Girls experience first periods in a variety of ways, as do women experiencing last menstrual cycles. Biology contributes to these variations, but so do the place, time, and culture in which we live. During puberty, we make the transition from childhood to physical maturity. In women,

puberty is characterized by growth of the breasts and the pubic and armpit (axillary) hair, and a growth spurt that results in increased height and weight. Bone size and strength stop increasing around puberty, but bone mass continues to grow through the twenties. The reproductive process is regulated by hormones, which are chemicals in the bloodstream and brain that relay messages from one part of the body to another. The levels of sex hormones are low during childhood, increase tremendously during the reproductive years, and then become lower and balance differently after menopause. The changes we experience around menarche and menopause (and during our entire menstrual lives) are thought to be caused primarily by changing levels of hormones.

Ovulation and menstruation start near the end of puberty, on average at about twelve and a half,[4] though any age from nine to eighteen is normal. The age of menarche varies depending on many factors. (Menarche, pronounced *men-ar-kee*, is when we get our first period.) Some factors are biological; for instance, a girl needs her body fat to be about one quarter of her total weight in order to menstruate. To sustain regular cycles, we also need to eat a balance of fat, carbohydrates (sugars and starches), and protein. Some factors are due to our environments. Women in different cultures may enter puberty at different times. For example, girls in Taiwan have a different average age of menarche than girls in the United States.[5] Girls living in the same country may have different average ages of menarche depending on factors such as diet, weight, race, environment, and family history.[6,7]

In class, I got up to go to the bathroom. Inside, I noticed that my panties had a funny discharge on them. Then suddenly it hit me: I'd gotten my period! I was so excited and could hardly wait to tell my friends. . . . They were all excited and very happy for me. . . . Nobody I knew was embarrassed about my getting my period.

I was born in 1944 and had my first period at 11, while still in the 6th grade. My mother had "left out" a book called On Human Growth, *which I had read, so I knew what it was when I had my first period. But it embarrassed me. I put lots of toilet paper in my crotch and walked around for a couple of hours before going home and forcing myself to tell mom. She was very apologetic. She hadn't expected it to happen so soon and had planned to take me through the pads information later.*

During the reproductive years, cycles of hormone rhythms determine the timing of ovulation and menstruation. This cycle, the menstrual cycle, regulates our fertility, allowing for the possibility of pregnancy a number of days every month. Many women also experience more outward signs of this rhythm—changing emotions, changes in our breasts, variation in foods we enjoy eating at different times over a month.

Menstruation and ovulation continue until age fifty (on average), but anytime between forty and fifty-five is normal.[8] When periods stop, *menopause* has occurred. The body changes that occur between the reproductive and postreproductive phases of our life often take place over as many as fifteen years. (For more information on menopause, see Chapter 26, "Midlife and Menopause.")

THE BASICS OF EGGS AND BLEEDING

Understanding the biological basics of the menstrual cycle can help us when we face decisions about menstruation, such as what to do if we have severe cramps. As you are reading about this biology, you can refer back to the anatomy tables and pictures from earlier in this chapter to remind yourself of body parts and their roles.

PLAYER 1: THE OVARIES

At birth, both ovaries together contain about two million follicles, which are hollow balls of cells, each with an immature egg in the center. The ovaries absorb about half of these follicles during childhood. About 300 to 500 of the 400,000 follicles present at menarche will develop into mature eggs across the reproductive life span. For many years, reproductive biologists believed that women (and other female mammals) are born with a lifetime's supply of egg-producing follicles and do not grow new eggs after birth. However, recent research has found that female mice have a reserve supply of these follicles that are capable of generating new eggs during their lifetime. More research is needed to determine whether the same is true for women.[9,10]

DOUCHE: DO OR DON'T?

Our body secretions and smells are a natural part of us, and the vagina has a natural cleansing process. Unless you are instructed by a health care practitioner, you never need to douche (wash out the vagina). Douching and the use of vaginal deodorants, even occasional, can change the acid and alkaline balance in the vagina and lead to infections. Scents used in vaginal deodorants can also cause allergic reactions. You can keep your body clean by washing the genital area daily with warm water. See the Healthy Vagina Campaign (run by African American Women Evolving) at www.aaweonline.org/TheHVC Pamphlet.pdf, and "Resources" for more information about possible douching risks.

Each month during our reproductive years, ten to twenty follicles begin maturing under the influence of hormones. Usually, only one follicle develops fully. Our bodies reabsorb the others before they complete development. Some of the cells in the follicle secrete the hormone called estrogen. The follicle with the maturing egg inside moves toward the surface of the ovary. At ovulation, the follicle and the ovarian surface open, allowing the tiny egg to float out. About this time, some women feel a twinge or cramp in the lower abdomen or back (called *mittelschmerz*), usually accompanied by wet cervical fluid, discussed under "Player 2: The Cervix." The cervical fluid at this point is sometimes bloody. A few women experience headaches, gastric pains, or sluggishness. Other women feel especially well at the time of ovulation.

Just before ovulation, the estrogen-secreting cells in the follicle start secreting the hormone progesterone in addition to estrogen. After ovulation, the empty follicle is called a *corpus luteum* ("yellow body," referring to the yellow fat in it). If the cycle is interrupted by pregnancy, the corpus luteum produces hormones that help maintain the pregnancy. If no pregnancy occurs, the corpus luteum is reabsorbed. After ovulation, the released egg is swept into the funnel-shaped end of one of the fallopian tubes *(oviducts)* and begins its several-day journey to the uterus, moved along by wavelike contractions of the muscles in the tube *(peristalsis)*. Each tube is lined with microscopic hairs that constantly move back and forth. If sperm enter the vagina, pass through the cervix, and travel through the uterus into the fallopian tubes, these cilia propel the seminal fluid in the direction of the ovary, carrying the sperm toward the egg.

If fertilization (the union of an egg and a sperm, also called conception) occurs, it usually takes place in the outer third of the fallopian tube (nearest the ovaries) within one day of ovulation. It takes a fertilized egg approximately five to six days to travel to the uterus. If the egg is not fertilized, it disintegrates or flows out with the vaginal secretions, usually before menstruation. You won't notice it.

PLAYER 2: THE CERVIX

The kind of mucus or fluid produced by your cervix changes throughout the cycle in response to hormones. Although there are general patterns of fluid secretion, you can follow your own cycle to find out your pattern. You can track your vaginal wetness or dryness by feeling the entrance to the vagina with your finger and looking at and feeling the secretions. Try writing down these changes every day for several cycles to get a sense of the changes that your fluid undergoes during your cycle. (For more information, see the section on fertility awareness on p. 246.)

If you took a sample of your cervical fluid at a time in your cycle when you were not fertile, and looked at it under a microscope, it would probably resemble a maze of tangled fibers. As ovulation approaches under the influence of estrogen, the fluid changes to form longer, aligned strands that look like ferns and can guide sperm into the uterus. Thus, the fluid is a kind of gatekeeper for the uterus. Around ovulation, it is slick and thick enough to coat the vagina and protect sperm from the vagina's acid secretions. Sperm can live up to five days in fertile-quality cervical fluid. After ovulation, as progesterone counteracts estrogen, cervical fluid thickens, and your vagina gradually becomes drier. If you look at your cervix with a speculum, you may notice that at about the time of ovulation, the cervix is pulled up high into the vagina. It may also enlarge and soften, and the os may open a little.

PLAYERS 3 AND 4: THE ENDOMETRIUM AND UTERUS

Estrogen, made by the maturing follicle, causes the glands of the uterine lining (endometrium) to grow and thicken, and increases the blood supply to these glands. This thickening of the uterine lining is called the *proliferative phase* of the menstrual cycle, and it can vary in length from six to twenty days. Progesterone, made by the ruptured follicle after the egg is released, stimulates the glands in the endometrium to begin secreting embryo-nourishing substances. This is termed the *secretory phase* of the cycle. A fertilized egg can implant only in a secretory phase, not in a proliferative one.

If conception has not occurred, the postovulation follicle will produce estrogen and progesterone for about twelve days, with the amount lessening in the last few days. As the estrogen and progesterone levels drop, the tiny arteries and veins in the uterus close off. The lining is no longer nourished and is shed. This is menstruation: the menstrual period or flow.

Women are often taught about menstruation in a way that makes it seem like it's a bad process, driven by failure (i.e., that it's what occurs when conception fails to happen). But actually, menstruation may serve as a sign of good health and a way to cleanse our bodies.[11]

PLAYER 5: MENSTRUAL FLUID

During menstruation, most of the lining of the uterus is shed, but the bottom third remains to form a new lining. Then, as a new follicle starts growing and secreting estrogen, the uterine lining grows, and the cycle begins again. (It is possible to have anovulatory bleeding—what may appear to be a menstrual period without ovulation—even after cycles have been established. Anovulatory cycles become more frequent as menopause approaches.) It's not just blood that flows out of your vagina during menstruation. In addition to blood (sometimes clotted), your menstrual fluid contains cervical fluid, vaginal secretions, cells, and endometrial tissue. This mixed content is not obvious, since the blood colors the fluid red or brown.

Women's menstrual cycles vary widely. Many women's cycles range from twenty to thirty-six days. Often we think of periods as occurring once per month. (In fact, the word "menstruation" is from the Latin *mensis,* for "month.") While some women's periods do occur exactly every month, other women have cycles that are longer or shorter. Some women have regular cycles (they bleed every twenty-eight or forty days, for instance), while other women have alternating long and short cycles. There are spontaneous small changes, and there can be major changes when a woman is under a great deal of stress or loses a significant amount of her body fat. As you get older, or if you have a baby, you may notice more significant changes in your cycle length.

The number of days we bleed also varies. Many women's periods last between two and eight days, with four to six days being the average. The flow stops and starts, though this may not always be evident. A usual discharge for a menstrual period is about four to six tablespoons (a quarter cup), or two to three ounces, though many women are surprised to hear this, as it often *looks* like more.

MENSTRUAL CYCLES AS A VITAL SIGN

You may want to get to know your menstrual cycle, if you haven't already. By keeping track of what's normal for you, you will get a strong sense of your unique health pattern. For instance, if you suddenly stop your periods, have much heavier bleeding, or experience very irregular spotting, you should see your health care provider. Marked changes in our cycles may signal things such as weight change, emotional stress, pregnancy, menopause, thyroid disease, or cancer.[12]

Many women find it helpful to keep track of cycles on a menstrual calendar or a special fertility awareness chart. We can chart when we bleed, whether we have vaginal secretions, and whether we have a range of physical or emotional experiences (including changes in energy level or mood, pain or cramps, heavier or lighter flow, sexual desire, and general physical health). We can track this in a calendar, day book, computer, or diary. (For specific menstrual calendar charts, see "Resources.") Like the self-guided tour of our sexual anatomy, keeping a menstrual calendar will help us get to know our bodies, learn what is normal for us, and be advocates for and authorities about our own health.

FERTILITY AWARENESS

One particular way of charting your menstrual cycles is to use the fertility awareness method (FAM). FAM is an excellent tool for assessing gynecological health and understanding your body. It is also a scientifically validated method of natural birth control and pregnancy achievement. It is based on the observation and charting of body signs that reflect whether a woman is fertile on any given day. In order to use the method effectively, you need more information than is provided here; you can learn more about FAM by reading a book or taking a class (see "Resources").

Your menstrual cycle can basically be divided into three phases: the pre-ovulatory infertile phase, the fertile phase, and the post-ovulatory infertile phase. You can determine which of the phases you are in by observing the three primary fertility signs: waking temperature, cervical fluid, and cervical position.

WHAT ARE THE SCIENTIFIC PRINCIPLES UPON WHICH FAM IS BASED?

- The menstrual cycle is under the direct influence of estrogen and progesterone, and a woman's body provides clear signs about the status of these hormones on a daily basis. Estrogen dominates the first part of the cycle; progesterone dominates the latter. Another hormone, called luteinizing hormone, is the catalyst that actually propels the egg out of the ovary.
- A woman produces three conspicuous fertility signs that signal ovulation is about to take place or has already taken place: waking temperature, cervical fluid, and cervical position.
- A woman ovulates (releases an egg) once per cycle. During that twenty-four-hour time, one or more eggs are released. An egg can live twelve to twenty-four hours. If a second egg is released in one cycle (as in the case of fraternal twins), it will be released within twenty-four hours of the first.
- The time from the woman's period until ovulation often varies, but the time from ovulation to the woman's next period is typically about two weeks.
- Sperm can live in a woman's fertile-quality cervical fluid for up to five days, though typically, they live only about two days.
- The corpus luteum (the remnant of the egg's follicle) releases progesterone, which prevents the release of any more eggs until the following cycle.

THE PRIMARY FERTILITY SIGNS

Waking or Basal Body Temperature (BBT)

Before ovulation, waking temperatures will typically range from about 97.0 to 97.5 degrees

Fahrenheit, and after ovulation, they will rise to about 97.6 to 98.6 degrees. They will usually remain elevated until your next period, about two weeks later. But if you were to become pregnant, they would remain high for more than eighteen days after ovulation.

The important concept to understand is the *pattern* of lows and highs that your temperatures exhibit. You will find that your temperatures before ovulation fluctuate in a low range, and the temperatures after ovulation fluctuate in a higher range. The trick is to see the whole, and not to focus so much on the day-to-day changes. Temperatures typically rise within a day or so after ovulation, indicating that ovulation has already occurred.

The sustained rise in waking temperature almost always indicates that ovulation has occurred. It does not reveal impending ovulation, as do the other two fertility signs, which are the cervical fluid and cervical position. It is commonly believed that most women ovulate at the lowest point of the temperature graph, but this is true for only a minority of women. In order to record the most accurate temperatures, you will need to use a special basal thermometer or digital thermometer that shows temperatures in increments of $\frac{1}{10}$ rather than $\frac{2}{10}$.

Factors that can disrupt your waking temperature include:

- fever
- alcohol intake the night before
- less than three consecutive hours of sleep before taking it
- taking it at a substantially different time than usual
- an electric blanket that you normally don't use

Cervical Fluid (CF)

Cervical fluid is the secretion produced before ovulation that allows sperm to reach the egg. In essence, fertile cervical fluid functions like seminal fluid: It provides an alkaline medium to protect the sperm in an otherwise acidic vagina. In addition, it provides nourishment for the sperm, acts as a filtering mechanism, and functions as a medium in which to move.

After your period and directly under the influence of rising estrogen, your cervical fluid typically starts to become wetter and wetter as you approach ovulation. After your period ends, you may have several days of nothing, followed by cervical fluid that evolves from sticky to creamy and finally to clear, slippery, and stretchy, similar to raw egg white.

The most important feature of this extremely fertile cervical fluid is the lubricative quality. After estrogen has peaked and dropped, the cervical fluid abruptly dries, often within a few hours. This is due to the surge of progesterone following ovulation. The lack of wet cervical fluid will usually last the duration of the cycle.

A trick to help you identify the quality of the cervical fluid at your vaginal opening is to notice what it feels like to run a tissue (or your finger) across your vaginal lips. Does it feel dry? Is it smooth? Does it glide across? When you are dry, the tissue won't pass across your vaginal lips smoothly. But as you approach ovulation, your cervical fluid gets progressively more lubricative, and the tissue or your finger should glide easily.

You should also be aware that, as with temperature, there are certain factors that can mask or interfere with cervical fluid. These include:

- vaginal infection
- seminal fluid
- arousal fluid
- spermicides and lubricants
- antihistamines (which can dry it)
- cough medicine (which can increase it)

In addition, if you have recently stopped taking birth control pills, you may notice one of two very different patterns: Either you may not produce much cervical fluid at all, or you may tend to have what appears to be continuous creamy cervical fluid for several months. In addition, you may experience midcycle spotting or bleeding during your first few pill-free cycles.

Cervical Position (Optional Sign)

Your cervix, the lower part of the uterus that extends into your vagina, goes through changes throughout your cycle. These changes can be felt by inserting a clean finger into your vagina (your middle finger is usually easiest). Your cervix is a wealth of information about your fertility, literally at your fingertips.

As with the cervical fluid, the cervix itself prepares for a pregnancy every cycle by becoming soft, open, and high around ovulation in order to allow the sperm passage through the uterus and on to the fallopian tubes.

The cervix is normally firm, like the tip of your nose, and becomes soft and rather mushy, like your lips, only as you approach ovulation. In addition, it is normally fairly low and closed, feeling somewhat like a dimple or rosebud, and rises and opens only in response to the high levels of estrogen around ovulation. The angle of the cervix also changes, becoming straighter when estrogen levels are high. And finally, it is the cervix that emits fertile-quality wet cervical fluid when the egg is about to be released.

SECONDARY FERTILITY SIGNS

Many women experience other signs on a regular basis, referred to as secondary fertility signs, because they do not necessarily occur in all women, or in every cycle in individual women. Still, they can offer additional information to help us identify our fertile and infertile phases.

Secondary fertility signs around ovulation may include:

- Midcycle spotting
- Pain or achiness near the ovaries
- Increased sexual feelings
- Fuller vaginal lips or swollen vulva
- Abdominal bloating
- Water retention
- Increased energy level
- Heightened sense of vision, smell, and taste
- Increased sensitivity in breasts and skin
- Breast tenderness

USING THE FERTILITY AWARENESS METHOD FOR NATURAL BIRTH CONTROL OR PREGNANCY ACHIEVEMENT

By charting your fertility signs every day, you can use the fertility awareness method (FAM) either to avoid or to achieve pregnancy naturally. If you want to use FAM for either of these purposes, you will need to take a class or get a book that teaches you specifically how to identify your fertility on a day-to-day basis, and provides you with a special FAM chart on which to record. (For information about books, see "Resources.")

FERTILITY AWARENESS METHOD FOR NATURAL BIRTH CONTROL

When you're using FAM to avoid pregnancy naturally, four rules will identify your infertile phase. The rules are conservative enough that they offer a buffer zone on either side of your fertile phase to be sure you don't have an accidental pregnancy. (To learn more about FAM for birth control, see p. 369 in Chapter 18, "Birth Control.")

FERTILITY AWARENESS METHOD FOR PREGNANCY ACHIEVEMENT

When you're trying to get pregnant, the most important points are probably the following:

1. Take your waking temperature to determine if you are indeed ovulating. You should notice a pattern of low temperatures before ovulation, followed by about twelve to sixteen days of high temperatures after. If you don't see an obvious biphasic pattern, or if your high temperatures after ovulation last under ten days, you should seek medical consultation to make sure you are indeed ovulating, and that the latter phase of your cycle is long enough to sustain a pregnancy.

2. Have intercourse or inseminate on all days of wet, slippery cervical fluid. The most fertile day of your cycle will be the last day that you have this slippery-quality cervical fluid. So, for example, if you have wet cervical fluid on Monday, Tuesday, and Wednesday, you should ideally have intercourse or inseminate on each of those days. That Wednesday, though, will be your most fertile day, since it will be the closest day to ovulation. (If your partner's sperm count is marginal or low, you should have intercourse or inseminate every other day that you have wet cervical fluid.)

3. If you conceive, your temperatures following ovulation will remain high for at least eighteen days.

4. If you don't get pregnant within six months of timing intercourse or insemination during days of wet cervical fluid followed by a sustained temperature shift of at least ten days, seek a fertility consultation.

WHAT DO WE DO WITH OUR MENSTRUAL FLOW?

Across time and cultures, women have used and continue to use a variety of products for catching menstrual flow. What we use depends on what we like, what is comfortable, and what is available, convenient, or affordable. Just as some of us like one style of underwear, some of us are loyal to one type of menstrual product. Others of us constantly change, looking for new options and a better fit.

MAINSTREAM

Many women use commercial tampons or pads (also called sanitary napkins) to catch menstrual blood. Often, those are the products most easily available. They line supermarket shelves and public restroom vending machines. They are the products we see advertised on television and in magazines. Whether you use a product worn outside your body (such as a pad) or a product worn inside your body (such as a tampon) is a personal choice.

Common questions about tampons:

1. **Will a tampon get lost inside me?** No, absolutely not. Your body is smart, and your cervix (that wonderful gatekeeper to the uterus) won't let a tampon go anywhere it shouldn't.

2. **Will tampons make me sick?** No, most likely not, if you use them correctly and change them often. You may not want to wear a tampon for extended periods of time (such as overnight) or use a higher-absorbency tampon than you need, since this may increase your risk of developing toxic shock syndrome (TSS). This issue is very controversial. Tampon manufacturers claim that their products are completely safe. Others are not convinced and cite the small but

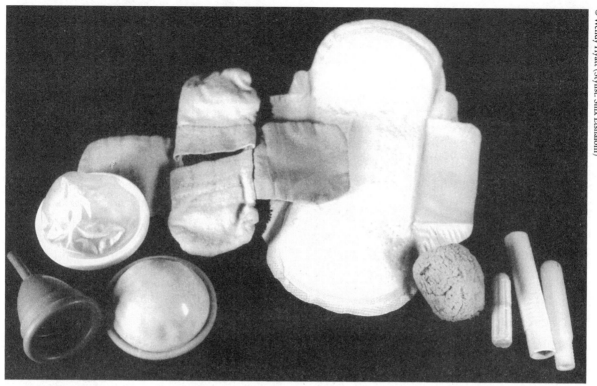

(L-R) The Keeper; diaphragm (to the right); INSTEAD Softcup; cloth pad; "mainstream" maxi pad; Sea Pearls sea sponge tampon; Natracare 100 percent organic cotton tampon; "mainstream" tampon applicators.

real risks of TSS and the hazards of chemical residues and irritating materials interacting with our bodies. (For more information about toxic shock syndrome and dioxins, see "The Truth About TSS and the Dish on Dioxins," p. 251. To find out more about why some folks are concerned about tampon safety, see "Menstrual Activism," p. 253.)

3. **If I use a tampon, does that affect my virginity?** No. "Virginity" is a term that refers to whether or not someone has had sexual intercourse, not to menstruation or tampons. Tampon use may play a role in the disintegration of your hymen. Whether you have a visible hymen says nothing about whether you have had sex.

SIDESTREAMS

For many reasons, including environmental concerns (desire to use reusable products), comfort, and fear of toxic shock syndrome (TSS) and chemical residues, many women use alternative products. These include all-cotton (preferably organic) chlorine-free tampons, chlorine-free disposable pads, washable cloth pads, and devices that collect rather than absorb the menstrual fluid. All-cotton and all-organic cotton, chlorine-free tampons are often sold in health food stores, online, and by mail. Also, you can make your own cloth pads: There are make-your-own sites online (see "Resources"), or you can use cotton handkerchiefs or old flannel shirts or T-shirts (very economical alternatives!).

Some women use natural sponges that work like tampons. Sea sponges often are available in health food stores. They are reusable and relatively inexpensive. Unfortunately, many pollutants are dumped into the oceans from which sponges are taken, and it's possible that sponges may absorb some of these pollutants and cause us problems. Therefore, some women boil a sponge for five to ten minutes before using it for the first time and between uses. Doing so, however, shrinks and toughens the sponge and reduces its lifetime. [14]

Some women prefer products that collect rather than absorb the menstrual fluid. The Keeper, one example of a menstrual cup, is an elongated cup made of gum rubber, held in place by suction in the lower vagina, to collect menstrual fluid. [15] It can be worn during swimming and other physical activities but not during intercourse or other penetrative sex. Some women use a diaphragm or a cervical cap in the same way as a Keeper. Instead is a disposable device worn in the upper vagina to collect menstrual flow. The rim softens in response to body temperature and creates a seal to protect against leakage and slipping. [16] (For more information, see "Resources.")

Those of us with disabilities that limit our mobility and our ability to do self-care often find all of these methods frustrating or difficult to use. As best we can, we adapt existing products to our needs. We may use very large pads, diapers, and panty liners designed for urinary incontinence. However, these often contain plastic, which can be a skin irritant, and most are bleached with chlorine. We hope to find products we can use with more satisfaction. All menstruators need to use consumer power to influence the industry that brings us the products we use. We should not have to settle for options that don't meet our needs.

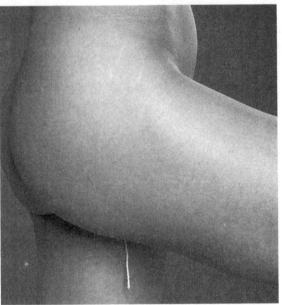

© Robin Holland

This photo appeared on the cover of *The Village Voice* on February 7, 1995, accompanying an article on the dangers of tampons. The visible tampon string caused quite a stir in New York City. "People were horrified," says photographer Robin Holland. "I think the reaction today would be similar. People are perfectly happy to see women as sex objects, but the actual biology of our bodies is apparently gross and unmentionable."

THE TRUTH ABOUT TSS
AND THE DISH ON DIOXINS

TSS*

Toxic shock syndrome is a rare but life-threatening blood infection that women, men, and children may contract in various ways. (For more information, see "Toxic Shock Syndrome" [W32] on the companion website, www.ourbodiesour selves.org.) In women, it has been linked to the use of tampons, especially to high-absorbency tampons made with rayon and other synthetic ingredients. Such tampons provide an inviting environment in which TSS-causing bacteria can flourish. In the past, tampon manufacturers were not held to a universal guideline that defined terms such as "super absorbent." Now there are standard definitions for "light," "regular," and "super." All-cotton tampons have not been associated with TSS, but TSS has been associated with diaphragms, the Keeper, and sponges, though quite rarely. Teenage girls and women under thirty are more susceptible to TSS. Warning signs include sudden fever (usually 102 degrees Fahrenheit or higher), vomiting, diarrhea, dizziness, fainting or near fainting when standing up, or a rash that looks like a sunburn. If you experience these symptoms while you are menstruating, con-

tact your health care practitioner immediately.[17]

The good news is that you can reduce your risk. If you use tampons, make sure to change them regularly (every four to six hours; check the box on the products you use). To avoid TSS, do not use tampons between your periods, and do not use tampons that are more absorbent than you need during your period. For instance, if you are having a light-flow day, do not use a super tampon. Likewise, if you take a tampon out and it hurts to remove it (or there is a lot of resistance), that may be a sign that you should be using a less absorbent tampon.

Dioxins

A separate and unrelated concern involves chemicals called dioxins. Most commercial pads and tampons are bleached to purify the wood pulp used to make them. The bleaching takes place either through elemental chlorine-free processes (which use chlorine dioxide for bleaching) or totally chlorine-free bleaching (which may use hydrogen peroxide). Chlorine bleaching leaves residues of dioxins in tampons and pads, as well as in the environment, through waste water and landfill disposal. According to the Food and Drug Administration, "While the methods used for manufacturing tampons today are considered to be dioxin-free processes, traces of dioxin may still be present in the cotton or wood pulp raw materials used to make tampons."[18] This means that while the menstrual product industry says that tampons and

* Much of what we know about TSS we owe to the late Esther Rome, one of the original authors of *Our Bodies, Ourselves*, who was an activist around this issue. Due to the work of Esther and others, tampons are much safer now than they once were, and TSS is extremely rare. Still, it is important to be an informed consumer and a savvy user.

pads are dioxin-free, the FDA doesn't make that claim.

There is ongoing scientific debate about possible connections between dioxins and health problems such as endometriosis and cancer.[19] We absorb dioxins in other ways besides through menstrual products (in the air and water, for example). However, dioxins are worrisome in menstrual products, because the vaginal lining is much more absorbent than skin, and because women wear tampons and pads for hours at a time. There are alternatives to chlorine-bleached menstrual products. Unfortunately, some products like the Keeper and cloth pads are more expensive in the short term and not as likely to be stocked at your local grocery or drugstore. But if you can make the investment, you will save money in the long run. Be a vocal consumer if you want more alternatives (see "Resources").

IT'S YOUR PERIOD— HOW DO YOU OWN IT?

For many women, there is much more to the menstrual experience than bleeding. Women's experiences, both physical and emotional, range widely. How does your period make you feel?

In mainstream Western culture, menstruation is largely taboo. We may hear jokes about it on television, or we may see advertisements for menstrual products, but rarely is bleeding talked about (is the word "blood" ever mentioned? Is menstrual blood ever seen?). Being "fresh" or "clean" is emphasized, and the fact that we bleed is hidden.

Many factors can influence how we feel about our periods and about menstruation in general. Some of these factors are religious or cultural—we may have certain traditions around menstruation, passed down through our families (even if the tradition is as simple as what kind of product to use or how to best wash out a bloodstain). Women's experiences with menarche, our first periods, may affect how we view and experience our periods years later. Do you remember how you first learned about menstruation? Did you know what your period was when you first got it?

What would you tell your daughter about menstruation? It's your body and your period, so own it in a way that is right for you. It's your choice to love it, hate it, or be indifferent to it.

When I first got my period at the age of 11, I thought I was just messing my pants; it didn't really scare me or anything like that. Now it surprises me when I get it, because I don't prepare beforehand, but otherwise I don't have any bad feelings about it or get upset when I get my period, because I know I can get pregnant when I have my period regularly, but at the same time it's also a sign that I'm not pregnant, which makes me happy, because I'm in college right now and I'm not at the stage where I want any kids yet.

MENSTRUAL CHANGES, INCLUDING PMS

The menstrual cycle is governed by hormones that rise and fall in rhythmic patterns. These hormones influence the physical and emotional changes we may experience during our cycles. We experience these changes in many different

MENSTRUAL ACTIVISM

The deaths of dozens of U.S. women from toxic shock syndrome in 1980 mobilized a small but spirited group of activists to press tampon manufacturers to regulate the safety of their products. Esther Rome, Jill Wolhandler, Nancy Reame, and others pushed the FDA to require the standardization of absorbency ratings of tampons. They also insisted that packages carry a TSS warning and advice for consumers to use the lowest possible absorbency necessary.

In 1989 the British Women's Environmental Network exposed the lack of regulation governing the so-called feminine protection industry in the book *The Sanitary Protection Scandal*. The book stimulated a campaign to persuade British manufacturers to reduce chlorine bleaching in diapers, sanitary napkins, and tampons. And it worked! Since then, a North American movement of menstrual activists has continued to question the health and environmental hazards associated with conventional products and more generally challenge the "culture of concealment" surrounding menstruation.[20]

Menstrual activists like New York Representative Carolyn Maloney are not convinced that conventional pads and tampons are risk-free. Maloney proposed HR 373, the Robin Danielson Act, to establish a research program investigating the risks associated with tampons and to collect and analyze data on toxic shock syndrome.[21] Other activists, such as the Montreal-based Bloodsisters (http://bloodsisters.org/bloodsisters/), the Student Environmental Action Coalition's "tampaction" campaign (www.seac.org/tampons), and filmmakers Teresa MacInnes and Penny Wheelwright, who co-produced the film *Menstruation: Breaking the Silence*, lead the menstrual underground activist movement. Together with many loosely connected individuals, they get the word out that menstruation is *not* a dirty word and that multiple safe and eco-friendly ways to deal with our flow do indeed exist.

Watch for menstrual health and do-it-yourself pad-making workshops, websites, zines, selected books and other consciousness-raising actions that challenge the menstrual status quo. (For more information, check out "Resources.")

---

ways. Some women notice few changes; some women experience times of increased energy and creativity; other women experience mood changes (some positive, some negative) and body changes (breasts may swell, for example). Some women experience cramps, while others do not. A table at the end of this section presents information on menstrual health care and home remedies.

I wasn't the biggest fan of my period, but then I discovered that I have the most incredible orgasms while I'm menstruating!

PREMENSTRUAL CHANGES

The term "PMS" (which stands for "premenstrual syndrome") is often used with words like "symptoms" and "treatments," as though pre-

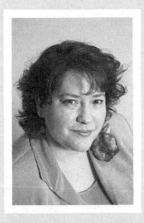

© John Lucassian

"JUST ONE DAY OUT OF LIFE"

GENEVA KACHMAN

Back when I had PMS and cramps, I would wonder about a line from the Madonna song "Holiday": "Just one day out of life. / It would be so nice." Why couldn't the first day of my period be that "one day"? By the year 2000, having healed from my menstrual difficulties, I was ready to turn the Monday before Mother's Day into that "one day"— Menstrual Monday.

Filmmaker Molly Strange wrote a visualization and poem; I took care of publicity, recipes, party suggestions, and favors. (Most popular party favor? The UFO, or "Uterine Flying Object." Most controversial? "Menstrububbles.") Astounding to both Molly and me, as of 2004, close to two thousand Menstrual Monday starter kits have been distributed worldwide.

Menstrual Monday is still evolving, moving from shared celebration to shared transformation: of tampon dispensers transformed into interactive sculpture; menstrual product ads from objects of ridicule to sites of redefinition and affirmation; and menstruation itself from burden into self-care opportunity.

Menstrual Monday has a new home—MOLT: the Museum of the Menovulatory Lifetime (www.moltx.org). I chose MOLT as the museum acronym because the natural process of molting—messy, intense, slow—best captures the transformation in menstrual attitudes now under way.

MENSTRUAL SUPPRESSION

Much attention has recently focused on menstrual suppression—using hormones or drugs to reduce the number of menstrual periods or to stop bleeding altogether. Some women suppress periods using birth control pills (oral contraceptives); women using Depo-Provera, an injected form of birth control, often experience the side effect of not menstruating. Some oral contraceptive pills provide continuous hormones for three months, leaving only four hormone-free times a year that the woman will bleed. Both popular culture and scientific research have asked whether it is safe and/or desirable to menstruate less.

The controversial book *Is Menstruation Obsolete?* describes how women living in industrialized countries today experience significantly more periods over our lifetimes than did our hunter-gatherer foremothers.[22] This is due to fewer pregnancies and less time spent breast-feeding, both of which temporarily suppress ovulation and therefore menstruation. The authors posit that menstruation is unnatural and that menstrual suppression is desirable. The book sparked numerous follow-up pieces and rebuttals.[23]

Health care providers have used menstrual suppression for years to treat women with very painful or problematic periods. The recent debate centers around a separate issue: the suggestion that healthy women should take medication to regulate our periods. Almost all medication has risks and side effects, even if they are small ones.

The menstrual suppression debate currently is just that—a debate. Researchers are in the process of collecting scientific data on the safety of menstrual suppression. More long-term safety data are needed. Until there is a body of evidence, based on large numbers of women over the long term, supporting the safety of menstrual suppression, products or practices to stop menstruation should be viewed with significant caution. For the most current information, contact the Society for Menstrual Cycle Research (see "Resources").*

The desirability of menstrual suppression is a different but related question. Some of us believe our monthly cycles to be signs of our health, while others of us experience them as painful or bothersome. Our experiences with menstruation are influenced by our environments, and in many places, menstruation remains a taboo subject. Are drug companies profiting from a cultural taboo? How can we make informed choices about menstruation in a culture that tells us that we are dirty when we bleed?

* The Society for Menstrual Cycle Research is a group of women's health researchers who believe that menstrual health should be studied within the bigger picture of a woman's life and health. SMCR members study all aspects of menstruation (including physical, emotional, psychological, cultural, and historical viewpoints) from before menarche through post-menopause, and provide women-centered perspectives on menstrual experiences.

menstrual changes are an illness. Some women do experience debilitating discomfort, cramping, or pain in the days before menstruation. But the label suggests that most women come down with a syndrome each month before we bleed. This does not reflect the real and significant variation in women's experiences. For that reason, this chapter does not use the term PMS.

Women can have a variety of sensations or experiences for several days before and sometimes during the first few days of menstrual bleeding. Among the more negative experiences are mood swings, fatigue, depression (frequently mild but occasionally severe), bloating, breast tenderness, and headaches. Sometimes these premenstrual experiences disrupt our lives significantly. Sometimes they are mild. For example, some women report feeling more energetic and creative premenstrually, and some find that it widens the range of emotions we feel and express. When we have negative changes, however, they may be extremely difficult to tolerate and should be taken seriously.

PREMENSTRUAL DEPRESSION: HOW MUCH IS TOO MUCH?

I get upset—sad about simple things—when I get my period.

Some of us experience mood changes premenstrually, and we may experience some level of depressed mood and emotion. Some of us find that our premenstrual moods are exaggerations of issues that have been with us all along, but become more pronounced at this time. Others see our moods as authentic expressions of feelings we didn't feel able, comfortable, or safe to show until this point in our cycles. Some women are better able to deal with problems premenstrually, while others find that problems grow more intense and frustrating. If, in addition to or instead of feeling depressed, you feel extremely tired and are quite pale, you may have anemia, and you should have your blood iron level checked.

When premenstrual depression is more than the blues and interferes noticeably with your daily life (you can't get out of bed, you miss work, or you have suicidal thoughts), seek advice from a mental health professional. A skilled provider can distinguish serious premenstrual problems from other emotional problems. (For more information about finding a counselor, see Chapter 6, "Emotional Well-Being.")

There is ongoing debate in the mental health community about premenstrual dysphoric disorder (PMDD), a very extreme form of premenstrual depression. People on one side of the debate argue that when you pathologize menstrual changes (by giving them the label of a specific disorder), you pathologize menstruation itself. That view may reinforce an idea that women are crazy once a month and perhaps should not be in positions involving great authority or stress. On the other side of the debate, people argue that some women do experience extreme premenstrual changes and depression. Some women have symptoms of clinical depression premenstrually, and that experience is undermined if society fails to acknowledge the seriousness of our premenstrual depression. An additional layer of this debate deals with controversy around the marketing of medications specifically for PMDD.[24] (For more information, see Chapter 6, "Emotional Well-Being," p. 91.)

SEVERE CRAMPS (DYSMENORRHEA)

Women experience many different levels of menstrual-related cramping, from no cramps to severe ones. A particular constellation of symptoms, including cramping and often nausea and diarrhea, may be caused by excess production and release of prostaglandins.[25] (One form of prostaglandins, which are hormonelike chemicals found throughout the body, causes contractions of the uterine and intestinal muscles.) With too many prostaglandins, the usually painless rhythmic contractions of the uterus during menstruation become longer and tighter at the tightening phase, keeping oxygen from the muscles. It is this lack of oxygen that we experience as pain. Anticipation often worsens the pain by making us tense up. It's not clear why some of us

HOME REMEDIES

The following table lists a few suggestions for menstrual health care and home remedies. Refer to "Resources" for information on where to find exact dosage amounts or specific types and dosages of herbs. A few sources that provide this information include:

- Feminist Women's Health Center, "Menstrual Cycles" website: www.fwhc.org/health/moon.htm
- D. Soule, *A Woman's Book of Herbs: The Healing Power of Natural Remedies* (Secaucus, NJ: Carol Publishing Group, 1998).
- Women's Health Specialists/Feminist Women's Health Center Home Remedies Index: www.womenshealthspecialists.org/selfhelp/selfhelphomeremedies.html.

MENSTRUAL HEALTH CARE AND HOME REMEDIES

IF YOU EXPERIENCE ...	CONSIDER TRYING ...
Amenorrhea	• Herbs
Breast tenderness	• Essential fatty acids (such as omega-3 fatty acids) • Vitamins: B_6, multivitamin • Water
Fatigue	• Exercise • Extra sleep • Ginger root tea • Vitamin B_6
Fluid retention/bloating	• Vitamin B_6 • Water • Foods to try: whole grains, whole flours, beans, vegetables, fruits, brewer's yeast (avoid caffeine, alcohol, and foods high in salt)
Heavy bleeding (to decrease)	• Herbs • Vitamins: A, C, E, multivitamin
Irregular cycle	• Acupuncture • Essential fatty acids (such as omega-3 fatty acids) *(continued)*

IF YOU EXPERIENCE...	CONSIDER TRYING...
Irregular cycle (*cont.*)	• Herbs • Meditation • Multivitamin • Relaxation techniques
Menstrual cramps or pain (dysmenorrhea)	• Acupuncture • Calcium, magnesium • Essential fatty acids (omega-3 fatty acids) • Exercise • Foods to try: fresh vegetables, whole grains, nuts, seeds, fruit (limit refined carbohydrates, caffeine, red meat) • Herbs • Massage • Nonprescription drugs (ibuprofen [Advil] or acetaminophen [e.g., Tylenol]) • Orgasm • Reflexology • Vitamins: B_6, E, multivitamin • Yoga or Pilates
Mild depressed mood	• Exercise • Meditation
Mood swings	• Exercise • Herbs • Vitamin B_6
Sugar cravings	• Vitamin B_6 • Magnesium

have more prostaglandins in our uteruses than others.

You can do something about primary dysmenorrhea, the sometimes incapacitating cramping during your period. (There are two types of dysmenorrhea: *primary dysmenorrhea* is pain not associated with any other pelvic disorder; *secondary dysmenorrhea* is painful cramping associated with another pelvic problem such as endometriosis or pelvic inflammatory disease.)[26] The home remedies in the menstrual health care table (p. 257) may help alleviate your cramps. If these methods do not work, you might consider acupuncture or a visit to your health care professional. Some providers prescribe birth control pills to help women with severe menstrual cramps. Your provider will help determine whether you're experiencing primary or secondary dysmenorrhea.

VERY HEAVY PERIODS (MENORRHAGIA) AND/OR IRREGULAR BLEEDING

You may experience a very heavy period if you did not ovulate during a cycle (which happens to all women occasionally, and more often in perimenopause or menopause), if you are under severe stress, if you are using an IUD for birth control, if you are having a miscarriage, or if you have fibroids or a tumor in your uterus. Irregular bleeding—off-schedule menstrual flow—can be caused by entering menopause, by recent sterilization surgery, or by a health problem. If you have an inherited bleeding disorder, you also may experience irregular bleeding. The most common inherited bleeding disorder, Von Willebrand Disease (VWD), affects about 1 to 2 percent of the United States population (people of all racial/ethnic backgrounds).[27,28] While it is often difficult to diagnose, and there is no cure, VWD can be treated. (For more information on VWD, see Chapter 29, "Special Concerns," p. 696.)

Because heavy periods and irregular bleeding can signal serious health problems, it's a good idea to talk with a health care provider. This is another reason to keep a menstrual calendar—it helps you develop awareness of what a "normal" or "typical" flow is for you (see "Menstrual Cycles as a Vital Sign," p. 244).

VERY LIGHT OR SKIPPED PERIODS (AMENORRHEA)

Some women experience the absence of menstrual periods or extremely light periods; this is called *amenorrhea*. Primary amenorrhea is the condition of never having had a period by the latest age at which menstruation usually starts (age eighteen). Secondary amenorrhea is the cessation of menstruation after at least one period. Some causes of amenorrhea are pregnancy; menopause; breast-feeding; heavy athletic training; emotional factors; stress; previous use of birth control pills; excessive dieting or anorexia; starvation; use of some drugs; a congenital defect of the genital tract; hormone imbalance; cysts or tumors; chronic illness; and chromosomal abnormalities. Often amenorrhea is caused by a combination of several of these factors. Because amenorrhea is a frequent symptom of infertility, medical textbooks and practitioners pay considerably more attention to it than to premenstrual changes or painful periods, although the latter two are far more common.

NOTES

1. American College of Obstetricians and Gynecologists, "Vulvar Problems," November 2001, accessed at www.medem.com/MedLB/article_detail1b.cfm?article_ID=ZZZQX9DQA7C&sub_cat=9 on October 13, 2004.
2. T. Conforth, "Vulva Self-exams," accessed at http://womenshealth.about.com/cs/vaginalinfections/a/vulvarcanhealth.htm on October 13, 2004.
3. Angela Moreno, "In Amerika They Call Us Hermaphrodites" in *Intersex in the Age of Ethics*, A. D. Dreger, ed. (Hagerstown, MD: University Publishing Group, 1999), p. 137.
4. S. E. Anderson, G. E. Dallal, and A. Must, "Relative Weight and Race Influence Average Age at Menarche: Results from Two Nationally Representative Surveys of U.S. Girls Studied 25 Years Apart," *Pediatrics* 111 (2003): 844–50.
5. Z. J. Lu, "The Relationship Between Menstrual Attitudes

and Menstrual Symptoms Among Taiwanese Women," *Journal of Advanced Nursing* 33 (2001): 621–23.

6. G. C. Windham, C. Bottomley, C. Birner, and L. Fenster, "Age at Menarche in Relation to Maternal Use of Tobacco, Alcohol, Coffee, and Tea during Pregnancy," *American Journal of Epidemiology* 159 (2004): 862–71.

7. W. C. Chumlea, C. M. Schubert, A. F. Roche, H. E. Kulin, P. A. Lee, J. H. Himes, and S. S. Sun, "Age at Menarche and Racial Comparisons in U.S. Girls," *Pediatrics* 111 (2003): 110–13.

8. See the National Women's Health Resource Center's website on menopause (www.healthywomen.org/Content.cfm?L1=3&L2=52.0) or the Canadian Women's Health Network (www.cwhn.ca/publications.html#aging) for updated information.

9. J. Johnson, J. Canning, T. Kaneko, K. J. Pru, J. L. Tilly, "Germline Stem Cells and Follicular Renewal in the Postnatal Mammalian Ovary," *Nature* 428 (2004): 145–50.

10. J. Warner, "Women Not Born with Lifetime Supply of Eggs? Animal Study Shows Mammals Have a Reserve of Egg-Producing Follicles," March 10, 2004, WebMD.com, accessed at http://my.webmd.com/content/article/83/97808.htm on October 13, 2004.

11. K. O'Grady, "Is Menstruation Obsolete?," *Thirdspace*, November 2002, accessed at www.cwhn.ca/resources/menstruation/obsolete.html on October 13, 2004.

12. For more on menstrual cycles as a vital sign, see the Pituitary Network Association, www.pituitary.com/news/PituitaryNewsUpdates/PressReleases/MenstrualCycle.php.

13. A. DiFranco, "Blood in the Boardroom," *Puddle Dive*, Righteous Babe Records.

14. See www.jadeandpearl.com/sea_pearls.html.

15. See www.thekeeperinc.com or call 1-800-500-0077 for product information.

16. See www.softcup.com for product information.

17. *FDA and You: News for Health Educators and Students* (Fall 2003), accessed at www.fda.gov/cdrh/fdaandyou/issue01.html on October 13, 2004.

18. FDA's Center for Devices and Radiological Health (CDRH): www.fda.gov/cdrh/consumer/tamponsabs.html.

19. L. S. Birnbaum and A. M. Cummings, "Dioxins and endometriosis: A Plausible Hypothesis," *Environmental Health Perspectives* 110 (2002): 15–21; also A. R. Scialli, "Tampons, Dioxins, and Endometriosis," *Reproductive Toxicology* 15 (2001): 231–38; and P. Cole, D. Trichopoulos, H. Pastides, T. Starr, and J. S. Mandel, "Dioxin and Cancer: A Critical Review," *Regulatory Toxicology and Pharmacology* 38 (2003): 378–88; and L. Hardell, "From Phenoxyacetic Acids to Cellular Telephones: Is There Historical Evidence for the Precautionary Principle in Cancer Prevention?," *International Journal of Health Services; Planning, Administration Evaluation* 34 (2004): 25–37.

20. Karen Houppert uses this phrase in her book *The Curse: The Last Unmentionable Taboo: Menstruation* (New York: Farrar, Straus and Giroux, 1999).

21. At the time of publication, the bill was still under review. Check this website to track its status: http://thomas.loc.gov. (This is a useful tool for checking any bill's status.)

22. E. Coutinho and S. Segal, *Is Menstruation Obsolete?* New York: Oxford University Press, 1999.

23. Examples of rebuttal pieces include: S. Rako, *No More Periods?: The Risks of Menstrual Suppression and Other Cutting-Edge Issues About Hormones and Women's Health* (New York: Harmony Books, 2003); and K. O'Grady, "Is Menstruation Obsolete?," *Thirdspace* 2 (November 2002), accessed at www.thirdspace.ca/articles/ogrady.htm on October 13, 2004.

24. J. Daw, "Is PMDD Real?," *Monitor on Psychology* 33 (2002): 58.

25. K. J. Sales, H. N. Jabbour, "Cyclooxygenase Enzymes and Prostaglandins in Pathology of the Endometrium," *Reproduction* 126 (2003): 559–67.

26. A. E. Jones, "Managing the Pain of Primary and Secondary Dysmenorrhoea," *Nursing Times* 100 (2004): 40–43.

27. See the Centers for Disease Control and Prevention website for National Center for Birth Defects and Developmental Disabilities, hereditary bleeding disorders: www.cdc.gov/ncbddd/hbd/hemophilia.htm.

28. See Hemophilia.org, a bleeding disorders information center, at www.hemophilia.org/bdi/bdi_types3.htm; or the Canadian Hemophilia Society, at www.hemophilia.ca/en/2.2.php.

CHAPTER 14

Sex can be pure pleasure. When we make love with a part-ner, we can express our desire, playfulness, passion, and trust. We can experience an ecstatic, erotic connection with another human being.

We can also expose ourselves to a nasty disease, with poten-tially fatal consequences.

How do we get the pleasure without the pain? How can we explore our sexuality safely? Many of us know the basic an-swers: Use protection such as condoms, and prevent transmis-sion of bodily fluids. But in the heat of the moment, we may fail to act in our best long-term interests.

It's one thing to talk about "being responsible about STIs" (sexually transmitted infections) and a much harder thing to do it at the moment. It's just plain hard to say to someone I am feeling very erotic with, "Oh, yes, before we go any further, can we have a conversation about STIs?" It is hard to imagine murmuring into someone's ear at a time of passion, "Would you mind slipping on this condom just in case one of us has an STI?" Yet it seems awkward to bring it up any sooner if it's not clear between us that we want to make love.

Whether we are entering a new relationship or negotiating sexual choices in a long-term partnership, we face the same questions: When and how can we talk with our partners about sexually transmitted infections? What can we do that will be safe but won't kill the mood? Which activities are risky, and which ones are less likely to expose us to disease? How can we inform ourselves, decide what we want to do—even practice in advance—and then follow through with our decisions?

Thinking about these questions before we get hot and heavy is the first step toward staying safe and having fun while we do it.

WHY SAFER SEX?

Many of us have heard of sexually transmitted infections (STIs, sometimes called sexually transmitted diseases, or STDs). We may know of HIV/AIDS, gonorrhea, chlamydia, HPV, and others. But we may not realize how many people have them. About 65 million Americans currently have an incurable sexually transmitted infection, and approximately 18 million Americans get one or more STIs every year.[1] That's a lot of potential sex partners who could give you an STI if safer sex isn't on your agenda.

Preventing sexually transmitted infections is more important today than ever because of the increase in the ones that are viral and incurable. Even curable and treatable STIs can cause serious health problems if they aren't found and treated in time. Also, if you have one STI, the symptoms of a second STI may be more serious. (To learn more about STIs, see Chapter 15, "Sexually Transmitted Infections," and Chapter 16, "HIV and AIDS.")

Those are the negative reasons that motivate us to have safer sex, and they're good ones. Who wants to get itchy, painful sores, or worse, when they can be prevented? But there are also positive reasons to take the safer path. Talking with a partner and agreeing to protect yourselves can help both of you feel more comfortable, relaxed, and intimate. Rather than being boring or limiting, safer sex can open new doors. We often find that we are better able to explore and enjoy sex when we are more confident that we will not get a sexually transmitted infection.

TALK THE TALK

Talk with your lover(s) about STIs before having sex. It may be hard to do, but it is important to protect your health and theirs. If you think you

---

MYTHS ABOUT STIS:
DON'T BELIEVE THEM!

1. You can tell by looking if someone's infected.
2. Being faithful to one partner will keep me safe.
3. If he pulls out before he comes, I won't be exposed.
4. My birth control pills or my diaphragm will protect me.
5. Lesbians don't get STIs.

or your partner may have an infection, don't touch any body parts that might be infected. You may be able to do other things, such as massage and caressing other parts of the body, until you and your partner can get tested for STIs.

SOME IMPORTANT TOPICS

- Has either of us, or any of our partners, ever had an STI? When? What was it? Did it ever come back?
- Does either of us have (or have we ever had) any unusual sores, bumps, discharge from the genitals, or other symptoms? Where?
- Have we or any of our other partners ever been exposed to an STI, been tested for an STI, or had an abnormal Pap test?
- What do we usually do to make sex safer?
- What are we going to do right now to prevent disease?

Using humor can be a good way to bring up the subject of protection. If you or your partner feel uncomfortable talking about safer sex, lightening the mood a little might help you relax and pave the way for more serious discussion. (For ideas on how to talk about sex more comfortably with a lover, see Chapter 12, "Sexuality.")

SAFER-SEX GUIDELINES

The safest sexual behavior is having only one partner—someone who is not infected with an STI and who is having sex only with you. But we can't always be sure of our partner's sexual practices. If you are having sex with only one person but that person has other partners, you can be exposed to STIs from those other people. Each new partner can expose us to common STIs. No method of prevention is 100 percent effective, but the following strategies can reduce your chances of getting an STI.

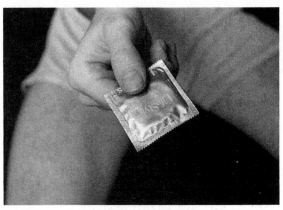

© Donna Alberico

SAFER-SEX PEARLS OF WISDOM

1. Barrier methods rule the day (and the night). Use barrier protection for sex, even when you and your partner(s) have no symptoms; you may not realize you have an infection. Latex condoms (rubbers), used during vaginal, oral, and anal intercourse, are the safest and best-known barrier protection. Other barrier methods can be used for mouth-to-vagina or mouth-to-anus contact, or to protect infected areas not covered by a condom. Squares of latex (dams) made especially for sexual activity are available from erotica stores (see "Resources"), and dental dams are found in some drugstores. **Remember, condoms and other barriers don't protect you from getting infected in places they don't cover.**

2. Use protection even if you don't need birth control. Women who have had a hysterectomy or a tubal ligation, or who have gone through menopause, can't get pregnant but still need to use protection to reduce the risk of getting an STI. If you are using an IUD, a diaphragm, or hormonal methods of birth control to prevent pregnancy, you can still get an STI if you don't use a barrier method of protection.

3. Lather up, then cover up. Washing the genitals, anal area, and hands before and after sex, and between anal and vaginal contact, is good hygiene and may cut down on urinary tract infections, but **washing or douching will not prevent STI transmission.** Douching may even push infections higher up in our vaginas and affect our other reproductive organs. After you wash, don't forget to reach for that condom or dental dam.

4. Watch out for blood. Be careful during sexual activities that may involve blood. Direct contact with blood—including menstrual blood—of an infected person can transmit infections, including HIV or hepatitis.

5. Know your risk. If you're having sex that puts you at high risk for getting an STI, make sure you're well protected. Anal and vaginal intercourse are high-risk sexual activities for STI transmission; kissing and massaging are not. If you know what kinds of sex put you at higher risk, you can protect yourself accordingly.

6. It's never too late for safer sex. If you haven't been safe in the past, that doesn't mean being safe won't help you in the future. There's no better time to start than the present. If you don't have an STI, practicing safer sex will help ensure that you don't get one. If you do have an STI, safer sex protects your future partners and prevents you from getting another STI.

In my youth, I was extremely experimental and reckless. I discovered I was bisexual, enjoyed having multiple partners at one time, and had a few one-night stands and didn't use condoms. . . . At the age of 28, I decided that I would have sex only with people who would agree to celibacy for six months and then get pre-sexual testing. I found that I was clean despite the chances I took earlier.

7. Make foreplay the main course instead of just the appetizer. Touching, stroking, and ca-

ressing each other can be very erotic and fulfilling. If you don't have a condom and you want to make love, this kind of contact (sometimes called *outercourse*) is a good way to get off while being safe. It's low-risk and feels great. If you do want to have intercourse, good foreplay will help make sure your vagina is lubricated so that a condom is less likely to tear during sex.

ACTIVITY-SPECIFIC SAFE SEX TIPS

- *Vaginal intercourse:* For the best protection, use a lubricated latex or polyurethane male condom (not lambskin) or the female condom. No other method of protection has been conclusively proved to prevent HIV transmission. Polyurethane condoms for men are more likely to break than latex ones, but you may want to use them if you are sensitive to latex.[2] With latex condoms, use a water-based lubricant like K-Y jelly, Astroglide, or Probe. Any oil-based substances, like Vaseline or lotion, will damage a latex condom within minutes. You can also hold the condom rim while you're having sex; visually check the condom during sex; change the condom when changing activities or if the sex lasts a long time (condoms are intended to last for approximately ten minutes during sex); and use your own condom so you will know it was stored correctly. (For specific tips on proper condom use, see "Condoms 101," p. 266.)
- *Anal intercourse:* This is a high-risk activity, even more so than vaginal intercourse, because the fragile tissue in the rectum tears easily and may allow HIV or other infectious agents directly into the bloodstream. Lack of natural lubricant makes the rectal lining more susceptible to tearing. For sufficient protection, your male partner should use a strong latex condom with plenty of lubricant. Poly-

urethane condoms are another option, but studies suggest that they are more likely to break. Massaging the anus with a finger or sex toy can be a pleasurable prelude to anal sex, and it may help relax the muscles so that the condom is less likely to break during sex. (For information on how to protect yourself during anal massage, see finger play, next page.)

- *Oral sex on a man:* This is not as risky as vaginal or anal sex, especially if the man doesn't come in your mouth. However, it still carries some risk for transmitting STIs. For maximum protection, use a nonlubricated latex condom as soon as the penis is erect, since the pre-cum (drops of fluid that the penis discharges during arousal) can contain HIV. Use a new condom each time. If licking plain latex doesn't do it for you, try using a flavored condom.

- *Oral sex on a woman:* This carries some risk, especially if the woman has her period or an STI with open sores. For maximum protection, cover your partner's vulva and anus with a dental dam, a cut-open latex glove, a nonlubricated condom, or nonmicrowaveable plastic wrap (which does not have microscopic holes). Dental dams used by dentists are small and thick, but some sex boutiques carry ones that are larger, thinner, and flavored. To turn a latex glove into a barrier, wash out the powder, cut off the four fingers, and slit it up the side, leaving the thumb intact. Try lubricating the side that touches your partner. Be sure to keep the same side against her vulva, and keep track

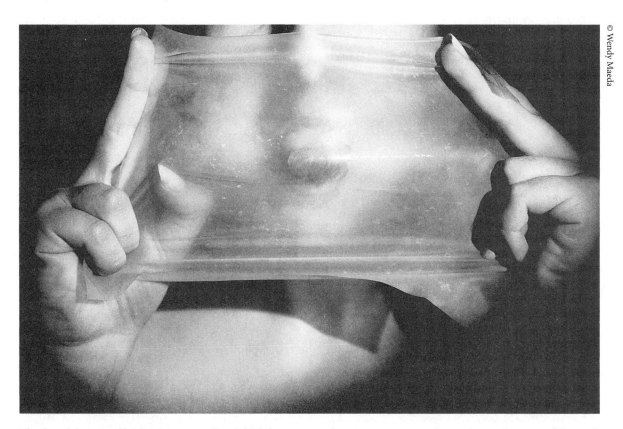

© Wendy Maeda

The dental dams used by dentists are small and thick, but some sex boutiques carry ones that are larger, thinner, and flavored.

of which side is which so you don't touch the body fluids you are trying to avoid.

- **Fisting and finger play:** Fisting (putting a hand or fist into the rectum or vagina) carries some risk because the internal tissue can be easily bruised or torn. Finger play (playing with the vagina or labia or touching your partner's anus) is much less risky, although HIV can travel into the bloodstream through cuts on your fingers, or cuts in his or her membranes. For protection, use latex gloves (or finger cots, which cover only a single finger, for finger play), and change them with each use. If you have any sores, cuts, or cracks on your hands or fingers, a latex glove will protect you from your partner's body fluids.
- **Rimming (mouth-anus contact):** Rimming has some risk of HIV transmission if there is blood in the partners' feces or saliva. Rimming can also spread hepatitis A and intestinal parasites. For protection, use nonmicrowaveable plastic wrap or a dental dam.
- **Dildos, sex toys, vibrators:** If shared, toys can transmit STIs from one partner to another. Put a condom on a dildo before use, and do not share a dildo without washing it thoroughly in hot soapy water after each use. Let the dildo dry completely before you use it again. For extra protection, you can clean a sex toy with 10 percent hydrogen peroxide, or soak it for twenty minutes in a bleach solution (one part household bleach, nine parts water). Make sure to rinse the toy with water after cleaning it with chemicals, and let it dry completely before using it again.
- **Bondage or S/M (sadomasochism):** Negotiate first with your sex partner(s) that no blood, semen, or vaginal fluids will get inside you or onto irritated or cut skin. If an abrasion or cut does happen, clean it well, cover it with a bandage, and keep it away from body fluids. Clean any S/M gear after use (see dildo cleaning, above).

- **Fluid bonding:** This means sharing body fluids with only one person, and using condoms with all others. This reduces risk only if you both use protection consistently and never have unprotected sex with anyone else, not even "just this once." Exposure to several partners, either your own or your partner's partners, increases your chances of getting an STI.
- **Water sports (sex partners urinate on each other):** This is relatively low-risk, as long as there is no blood in or mixed with the urine. Protect your eyes, and avoid any broken skin or cuts.
- **Least risky sexual activities (outercourse):** Intimate touching and pleasuring that do not include vaginal, anal, or oral penetration are less likely to spread STIs. This includes kissing (unless you have cuts in your mouth, gum disease, or bleeding cuts in your gums from flossing), hugging, rubbing, hand jobs, mutual masturbation (avoid getting the ejaculate or vaginal fluids of your partner on your skin if you have small cuts or sores), fantasizing, and massage.

(To learn more about safer-sex activities, see "Resources" and Chapter 12, "Sexuality.")

CONDOMS 101

The following guidelines provide basic information on condom and lubricant use. (For more guidelines on condom use, see Chapter 18, "Birth Control.")

- For sex with a man, the condom has to be on his penis when it's erect and before it touches your body, especially the vulva, mouth, or anus. Roll the condom over your finger first to see which way it unrolls. If you put the wrong side against the penis by mistake, it might touch fluid, so don't reverse it—use a new

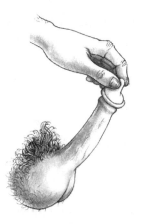 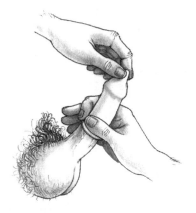 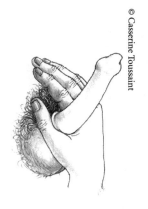

How to put on a condom:

1. Put the condom on your partner as soon as his penis is hard/erect, before his penis gets near your vagina, anus, or mouth. Be sure the rolled-up ring is on the outside. Leave space at the tip to hold semen; squeeze the tip gently so no air is trapped inside.

2. Hold the tip while you unroll the condom all the way down the shaft of the penis, smoothing out air bubbles as you go.

3. During sex and after ejaculation, while the penis is still erect, hold the condom firmly at the base of the penis to keep it from slipping off while the man withdraws.

one. Be careful not to rip the condom with rings or fingernails. Most condoms have a reservoir tip for the semen. Pinch this tip with your other hand to get air out while you roll the condom onto the penis, or have your partner do it. This keeps the condom from breaking when he comes. One of you needs to hold the base of the condom when he pulls out, so it doesn't come off and leave sperm in or near your vagina.

- Use a new condom each time you have sex, and have more than one with you just in case.

- If you or your partner(s) experience irritation with latex condoms, don't despair! The irritation may be due to spermicide (chemicals that kill sperm) on the condom, so try a brand without spermicide—don't stop using condoms. If you experience itching, rash, or dryness, you might be sensitive to latex: Try using a polyurethane condom.

- Flavored condoms may be more pleasant to use for oral sex, but the flavoring may contain sugars, which could encourage bacterial infections in the vagina if you use these condoms for intercourse. So it's best to save those yummy chocolate-mint and strawberry condoms for going down on him.

- For extra sensation, try using a ribbed condom.

- Use a lubricant if you are dry, because dryness can cause condoms to break. Lubricant can be put directly into your vagina. Putting a tiny amount in the tip of the condom may give the man extra pleasure—which could be a plus in persuading him to use condoms. Be careful to use only a tiny drop, and only in the tip, not the sides, so the condom won't get loose and slip off. **Use only water-soluble lubricants, such as K-Y or Astroglide. Never use an oil-based product with latex.** Vaseline, baby oil, or baby lotion will damage the rubber and destroy its protection (see Chapter 18, "Birth Control"). Using spermicide for lubrication is also not recommended (see information on nonoxynol-9 on p. 269).

TEN WAYS TO MAKE IT SAFER

1. Practice putting a condom on a banana or a cucumber.
2. Role-play with your friends what you will say with a partner.
3. Create some rules for yourself about what you will and will not do—such as "Safer sex until we test"—and follow them.
4. Avoid getting so high or drunk that you can't control your actions.
5. Talk with your partner about how to make using condoms or dental dams sexy.
6. Put the condom on together.
7. Explore lovemaking that doesn't include penetration. (You're more likely to have an orgasm, too. See Chapter 12, "Sexuality.")
8. If you have a history of sexual abuse, seek a supportive therapist who can help you heal.
9. Tell a man who resists using a condom, "I'm so hot for you, and a condom keeps you hard longer."
10. Try a female condom. Tell a man, "There's more room to move," since it's not as tight on his penis.

• The female condom can be useful if your male partner(s) can't or won't use other condoms. Once you try it and get used to it, you may find it as convenient as the male condom. Some women like it even better. It's a good idea to practice inserting a female condom before you use one during sex. You can use small amounts of any lubricant, including oil-based ones, inside the pouch or on the penis, but don't use a spermicide as lubricant (see information on nonoxynol-9, next page). If your drugstore doesn't carry the female condom, you can order it from the pharmacy, your health care provider, or by mail (see "Resources"). Some sex stores also carry female condoms.

CAN'T I JUST USE MY DIAPHRAGM OR BIRTH CONTROL PILLS?

No. Most birth control methods—such as the pill, Norplant, the diaphragm, and the IUD—**do not** protect against STIs. You may have a slightly higher risk of pelvic inflammatory disease (PID) at the time of insertion of an IUD, but this risk is greatly reduced if you are tested and treated for STIs at the time. In addition, at least one research study has shown that IUD use may be associated with an increased risk of developing bacterial vaginosis (BV). Birth control pills are linked to changes in the cervix that may also increase risk for certain STIs, particularly chlamydia (see Chapter 18, "Birth Control"), and possibly HIV.

For women having sex with men, the safest protection against STIs and pregnancy together is condom use without spermicides (chemicals that kill sperm). Nonoxynol-9 (N-9), the main ingredient in most spermicides, is still used for birth control but may cause irritation and is not recommended for protection against STIs. Many condoms are available without added N-9; take a stroll in your local pharmacy to find a brand that works for you.

STI prevention approaches currently being explored internationally include adult male circumcision, for hygienic reasons, and involving men more actively in preventing pregnancy and HIV. In the United States, self-tests for STIs appear to improve the chances of early detection, especially for teens. Microbicides—gels or creams applied directly to the vagina or rectum—are being developed and may soon offer an important new approach to STI prevention.

NONOXYNOL-9: NOW NOT FOR EVERYONE

Nonoxynol-9 (also called N-9) is the sperm-killing ingredient in most over-the-counter contraceptive creams, foams, jellies, films, and sponges. Although it's an effective spermicide, it has been proved ineffective for stopping HIV transmission and may actually increase risk, because it can cause irritation in the vaginal and rectal linings. Irritation is most common among women who use N-9 products more than once daily.

N-9 contraceptive products (used alone or with a diaphragm or cervical cap) are still an option for women who choose not to use hormonal birth control methods and who are at low risk for HIV and other STIs. If you have intercourse more than once a day, however, or know you may be at risk of HIV infection, you are advised to choose another birth control method.

Recent studies also show that even very low doses of N-9 can be far more damaging to the rectal lining than to the vaginal lining. "Spermicidally lubricated" condoms, coated with N-9, are no safer than condoms lubricated without N-9 but can increase your risk if you use them rectally. Condoms without spermicidal lubrication are the best type of condom for both vaginal and anal intercourse.

(For more information, see "Nonoxynol-9 and Risk Reduction" [W33] on the companion website, www.ourbodiesourselves.org.)

CHALLENGES TO USING PROTECTION

Condoms, gloves, dental dams, and plastic wrap are known to stop the transmission of HIV and other STIs. Yet many of us are not protecting ourselves consistently or effectively. Why?

OUR OWN ATTITUDES

Who, me? I'm not a gay man or a junkie . . . I'm too young . . . I can tell who's infected . . . I love him so much—he'd never do anything to hurt me . . . If I bring a condom, he'll think I'm a sleaze . . . I'm a lesbian and don't need to use protection . . . I'm afraid he'll refuse . . . He's too important to risk losing . . . I need the drugs, and he won't give them to me if I make trouble . . . I can't carry condoms around—my mother would find them . . . He'll get mad . . . I'm not worth protecting . . . Talking about sex is too embarrassing . . . I just can't deal . . .

That condom seems to pour cold water on the romance by saying, "OK, to be brutally honest, we've both slept with other people." The condom seems like a statement of distrust: "You could give me a disease; you could kill me."

OUR PARTNER'S ATTITUDES

Some men and women complain that sex isn't as good with condoms. Some men are afraid they won't stay hard. If men are used to being in charge sexually, they may resent it when women initiate safer sex. Many sex workers' clients refuse to pay for protected sex, or they pay more for sex without condoms. A lesbian may believe there's no HIV risk for lesbians, or may resist cleaning sex toys. If we suggest using protection, our partners may feel that we're accusing them of sleeping around or of using drugs.

A woman from Chicago writes:

If you're "poor" and Latina, sexuality is one area over which men still feel like they have some control in their lives. If the women bring home the safer sex message, we may become lightning rods for the frustration and anger the men feel as a re-

sult of racism, unemployment, and poverty. The educational strategy has to be developed by the community itself.

Suggesting safer sex can sometimes provoke a response we didn't anticipate. One woman's partner poked a pencil through the six condoms she brought home from a clinic, saying, "I'll show you what I think of this shit." For some of us, the choice may seem to be unsafe sex or no sex.

DRUG AND ALCOHOL USE

When we get drunk or high, we compromise our judgment and weaken our power to protect ourselves. If our sex partners are also under the influence of drugs or alcohol, we may be even less likely to practice safer sex.

LACK OF INFORMATION

If we don't have opportunities to learn how to protect ourselves, we may be more likely to have unsafe sex. We may get incorrect information from our friends, family, or health care providers about the risk involved with different sexual activities.

If you have an STI, you might think that safer sex with your current partner(s) is no longer helpful because he or she has already been infected. This is not necessarily the case; it is still best to practice safer sex in case your partner has not yet been infected. Using protection will also prevent you from being reinfected if your partner has the infection.

There is a lot of rhetoric about how lesbians don't need to be so hyper about safe sex, etc. but in my experience, this is not true. Nearly every lover I had was asymptomatic for BV [bacterial vaginosis, a common vaginal infection often transmitted through sex] (no odor or discharge) but was a carrier, because I would have the symptoms after sexual activity.

I've been with my [lesbian] partner for over two years. A year ago I found out I had genital herpes. . . . [Now] we have oral sex but are careful about washing our hands and do our best to make sure that none of my cum ever gets near her vagina, whether through direct contact or orally.

Even if both you and your partner(s) are HIV-positive, it's best to practice safer sex, as it is possible to be reinfected with a different strain of HIV that may make you resistant to certain antiviral drugs.

OTHER FACTORS

- We may want to have a baby, so we don't want to use a condom.
- Safer-sex supplies may be too expensive or too difficult to get.

(For more information about political and social influences on using protection, see Chapter 18, "Birth Control.")

I HAD UNSAFE SEX– WHAT SHOULD I DO?

STI DIAGNOSIS AND TREATMENT

If you have been raped, had a condom break, or engaged in unprotected sex with someone whom you either know or think might have HIV, you may be able to get medication from your health care provider that will prevent infection from developing.

(For more information on preventing HIV infection after exposure, see Chapter 16, "HIV and AIDS," p. 296.) If you suspect that you have been exposed to another type of STI, consult a health care provider for information on diagnosis and treatment options. (For more information, see Chapter 15, "Sexually Transmitted Infections.")

FUTURE PREVENTION METHODS

Because many women lack the power to negotiate safer sex and condom use, there is an urgent need for a discreet, female-controlled means of prevention, one that could be used even without a partner's knowledge. For years, scientists have been developing one such prevention method, called *microbicides*. These substances can be inserted into the vagina or rectum in a gel or cream; they will help reduce the risk of HIV transmission and other sexually transmitted infections. While microbicides aren't likely to be as effective as condoms, they will offer urgently needed protection to women who, for whatever reasons, currently can't insist on condom use or refuse unprotected sex. New cervical caps and diaphragms are also being tested for effectiveness in HIV prevention, and researchers are trying to develop an effective vaccine. Although there are many products currently in various stages of development and testing, the first microbicides probably will not be on the market before 2010. (For more information, see "Microbicides" [W34] on the companion website, www.ourbodies ourselves.org.)

THE MORNING-AFTER PILL

If you have unprotected sex and are worried about getting pregnant, you can take medication to help prevent conception. This pill, which contains large concentrations of hormones, is available from hospital emergency rooms and clinics. It's best to take the morning-after pill within seventy-two hours of having unprotected sex. (For more information on the morning-after pill, see page 374 in Chapter 18, "Birth Control.")

JUST USE IT

The "just do it" message of popular culture suggests that sex should be completely spontaneous. We rarely see couples in sitcoms and movies discussing sexually transmitted infections or reaching for the condoms before the lights go down. But in the real world, lovers are talking, planning, and taking precautions to protect each other's health. With knowledge, communication, and just the right well-placed piece of protection, we know we can avoid suffering a whole lot of headaches tomorrow—and that makes sex a lot more fun today.

NOTES

1. H. Weinstock, S. Berman, and W. Cates, "Sexually Transmitted Diseases Among American Youth: Incidence and Prevalence Estimates, 2000," *Perspectives on Sexual and Reproductive Health* 36, no. 1 (January/February 2004): 6–10.
2. M. F. Gallo, D. A. Grimes, K. F. Schulz, "Non-latex Versus Latex Male Condoms for Contraception," *Cochrane Review* (2003, Issue 2: CD003550).

CHAPTER 15 ■ ■ ■ ■ ■ ■ ■ ■ ■ ■ ■ ■ ■ ■ ■ ■ ■

Every woman has a right to enjoy her sexuality without fear of disease. That means we need to know how to protect ourselves from sexually transmitted infections (STIs), how to be treated if we get one, and how to avoid spreading an infection without giving up our sex lives.

Because the AIDS epidemic has raised public awareness, more people are willing to talk about using condoms and other barriers to avoid getting a life-threatening virus. But talking about the risk of disease and negotiating safer sex is still hard to do. Many people know about the dangers of STIs and still don't use condoms or other forms of protection. Because STIs are so common, and because many cause no symptoms, people may not be aware that they are carrying an infection. Also, because of social attitudes toward sex, having this kind of disease can bring up embarrassment, shame, anger, and depression. We may feel responsible and blame ourselves unfairly. It can help to remember that STIs are a health problem like any other.

When I found out that I had HPV [human papillomavirus] I was devastated. . . . I remember how scared I was, telling my next new partner about it. He said, "That's a risk I'm willing to live with." It didn't end my chances of connecting with him. That was very reassuring to me—it made me feel that I could still have the kind of sex life I wanted, even with this health issue.

If one person in a supposedly monogamous couple gets an STI, it may be from sexual contact outside the relationship. In that case, the infection may bring up other problems the couple might have.

My husband told me he'd slept with someone else and might have gotten an STI. I didn't know what to do. . . . I saw an ad yesterday for an STI hotline, and after a lot of hesitation, I called. It was a relief to get information without anyone knowing who I was.

WHAT ARE STIS?

Sexually transmitted infection (STI) or sexually transmitted disease (STD) is a term applied to a variety of infections (diseases) that are passed from one person to another primarily through vaginal, oral, or anal sex. Many infections can be

caught through sex, but only some are common in the United States. In addition to HIV, these are chlamydia, gonorrhea, syphilis, genital herpes, human papillomavirus (HPV), hepatitis B, trichomoniasis, and bacterial vaginosis (BV).

HOW ARE STIS TRANSMITTED?

STIs are spread primarily through blood, semen, vaginal secretions, and the discharge from sores or lesions caused by STIs. The most likely way to get an STI is to have vaginal, oral, or anal sex without any protective barrier between the body parts involved. You can also get infected through contact with sores or lesions on other parts of the body, or through sharing razors, needles, or an object like a sex toy, if body fluids from another person are on it. Some STIs, like herpes, can pass from one person to another through skin-to-skin contact. Getting STIs from toilet seats or towels is not likely. Transfusions or transplants can infect someone if blood and organs are not carefully screened for disease, but screening is now strictly instituted in the United States.

WHAT'S THE CONNECTION BETWEEN HIV AND OTHER STIS?

Infection with any STI makes us much more vulnerable to HIV, the virus that causes AIDS, if we are exposed to it. Why? The other infection may cause skin cracks, sores, or lesions in the same body parts that can be exposed to HIV—such as the vagina—making it easier for HIV to get into our bloodstream. HIV targets white blood cells, which are supposed to fight infection, so having an STI mobilizes more white blood cells for HIV to infect. Finally, the same risky behaviors that expose us to one infection can expose us to others, and a partner with one STI may have others,

To learn more about preventing the transmission of STIs, see Chapter 14, "Safer Sex."

• *I can get an STI through oral sex.*

Reality. Oral sex involves exchange of bodily fluids, which can transmit infections. When your partner performs oral sex on you, or you perform oral sex on a woman, you should use a dental dam to prevent transmission of bodily fluids. If your partner is a man, he should put on a condom before your mouth touches his penis.

• *If I get an STI, medicine will easily cure it.*

Myth. Viral STIs, such as herpes, hepatitis B, HPV, and HIV can be treated to relieve symptoms and slow infection progression, but the infection will never be cured. STIs such as chlamydia, syphilis, and gonorrhea that are caused by bacteria, protozoa, and other small organisms can be cured with antibiotics or topical creams/lotions. However, "curable" means that the progression of the infection can be stopped; the damage already done to your body can't be reversed.

too. So, practicing prevention for *all* STIs helps prevent HIV. (For more information on HIV, see Chapter 16, "HIV and AIDS.")

WHAT ARE THE SYMPTOMS OF STIS?

The most common symptoms of sexually transmitted infection are:

• Pain or burning while urinating
• Itching, discharge, or an unusual smell from the vagina, penis, or anus

• For women, sharp pains in the lower belly
• Growths, bumps, sores, or rashes, often around the genitals or anal area

Symptoms are usually found in the genital area. Sometimes they also affect the thighs, throat, and eyes (common in gonorrhea), mouth (common in syphilis or herpes), or, less frequently, the nose or hands. The early symptoms of syphilis are painless (sores) or nonspecific (like the rash, which occurs in the second stage). Because they don't hurt and don't persist, many of us may not be aware of them. Symptoms may disappear on their own before we get worried about them, while the infection continues to spread in our bodies.

SOME STIS HAVE NO SYMPTOMS

Most women with a chlamydia infection don't realize that there is anything wrong. Similarly, gonorrhea often has no symptoms. If not treated, both chlamydia and gonorrhea can result in a serious infection of the reproductive tract called *pelvic inflammatory disease* (PID). However, these bacterial infections are completely curable, and damage from them can be prevented (see Chapter 28, "Unique to Women").

IF I HAVE ANY OF THOSE SYMPTOMS, DO I HAVE AN STI?

Not always. It's important to find out what's causing them, though. It might be something else, but don't ignore the symptoms. These infections need to be checked and treated.

Vulvovaginitis, inflammation of the vagina and vulva (external female genitals), may be caused by various things. One is a change in the pH (balance of acidity and alkalinity) inside the vagina. Things that can affect the pH include semen (which lowers acidity in the vagina), douching, menstruation, and other kinds of infection. Antibiotics may kill some beneficial organisms, allowing an overgrowth of other organisms such as yeast. Some women have vaginal discharge (dripping) with no clear cause. Having frequent intercourse can make vaginitis worse, because germs get pushed farther up into the vagina. Chemicals in creams, sprays, or even clothing can cause irritation.

Urinary tract infections (UTIs), including cystitis, may also account for symptoms. UTIs can occur with or without sexual contact. We can get them when germs travel from the anus or anal area to the urethra and bladder—when we have vaginal contact after anal contact, or when we wipe ourselves from back to front. "Honeymoon cystitis" occurs when having sexual intercourse pushes germs up into the urethra (for more on UTIs, see Chapter 29, "Special Concerns," p. 692).

CAN STIS BE CURED?

Many STIs are curable. STIs that are caused by bacteria, protozoa, and other microorganisms can be cured with antibiotics or topical creams and lotions. STIs of this kind include syphilis, chlamydia, gonorrhea, and trichomoniasis. The list also includes skin parasites like mites, crabs, and scabies, which cause itching and rash and can be passed along through sexual contact. "Curable" means that the organisms can be killed and progression of the infection can be stopped. It does not mean that damage already done to your body can be undone. An unidentified and untreated infection can have serious consequences. Prevention is better than taking risks, and quick response to symptoms can avoid long-term consequences.

Viral STIs can be treated but cannot be cured. Common viral STIs include herpes, hepatitis B, human papillomavirus (HPV), which causes genital warts and other changes in cervical cells,

and human immunodeficiency virus (HIV), which causes AIDS. Treatment may help relieve the symptoms and slow the progression of viral infections.

HOW LIKELY AM I TO GET AN STI?

STIs are among the most common contagious diseases in the United States today. More than 65 million people in this country currently have an incurable sexually transmitted infection. Each year an additional 18 million people will get one or more STIs, and more than half of all new STI cases occur in people ages fifteen to twenty-four.[1] If we have unprotected sex with someone who has an STI or we already have one, we are more likely to get or transmit another one, including HIV.

BIOLOGICAL FACTORS

Women can catch an STI from infected men more easily than men can from us, because germs can get inside our bodies more easily. We may not even realize we have been exposed. Once germs are inside, the warm, moist body provides a good place for them to grow.

A young woman's cervix is not fully developed until the late teens, and it may be more vulnerable to infection, yet many of us engage in sexual activity earlier than that. After menopause, the vaginal lining gets thinner and possibly drier, so older women can get small breaks in the skin during sex that leave us open to infection. Health care providers are also less likely to give older women prevention messages and screening tests. We may even think our risk is lower "at our age." If we have sex exclusively with other women, our chances of getting an STI are significantly lower, but women *can* transmit STIs to other women. Many of us who consider

TAKING CARE OF YOUR SEXUAL HEALTH

1. The best way to deal with an STI is to avoid getting it in the first place. Many women now find that having sex is an expected part of a new relationship, often before the individuals know very much about each other. At any age, we may want to delay sex until we know our partner(s) well enough to talk about the risks of disease and ways to protect ourselves. Willingness to talk about safer sex and STI prevention may be a good indicator of whether both partners are really ready to have sex. It's your decision. Other people have to respect your choice and your feelings about it. **Don't let anyone pressure you into having sex if you don't want to.**

2. If you want to have sex, be prepared to protect yourself. Keep your safer-sex supplies within easy reach. Get them out before you start playing, since once you're aroused, it may be harder to stop and look for them. (For more information, see Chapter 14, "Safer Sex.")

3. If you find it hard to talk to your partner about safer sex, you can practice what to say and how to say it with a friend, or with a counselor at a health care or family planning clinic.

4. If you think there's a chance you or your partner(s) have been exposed to an infection, go for testing and treatment right away. **Remember, you might have an STI and not have any symptoms.**

5. You can get screened (tested when you don't have any symptoms) for some STIs that don't always have visible symptoms. It's smart to do this if you are starting a new sexual relationship, have sex with more than one person, or think or know your partner has another sex partner. Ask exactly which STIs you are being tested for—some have to be diagnosed from symptoms because there's no reliable screening test. Current guidelines recommend screening sexually active women who are age twenty-five and under every year for chlamydia, which is very common and may cause serious health problems if not treated.

6. If you or your partner has an STI, sex is risky until you and all your current partners (and their partners) have been tested, treated, and cured. Ask your health care provider how long you need to wait to be sure it's safe.

7. Before accepting treatment, make sure you understand what you are taking and for how long, the side effects of medication, and any follow-up tests or treatment required. **Don't be embarrassed about asking questions.**

8. Ask your health care provider about getting a vaccination against hepatitis B.

9. Regularly examine your body, especially your genitals, to see how everything looks normally (see Chapter 13, "Sexual Anatomy, Reproduction, and the Menstrual Cycle"). You may want to use a speculum to look inside at your cervix.

(To order one, see "Resources.") If anything looks or smells different, you can ask your provider for a test. Even if a sore goes away, it may still be a sign that you have been infected.

10. Get regular pelvic exams, routine Pap smears, and STI screenings.

11. Find a health care provider who is comfortable discussing sexual health. Look for someone who gives you complete and understandable information, encourages and answers questions, and accepts your sexuality. Don't wait for your provider to bring it up. If you need help, ask for it!

ourselves lesbian may also have had sex with men, recently or in the past. During those contacts, the risk for infection is the same as for women who usually have sex with men.

Where does the trade-off between "fun" and "being safe" become unacceptable? There is no such thing as risk-free sex anymore. This is very different from when I grew up.

SOCIAL AND CULTURAL FACTORS

Women who are fifteen to twenty-four years old, sexually active with more than one partner, or living in an urban setting—where the number of people with STIs is greater and other risk factors are multiplied—are at highest risk. For many of us, poverty may contribute to a higher risk of getting an STI. Not having enough money can mean lack of access to prevention and treatment, economic dependence on a partner who may be exposing us to infection, or just being preoccupied with day-to-day survival more than anything else. Some experiences in childhood, including emotional and sexual violence, increase the likelihood of exposure to an STI then or later in life (see Chapter 8, "Violence and Abuse"). If our cultural tradition values passivity and submissiveness in women, it may be difficult to refuse unwanted sex and to negotiate safer-sex protection. If our culture discourages

us from touching or looking at our genitals, we may not notice early signs of an STI.

STIS AND FEMALE GENITAL CUTTING (CIRCUMCISION)

Women whose genitals have been cut may have a higher risk of catching an STI from an infected partner because of unhealed ulcers, inflamed vulval membranes, or small wounds resulting from intercourse. Infibulated women or women whose vaginal opening has scars from the circumcision may have trouble getting rid of the infection, even with treatment, because vaginal secretions aren't draining. In some cases, surgical opening of the scar may be necessary before the infection can be cleared completely. A gynecologist or a support group that helps circumcised women with physical and emotional needs can give more advice about this (see also p. 643 in Chapter 28, "Unique to Women.")

WHAT CAN I DO IF I THINK I HAVE AN STI?

Get a diagnosis as early as possible. If you are under eighteen, you can get examined and treated without your parents' permission. in every state.

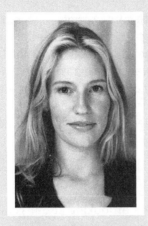

"MY GIFT OF A LIFETIME"

JENNIFER BAUMGARDNER

When I was twenty-six, I got herpes from a lovely guy on our first real date. At first I held out hope that the searing pain in my vulva, fever, and chills were just signs of a bad urinary tract infection, but a trip to my gynecologist confirmed otherwise. I had HSV-1, more commonly known as oral herpes, but I had it on my genitals. Because of the popularity of oral sex, having this variety was becoming as common as having genital herpes on one's genitals.

To be honest, I was initially very depressed after diagnosis. I pored over my Mayo Clinic health book and Our Bodies, Ourselves *for days, wondering what my future held. The books sort of scared me, actually, because (for good reason) they mention all of the more dangerous possibilities that might come with herpes. For instance, I might have many outbreaks each year, and it appeared likely that I would have to have a C-section if I ever got pregnant. If a lesion infected the baby during delivery, he or she would be made blind. I also felt sort of trapped in the relationship with the carrier—although I really did like him—because I feared telling other lovers or being rejected. As it turned out, I haven't had any other outbreaks in the eight years since diagnosis, and I'm currently seven months pregnant. My doctor says that most women can have vaginal births as long as they aren't having an active recurrence. She's putting me on a drug that suppresses outbreaks (acyclovir) for the last month or so of my pregnancy, as a precaution.*

As for telling lovers, I have had three since that lovely guy who gave me my gift of a lifetime. Breaking the news is a little excruciating—and one person was really upset to hear it—but it has never derailed my love life. I went on to have a long relationship with the guy who was so upset, so he eventually got over his fears. The worst thing that has happened was that I did give it to someone once. I had no symptoms but must have been shedding the virus, and I have tended not to use condoms after the relationship gets serious and committed. He had one bad outbreak, the initial one, but has never had a problem since. One thing that helped me to deal with having an STI was to realize that I was part of a mighty big club: 40 million strong. Another thing that helped was telling my dad, a doctor in my hometown of Fargo, ND. The first thing he said was "Hey, it's not going to be a big deal. Herpes is one of the least serious medical conditions you are going to have." He was right.

WHERE TO GO FOR CARE

- **Public health clinics.** Government-funded sexually transmitted disease clinics are free to teens and provide services regardless of ability to pay. STD clinic staff are likely to have the most expertise in testing, diagnosing, and treating such diseases, and the setting offers more privacy than your usual provider's office. To find the nearest walk-in facility, call the Centers for Disease Control's national STD hotline: 1-800-227-8922.
- **Family planning clinics.** Many family-planning providers also offer STI counseling and testing or referral. Even if they don't, they'll know where you can get them. They are also likely to treat you with sensitivity and respect. Many are low-cost and also have sliding-scale fees.
- **Primary care clinician.** Go to your regular health care providers if you feel comfortable talking to them and they offer clear, understandable responses to your questions. However, not all providers have the right equipment to do routine STI testing, and they may not know enough about these diseases. You may want to ask whether your treatment

follows the most recent Centers for Disease Control treatment guidelines, which are available online (see www.cdc.gov/std/treatment/).
- **ER.** This isn't the best place to go, because a hospital emergency room won't give you the time, expertise, and sensitivity that you need to deal with STI issues, unless you really need emergency care. However, if you have been forced to have sex and you're afraid you've been exposed to a disease, most emergency rooms can give you preventive treatment for STIs, including HIV. Tell the ER staff if you need emergency treatment (see p. 131 in Chapter 8, "Violence and Abuse").

Information from the National Women's Health Network may help you choose the right provider (see "Resources").

PREPARE FOR YOUR HEALTH CARE VISIT

- **Call ahead** to find out what services are offered and how much you'll have to pay. Tests are often free, but there may be a fee for the visit. If you are a minor and you don't want your parents to be notified or to receive a bill or statement, ask about your provider's policy. Ask how she or he deals with billing, and find out if she or he knows how your health plan handles it.

- **Get seen right away,** even if the symptoms are not painful. Many STIs can be diagnosed more accurately if you have symptoms. Providers can usually diagnose herpes by sight, and lab tests are more accurate with samples from active sores. A blood test to distinguish Type I from Type II herpes is now available.
- **Try to relieve discomfort** while waiting for your appointment. (See "Self-Help Treatment for Herpes," p. 288.) However, don't put any cream or ointment on a painless sore, as that could destroy bacteria and make tests less accurate.
- **Do not have sex or douche** before your appointment. That, too, can make tests less accurate and confuse the diagnosis.

GETTING CARE AND TREATMENT

Wherever you go for care, you have a right to courteous and thorough treatment. It's always a good idea to take someone with you to write down information and give you emotional support.

- Expect to have a medical history taken and to undergo a pelvic exam (see Chapter 28, "Unique to Women").
- Ask the health care provider to explain any tests, treatments, and negative side effects in a way you can follow. Make sure you understand all your choices.
- Before leaving, find out what your follow-up care will be. If your doctor is too busy to answer questions, ask to speak to someone else. Don't leave before your questions have been answered. Ask how long your symptoms should take to clear up. If they don't, go back for another examination.

- If you have more questions after your visit, call back and ask for the information you need.
- Take all prescribed medication for the STI, even if you feel better or the symptoms disappear. Never share your dose of medication with anyone else. Each person needs to have individual treatment.
- **You and all your partners (and their partners) must be treated, and take all medication as prescribed, before you have sex again.** If not, you can keep reinfecting each other. Wait until you complete treatment or your doctor says it's okay.
- If you have trouble with urination, avoid drinking alcohol until the infection has cleared up. Alcohol may irritate your urinary tract.

You may still feel uncertain about your treatment. Sometimes tests are not accurate; sometimes treatments are a burden or they don't work, and that means more medical visits, time, and money. But the alternative—not getting treatment—is worse.

OBSTACLES TO OVERCOME

Any kind of discrimination in the medical system makes it harder to discuss sexual behavior, STI risk, and infections. Many medical providers still express negative attitudes toward women's sexuality. Some may be racist or homophobic. They may make assumptions about women of color and women with low incomes, but they may not bother to test a white, middle-class, or older woman, or a "nice" married woman, even when she has symptoms.

The first time I asked a gynecologist for a routine gonorrhea culture, he smiled with a comradely look in his eye. "But I'm sure no man you'd be involved with would have gonorrhea."

It started out as cystitis. A few months later, I started having fever, chills, and a lot of pain in my lower abdomen. . . . After nine months, I had a good case of PID [pelvic inflammatory disease], which they called "a little pelvic infection." It wasn't until my husband came down with symptoms that they took me seriously and treated us both with the right drugs.

For lesbians, "coming out" to a health care provider may be necessary to make sure appropriate information, tests, and treatment are given for STI symptoms. However, even when we explain our sexual behavior, some providers may still not be trained to understand the needs of women who have sex with women.

Recently, I met with a new gynecologist, and I told her I was sexually active with women. . . . Later, during the exam, she said we wouldn't need to bother with tests for STIs. I was really surprised. She assumed I couldn't get an STI because my partners are women. Fortunately, I knew that wasn't accurate. . . .

Try to find a well-informed doctor or nurse with whom you can talk freely about your sexual health, before you have any problems. Then you'll know where to go for care if you need it.

STIS AND THE LAW

Physicians and clinics are required by law to report all cases of gonorrhea and syphilis, along with AIDS, to the state or local health officer. Chlamydia and chancroid (a bacterial disease with painful sores) are reportable in most states. HIV infection is reportable in many states. Granuloma inguinale (a chronic inflammation of the genitals) and lymphogranuloma venereum (caused by another type of chlamydia), usually seen in tropical and subtropical climates, are also reportable in most states.

If you have gonorrhea or syphilis, a social worker may ask you for the names of your sexual contacts (people you may have caught the disease from or given it to). They should be notified without your name being mentioned, to protect your confidentiality. If you don't want to give their names, say you will contact them yourself. Then it is your responsibility to contact each person you've had sex with and urge him or her to seek treatment. Doing so may save their fertility or even their lives, as well as that of their other or future partners.

You are also entitled to confidentiality regarding your STI medical care and records (see Chapter 30, "Navigating the Health Care System").

PREGNANCY AND STIS

STIs may reduce or endanger our ability to become pregnant and make pregnancy complications more likely. They may also infect a fetus or infant.

RECOMMENDED PRENATAL SCREENING

Screening means testing people without symptoms to check for disease. All pregnant women should be offered HIV screening and tested for syphilis, hepatitis B, chlamydia, and gonorrhea. A test for hepatitis C is recommended for women who use IV drugs or have received blood products, transfusions, or transplants. An early prenatal visit is also a good time to check for bacterial vaginosis (BV) and to have a Pap smear if it wasn't done during the previous year. For more about screening and tests during pregnancy, see chapter 21, "Pregnancy," and read the CDC Treatment Guidelines (see "Resources").

If you have sex during your pregnancy, you

MAJOR BACTERIAL STIS

(Can be cured if caught in time and treated with antibiotics)

CAUSE	HOW SPREAD	SYMPTOMS APPEAR	COMMON SYMPTOMS	TESTING/TREATMENT	COMPLICATIONS
Chlamydia	Vaginal, oral (less likely), anal sex Touching hand with infected fluid to eye Mother to baby at birth	PID: time unknown Other symptoms 7-14 days	Women: No symptoms in 4 out of 5 women. If cervix infected, vaginal discharge, painful urination, unusual vaginal bleeding, bleeding after sex. If pelvic inflammatory disease (PID): bleeding and low abdominal pain. Cervix may look inflamed. Inflammation of the rectum (proctitis). Men: Burning, discharge from penis. May cause inflammation of urethra (urethritis).	Women: Specimen from pelvic exam; urine test Men: Urethral sample, urine test May be confused with gonorrhea—get tested for both. Meds: pills	Women: PID can result in chronic pelvic pain, infertility, pregnancy complications (ectopic pregnancy). Men: Inflammation of epididymis, testicles, and prostate. Infant: May infect baby at birth, causing eye infection and pneumonia.
Gonorrhea ("clap")	Vaginal, anal, and oral sex Touching hand with infected fluid to eye Mother to baby at birth	2-30 days (average 3-7 days)	Women: No symptoms in most women. If cervix infected, thick discharge (pus) from vagina or bleeding; sore throat, painful urination, swollen glands (near genitals), rectal pain or inflammation (proctitis), anal discharge, eye infection that can cause blindness in adults and infants. Men: Thick discharge (pus) from penis; frequent and burning urination.	Women: Specimen from pelvic exam; urine test Men: Urethral sample; urine test May be confused with chlamydia–get tested for both. Meds: pills or injection	Women: PID (see above) Men: Inflammation of testicles, prostate; sterility (rare). Women and men: If untreated, widespread infection (rare but serious) when bacteria travel through blood-stream; causes pustular skin rash, painful swollen joints; rarely, infection of heart valves, arthritis, or meningitis.

CAUSE	HOW SPREAD	SYMPTOMS APPEAR	COMMON SYMPTOMS	TESTING/TREATMENT	COMPLICATIONS
Gonorrhea ("clap") (*continued*)			Other symptoms similar to women (sore throat, rectal pain or discharge, eye infection).		Infant: May infect newborns, causing blindness if preventive treatment not given at birth.
Syphilis	Sexual/skin contact with infected person Spreads via open sores or rashes anywhere on the body May infect baby before birth Not contagious after first few years of latent stage	Primary stage: 10–90 days (average 3 weeks); second stage: 1–6 months	Women and men, *primary*: painless sore on or around vagina (labia or inside), penis, mouth, and anus; on body wherever bacteria entered (fingertips, lips, breast). Sores heal in 1–5 weeks, but bacteria stay in body. *Secondary*: non-itchy rash on face, body, palms, soles; flu-like symptoms, swollen glands, hair loss, wart-like growths. All secondary symptoms clear up w/o treatment after about a month. *Latent*: up to 20 years with no outward signs; bacteria may be invading inner organs, including the heart and brain. *Tertiary*: see complications.	Blood test; meds: injection	Women and men: If untreated: blindness, brain damage, heart disease, crippling arthritis, paralysis. Infant: Damage to baby's bones, eyes, skin, teeth, and liver at birth. Death.

MAJOR VIRAL STIS

(Not curable, but treatments available)

CAUSE	HOW SPREAD	SYMPTOMS APPEAR	COMMON SYMPTOMS	TESTING/TREATMENT	COMPLICATIONS
Herpes I and II Type I is more often on mouth; however, both Type I and II may infect the genital tract. Type II, known as genital herpes, is more serious	Sexual contact Most often transmitted when no symptoms present–infected person may not be aware of having the virus. Virus will be shed at same spot(s) where original infection occurred.	First outbreak: usually 2-10 days; symptoms may recur often, usually within 3-12 months	None in majority of those infected. Cluster of ulcerated painful blisters in genital area. Painful urination, discharge, swollen glands, fever, body aches. Symptoms usually recur at same spot(s) where virus originally entered the body. More likely if first episode was severe and caused by HSV II. Repeat episodes usually milder; may be triggered by stress or lowered resistance. Some people never have recurrence.	Visual exam and lab exam of sample from blisters New blood tests can find Type I and Type II Antiviral medications (pills) can reduce symptoms and frequency of repeat attacks.	Person remains infected for life. Symptoms vary with individual. Can cause emotional as well as physical stress, including inability to pass urine, but many people cope well. Support groups available. May infect baby at birth (serious illness). More likely to pass to infant if mother infected close to time of delivery. Only 1 percent of women with repeat attacks transmit to infant. Cesarean delivery (C-section) may be needed to avoid newborn coming into contact with blisters.

CAUSE	HOW SPREAD	SYMPTOMS APPEAR	COMMON SYMPTOMS	TESTING/TREATMENT	COMPLICATIONS
Human Papilloma-virus Of 100 types, 30 are sexually transmitted.	Sexual contact with infected person	Several months to years for cervical lesions	*Virus* not visible; small painless lesions on cervix.	*HPV:* Annual Pap smears to find any abnormal cells on cervix. Colposcopy (painless exam with magnifying lens) to confirm abnormal Pap. Biopsy (small sample of cells) tests lesions for cervical cancer.	Certain types of HPV associated with increased risk of cervical cancer (different type causes warts).
Genital Warts (an STI caused by HPV)	Contact with warts (may be inside vagina) After warts are removed, virus may still be shed from area of original infection	3 weeks to several months for warts	*Wartlike* growths, sometimes with itching, irritation, bleeding. Warts may grow during pregnancy, appear cauliflower-like as they grow larger. Around anus, can be mistaken for hemorrhoids. Warts may come back after treatment.	*Warts:* diagnosed on visual exam. Warts can be removed with topical solutions, freezing, surgery, and laser.	*Warts:* Can block vaginal, penile, and rectal openings. During pregnancy, warts inside vagina may grow larger, making vaginal wall less elastic and delivery difficult. Some women report discomfort during sex at the place of infection even after warts have been removed. May infect baby's throat at birth (rare)
Hepatitis B	Sexual contact and needle sharing; may infect baby before or at birth	6 weeks–6 months	Loss of appetite, weakness, muscle pain, headache, fever, dark urine. Symptoms may be too mild to notice.	Blood test	Some infected people can become chronic carriers. Can lead to chronic liver problems, liver cancer.
Human Immunodeficiency Virus (HIV) (see Chapter 16, "HIV and AIDS")	Sexual contact with infected person (blood, body fluids); sharing needles; breast-feeding; may infect baby before or at birth	Blood test for HIV; usually positive at 6 weeks to 3 months It may take 10 years or more for AIDS to develop.	Often no symptoms or very mild symptoms. Symptoms may include swollen glands, sore throat. Also may get night sweats, weight loss, and sores in mouth.	Blood tests; pregnant women offered testing and treatment to prevent transmission to baby Complex medications	Virus associated with development of AIDS; pneumonia and other infections; Kaposi's sarcoma (tumors). May be transmitted to baby, but medicine available to prevent in most HIV-positive women. Some AIDS medications have serious side effects.

OTHER COMMON CONDITIONS

CAUSE	HOW SPREAD	SYMPTOMS APPEAR	COMMON SYMPTOMS	TESTING/TREATMENT	COMPLICATIONS
Trichomonas Vaginalis	Sexual contact, contact with sexual fluids (can live in warm, wet environment outside body)	Within 6 months of exposure, usually sooner	**Women:** Frothy, bad-smelling greenish-yellow discharge, vaginal itching, irritation, or redness. Can include painful intercourse, lower abdominal discomfort, and urge to urinate. **Men:** Often no symptoms. Sometimes puslike discharge; urination frequent and painful.	Office exam of vaginal/penis discharge under microscope, lab culture Meds; pills; must avoid alcohol	May lead to problems with pregnancy (only if infected while pregnant).
Bacterial Vaginosis **Yeast Infection (Candida, Monilia)**	May or may not involve sexual contact, including with women	When pH and vaginal flora change as result of premenstrual changes, menstruation, birth control, intercourse, douches or other chemical products, antibiotics, other infections.	BV: Up to 50 percent of women have no symptoms. If symptoms: vaginal discharge, may be bad-smelling. May include itching, but not always. Yeast: clumpy discharge ("cottage cheese"), mild yeasty odor. Usually itchy. Sometimes vaginal redness, swelling. Odor worse after sex.	Vaginal sample, microscopic exam, test of pH, odor of discharge upon testing Prescription pills or medicinal cream in vagina	BV during pregnancy linked to miscarriage, waters breaking early, preterm labor, preterm birth, and postpartum endometritis. BV may cause PID or post-op infection. Treatment to prevent infection can benefit women w/o symptoms during pregnancy and when undergoing abortion or hysterectomy.
Scabies and Crabs (Mites and Lice)	Sexual and other close body contact. Sometimes from clothes or bed.	2–4 weeks	Severe itching. Mites burrow under skin. Crabs and eggs attach to hair.	Visual exam, skin sample Topical treatments (apply to skin)	Scratching can lead to infections.

could be exposed to a new STI. Infections acquired during pregnancy are the most likely to be passed to the baby. You may need more testing if you are at risk of exposure during your pregnancy. Also, keep using condoms and other barriers to protect yourself from another infection.

HERPES AND PREGNANCY

Herpes is a serious condition in a newborn baby. Pregnant women who don't have herpes should avoid unprotected sex with partners who have herpes. Tell your health care provider if you have herpes flare-ups. If you have prodromal symptoms or active sores at the time of delivery, a cesarean (C-section) may be recommended. After birth, take care not to infect the infant. Don't touch sores, and wash your hands thoroughly before touching the baby.

SYPHILIS AND PREGNANCY

A pregnant woman with syphilis can pass it to her fetus, especially during the first few years of her infection. If treatment is given early in the pregnancy, the fetus probably won't be affected. Later on, medication can stop the disease, but it cannot repair damage already done (a child may be stillborn or have serious abnormalities at birth). Every woman should get a blood test for syphilis as soon as she knows she is pregnant, before delivery, and anytime she may have been exposed.

LIVING WITH HERPES

Many people experience early-warning ("prodromal") signs of an outbreak: tingling, itching, pain, burning, or pressure in the infected area. Later, the sores appear, starting as red bumps and changing to watery blisters within a day or two. After a few days, scabs form and the sores heal. In addition to symptoms listed in the chart on p. 284, women with severe outbreaks may be unable to pass urine. *Call your health care provider if this happens.* The initial outbreak is usually the most painful and takes the longest time to heal.

Accepting herpes as a permanent part of your life may be difficult. You may feel shocked when you discover you have herpes and it cannot be cured. You may feel isolated, lonely, and angry, especially toward the person who gave you the infection. You may become anxious about staying in long-term relationships or having children. But not everybody experiences herpes in these ways, and these feelings may not last forever.

After the first big episode of herpes, I felt distant from my body. When we began lovemaking again, I had a hard time having orgasms or trusting the rhythm of my responses. I shed some tears over that. I felt my body had been invaded.

Herpes attacks can be triggered by getting your period, emotional or physical stress, sexual intercourse, or exposure to sunlight. Oftentimes the trigger is unknown. It may be easier to cope with herpes if you feel comfortable enough to talk about it openly. Identifying what triggers your flare-ups and reducing tension in your life, if you can, may lead to fewer herpes attacks.

Herpes is an inconvenience and a pain, but it's something you learn to live with.

When I feel my vulva start to tingle and ache, it's immediately a reminder to slow down. . . . I try to think relaxing, releasing thoughts and send healing, calming energy to that area. Sometimes I meditate.

EXTRA PRECAUTIONS TO KEEP HERPES FROM SPREADING

There is no cure for herpes, and efforts to develop a vaccine against it have been unsuccessful so far. Besides practicing safer sex, avoid all contact (including any kind of sex) with active sores on mouth or genitals, and with places where the sores were, even after they dry up (you can still spread herpes to sexual partners even if you have no open sores). If you have fever blisters or cold sores on your lips or in your mouth, avoid oral sex. If your hands touch the sores, wash carefully, especially before touching yourself and before putting in contact lenses. Be especially careful not to touch your eyes. Blood or sperm should not be donated during a herpes flare-up.

SELF-HELP TREATMENT FOR HERPES

The remedies described on p. 289 seem to work for some women, though there isn't much scientific evidence for them. Also, treatments that keep sores moist may actually delay healing. You may need a trial-and-error approach to find something that's helpful for you.

The National Herpes Resource Center (HRC), run by the American Social Health Association (ASHA), provides support, information, a quarterly newsletter called *The Helper,* and self-help groups for people with herpes (see "Resources").

LIVING WITH HPV AND GENITAL WARTS

There are more than a hundred varieties of human papillomavirus (HPV), but only thirty are sexually transmitted. Genital warts, a visible infection caused by HPV, are not associated with cervical cancer. However, having any kind of HPV may mean you have been exposed to other kinds. They can never be cured, and some can be difficult to live with, given the uncertainties. Take care of yourself by getting regular gynecological care, including Pap smears to screen for abnormal cells on the cervix. It's also a good idea for you and your sex partners to use barrier protection (see Chapter 14, "Safer Sex"). Warts may reappear even after treatment, so you may need to have them removed more than once. Virus can be shed from the area originally infected, even after the warts have been removed. Support services are available from the American Social Health Association (see "Resources").

OTHER STIS

Besides the STIs described here, there are others such as hepatitis C, cytomegalovirus (CMV), and molluscum contagiosum. If you have sexual contact outside the United States or with someone here who is from another country, you might be exposed to STIs that are not common in the United States. These include lymphogranuloma venereum (LGV), granuloma inguinale, chancroid, and a type of gonorrhea that's resistant to treatments used in this country.

Some STIs are more easily transmitted through anal sex. You can get an infection in the rectum from gonorrhea, chlamydia, LGV, syphilis, or herpes. Other organisms, such as shigella, can cause diarrhea and cramping. Oral-fecal contact may also transmit hepatitis A and giardia, a parasite. Although many women engage in oral or anal sex, your health care practitioner may not think to ask you about these activities. You'll find more information on these STIs in the CDC treatment guidelines (see "Resources").

SELF-HELP TREATMENT FOR HERPES (see p. 288)

REMEDIES TO RELIEVE SORES	HOW TO USE
Clove tea, black tea	Compress on sores
Uva ursi (bearberry, kinnikinnick)	Sitz bath (fill bath with 3-4 inches of warm water and sit with only your buttocks and hips in the water; you can rest your legs and arms on the sides of the tub)
Pulverized calcium tabs, powdered slippery elm, goldenseal, myrrh, comfrey root, cold milk	Poultice on sores
Aloe vera gel, Neosporin, camphor-phenol, povidone iodine (Betadine)	Apply to sores to dry and heal

STRATEGIES TO SHORTEN/ PREVENT HERPES FLARE-UP	WHY	HOW TO USE
Avoid foods high in arginine (peanuts, chocolate, rice, cottonseed meal)	Arginine stimulates herpes virus	Eat less or not at all
Eat foods high in lysine (potatoes, meats, milk, brewer's yeast, fish, liver, eggs), or take lysine capsules	May keep virus from becoming active	Add to diet 750-1000-mg capsules if sores, 500 mg capsules daily for prevention
Echinacea (capsules, tincture, tea)	May shorten flare-up	2 capsules every 3 hours, 1 tsp. tincture every 2 hours on sores for 3-4 days, or 4 cups of tea daily
Chlorophyll (powder), red grapes, wheatgrass	May have antiviral effect	Add to diet
Vitamins A, B, C, E; minerals iron, calcium, zinc	Antioxidant, strengthen immune system, calm nerves	Take daily supplements in moderate doses; more than 10,000 IU of vitamin A can be toxic
Acupuncture, acupressure on feet	Stimulates immune system, may shorten or prevent flare-up	Press the point three thumb widths forward of the ankle bulge, along the line between the ankle bulge and little toe

NONGONOCOCCAL URETHRITIS (NGU)

Any discharge from the urethra not caused by gonorrhea is called NGU. The term usually refers to infections in men. This is not a precise medical diagnosis. The infection could be caused by chlamydia, ureaplasma urealyticum (which is found in many people with no symptoms), or mycoplasma genitalium. These are possible causes of cervicitis, PID, infertility, miscarriage, and premature birth, so a woman with infertility or a history of miscarriages may wish to be tested for them.

SOCIAL AND POLITICAL ISSUES

Preventing infection is urgent, because viral and incurable STIs are on the rise. Even curable STIs can cause serious problems if not found in time. However, the social stigma attached to STIs can make it difficult to find the care we need. Some people still believe that STIs are a just punishment for "immoral" sex.

Until recently, medical schools virtually ignored STIs. Even today health care providers may have limited training in diagnosing and treating STIs, especially when there are no symptoms.

WE NEED BETTER PROTECTION

Women everywhere need access to contraceptive and STI prevention methods that work. We're at greater risk than men for cultural, economic, and biological reasons, so protecting us from these infections should be a high priority. Women's health advocates are working to promote the development of products such as microbicides, which are gels or creams applied directly to the vagina or rectum that prevent or reduce the risk of transmitting infections. However, many substances that could kill STI germs are not developed into drugs because there isn't enough funding, and pharmaceutical companies put profits first. Also, research has been slowed by ethical concerns about testing experimental products that may not work. (To find out more, see p. 271 in Chapter 14, "Safer Sex.")

WE NEED STI EDUCATION
AND SERVICES

Even though rates of STIs among American adolescents are higher than among adolescents in most other developed countries, there's not enough political drive to improve education and prevention. Pressure from religious groups opposed to sex education and condom distribution has limited prevention efforts, particularly in schools and clinics used by teens and young women. Studies show that accurate sex information does not increase sexual activity among young adults, and that STIs *can* be prevented. STI education programs in schools work—if they are supported. Condom distribution has proved effective for protection. Schools that make condoms available report fewer students having intercourse, compared to schools without this program, and more safer-sex practices among students who are having sex. However, because of public attitudes, change comes slowly, and funding is being limited or even cut back. We urgently need to keep developing and providing culturally relevant education, prevention, and treatment for everyone, especially young women whose risk is highest. (For more information, see Chapter 32, "Organizing for Change.")

NOTE

1. H. Weinstock, S. Berman, and W. Cates, "Sexually Transmitted Diseases Among American Youth: Incidence and Prevalence Estimates, 2000," *Perspectives on Sexual and Reproductive Health* 36, no. 1 (January/February 2004): 6–10.

CHAPTER 16

After [my boyfriend] picked up his results, he sounded funny on the phone. Then he told me that the test came back positive. I was stunned and upset. . . . I was just thankful that I had used condoms. . . . At this point, I've already been tested several times, and I'm negative. It definitely served as a wake-up call for me and my girlfriends. A lot of them got tested and started being more careful, too.

Having AIDS is like continually having to put out brush fires in my body.

We must advocate for ourselves. You are not alone. . . . We have no reason to be ashamed. It is time we run our lives.[1]

The HIV/AIDS epidemic is a global crisis. Those of us who are not infected with HIV need to protect ourselves from infection. Those of us who are living with HIV/AIDS need vital care and support networks, more effective treatments, and government assistance to live as well and as long as we can and to prevent infection of our partners and babies. We all need to advocate for public health initiatives, increased funding for research, and better health care.

Information about HIV/AIDS changes rapidly. Please use this chapter as a springboard for locating the most current treatment and wellness information.

THE HIV/AIDS EPIDEMIC

AIDS (acquired immunodeficiency syndrome) was recognized by health care professionals in the United States in the early 1980s. It currently exists throughout the world. HIV (human immunodeficiency virus) causes AIDS by attacking T cells (CD4 lymphocytes), which are central to a healthy immune system. Because this process happens gradually, many people have HIV in their bodies for eight to ten years before they develop AIDS. Signs that AIDS has developed include opportunistic diseases and a T-cell count below 200.

In the past few years, advances in antiretroviral drug treatments have allowed people to live longer with HIV/AIDS. For people with access to such treatments, death rates have plummeted, and HIV infection is becoming a manageable chronic disease. Despite intensive research efforts, there is currently no vaccine or cure for HIV.

Increased awareness of HIV/AIDS has decreased its spread in some areas, but some forty thousand new infections still occur each year in the United States, and the epidemic continues to devastate many resource-poor regions of the globe, especially sub-Saharan Africa, Southeast Asia, Eastern Europe, and the Caribbean. Since the last edition of this book was published in 1998, the number of people worldwide living with HIV/AIDS increased from 10 million to approximately 37.8 million adults[2] and from 1 million to an estimated 2 million children.[3] Over 20 million people have died of HIV/AIDS in the past twenty years, and by the end of 2003, an estimated 15 million children had lost one or both parents due to AIDS.[4] The epidemic has taken a heavy toll on the health care services, social structures, and economies of developing nations that can little afford it, and there is no end in sight.

WOMEN AND HIV/AIDS

As of December 2003, nearly 50 percent of people living with HIV/AIDS worldwide were women.[5] In the United States, about 25 percent of people with HIV/AIDS are women.[6] Between 1998 and 2002, new AIDS diagnoses increased 7 percent among U.S. women, compared to a 5 percent decline in diagnoses among U.S. men.[7] In the United States and worldwide, the majority of women are infected through heterosexual sex, and women of color continue to be disproportionately affected. While representing only 12 percent of the U.S. population, African-Americans account for half of new infections in the country, and that proportion is increasing.[8] Overall HIV/AIDS death rates for women have

MYTH OR REALITY?

• *Most women get HIV through IV drug use.*

Myth. Over 70 percent of HIV infections among U.S. women are due to heterosexual transmission.

decreased since the mid-1990s, but death rates among African-American and Latina women remain much higher than among white women.[9] (For more information, see "HIV/AIDS Among Asian/Pacific Islanders and Latinas" [W35] on the companion website, www.ourbodiesour selves.org.)

Thankfully, physicians, scientists, and activists are paying more attention to women's experiences of HIV/AIDS. Women are being included in more clinical trials, including a huge national group called the Women's Interagency HIV Study, which is investigating how HIV progression and treatments affect women. Health care providers are better equipped to diagnose the gynecological symptoms of HIV/AIDS and use routine Pap smears and colposcopy to prevent invasive cervical cancer, a female-specific indicator of AIDS. New treatments have reduced the number of babies born with HIV infection (see "HIV and Pregnancy," p. 304). And in many communities, women with HIV infection and AIDS are supporting one another, doing outreach, teaching prevention, getting into recovery from substance abuse, and finding hope.

Women may be biologically more vulnerable than men to contracting HIV through heterosexual intercourse because infected semen stays in contact with the vaginal lining and cervix longer than infected vaginal secretions remain on the penis. Other factors increase our risk as well. Even if we are in monogamous relationships with male partners, we may still be at risk for getting HIV. Sometimes men pressure or force women into unprotected sex, and sometimes women may be hesitant to talk about safer sex with a partner because we are afraid of being hurt or abandoned. Fear of sexual violence and/or dependence on a male partner may make us less likely to protect ourselves during sex. A study among African-American women in Los Angeles showed that straight couples were less likely to use condoms if the woman was dependent upon her male partner for rent money.[10]

Intravenous drug use—both directly, through shared needles, and indirectly, through unprotected sex with male users—plays a significant role in transmitting HIV infection to women in the United States. At the end of 2002, 26 percent of U.S. women living with HIV/AIDS had contracted the disease through personal IV drug use. Of the 72 percent of U.S. women exposed through heterosexual contact, a significant percentage most likely contracted HIV from a male partner who used IV drugs.[11] Quality treatment programs can be less accessible to women of color, women who live in poverty, and those of us who are pregnant or have dependent children. Even when we have access to effective combination therapies (see "Treatment Options," p. 302), their required dietary schedules and side effects can make them challenging to use if we have an addiction. However, recent advances in drug therapies, including some once-a-day regimens, have made treatment easier.

Another issue is that we often don't know whether our male partners have sex with men. A recent study by the Centers for Disease Control found that over one third of HIV-positive African-American men said they had sex with both men and women, but only a small fraction of HIV-positive African-American women reported knowing that their partners had sex with men.[12]

TAKING CARE OF OURSELVES

For various reasons, taking care of ourselves often comes last. The insensitivity of some medical institutions to women—especially to women of color, poor women, uninsured women, and women who don't speak English—still drives many of us to delay seeking care or testing. We may go without treatment for sexually transmitted infections (STIs, also called sexually transmitted diseases or STDs) or vaginal irritations, which can increase our risk of being infected by

HIV if we are exposed. On average, women have fewer financial resources than men; we are also more likely to be single parents and major caregivers for those who are ill. Some of us get treatment only when our children are found to be infected.

Yet it is crucial that we take care of ourselves and work to change the systems that make it so hard for us to do so. Improving women's experiences with HIV/AIDS in the United States will depend on fundamental social changes that address poverty, racism, and sexism. Too often, public support is lacking for the tools that we need: drug treatment programs, housing, adequate nutrition, health care, and child care. We all have a right to be healthy, to enjoy sex without risking our health, to care for ourselves and one another, and to get the medical care we need. HIV/AIDS activists can help make this right attainable for every woman. (For more information, see "Taking Care of Ourselves" [W36] on the companion website, www.ourbodiesourselves.org.)

HIV TRANSMISSION

Two conditions must be met for HIV to pass from one person to another:

1. *The virus must be present in sufficient quantity.* Five bodily fluids—blood, pre-ejaculate (pre-cum), semen (cum), vaginal fluid, and breast milk—can carry enough virus to cause infection. Saliva, tears, sweat, urine, feces, and vomit (unless they are mixed with blood) do not contain enough virus to infect you.

2. *The virus must have a way to get into your bloodstream.* HIV can enter your body through the mucous membrane that lines the vagina and rectum; it can enter directly into the blood via a shared IV-drug or tattoo needle; through the

skin via any open cut, wound, or scratch; or through the mucous membrane in the eyes, the nose, and the foreskin and opening of a man's penis. Oral sex, rimming, fisting, finger fucking, and deep kissing are considerably lower-risk activities for HIV transmission unless blood is involved.

The virus can enter mucous membranes more easily if there are tiny tears, inflammation, or open sores due to an STI or untreated vaginal infection. Therefore, your risk of becoming HIV-infected, or potentially infecting your partner, is increased if you have any STIs.

(For more information, see "Terms Related to HIV/AIDS" [W37] on the companion website, www.ourbodiesourselves.org.)

PROTECTING OURSELVES FROM HIV

It is possible to live with HIV for many years without any outward symptoms, which is why it is so important to use condoms every time you

MAIN WAYS HIV CAN BE TRANSMITTED:

- Sharing needles that contain blood, including works for IV drugs (heroin, cocaine, speed) or needles shared for tattooing or body piercing
- Unprotected vaginal and anal sex
- During pregnancy, childbirth, and breast-feeding, from mother to child (see "HIV and Pregnancy," p. 304)
- Receiving a transfusion of HIV-infected blood and blood products (these are now fully screened in the United States, so risk is negligible)

have intercourse, and to know your status and the status of anyone you have sex with. Open communication with our partners is vital, but even in long-term relationships, our lovers may be having sex with other women and men or injecting drugs without our knowledge. They also may have been infected long before they met us.

Even for couples in which both partners are HIV-infected, medical professionals advise safer-sex practices to prevent "mixing" of HIV strains and transmission of other sexually transmitted pathogens that may be present, especially when your immune system weakens as HIV disease progresses. If one member of a couple is infected and the other is not, using a barrier method can prevent infection of the uninfected partner. (For more information and guidelines on practices to prevent HIV transmission, see Chapter 14, "Safer Sex.")

NONOCCUPATIONAL POST-EXPOSURE PROPHYLAXIS (NPEP)

If you think you might have been exposed to HIV, you may be able to obtain treatment immediately, without waiting for tests to show the presence of HIV antibodies. People who have accidental needle sticks in health care settings use such treatment, called post-exposure prophylaxis (PEP). This involves taking medications that are used for people with HIV but may prevent HIV infection in early exposure. You can go to an emergency room within seventy-two hours (the sooner the better) of suspected exposure to HIV and get access to this treatment. The drugs used in the twenty-eight-day regimen may cause serious side effects and can cost around $1,000, but they have the potential to prevent you from becoming infected with HIV. Insurance may cover some of the costs of NPEP.

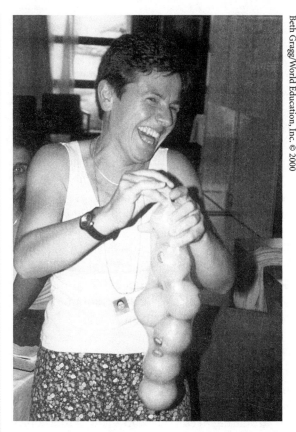

Some say that condoms are not strong enough—or big enough. Trainees in the Public Health in Complex Emergencies course in Bosnia-Herzegovina learned differently by playing a game to see how many oranges they could stuff into a condom.

HIV-SAFE IV NEEDLE USE

Sharing needles, like having unprotected sex, does not automatically transmit HIV. Your risk level is determined by the context of your behavior. For example, if you share needles with a monogamous partner and you have both tested negative for HIV and hepatitis C, there is no inherent risk. Sharing needles with people you don't know or whose HIV status is unknown increases risk for both HIV and hepatitis B and C transmission.

If you inject drugs, think about changing to a

LESBIANS: AT RISK?

Those of us who are lesbians have been told we're a low-risk group, yet some of us have sex with men, some use IV drugs, some are sex workers, some are raped, and some engage in risky behavior, like sharing sex toys with partners of unknown HIV status. Our risk for HIV infection depends on what we do, not how we identify ourselves. Defining risk in terms of groups rather than behavior can be fatal.

For those of us who are living with HIV or AIDS, it is essential that programs and services provide environments that are safe and supportive, displaying information and resources specific to lesbians.

non-IV drug (sniffing or smoking) or getting into treatment. If you continue to use IV drugs, avoid sharing needles or works (including cookers and cotton) with anyone. Try not to reuse needles or syringes, and if you do, clean them and the cooker with full-strength household bleach (three rinses of bleach is best, followed by three rinses of clean water). In an emergency, rubbing alcohol, vodka, or wine can also be used, but they are not as effective as bleach. (Note: Bleach will not kill hepatitis C.) Use fresh cotton and water each time. Take advantage of needle exchange programs that exist in some areas, and advocate for them if they do not exist. Such programs have been highly successful in decreasing HIV transmission among injection drug users.

Acceptance was the key for me. I had to accept that I had this virus and there was nothing I could do to make it go away. . . . My worst day with HIV is ten times better than my best day in active addiction.

HIV SYMPTOMS AND TESTING

According to the Centers for Disease Control, an estimated 180,000 to 280,000 people in the United States—about one quarter of those infected with HIV—don't know they are infected. This is why testing is so important. Even though it can be scary to get tested, the sooner HIV is diagnosed, the sooner we can begin treatments that may protect our immune systems from serious damage and extend our lives by years.

Many people who are infected with HIV experience a set of flu-like symptoms—such as high fever, sore throat, swollen glands, extreme fatigue, and rash—within one month of infection. If you have these symptoms and think you might have been exposed to HIV, it is important to get tested. Some clinical trials at hospitals can place you on medications to help slow the disease process.

After the initial reaction to HIV infection (called *acute seroconversion*), most people feel fairly healthy for several years. But as immune function begins to break down, symptoms of AIDS start to appear. These include weight loss, fatigue, swollen glands (lumps in the neck, armpits, or groin), and skin rashes. Night sweats, fevers, thrush, headaches, diarrhea, and loss of appetite can also occur. Recurrent vaginal yeast infections, chronic pelvic inflammatory disease, frequently recurring severe genital herpes, or human papillomavirus (HPV)—the virus that causes venereal warts (condyloma)—can also indicate that HIV infection has progressed to AIDS. Opportunistic infections, such as *Pneumocystis carinii* pneumonia (PCP), severe thrush, or lymphoma often occur when the immune system has been severely damaged by HIV.

Finding out that you are HIV-positive is life-changing and can be traumatic. Check to see if there are support groups or counselors in your

WHO IS PARTICULARLY VULNERABLE?

Teens

People under twenty-five now carry the highest risk of contracting HIV worldwide.[13] It has been estimated that approximately half of all new HIV infections both worldwide[14] and in the United States are among people under twenty-five.[15] In 2003 approximately 2,000 children under age fifteen and 6,000 people between fifteen and twenty-four years old worldwide became infected with HIV each day.[16] In the United States, as in many developing countries, the primary cause of HIV infection in children under age thirteen is mother-to-child transmission. However, such transmission is relatively rare in the U.S. because of widespread HIV screening and treatment for pregnant women.[17] As a result, adolescents bear the brunt of the epidemic in people under twenty-five in the United States.

The majority of young women in the U.S. are infected through heterosexual sex.[18] Unfortunately, conservative religious and political groups in many areas of the country have fought for "abstinence only" education and against comprehensive sexuality education and HIV/AIDS prevention. Without knowledge of safer-sex practices and the skills to use them, young people put themselves at risk. To prevent pregnancy or to maintain a type of virginity, some will have unprotected oral or anal sex, both of which can transmit HIV.

IV Drug Users

In the United States, IV drug use has contributed to HIV infection for a larger proportion of HIV-positive women than men. Since the AIDS epidemic began, 57 percent of all AIDS cases among U.S. women have been attributed to injection drug use or sex with partners who inject drugs, compared to 31 percent of cases among men.[19] Women of color are disproportionately affected; in 2000, 26 percent of AIDS cases among African-Americans and 31 percent among Latinos were attributed to IV drug use, compared to 19 percent of cases among whites. Once diagnosed with AIDS, women who became infected with HIV through IV drug use generally die sooner than women who were infected in other ways.[20]

Sharing contaminated needles and having sex with infected partners are the main ways that women get HIV due to IV drug use. Injectable drugs often impair our judgment, which may make us less likely to inject safely or to practice safer sex while high. If we do not use IV drugs ourselves, we may still be at risk for getting HIV by having unprotected sex with an IV-drug-using partner. This is a significant problem, especially if we do not know that our male partners inject drugs.

Sex Workers

The U.S. public, media, police, and courts tend to accuse sex workers, but not male clients, of spreading HIV. In fact, because women are more biologically vulnerable to HIV infection, an uninfected female sex worker may be more likely to contract HIV from an infected male client than an infected sex worker is to give an uninfected male client the virus. Many men will pay more for unprotected sex, and some men—believing that younger women are infection-free or that having sex with a virgin cures STIs—seek out the youngest and most vulnerable sex workers.

Many states require mandatory HIV testing of sex workers who are arrested, with no similar mandates for testing clients. This is a human rights violation. Sex workers need legal protection and access to confidential client-centered health care that includes HIV and STI screening and treatment, not harassment and mandatory testing. Happily, some female sex workers in the United States overcome these obstacles, building on years of experience in using condoms as protection from STIs. In some communities, sex workers have helped train AIDS educators to teach more effectively.

Women in Prison

Women in United States prisons are three times more likely than incarcerated men to be infected with HIV, and HIV infection is much more common among female prisoners than in the general population.[21] The HIV/AIDS death rate is two times higher for prisoners than for the general population.[22] In some prisons, unhealthy living conditions and inadequate health care may make HIV-infected women more likely to develop complications. Many HIV-positive women in prison are also infected with hepatitis C, which can exacerbate HIV infection.[23] In prisons with sufficient health care, wellness programs, and HIV education, a woman may receive higher-quality care and be more likely to follow treatment plans than she would outside the prison.

area to help you with testing decisions, and find a testing site that provides good counseling.

I had engaged in many risky behaviors, particularly a number of unprotected sexual encounters while I was heavily intoxicated. . . . The night before I was to get tested, I prayed to God that I would help people with HIV/AIDS if he would only see to it that my tests came out negative. . . . A very long two weeks later, I found out that I was negative. . . . For the past year, I have volunteered every Wednesday night at AIDS Action Committee.

WHAT IS THE HIV ANTIBODY TEST?

There are several types of HIV tests available: conventional and rapid tests using blood, oral testing (which uses a small sample of mucosal cells from the inside of your cheek and gum), or urine testing. All methods test for antibodies to HIV, which are produced by the body's immune system in response to the virus. An initial positive result is always confirmed by a more specific test (i.e., Western blot).

WHEN SHOULD I TAKE THE TEST?

It's recommended that you take the test approximately three months after your last possible exposure to HIV. This is sometimes called the "window," the period between the time when a person is infected with HIV and when she has built up a level of antibodies in her bloodstream that is high enough to be detected by the test. According to the Centers for Disease Control, testing is now 100 percent sensitive twelve weeks post-exposure. However, if you think you are

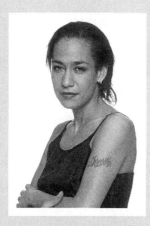

© Robin Holland

"THERE IS NO TURNING BACK"

MARLENE DIAZ

In one day, my life changed completely. I was no longer Marlene Diaz; I became Marlene Diaz, HIV-positive female.

In 1992, I survived a five-hour ordeal of rape. I was two months pregnant. Six months later, I was able to be tested. When I got a call saying the results were in, I phoned my friend and said, "I have a bad feeling. It can't be good if they have to tell me in person." I was right. My aunt, a health professional, asked me to have my baby at another hospital from the one she worked at, because she didn't want anyone to know I was positive. I was twenty-nine.

I started fighting back against the stigma and injustice, and activism has given me strength. One of my biggest battles was against mandatory testing for babies, which means that the mothers are tested without their consent. But although that fight consumed two years of my life, I lost. A battle we did win was establishing a definition of full-blown AIDS that included symptoms common to women and that let them get treatment and financial entitlements, such as disability, available to men.

But even some of the victories have not turned out right. Because of new drugs, the good news is that there are fewer infants born with HIV. The bad news is that now there is not a big enough market [of children], so drug companies base dosage on a 150-pound male and are not even trying to figure out a dosage for a child. Figuring out what to give my daughter is like consulting a Ouija board.

Last year for Margaretha was horrible. She was ten then and almost five feet tall, but her weight went down to 59 pounds. She had shingles. This year she is Lazarus; her viral load is not detectable, she takes horseback riding and, after school, participates in ballroom dancing and hockey.

I was mugged last weekend by some young guys in my neighborhood. As they beat me, I could hear them yelling "El monstro," slang for AIDS. Afterward, I was upset not only for myself but for Margaretha. In the writing samples she had submitted to get into her middle school, she talked about being HIV-positive. It was her way of saying: "This is who I am, take it or leave it." I am so extremely proud of her bravery, but worried, too. She has known the word "AIDS" for years, but when I was attacked in that hate crime, she began to understand the stigma.

Still, I know we are among the lucky ones. The international work I did was very humbling. I admire the women from South America, the Caribbean, Africa. What they have survived and challenged is amazing: They confront hate on a daily basis.

There is no turning back. I don't have it in me to shut up. I feel if you shut up—how do I explain it to you?—it won't make change.

having symptoms of acute seroconversion (initial infection) and want to be considered for trials that provide access to new drug therapies, you may want to take the HIV test before the three-month period is over.

WHAT KIND OF TEST SHOULD I TAKE?

- *Blood:* This is the most common test. Blood is drawn from your arm (or finger) and tested for antibodies. The test results are available approximately one week from the time you are tested. Testing for hepatitis C can also be done using the same blood sample, as can HIV-2 (a less virulent form of HIV present in western Africa, Brazil, and parts of Europe).
- *Oral (OraSure) or Urine Testing:*[24] Like the blood test, both the oral test and urine test are extremely accurate, quick, and painless. With the oral test, a small quantity of mucosal cells is collected from the inside of your cheek and gum, using a toothbrush-like wand. (It does contain gelatin, so if you are vegetarian, you might prefer to have the blood or rapid test.) Your results are available approximately one week from the time you are tested. Urine testing is less widely used and requires a blood test to confirm a preliminary positive.
- *Rapid (OraQuick or Reveal):* Two versions of this test, which requires just a drop of blood or saliva, were approved by the FDA in 2003 and 2004, respectively. The test's results are very accurate and can be determined twenty minutes after your sample has been collected. As with all testing methods, further testing is required to confirm an OraQuick preliminary positive. Still, rapid testing can be invaluable

in preventing mother-to-child HIV transmission for women in labor who have not been previously tested.

WHERE SHOULD I TAKE THE TEST?

Testing is available in many hospitals, clinics, test sites, and doctors' offices. First decide if you want anonymous testing (in which you are identified by number, not name). Your local department of public health or AIDS agency can tell you about the laws in your state and anonymous test sites nearest you. In general, public health clinics are a good place to get tested because they are experienced and often offer post-testing counseling, which your doctor or local hospital may not. You should be aware that "confidential" testing is not anonymous—your test result can go into your medical record, which may be available to courts and insurance companies. Many of us worry that having our HIV status in a medical record could prevent us from getting health insurance or proper care for health problems in the future. While these fears are not unfounded, recent protections on medical records have made the possibility of disclosure of HIV status less likely.

HOME TESTING

Home test kits, which are available in most pharmacies, make it possible to collect a blood sample in privacy. You prick your finger, place a smear of your blood on the piece of filter paper provided, and send it to a specified lab. The smear is identifiable only by an identification number. You then call a toll-free number seven days later to hear the results. For best reliability, look for an FDA-approved test, such as the Home Access Express HIV-1 Test System.

COPING WITH YOUR TEST RESULTS

If your test result is negative for HIV (and you have closed your "window"), you may find that relief and gratitude are mixed with other feelings. You may ask "Why not me?" as you watch friends suffer from the disease. Or you may find, as some people do, that it is difficult to keep practicing safer sex or using clean needles. A support group, counselor, or friend may help you find your balance.

If your test result is positive for HIV, keep in mind that people are living longer and better with HIV. We can have the infection for ten years or more without having any noticeable symptoms or effect on quality of life.

LIVING WITH HIV/AIDS

Most important, at least for me, is learning to live with the AIDS virus—learning how to put myself first.[25]

We all have to die from something, but why die before you're dead? Life is what you make of it. . . . Personally, I do not consider HIV a death sentence. I know that as long as I take care of myself through good nutrition, proper sleep, attending support groups, visiting my physician, and keeping up with my recovery from drug use, I will be all right. . . . I was so convinced I was going to die that I didn't pay taxes for four years. Now the IRS is saying, "You're gonna live, and you're gonna pay us."

If your test result is positive for HIV, remember that this does not mean you have AIDS. It is a time to take particularly good care of your health, if you can, by eating better, resting more, and protecting yourself from other STIs. There are promising new combination treatments, or "cocktails" (see p. 303), which may make a difference in how soon you develop AIDS. Finding health care is a crucial step—especially finding a provider experienced in treating HIV infection. So is negotiating whatever insurance or disability benefits might be available to you. Finding emotional support is important, too. Seek out groups in your community for people who are HIV-positive.

GETTING THE BEST HEALTH CARE POSSIBLE

The quality of health care in the U.S. is unfortunately not consistent, and we often don't have access to the best care if we are poor, if we are women of color, or if we are undocumented. Still, there are highly dedicated health care providers at every level of the system. An AIDS hotline or agency may be able to help you find the best care possible in your area (see "Resources").

The best health care means frequent visits for physical exams and laboratory tests. What follows is what should be the basic, minimal standard of care for all people with HIV or AIDS:

1. Evaluation: Frequent CD4 cell (or T-cell) monitoring and viral load testing to help you plan and assess treatment. T-cell monitoring will show how well your immune system is doing, and viral load testing will show how much HIV is in your body at a given time.

2. Vaccinations: Vaccinations should be brought up-to-date, especially for pneumonia, hepatitis B, tetanus, and flu.

3. Treatment: HIV disease can be treated in many different ways: treating the virus itself with antiviral medications, treating or preventing the opportunistic infections, taking care of overall health, and boosting the immune system (through self-care and nonmedical alternatives). See "Treatment Options," this page.

4. Support: Our emotional well-being is important, as is nutritional advice and the assistance of a social worker.

5. Female-specific care: HIV-positive women often have specific problems that should be addressed, including chronic vaginitis, pelvic infections, vaginal and cervical diseases, and bacterial lung infections. HIV-positive women are also at higher risk for the human papillomavirus (HPV), which may increase risk of cervical cell changes that can lead to cancer. A Pap smear every six months is advised.

TREATMENT OPTIONS

Treatment for HIV/AIDS is constantly changing as science delivers more information and new drugs, and as we learn more about the effects of nonmedical therapies. Many AIDS service organizations hold strategy sessions for treatment issues, and there are some great treatment hotlines and helpful publications (see "Resources"). Sometimes we feel better than ever before, because we are paying closer attention to our own well-being. We may qualify for government aid and have access to financial and medical support for the first time in our lives. We may access treatment for drug or alcohol addiction. Those of us who find a support or activist group often find that we are less alone. Helping others protect themselves against HIV can also make us feel better. More than one woman has said, "The virus gave me my life."

MEDICAL (ALLOPATHIC) TREATMENT

While the strategy used to be "hit hard, hit early," now antiretroviral therapy is initiated only when T-cell count is low and the viral load is high.[26] Antiretrovirals include many different classes of drugs, and new classes are being developed every year. As of 2004, the four main classes of antiretrovirals are nucleosides (nukes), non-nucleosides (non-nukes), protease inhibitors, and fusion inhibitors. There are currently some nineteen different drugs and more than one hundred combinations (sometimes called *cocktails*) to keep viral load as low as possible and maintain immune function. These therapies have dramatically reduced death rates and improved quality of life, so HIV is often a manageable long-term illness.

Still, therapy can cause side effects, ranging from mild to debilitating. These include nausea, severe diarrhea, fatigue, bone loss, and fat redistribution. Some drugs have been associated with diabetes and liver disease. It is important to make sure your HIV medicines are compatible with the other medications you may be taking (for seizures, asthma, or cholesterol) as well as with birth control pills and that you follow dietary requirements. For those of us with limited financial resources, eating the right foods can be difficult.

How many people do you know [who] eat three full meals a day? On my budget, let's be realistic.

It is important to find a medical regimen that you are able to follow and tolerate so you can have the complete benefit of the medicines yet still live life to the fullest. HIV mutates very fast and can become drug-resistant if it replicates in the presence of low levels of antiviral drugs. Therefore, **if you don't take the drugs consistently, you may develop HIV strains that are drug-resistant, and you may not be able to use the drugs later in the course of the illness.** Although it can be hard to take medicines daily, many women learn to make the medicines part of daily life with support from others who have HIV, families and friends, and health care providers.

Every woman who wants antiretroviral therapy should have access to it. Many of us with low incomes, who are homeless, or who use IV drugs worry that doctors may not offer us the latest cocktails because they think we might not take the medications as directed.

You know people look at you, see you're black or Latina, and think you must be a welfare mom, or an addict and stupid.

Studies have indicated that doctors are often wrong when they try to guess how likely patients are to comply with antiretroviral therapy.[27] Try talking with your health care provider about how to make the most effective treatments work for you.

Your health care provider may also want to protect you against tuberculosis, herpes simplex virus, yeast infections, and other opportunistic infections. You may be offered a place in a clinical drug trial. Participating in a clinical drug trial, which is the last stage of testing to prove drug safety, efficacy, and appropriate dosage, is one way to benefit from the latest research and receive free medicine and medical attention. It involves risks, but some people prefer the risk of taking a new drug that might help, to the near certainty of suffering without it, especially if they have a virus that is resistant to approved treatments. For information about clinical trials, you can contact the National Institutes of Health (NIH) at 1-800-TRIALS-A (1-800-243-7012 TTY/TDD) or visit www.actis.org.

HOLISTIC (NONALLOPATHIC) CARE

Alternative treatments, used in conjunction with more common, allopathic medical treatments such as drugs, may reduce the severity of symptoms associated with HIV disease and bolster the immune system. The use of Chinese medicine—both acupuncture and Chinese herbs—may improve CD4 cell counts and immune system functioning, abate drug side effects, and relieve some symptoms, such as night sweats, nausea, diarrhea, and neuropathies (pain or lack of feeling in the extremities).[28,29] However, be aware of drug interactions and toxicity, especially if you are taking multiple drugs.

Visualization, relaxation, exercise, yoga, massage, and cognitive therapy may help to improve immune system functioning and enhance quality of life.[30,31] Both acupuncture and chiropractic care may reduce stress and muscle tension and can be helpful for insomnia, neuropathies, and headaches.[32] Recent clinical trials have indicated that homeopathy may help reduce viral loads and improve lymphocyte counts.[33]

Some AIDS service organizations, hospitals, and clinics provide alternative therapies regardless of an individual's ability to pay. If you have health insurance, some complementary treatments may be covered. For more on complementary health care, see Chapter 5, "Complementary Health Practices."

HIV AND PREGNANCY

I have had patients with HIV infection who were not so gently pushed to have tubal ligations that they have come to regret, since the chances of having an infected baby have decreased in this country over the years.

HIV can pass from mother to fetus (called *vertical transmission*) during pregnancy and childbirth. If you want to have a child and think you might have been exposed to HIV, it is a good idea to get tested before you become pregnant. For those of us who know we are HIV-positive and want to bear children, antiretroviral drugs offer more choices and increased hope. In some clinical studies, antiretroviral drugs taken before and/or at the time of birth and elective cesarean section have reduced the rate of vertical transmission to under 2 percent.[34] The introduction of rapid HIV testing during labor and delivery

has allowed women who were previously unknown to be HIV-positive to receive short-course antiretroviral therapy to reduce the risk of transmitting HIV to babies.[35] Since HIV can pass to the infant through breast milk, it is safest for HIV-positive mothers not to breast-feed. Researchers are currently investigating whether certain types of antiretroviral therapy may help prevent transmission from mother to baby in cases where breast-feeding is necessary.[36]

HIV-positive women and women with HIV-positive partners who desire children have a few options. Adoption is the lowest-risk option for preventing HIV transmission from parents to children. Artificial insemination with semen from an HIV-negative donor is also a safe option for HIV-negative women with HIV-positive partners. Also, a new (still experimental) sperm wash method removes most of the HIV from the semen of infected men so that it is safer for insemination of HIV-negative women.[37] This method may allow women to have children fathered by HIV-positive male partners. If you would like to become pregnant and you have an HIV-positive partner, seek a consultation with a fertility expert to learn what your options are.

Some HIV/AIDS policy makers have actively discouraged all HIV-positive women from becoming pregnant, and encouraged pregnant HIV-positive women to terminate pregnancies. Ironically, if you are HIV-positive and pregnant and wish to abort, you may find that abortion clinics will refuse to take you or will charge extra. Advocates are fighting to preserve the reproductive rights and freedom of HIV-positive women, including access to nondiscriminatory health care.

PERSONAL ISSUES

The list of personal dilemmas and questions for women with HIV or AIDS and our families is long. What about my sex life? Who will care for my children if I get too sick? Will I tell my family and friends I have HIV? My coworkers? My children? What if people find out? How do I deal with health care providers who don't respect me? How do I get on public assistance? What legal protections are there if I feel I am being discriminated against because of HIV? How do I face the possibility of my death? (For more on hotlines, organizations, books, and magazines, see "Resources.")

PREPARING FOR OUR CHILDREN'S CARE

Although more people are now living longer with HIV, it remains a life-threatening disease. If we are mothers, the thought of getting too sick to care for our children, or dying while they are young, is often the hardest thing to bear. Many states have enacted important "standby guardianship" laws that allow us to decide in advance who will become guardians of our children in the case of incapacitating illness, while still caring for them ourselves for as long as we are able.

GETTING INVOLVED

Many women have found that getting active in the community helps us feel better emotionally and spiritually while living with HIV or AIDS. During the periods when we're not feeling sick, we might join a group to pressure a hospital to improve its treatment of people with AIDS, to lobby the city council or Congress for better AIDS legislation, to convince a church or other religious group to open up about HIV, or to advocate for more resources for vaccine and microbicide research and development. Many women become peer counselors, educating people in our communities about preventing HIV.

Or we can get involved in a recovery program, become a sponsor, and encourage other women in recovery from drug or alcohol use. As one woman from the AIDS Action Committee in Massachusetts said, "If I can save one more person, it's worth it."

NOTES

1. Elizabeth Banks, "Living with HIV," *Sojourner: The Women's Forum* 22, no. 7 (March 1997): 20.
2. Joint United Nations Programme on HIV/AIDS (UNAIDS) and World Health Organization (WHO), 2004 report on the global AIDS epidemic, July 2004, accessed at www.unaids.org/bangkok2004/report_pdf.html.
3. Ibid.
4. Ibid.
5. National Institute of Allergy and Infectious Diseases, "HIV Infection in Women," National Institutes of Health, U.S. Department of Health and Human Services, May 2004, accessed at www.niaid.nih.gov/factsheets/womenhiv.htm on May 20, 2004.
6. Centers for Disease Control and Prevention, "HIV/AIDS Surveillance Report" 14, no. 6 (2002). Also available at www.cdc.gov/hiv/stats/hasrlink.htm.
7. Ibid.
8. Joint United Nations Programme, report on the global AIDS epidemic.
9. Centers for Disease Control, National Center for Health Statistics, "Table 42: Death Rates for Human Immunodeficiency Virus (HIV) Disease, According to Sex, Race, Hispanic Origin, and Age: United States, Selected Years 1987–2001," *Health United States* (2003): 177–78, accessed at www.cdc.gov/nchs/data/hus/tables/2003/03hus042.pdf.
10. Gail Elizabeth Wyatt, "Transaction Sex and HIV Risks: A Women's Choice?," *HIV Infection in Women: Setting a New Agenda*, Washington, D.C. (February 22–24, 1995): S2, abstract Number WA1-1.
11. Centers for Disease Control and Prevention, "HIV/AIDS Surveillance Report."
12. Joint United Nations Programme on HIV/AIDS (UNAIDS) and World Health Organization (WHO). *AIDS Epidemic Update: 2003.* December 2003. Accessed May 20, 2004 at www.unaids.org/Unaids/EN/Resources/Publications/Corporate+publications/AIDS+epidemic+update+-+December+2003.asp.
13. World Health Organization, "Tuberculosis and HIV:

Questions and Answers," December 2003, accessed at http://w3.whosea.org/hivaids/faqchapter2.htm.

14. World Health Organization, "World Health Report 2004: Changing History," accessed May 20, 2004 at www.who.int/whr/2004/en/.

15. National Institute of Allergy and Infectious Diseases, "HIV/AIDS Statistics," National Institutes of Health, U.S. Department of Health and Human Services, January 2004, accessed May 20, 2004 at www.niaid.nih.gov/factsheets/aidsstat.htm.

16. Ibid.

17. Centers for Disease Control and Prevention, "HIV/AIDS Surveillance Report."

18. Ibid.

19. Centers for Disease Control and Prevention, "Drug-Associated HIV Transmission Continues in the United States," March 2002, accessed at www.cdc.gov/hiv/pubs/facts/idu.htm.

20. Centers for Disease Control and Prevention, "HIV/AIDS Surveillance Report."

21. Anne S. De Groot, M.D., "HIV Infection Among Incarcerated Women: An Epidemic Behind the Walls," *HIV Education Prison Project (HEPP) News* 3, no. 4 (April 2000): 1–4.

22. L. Maruschak, "HIV in Prisons, 2001," *Bureau of Justice Statistics Bulletin,* U.S. Department of Justice, January 2004, accessed at www.ojp.usdoj.gov/bjs/pub/pdf/hivp01.pdf.

23. Centers for Disease Control and Prevention, "Prevention and Control of Infections with Hepatitis Viruses in Correctional Settings," *Morbidity and Mortality Weekly Report* 52, no. RR-1 (2003): 3.

24. www.cdc.gov/hiv/pubs/faq/faq8.htm.

25. Elizabeth Banks, "Living with HIV."

26. U.S. Department of Health and Human Services, HIV/AIDS Bureau, ADAP Manual, 2003 version, accessed at http://hab.hrsa.gov/tools/adap/adapSecVIChap2.htm#SecVIChap2.

27. R. Murri, A. Antinori, A. Ammassari, S. Nappa, A. Orofino, N. Abrescia, C. Mussini, A. D'Arminio Monforte, A. W. Wu, AdICoNA Study Group, "Physician Estimates of Adherence and the Patient-Physician Relationship as a Setting to Improve Adherence to Antiretroviral Therapy," *Journal of Acquired Immune Defi-ciency Syndromes* 31, Suppl. 3 (December 15, 2002): S158–62.

28. J. Wang, Z. Yu, G. Li, Y. Zhang, C. Guan, W. Lu, "Clinical Observation on the Therapeutic Effects of Zhongyan-2 Recipe in Treating 29 HIV-infected and AIDS Patients," *Journal of Traditional Chinese Medicine* 22, no. 2 (June 2002): 93–98.

29. X. Chen, L. Yang, N. Zhang, J. A. Turpin, R. W. Buckheit, C. Osterling, J. J. Oppenheim, O. M. Howard, "Shikonin, a Component of Chinese Herbal Medicine, Inhibits Chemokine Receptor Function and Suppresses Human Immunodeficiency Virus Type 1," *Antimicrobial Agents and Chemotherapy* 47, no. 9 (September 2003): 2810–16.

30. S. C. Lechner et al., "Cognitive-Behavioral Interventions Improve Quality of Life in Women with AIDS," *Journal of Psychosomatic Research* 54, no. 3 (March 2003): 253–61.

31. Asian Community AIDS Service, overview of different forms of complementary therapies, 2003. Accessed at www.acas.org/treatment/pdf/english/ct.pdf on October 13, 2004.

32. Ibid.

33. D. Ullman, "Controlled Clinical Trials Evaluating the Homeopathic Treatment of People with Human Immunodeficiency Virus or Acquired Immune Deficiency Syndrome," *Journal of Alternative and Complementary Medicine* 9, no. 1 (February 2003): 133–41.

34. A. P. Kourtis, A. Duerr, "Prevention of Perinatal HIV Transmission: A Review of Novel Strategies," *Expert Opinion on Investigational Drugs* 12, no. 9 (September 2003): 1535–44.

35. M. Lampe et al., "Rapid HIV-1 Antibody Testing During Labor and Delivery for Women of Unknown HIV Status: A Practical Guide and Model Protocol," Centers for Disease Control and Prevention, January 2004, accessed at www.cdc.gov/hiv/rapid_testing/materials/Labor&DeliveryRapidTesting.pdf.

36. C. Thorne and M. L. Newell, "Prevention of Mother-to-Child Transmission of HIV Infection," *Current Opinion in Infectious Diseases* 17, no. 3 (June 2004): 247–52.

37. Y. Englert et al., "Medically Assisted Reproduction in the Presence of Chronic Viral Diseases," *Human Reproduction Update* 10, no. 2 (March–April 2004): 149–62.

Reproductive
Choices

CHAPTER 17

The last half of the twentieth century saw enormous changes in women's choices about motherhood. For our great-grandmothers, the lack of effective birth control, along with rigid societal expectations, meant that almost all women who were fertile had children. Today, however, more choices exist. Access to birth control, legal abortion, and reproductive technologies makes it possible for more of us to control whether and when to have children. In addition, changing laws and social mores have led to greater acceptance of women who decide not to have children, as well as single women, same-sex couples, and other nontraditional families who seek to conceive or adopt a child.

Some of us have always known we wanted children, while

others of us are sure that we don't. Many of us find ourselves, at some point in our lives, struggling with ambivalence. Life's realities often limit available choices: You may have so little money or other resources that you can't imagine taking care of a child. You may be single and not want to raise a child alone, or find yourself pregnant and raising children without having consciously made a decision to do so. You may be infertile, or have an illness or disability that prevents conception, pregnancy, or parenthood. Still, having more control of our fertility can give us time to think deeply and fully about becoming mothers.

The first section of this chapter explores some of the questions to ask yourself if you are considering becoming a parent. It provides tools to help you with this process. If you decide to have a child, further questions arise that our foremothers did not face: Should I pursue conception, adoption, or foster parenthood? The second section of the chapter addresses some of these issues.

MAKING A DECISION

MOTHERING TODAY

Like many of the personal choices we make, the decision whether to have children is influenced by our families, our culture, and the society in which we live. U.S. society presumes that motherhood is central to women's identity and fulfillment, yet our government provides little concrete support for children and families. The United States, unlike most other industrialized countries, has no paid family leave, no guaranteed health care, and little affordable high-quality child care.

In addition, a good mother/bad mother framework pervades public discussion and perceptions of motherhood. The media is full of stories about an alleged competition between women who "choose" to be "full-time" mothers (stay-at-home moms) and those mothers who "choose" paid employment (working mothers). This scenario would have us believe that women fall into one group or the other, with each group negatively judging the other. These so-called Mommy War stories invite us to take sides, to praise working mothers for keeping so many balls in the air or condemn them for neglecting their children; to praise the stay-at-home mothers for being so devoted to their children or condemn them for giving over so much of their identity to motherhood.

In fact, very few mothers' lives can be described in these polarized terms. According to the U.S. Census Report, in 2002 over 50 percent of women with infants and 72 percent of other mothers were in the labor force. Many mothers of small children work part-time, or wait until children start school before returning to work. Most mothers move in and out of full-time or part-time paid employment in response to changing family needs. The reality is that most of us have to work, whether we want to or not. This is particularly true for single mothers, of whom there are currently 10 million in the U.S.[1]

By and large, real-life mothers' experiences rarely make the news and don't figure significantly in public policy. For example, during the period of "welfare reform" in the 1990s, the media contained plenty of negative stories about mothers who had been on welfare for years, stories certainly not told from the perspective of the women. News articles abounded about a "typical" woman on welfare, called Denise M. or Letitia B., mother of five kids by four different men * who spent her days smoking cigarettes and barely tending to her most recent baby's needs. Despite the fact that the majority of welfare recipients are white, she was almost always a woman of color, usually African-American, and

* In actuality, the average woman on welfare has fewer than three children.

stereotypically depicted as a "bad mother." The repetition of stories like this encouraged readers or viewers to associate race and poverty with inadequate mothering, and to hold mothers in need responsible for failing to provide for our children. During the same years, "welfare reform" eliminated a financial and social support network that had been in place for sixty years. The message to women was clear: When it comes to your children, you are on your own.

Our culture idealizes some mothers, demonizes others, and takes the *work* of mothering largely for granted. Many mothers are caught off guard by the huge gulf between fantasies about motherhood and the daily reality of providing children with love, care, and a nurturing home.

CONSIDERING THE QUESTION

What does it mean to be a mother in today's world? What will it mean to *me* if I become a mother? It is hardly surprising that neither question has a straightforward or universal answer.

I hear two conflicting points of view. One, that it's terrific to be a mother; the other, "You'll regret it; your life will change."

I had a child at 46. Before that, although I loved being with other people's children, anytime something went wrong and the child irritated me, I would think to myself, How could I ever stand the full-time responsibility of being a mother? Somehow, becoming a mother changed that. There is an intangible, indescribable bond intrinsic to the relationship, that in the long run transcends the petty everyday irritating occurrences.

I love kids, but I've never had a strong urge to have them myself. I always wondered: How do you fit together the pieces of taking care of yourself and being a parent? I was single for most of my thirties, then got involved with someone who was sure he didn't want children. But I still felt it was important for me to make an active choice for myself—I didn't want to say no just because he said no. I talked with a lot of women, looked at both sides, then decided against having a child. . . . The hardest part was telling my parents, because I felt like they'd be so disappointed in me. But when I did, I felt a tremendous relief, and really, I haven't thought about it much since.

As you approach your decision, it helps to look at all sides of the question. Children are engaging, inventive, interesting, and funny. They

IF YOU HAD A PAINFUL CHILDHOOD . . .

Women who had difficult childhoods may find it particularly hard to make decisions about whether to have children. If you feel distressed or damaged by things that happened when you were younger, you may wonder if you will be able to nurture a child. Many women who have lived through incest or physical abuse fear the physical changes of pregnancy, and medical examinations or inseminations can feel invasive. Some women with abuse histories find that pregnancy and childbirth sometimes trigger flashbacks or feelings of helplessness.

It is often difficult to think seriously of having a child until you work through the issues of most concern to you. Counseling can help make your past less burdensome and give you the space to consider parenthood more comfortably. Some feminist counseling centers, family service agencies, community health centers, and other community organizations offer free or low-cost professional help.

can teach us much as they grow and change; we grow and change along with them. They challenge and inspire us to make the world a better place, and they give us a way to be part of the continuity of life. Many of us want to nurture and love children of our own, and experience parenthood as a tremendously moving and satisfying adventure.

At the same time, being a parent involves exchanging spontaneity and relative control of everyday life for a huge responsibility, complicated schedules, and relative chaos. You may not enjoy the day-to-day reality of being with children; you may love them without wanting your own. You may fear bringing children into a troubled world or want to pursue dreams incompatible with child-rearing. Being child-free often means more personal freedom and more time, money, and energy to invest in relationships, work, and other interests and passions.

Many of us are concerned about how the decision will affect our lives and relationships. If you have a partner, you may worry that a baby will change, stress, or hurt your relationship. Having children may interrupt your plans for career advancement, economic security, or professional growth. Your partner or others may pressure you to have children even though you don't feel interested or ready. On the other hand, you may fear that giving up motherhood means missing a wonderful lifelong experience.

Many questions arise. Some have straightforward answers; others are more complicated: Does my job give me financial stability? Do I have a stable household? Is my partner or any other household member abusive? What about alcohol and drugs in my life? Are there family medical problems that might be passed on genetically? Do I have parenting skills, or am I eager to learn them? How will I juggle work and child care? If I am single, how would having a child affect any new intimate relationships? Do I have adequate health insurance and accessible health care? What will the financial costs be? What kinds of values would I want to encourage in my child, and who could help me do this? What kind of community would I want to raise children in? Would I have support if I or my child developed a disability? Am I ready to prepare a child to deal with the difficulties in life, such as racism, sexism, and homophobia?

If you have a partner, talk about the kind and amount of involvement in child-rearing you each would want to have. Would one of you stay home with the baby? Would you find child care? If your partner is a man, you may want to be especially careful to talk about how he, too, and not just you, will be balancing parenting, work, or other priorities.

Try, too, to evaluate your emotional resources for parenting. Are there caring people around you to help you keep your perspective, your temper, your sense of humor, and your sanity in the

FERTILITY AND AGING

The media is full of scare stories about women and our ticking biological clocks. But these stories should be taken with a grain of statistical salt and common sense. Fertility does naturally decline as women age, but when this decline begins and the rate at which it progresses vary widely.

While it is important to have accurate information about the average woman's chances of conceiving and carrying a child to term at different ages, the fact that most women are less fertile at thirty-eight than at twenty-two should be one of the many considerations you take into account when deciding whether or when to have a child. (For more information, see "Fertility and Aging" [W38] on the companion website, www.ourbodiesourselves.org.)

midst of the emotional upheaval, changes, and chaos that occur with parenthood? As you consider whether you want a child, know that there will be times when you wish you had chosen differently, no matter what you decide.

Having a child is an irreversible decision. You are a parent forever. Even if we place children for adoption, we remember them in ways great and small. But if you decide not to have children at a certain point in your life, your choice is not necessarily a final one. If you are past childbearing age, you have opportunities to adopt, to become a foster parent, or, in a new relationship, to become a step-parent. At all times you can enjoy and love the children who become part of your life.

GUIDELINES FOR DECIDING

Making decisions is sometimes easier when you understand that:

- Choosing means letting go of other options
- You'll need time to reach a decision that is your own, that you are happy with
- You can't expect to be 100 percent certain
- The "wrong" decision won't ruin your life
- It's important to use logic *and* intuition when considering your options
- You can seek the support of family and friends
- You can consider nontraditional options for raising children

(For a further discussion of these issues, see "Guidelines for Decision-making" [W39] on the companion website, www.ourbodiesourselves .org.)

COMMON CHALLENGES

The decision of whether (and when) to have a child or children is important, yet many of us delay, deny, or avoid it altogether. Here are some common challenges and misconceptions:

1. *Avoiding a conscious decision.* Some women let nature "decide" by not using contraception. Others delay so long that the decision is made by default.

2. *Letting your partner decide for you.* He or she might be eager to have a child, or might want you to promise *not* to. You may go along with such a wish if you're afraid your partner will get angry or leave, or if you're uncertain and just want the decision to be over and done with. When you're newly in love, you may go along with your partner's wish to have a baby together, and then regret it later. It's crucial that you have a strong voice in any decision you make.

3. *Thinking your partner will change.* In your eagerness to form a family, you may ignore warning signs that your partner isn't ready for parenthood. If he or she has a drug or alcohol problem, or is explosive and violent, it is unlikely that he or she will change when the baby arrives.

4. *Thinking it's a decision between no children and two children.* Many of us assume that we must have two children, to provide the first child with a companion and as a hedge against having a "spoiled" only child. However, only children are no more or less spoiled, lonely, or malad-

justed than children with siblings. For many people, a one-child family is just right.

5. *Making the decision without knowing what children are really like.* How do you feel when you're with babies and children? Spending time with them may be one of the best things you can do. Get to know your friends' kids, your nieces, nephews, and cousins. Take them to the park. Have a sleepover. Spend an afternoon at the playground. Do you have a good time? Do you feel drawn to them?

6. *Worrying that you won't be a good parent.* Because of your parents' mistakes, or your own behavior, you may doubt your ability to parent. Be assured that you can learn, grow, and change by talking with supportive people in your life, reading parenting books or taking parenting classes, or getting some counseling.

IF YOU AND YOUR PARTNER DISAGREE

Don't panic if you and your partner seem to want different things. You both need time to listen to each other and sort things out.

During disagreements about something so important, it's easy to see your partner as the main obstacle in your path. It can be hard to hear what he or she is saying. But if you can get yourself to listen and not try to push your choice, you may find a solution that works for both of you.

Here are some helpful steps for working on a joint decision:

- First, let your partner express all of his or her ideas and feelings, so that you can better understand the objections to your desires and point of view.
- Brainstorm possibilities together. For instance, if one of you fears being overwhelmed

COUNTDOWN

One way to think about the decision is to consider how your everyday life would change. Make two columns on a sheet of paper. In the first, figure out how many hours a week you spend on each of your present activities, and in the second, the time you might spend on each if you had a baby.

- Work
- Recreation and socializing
- Hobbies
- Relaxation, e.g., yoga, meditation
- Sports
- Political activities
- Religious activities
- Time alone with partner
- Sleep

Are you willing to change your schedule in these or countless other unexpected ways? If such a prospect seems overwhelming or impossible, perhaps you shouldn't have a baby just yet.*

* Adapted with permission from *The Baby Decision* by Merle Bombardieri (New York: Rawson Wade, 1981).

by responsibilities, you might discuss having just one child, or finding out whether friends or family members could commit themselves to helping out. At the other extreme, if your partner doesn't want to miss the experience of loving closeness to children, explore ways of spending time with nieces or nephews, or doing volunteer work with children.

A good ground rule for communication is that you each agree to express both positive and negative thoughts and feelings. This openness prevents you from locking yourself into such a hard-and-fast role that you don't mention any of your own ambivalences, doubts, and fears. After doing so, if one of you winds up going along with a decision you didn't completely like, you will know that you made your best efforts to honor the other's needs and preferences.

Timing can be a crucial factor. One of you may want to finish school or career training, to save more money, to move to a better home, or to be further along in individual or couple counseling. Perhaps you can concentrate on negotiating the timing rather than the actual choice.

Your values may clash on issues such as how to discipline children, the place of religion in a child's life, saving for a child's education or future, baptism, circumcision, and the like. Know that even strongly held values do change over time. You might ask trusted family members or friends to help you sort out these issues. Parenting workshops, spiritual guides, financial counselors, and psychotherapists may also help.

If you're still stuck after a number of weeks or months, you may want to undergo some counseling sessions with a therapist specializing in short-term work about parenthood. Decisions about parenthood are tough and scary, but they can also clarify what's important to you, and help you realize what you most need and value.

IF YOU DECIDE NOT TO HAVE A CHILD

Once my husband and I had been married a few years, there were constant questions about when we would start a family—particularly from our parents, whose friends were all grandparents. Then there was additional pressure when our friends were all having children—this changed the dynamics of our friendships and was an unexpected result of deciding not to have children.

The societal and familial pressures on women to have children can be intense. Those of us who choose not to have children are often judged by those around us. Many of us find it helpful to join a support group or find others ways to connect with people who support and validate our choice. (For more information on child-free living, see "Resources.")

PATHS TO PARENTHOOD

In becoming parents, we embark on a transformative journey. Welcoming children into our lives brings moments of elation, fear, grief, frustration, and joy. This section offers a brief overview of several different paths to parenthood: conceiving and bearing a child, adopting, or caring for a foster child.

CONCEIVING A CHILD

FERTILITY AWARENESS/CHARTING YOUR MENSTRUAL CYCLE

It's amazing how little we are taught about our own bodies in health class. We get a few basic lessons on birth control, but that's it. Where is the detailed information on predicting the timing of ovulation and learning to monitor your own unique fertility patterns? It certainly wasn't covered in my high school health curriculum.

Once you decide to try to get pregnant, you may be surprised to find that you know much more about preventing pregnancy than about achieving it. Charting menstrual cycles is one useful way to learn about fertility "signals" and optimize your chance of getting pregnant. (To find out more, see Chapter 13, "Sexual Anatomy, Reproduction, and the Menstrual Cycle.")

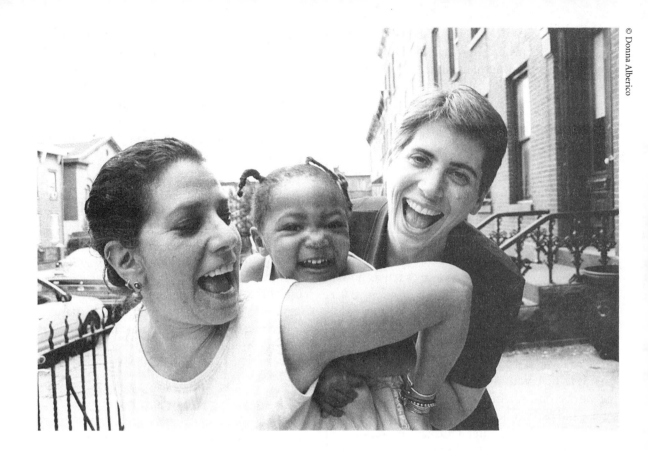

© Donna Alberico

CARING FOR YOURSELF AS YOU TRY TO CONCEIVE

While you are trying to conceive, care for yourself well: Eat healthy food, exercise, and avoid exposure to toxic substances. Many practitioners recommend taking prenatal vitamins (particularly folic acid) and stopping smoking or drinking alcohol. Some of us conceive right away, with no problem at all. Others of us must cope with the emotional roller coaster of trying to conceive: two weeks of waiting to ovulate, followed by two weeks of waiting to see if we are pregnant, then coping with the disappointment if it has not happened, and starting all over again. (For more information on taking care of yourself while trying to conceive, see Chapter 21, "Pregnancy.")

USING DONOR INSEMINATION TO CONCEIVE

As more single women and lesbian couples choose to have children, donor insemination (DI)—inserting from a known or anonymous donor into your vagina or uterus—has risen in popularity. It is estimated that in the United States alone, between 30,000 and 50,000 babies are conceived through DI each year. (For a detailed discussion about deciding whether DI is for you, choosing a donor, and inseminating, see "Donor Insemination" in Chapter 25, "Infertility and Assisted Reproduction.")

ADOPTION

Adopting Katy has been the greatest joy of my life. She is 11 months old now and was born in Kazakhstan. Since [I] adopt[ed], several people have said how lucky Katy is or how brave I am to be doing this alone. In all honesty, though, I am the lucky one to have such a fabulous daughter and courage has nothing to do with it. A mother's love and desire is what made (and continues to make) this family happen. I have never been more sure of anything and am thrilled that she is my daughter.

TYPES OF ADOPTION

- In a *kinship* or *relative* adoption, a child is placed with a relative. These are by far the most common kind of adoptions.

- A *public* adoption involves the placement of a child with adoptive parents by a public agency, such as child welfare or social services department of a state. Public agencies generally place children who have become wards of the state for reasons such as abandonment, abuse, neglect, or the death of one or both parents. Children who are still legally tied to their biological parents are available for *foster parenting,* while children whose legal ties are severed are available for adoption.

- A *private* adoption is facilitated by a private agency, often a charity or social service organization that is licensed or regulated by the state.

- An *independent* adoption is facilitated by someone other than an agency worker, such as a physician, an attorney, or an intermediary.

- Some private and independent adoptions are *open*. Others are *anonymous*. Open adoptions involve some amount of initial and/or ongoing contact between the birth and adoptive families. The adoptive and birth parents agree upon the birth parents' role, future communication, and the degree of openness prior to adoption. With anonymous adoptions, neither the birth parents nor the adopting parents know each other.

- In *domestic* adoptions, children are born and adopted in the United States. All domestic adoptions are governed by state laws, both in the state where the adopting parents reside and the state where the child is born.

- *International* adoptions are adoptions of children from a foreign country. They are subject to each country's requirements and regulations, as well as to U.S. Citizenship and Immigration Services laws. Usually, but not always, the adoptive parents adopt the child in the court of the country of that child's birth before being allowed to bring the child to the U.S. (For information to help you sort through the many complex rules and regulations surrounding adoption, see "Resources.")

The time between finding out you cannot or should not have a pregnancy and deciding to follow a new dream is the saddest time. In life there are no guarantees, but if you go with an adoption agency with a good reputation, you can be almost certain you will become a parent. And once you make the decision, it is as if a rainbow appears. We call this our paper pregnancy, a child born in our hearts. Instead of running out of stores at the sight of a pregnant woman and avoiding the baby-product aisle at the market, I smile, hold my head up. I am on cloud nine.

Adoption is another way to create or extend families. You may be unable to conceive, or you may have a medical condition that would make pregnancy and childbirth unsafe. Some women prefer not to become pregnant. Others choose adoption over giving birth out of concern for children who need loving families.

Adoption entails logistical, emotional, and financial challenges. While finances, the requirements of adoption agencies and foreign countries, or the availability of children to adopt often limit our options, learning about the various choices and being honest about whatever limits exist will help create a situation that will work for everyone.

My partner and I were present at the birth of our son, which we considered an incredible gift, after years of infertility and a long adoption process. After a difficult birth, I was allowed to carry the baby to the neonatal unit, where he was measured and tested. It was in this intense moment that we learned that our birthmom had tested positive to drugs, so they were going to test our baby too. I experienced an amazing tug of mixed emotions— I was furious at the birth mother for lying to us about her drug use and worried that the baby would have some problem that we weren't prepared to take on. . . . [The baby] also looked terrible—so huge and puffy from the birth mom's

untreated diabetes—and I worried whether I could love this ugly baby. Over the next few days, as it became clearer that the birthmom was going to follow through with the adoption, I still freaked out about my mixed feelings about the baby. Ironically, my partner, who had always been more ambivalent about being a mother, was the one who immediately and fiercely bonded with the baby. My feelings gradually resolved themselves, as I spent time holding and talking to this little person in the NICU [neonatal intensive care unit], where he spent six days. He began to lose his puffiness and turned into MY beautiful baby.

There are a number of things to think about in planning to adopt. How would you feel about having and maintaining contact with your child's birth parents? Would you want to have a child who resembles you as much as possible, or do you want a child of another race or ethnicity? Do you want to adopt a newborn baby or an older infant or child? Are you willing to welcome a child with medical or emotional challenges? Are you open to parenting any child you are able to adopt? How will you finance the adoption?

It may be helpful to find a community of other adoptive and prospective adoptive parents. They can answer questions, direct you to resources, and support you in the joys and frustrations of the adoption process. These groups are available in many cities, and many adoption websites offer online support.

FINANCES

Adoption is often an expensive process. To help offset the cost, the federal government provides a tax credit of up to $10,160 per child to adoptive families; many states also provide tax credits or deductions. The military provides some reimbursement for adoptive families. Low- or no-interest loans are also available for adoptive families, and many employers offer adoption

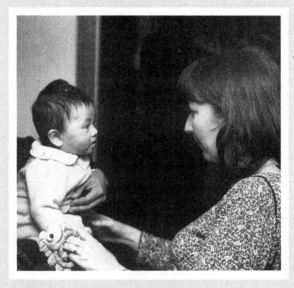

"THEY JUST HANDED JESSICA TO ME"

RACHEL GINGOLD

It was an unbelievable moment. All these American parents with cameras and all these Chinese caretakers in a meeting room in a hotel in Fujian Province, China. The babies were crying and the parents were crying. It was noisy and emotional and overwhelming. And then somebody came out, called our names, and they just handed Jessica to me. I thought, Oh my gosh, what am I getting into? Here's my baby, right here in my arms. Now I'm this child's mother. Even though it took a year of paperwork and planning, it all seemed a big surprise. I worried: Will she take to us? Will she scream a lot? Is she healthy?

Then I carried her to meet her dad and her new sister (who was also adopted from China), and Jessica looked a little shell-shocked, too. She cried a little the first couple of days and was latched on to me like Velcro, but once she realized we were going to take care of her, she warmed up to us all.

China has a preference for sons, and people can have only one or two children. Since there is no policy to allow people to put children up for adoption, they have to abandon them. They have too many abandoned baby girls. It's a heart-wrenching problem.

We are all interested in Chinese culture. We are hoping to take Mandarin classes and, when they are older, take them back to China. People are curious and have questions because we don't look like all other families, but we are fortunate to live in a cross-cultural community.

ETHICAL CONSIDERATIONS IN ADOPTION

The process of adoption can force us to confront complex ethical questions rarely considered by those who produce biologically related children. Why are home studies and other measures of parental fitness reserved only for adoption? How much control should we be allowed to exercise over the selection of a child? How can we be aware of, avoid, and work to prevent situations that might exploit or coerce birth mothers? How do we balance the potentially different needs of the child, birth parents, and adoptive parents regarding the degree of openness in adoption? Are those of us who live in wealthier nations "entitled" to raise children left homeless in other parts of the world by poverty or social stigma? How can we help our children deal with the racial, cultural, and identity issues they may face?

(For a further discussion of the political, social, racial, and economic questions raised by adoption, see "Ethical Issues in Adoption" [W40] on the companion website, www.ourbodiesourselves.org.)

benefits. (For information about financing an adoption and locating employers who provide adoption benefits, see "Resources.")

EMOTIONS AND RELATIONSHIPS

The process of adoption can be an emotional journey. It is exciting to welcome our children, but there are also many times when we experience frustration, sadness, powerlessness, anxiety, and impatience. If you have been infertile, you may discover that adoption doesn't "fix" that experience. You may be elated at finally becoming a mother, yet still grieve for the pregnancies you will never have.

If you come to adoption purely through choice or preference rather than infertility, your primary struggles are likely to be logistical. The time it takes to find your child can feel as though it will never end, and it is difficult to plan ahead.

Women entering parenthood through adoption need as much support as women who are pregnant. The logistics of your life, your sense of identity, and your relationships will be changed as much as—or more than—if you were planning a pregnancy. In addition, you face challenges unique to adoption. You won't *look* pregnant, so you can choose not to discuss the ins and outs, ups and downs of your adoption process. On the other hand, others may discount your experience because they can't see that you are in the process of becoming a parent. In addition, some people still have misunderstandings and negative judgments about adoption.

FAMILIES AND PARENTS NEED A LOT OF SUPPORT

Parenting is hard work, both emotionally and physically. Our technological, fast-paced society does not serve the complex needs of parents and children, nor does it truly support and value caregiving within families. In order for women to balance the demands of family and work, we need a public commitment to family policies that make women's and children's needs a priority.

The Family and Medical Leave Act of 1993 mandates that companies with fifty or more employees allow workers to return to employment at the same level following a caregiving leave. Yet most women work in smaller companies; furthermore, mandated leaves for childbearing are unpaid. Some changes are in progress. Beginning in July 2004, California extended the federal Family and Medical Leave Act to enable

LESBIAN FAMILIES AND ADOPTION

While increasing numbers of lesbian, bisexual, and transgender women are choosing to adopt children, many of us still encounter discrimination as we expand our families. Although some adoption agencies will work with openly lesbian singles and couples, most of us are forced to adopt simply as "single, straight" mothers. However, once the adoption has taken place, several states allow a same-sex partner to be legally recognized as a parent through a second-parent adoption.

The Human Rights Campaign (HRC) website (www.hrc.org) has extensive material on the specific decisions and legal issues facing lesbians and bisexual women exploring adoption. HRC also maintains a database to help you search for LGBT-friendly adoption agencies.

employees of any size company in California to receive partial pay for up to six weeks (during any twelve-month period) to care for a new child or a sick family member. We need more policies like this throughout the country. All workers need paid parental leaves with job protection for parents; gradual return to work with no penalties; affordable quality day care; reentry programs at the same level for parents who take time off to raise children; parental leave for sick children; and part-time, flex-time, flex-place work, and job-sharing options.

Child rearing is important and valuable work that deserves social and economic support. Whether or not we individually choose to have children, we all have a shared stake in the next generation and must work together to advance better family policies.

NOTE

1. 2000 U.S. Census.

CHAPTER 18 ■ ■ ■ ■ ■ ■ ■ ■ ■ ■ ■ ■ ■ ■ ■ ■

As women, we have the right to make decisions regarding our bodies. These include decisions regarding the ability to control if and when we have children, regardless of whether we want several children or no children at all. Birth control is fundamental to our ability to have autonomy in our lives, and it helps us to understand our bodies and to enjoy our sexuality safely with men.

Today we have more choices than ever before. Advances in family planning technology have led to an increasing number of options to control our fertility. As new methods are developed, more women find an option that better meets our individual needs. The advent of the Pill, probably more than any other event, has enabled women the world over to prevent or delay pregnancy and, in doing so, to complete our educations, choose our careers, and create more egalitarian relationships.* The more recent development of emergency contraception has allowed women who have had unprotected intercourse to prevent pregnancy, an option that should be more readily available.

Most of us want contraceptives that are effective, have no harmful effects, involve no muss or fuss, protect us against sexually transmitted infections—including HIV/AIDS—and can be used before sexual intercourse. The perfect method does not exist, but we can choose the best available method to suit our needs, if we have unbiased, factual, and up-to-date information about all options. This chapter addresses questions and concerns that many women share—such as how to choose a method of birth control, how well each method works, safety concerns, and men's roles—along with a detailed description of each method.

REPRODUCTIVE RIGHTS NOT GUARANTEED

Our reproductive rights and our ability to decide if and when to become pregnant and bear children are not guaranteed. Conservative forces will always respond to advances in women's independence by reinforcing traditional gender norms. We need only study our history to know that we must be prepared for a prolonged battle.

If we look back over the past 150 years, we will see that there have been three significant periods of feminist activity, each followed by a conservative backlash:†

* Despite the advances in contraception over the past fifty years, an estimated 150 million women worldwide do not have access to appropriate birth control. For more information, see "Global Access to Birth Control" (W41) on the companion website, www.ourbodiesourselves.org.

† For more information, see "A Brief History of Birth Control" (W42) on the companion website, www.ourbodiesourselves.org.

- In the 1870s, the first major defense of birth control—called voluntary motherhood—emphasized the dignity of motherhood and women's right to refuse sexual activity. Branding birth control "race suicide," conservative opposition succeeded in criminalizing abortion and categorizing birth control as obscene.
- In the 1930s, Margaret Sanger inspired a resurgence of interest in birth control, fighting to make information and services available to every woman. At the same time, a broad-based feminist movement for legalization of birth control defended the separation of sex from reproduction and supported women's sexual freedom. By midcentury, the "birth control movement" had again died down, and a general conservative trend following World War II put women back into the home and fostered the "baby boom."
- By the 1960s, the new rise in feminism had defined birth control as a reproductive right and motherhood as a choice, leading the way to expanded access to contraception and the legalization of abortion. Since then, conservative forces have worked to deny access to reproductive health information and services and to recriminalize abortion. By defining both birth control and abortion as against religious teachings, they have further eroded women's access to reproductive health care.[1]

The conflict is focused on fundamental sexual, family, and gender issues. Thirty years after *Roe* v. *Wade* established a constitutional right to safe, legal abortion in the United States, our rights are once more at risk. So as not to repeat our history, we must remain organized, articulate, and vocal. The fight for women's true equality is still ahead of us.

NEW RESEARCH

Today there is more emphasis on developing methods that not only prevent pregnancy but also prevent sexually transmitted infections (STIs) and infertility. Examples of this new focus include new vaginal microbicides and human monoclonal antibodies (mAbs) that prevent both pregnancy and STIs, including HIV/AIDS. Noncontraceptive vaginal microbicides would allow women to conceive while preventing STIs, but they are still under development. (For more information on microbicides and other methods of preventing transmission of STIs, see Chapter 14, "Safer Sex.")

SOME OBSTACLES TO GETTING BIRTH CONTROL AND USING IT WELL

BIRTH CONTROL AND SEX INFORMATION

Negative attitudes toward pleasure and desire, and shame about sex, stop many of us from seeking information. On a wider scale, these same attitudes keep sex information from being distributed freely in schools and community organizations. Laws, medical practices, and public school policies continue to prevent us from getting the information and services we need, especially when we are young—in spite of many studies showing that giving birth control information to teenagers does not make them more likely to have sex.

WOMEN AND BIRTH CONTROL

Using birth control does not mean we always want intercourse. We need to be assertive about our desires and let our partners know that sex should be a mutual decision, not an obligation. Sometimes the fact that we are using protection makes it harder for us to say no when we really don't want to have sex.

Many of us have found that we resist using birth control. Sometimes this is because of social and political factors, such as poor sex education, a double standard concerning sex, or inequalities between women and men. For instance:

- We are embarrassed by, ashamed of, or confused about our own sexuality. We cannot admit we might have or are having intercourse, because we feel (or someone told us) it is wrong.
- We are unrealistically romantic about sex: Sex has to be passionate and spontaneous, and birth control seems too premeditated, clinical, and messy.
- We hesitate to "inconvenience" our partner. This fear of displeasing him is a measure of the inequality and our lack of control in our relationship.
- We think, It can't happen to me. I won't get pregnant.
- We hesitate to find a health care provider, who may turn out to be hurried, impersonal, or even hostile. If we are young or unmarried, we may fear moralizing and disapproval. We may be afraid the provider will tell our parents.
- We don't recognize our deep dissatisfaction with the method we are using, but we begin to use it haphazardly.
- We feel tempted to become pregnant just to prove to ourselves that we are fertile, or to try to improve a shaky relationship; or we want a baby so that we will have someone to care for.

WHAT CAN WE DO?

Each of us will have different opportunities for action, depending on where we live, how old we are, what resources are available to us, and how much political power we have. But all of us can learn for ourselves and teach one another about the available methods. By speaking openly, and by carefully comparing experiences and knowledge, we can guide one another to workable methods and good practitioners. We can recognize when a practitioner is not thorough enough in examinations or explanations and encourage one another to ask for the attention we need. By talking together, we can also gain an understanding of our more subtle resistances to using birth control. We can begin the process of talking with our male partners about birth control, encouraging them to share the responsibility with us. We can join together across state and national boundaries to insist that legislatures, courts, high schools, churches, parents, doctors, research projects, clinics, and drug companies change their practices and attitudes so that we can enjoy our sexuality without becoming pregnant. We can create self-help clinics and other alternative health care institutions where our needs for information, discussion, and personal support in the difficult choice of birth control will be better met. We can use the good clinics that do exist. We can campaign for decent housing, jobs, and child care for all, so that we can choose birth control freely instead of being forced to use it by our circumstances. We can insist that birth control methods meet the needs of all women, including women of color, women living in poverty, women with disabilities, and women in developing countries. Whatever we choose to do, we can act together.

BIRTH CONTROL—
WHO PROTECTS
OUR INTERESTS?

Women usually assume that when a birth control method is available through a doctor's office, a medical clinic, or a drugstore, its safety and efficacy have been proved. In the U.S., the

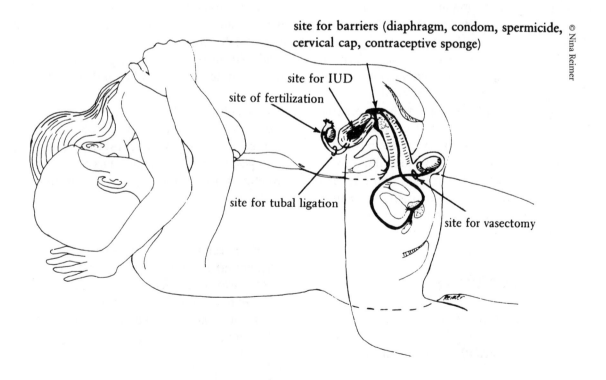

site for barriers (diaphragm, condom, spermicide, cervical cap, contraceptive sponge)

© Nina Reimer

site for IUD

site of fertilization

site for tubal ligation

site for vasectomy

Food and Drug Administration (FDA) regulates contraceptive devices and substances, deciding which ones are still experimental and which are legal to prescribe and sell. All birth control methods must be tested first on animals and then on women before the FDA approves them for marketing.

However, the recent history of women's contraceptives has shown that long-term complications and negative effects are rarely thoroughly understood at the point when methods are approved. Fulfilling FDA requirements takes up to ten years of work before a drug is marketed, but it takes twenty years or more for some complications to become apparent, especially those that may be serious but rare.

When we seek trustworthy advice about birth control in order to make careful choices, we often find conflicting information and false reassurances. Much information about contraceptives comes from drug companies and may be biased accordingly. Health care providers may be influenced by drug company literature and sales personnel and thus may recommend a method that is not the best one for us.

A number of other factors can undermine our choices, including substandard health services and, in some countries, the need to obtain a husband's consent before getting birth control. Thus, many of us find ourselves using inadequate methods or those that are risky for our individual situation. Some of us, unwilling to go through the hassle, end up using nothing at all. A method that sits in a drawer or that isn't used properly is not effective, no matter how technically sophisticated it is.

MEN AND BIRTH CONTROL

At first I was afraid to talk about birth control with my partner. I didn't think he would be interested. As we discussed it, however, I realized that he wanted to prevent unplanned pregnancy just as much as I did. We talked about ways that he could participate in the birth control process, and afterward we both felt more confident in our mutual choices.

It's really not discussed until the situation arises. It's kind of a non-issue because it's assumed that a condom will be used. Eventually, if you keep seeing each other, a deeper conversation takes place.

Birth control is not just a woman's issue. Men benefit from the use of birth control in many ways, including being able to decide when and if they will father a child, and being able to protect themselves and their partners from sexually transmitted infections. By leaving the decision about contraception up to the woman, the man not only creates an unfair burden for her, he also forfeits his ability to prevent an unplanned pregnancy. By failing to take responsibility for contraception, too many men become fathers before they are able or willing. By sharing decisions about birth control, a man increases the likelihood that his partner will be protected; he also shows that he cares about her and about her future.

Our culture and media rarely address male responsibility in the prevention of STIs and unplanned pregnancies. The prevailing societal messages about contraception target women but sometimes neglect the impact that unprotected

Many European countries are much more accepting of condom use and encourage both sexes to participate in reproductive health decisions. They boast much lower rates of unplanned pregnancies, STIs, and abortions.

For more information on male methods, see sections on condoms, p. 333; vasectomy, p. 367; withdrawal, p. 373; periodic abstinence, p. 368; and new methods, p. 368.

sex can have on men. Using condoms is the easiest way for men to get involved in the birth control process, but they must be willing to do so. Some men are not interested in using condoms because they have received messages that say it is unmasculine, or they have a preconceived notion that sex is not as good with condoms. These attitudes reveal both a lack of education and a lack of respect for women; they also free men from taking responsibility for their actions.

Taking responsibility for birth control can be a big task. Having a conversation with your male partner about birth control is a good way to learn of his interest in participating in the process. A man can share responsibility for birth control in many ways. In addition to buying and using condoms, men can help pay for doctors' visits and drugstore bills, remind us to take the Pill each day, help to put in the diaphragm or insert the foam, and check to see if supplies are running low. If you and your partner are sure that you will not ever want to have children, a vasectomy may be a suitable option (see p. 367). The future holds even more opportunities for men to participate actively in birth control, as several new hormonal methods for men are currently being developed and implemented around the world.

Regardless of a man's level of involvement, it is important that women's needs be met. Our sexual partners should be willing to listen to our concerns, and even if they won't participate directly, they should understand our need to protect ourselves from unplanned pregnancy and from contracting sexually transmitted infections.

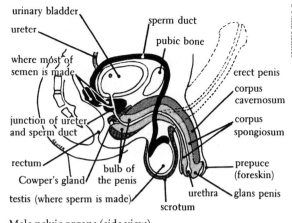

© Nina Reimer

Male pelvic organs (side view)

HOW PREGNANCY HAPPENS*

Pregnancy depends on a healthy egg, healthy sperm, and favorable cervical fluid. For birth control to work, the process of conception must be stopped at some point along the way (see illustration on p. 325). During sexual intercourse, sperm are ejaculated through the man's penis into the woman's vagina. In the presence of certain cervical fluid conditions, some of the sperm move, guided by the cervical fluid, through the cervical opening (the os), through the woman's uterus, and into the fallopian tubes. It is also possible for sperm to be deposited in or near the lips around the vagina during ejaculation, even without intercourse, and to travel up the vagina from there. If the sperm encounter an egg in the outer third of the fallopian tube, one may join with the egg. The process of an egg and a sperm uniting is called *conception* or *fertilization*. The fertilized egg takes several days to travel down the fallopian tube to the uterus, where, after one and a half to two days, it implants in the uterine lining and develops over the course of the next nine months.

* For more details, see Chapter 13, "Sexual Anatomy, Reproduction, and the Menstrual Cycle."

CHOOSING A METHOD OF BIRTH CONTROL*

DIFFERENCES AMONG METHODS

Because there is no one perfect method, our "choice" of a contraceptive will be something of a compromise. Safety and effectiveness are probably the most important factors. Convenience is also important to some. Those of us with medical problems, chronic illnesses, or disabilities may have additional needs to consider when seeking usable, effective contraceptives.

Birth control methods differ in how much protection they give against STIs (e.g., gonorrhea, herpes, chlamydia, and HIV) and pelvic inflammatory disease (PID). In general, barrier methods, especially male and female condoms, provide good protection against most reproductive tract infections. Inconsistent or incorrect use reduces the protection given by barrier methods.

The Pill provides some protection against PID; it may increase the risk of chlamydia. Its effect on other STIs remains uncertain. The IUD offers no protection against STIs. In women at risk for STIs, use of the IUD increases the chance of developing PID. (For more information on STIs and PID, see Chapter 15, "Sexually Transmitted Infections," and Chapter 28, "Unique to Women.")

HOW TO DECIDE WHAT'S RIGHT FOR YOU: PERSONAL CONSIDERATIONS

Recent developments have expanded the available birth control choices. Although health care providers and our partners, friends, or family members can offer advice about which methods might work best for us, the choice is ultimately ours. Factors we consider include: safety and effectiveness; how much we are willing to risk an

* See summary chart of types of birth control on p. 378.

unintended pregnancy; the type of relationship we are in; and the amount of money we can spend on birth control.

A FEW QUESTIONS TO CONSIDER AS YOU MAKE YOUR DECISION

1. Am I ready to have or interested in having sexual intercourse at this time in my life? So often we assume that a relationship must include intercourse, yet it need not.
2. How does this contraceptive method fit into my life and, more importantly, into my sexual lifestyle?
3. How involved will my partner be in this decision and with the use of the method?
4. How safe is this method for me and/or my partner? Do I have any medical or other reasons to not use the method?
5. What are the potential side effects of this method? Are these acceptable to me?
6. How effective is this method in preventing pregnancy? What would be the consequences in my life if I got pregnant?
7. How effective is this method in preventing sexually transmitted infections?
8. What are the noncontraceptive benefits to this method? Can it reduce menstrual cramps or help me in another way?
9. How much will this method cost?
10. What are my plans for a family? Am I using contraception to delay pregnancy? Am I done with childbearing? Am I choosing never to have children? *

* Adapted with permission from Planned Parenthood of Northern New England, "Birth Control," accessed at www.ppnne.org/site/PageServer?pagename-GTF#bc on October 28, 2004.

For some women, getting pregnant is absolutely unacceptable; for others, the timing may not be ideal, but the pregnancy may be desired. There is no method that is 100 percent effective in preventing pregnancy, so if you know that getting pregnant is not an option for you, you may want to abstain from sexual activity. If you choose to be sexually active, the effectiveness rating of each method may be your most important consideration. But keep in mind that effectiveness for most methods is connected to how consistently and correctly the method is used.

Of the methods currently available, IUDs are about as effective as sterilization, which is the most effective way to prevent pregnancy; hormonal methods are less effective. Many women who use IUDs or hormonal methods also use a condom or other barrier as an added safeguard against both unplanned pregnancy and sexually transmitted infections. You may want to try several different methods to determine which you most prefer.

SIDE EFFECTS AND CONTRAINDICATIONS

Sometimes the difference between side effects and contraindications is confusing. Side effects are the changes that can occur in our bodies as the result of using a particular medication or device. Side effects can be mild or severe and can vary greatly from person to person. For example, the side effects of hormonal methods may include mood changes, breast tenderness, and mild headaches. A side effect of some barrier methods may be an increase in urinary tract infections. Often it is the minor side effects that influence our choices in contraception.

Contraindications are the physical conditions or circumstances that put some people at risk of danger from using a particular medication or device. For example, it is *contraindicated* for a woman who is over age thirty-five and smokes to use birth control pills, because they will considerably increase her risk of stroke. As another example, having current breast cancer is a contraindication to using any hormonal method. A contraindication means that by using that particular method of birth control you may increase your risk of a serious problem. (For more information on how chronic diseases and disabilities can affect birth control options, see "Sex and Disability" chart, p. 218.)

TEENS AND BIRTH CONTROL

Teens have special needs for safe, reliable, and easy-to-use methods of birth control. Many teens do not plan in advance for sex; some have more than one partner. The lack of thoughtful discussion and information about healthy sexuality in our culture leaves teens vulnerable to high rates of early pregnancy and STIs.

Without an opportunity for open discussion with parents or other trusted adults, teens may have trouble obtaining family planning services. For example, lack of transportation, money, and/or health insurance may be obstacles to getting services. Although many teens think that parents must give consent in order for teens to obtain contraceptives, this is not true. (However, parental notification and consent laws for abortion vary by state. For information on the laws in your state, check out www.positive.org/Resources/consent.html.)

DUAL PROTECTION

Dual protection is defined as the simultaneous prevention of a sexually transmitted infection and unwanted pregnancy. This can be accomplished by the consistent use of condoms alone or by the simultaneous use of two methods at once, one of which must be condoms. Avoiding penetrative sex (penis-in-vagina intercourse) is

FOR TEENS

If you are a teenager, you may want to wait to start having sex (see "Abstinence," p. 368). If you have already made the decision to be sexually active and don't want to get pregnant, you need a safe and effective birth control method. Reading this book and, if possible, taking a comprehensive sex education course will help you to make healthy choices about if, when, and with whom to have sex, as well as how to protect yourself when you do decide to be sexually active.

If you have a family planning center nearby, you can go there and speak with a medical provider. Most family planning clinics, such as Planned Parenthood, will provide free or reduced-cost services and supplies to teenagers. They are also completely confidential. That means no one else will know you have an appointment or are using birth control.

If you do not know where there is a clinic, you can visit www.plannedparenthood.org/ZIP.HTM or www.teenwire.com (go to "Clinic Connections"), or call 1-800-230-PLAN.

Regardless of your age, you can also buy safe and reliable methods, such as condoms and contraceptive foam, in any drugstore. Condoms are sometimes given out in teen centers, clinics, or AIDS prevention programs. Whatever method of birth control you decide to use, always remember to protect yourself from STIs as well (see below).

The only way to be completely safe from STIs is either to abstain from sex or to be in a mutually monogamous relationship with a partner who has never had any other partners. If this is not your situation, there is some risk of either getting or giving an STI.

While injectable and implantable hormones, the Pill, IUDs, and sterilization are highly effective for pregnancy prevention, they do not provide protection against STIs, including HIV/AIDS.

Using two methods simultaneously can also increase the effectiveness of your birth control method. For example, if you are using both the Pill and condoms correctly and consistently, your method is as close to 100 percent effective in preventing pregnancy as you can get without using a permanent method, such as sterilization.

Many couples begin by using condoms, but after a period of time, when they feel that they trust each other, they stop using condoms. Unfortunately, trust has little to do with whether a partner is already carrying an STI. If either you or your partner has ever been with another partner, there is a possibility that one of you may be carrying an STI. It is best to continue to use dual protection until you have both been tested. (For information on testing, see Chapter 15, "Sexually Transmitted Infections.")

WOMAN-CONTROLLED METHODS FOR BIRTH CONTROL AND STI/HIV PREVENTION

When used correctly and consistently, condoms offer the best protection against STIs. However, some men and women are unwilling to use condoms, and even when a woman wants to use condoms, she may not be able to negotiate their use with her partner. For these reasons, there is

another means of achieving dual protection. So, too, is being in a monogamous relationship in which both partners are free of STIs and at least one partner is using effective contraception.

• *Teenagers who participate in sex education classes are more likely to have sex.*

Myth. Many studies have shown that providing birth control information to teenagers does not make them more likely to have sex. When teenagers do have sex, knowledge about condoms, hormonal contraceptives, and other forms of birth control helps prevent pregnancy and STIs.

• *If I miss a period while I'm on the Pill, it doesn't necessarily mean I'm pregnant.*

Reality. It is not uncommon to miss a period while on birth control pills. If you miss one period and you took all of your pills correctly and you don't have any signs of pregnancy, the chances of pregnancy are very low. If you often miss periods and are taking the Pill correctly, talk to your provider about whether you should change to a different pill.

growing interest in woman-controlled methods that prevent STIs.

The female condom, diaphragm, and other cervical barriers such as the cap and the sponge physically cover the cervix. Research suggests that protecting the cervix can reduce the risk of acquiring HIV and some other STIs, such as gonorrhea and chlamydia. Some of these methods, however, are less likely to provide protection from infections such as human papillomavirus (HPV) and herpes. Cervical barrier methods such as the diaphragm can be used without the knowledge or cooperation of the man. All of these methods can be inserted hours before sex and therefore need not interfere with intimacy.

For more information on protection from STIs, see Chapter 14, "Safer Sex."

EFFECTIVENESS AND SAFETY

WILL IT WORK?: EFFECTIVENESS OF BIRTH CONTROL METHODS

One of the first things we need to know about a contraceptive method is how well it works to prevent pregnancy—though choosing a method will involve consideration of many factors.

A method's effectiveness is based on the probability of unintended pregnancy in the first year of use. Effectiveness is usually presented with two numbers. The first reflects the effectiveness of the method when it is used perfectly, and the second is based on the effectiveness of the method with typical use. For example, the birth control pill has a "perfect use" effectiveness rating of 99.9 percent, which means that for every hundred women using the Pill for one year, fewer than one will become pregnant. In typical use, however—for example, when we forget to take a pill or don't get supplies in time—the effectiveness is only about 95 percent, or five women in a hundred becoming pregnant. (For information on perfect versus typical effectiveness of various methods, see p. 378.)

How well a method will work for you will be determined by a number of factors:

1. The expected effectiveness of your chosen method
2. How consistently and correctly you use your chosen method
3. How often you have intercourse (a woman who has sex every day is at greater risk of pregnancy than a woman who has sex only occasionally)
4. Your age and fertility (younger women are more likely to become pregnant from

a single act of intercourse than older women)

TO LOWER YOUR RISK OF UNPLANNED PREGNANCY

1. Be sure you have complete and correct information about the use of your method.
2. Use your method consistently and correctly.
3. Use two methods at once (dual protection) to lower your risk of pregnancy dramatically. If one of the two methods is a condom, this also provides protection from sexually transmitted infections.
4. Have an emergency method (see p. 374) available for backup if your method fails or if you have unprotected intercourse.
5. If your greatest concern is long-term protection, use a method such as long-acting injections, implants, or an IUD.

BUT IS IT SAFE?

"I heard that the Pill is dangerous, but my partner won't use condoms."

"Is it true that the IUD causes infertility?"

Birth control methods that are currently available have been tested for safety as well as effectiveness. If you are a healthy woman without preexisting health problems, contraception poses few serious risks. If you have a serious health problem, such as severe migraine headaches or hypertension, some methods can be unsafe for you. For most women, however, negative experiences are generally due to inconvenient side effects, such as breakthrough bleeding (spotting between expected menstrual periods), rather than harmful consequences. Perhaps the greatest obstacle to women's use of contraception is the fear of possible negative health effects from the use of hormonal methods or the IUD. Some women hear alarming stories from friends, trusted adults, or the media. These stories may be based on half-truths, isolated cases, or old information, so it is important to seek out accurate and balanced information before making a birth control decision.

GETTING PREGNANT LATER

You may have heard that using some methods of birth control can impair your ability to become pregnant even after you stop taking the contraceptive. Depo-Provera, for example, may continue to prevent pregnancy for up to eighteen months after the last injection, though it has no proven long-term effects on fertility. (Note: Do not rely on Depo to last longer than the prescribed three months.) Except for sterilization, none of the methods described here has proven effects on future fertility.

Sexually transmitted infections (STIs) are the cause of much infertility. Though methods such as the Pill or the IUD are very effective at preventing pregnancy, they do not protect against STIs. To avoid contracting an STI and to protect your health and future fertility, it is important to use condoms either alone or with another appropriate method.

BARRIER METHODS*

Barrier methods prevent pregnancy by blocking sperm from reaching the cervix. The effectiveness of barrier methods varies a great deal depending on how correctly and consistently they are used. Barrier methods usually have fewer side effects than many other methods, and most barrier methods, especially condoms, can help

---

* Some of the following information about birth control methods has been adapted with permission from the Feminist Women's Health Center's website, www.fwhc.org.

prevent the spread of sexually transmitted infections (STIs), including HIV/AIDS.

MALE CONDOMS (RUBBERS, PROPHYLACTICS, OR SAFES)

The condom is typically a latex sheath that fits over the erect penis and prevents sperm from entering a woman's body. It is sold rolled up and stored in a foil packet. For those who are sexually active, condoms offer the best protection against sexually transmitted infections (STIs); only abstinence protects you better. They are also the sole barrier method that has been proved to protect against HIV transmission during vaginal and anal intercourse. Condoms come in many different sizes, colors, and textures.

While most condoms sold are made of latex rubber, some are made from a thin polyurethane (plastic) material (sold under the brand name Avanti). They, too, protect against STIs; they may provide more sensation for men who have difficulty maintaining an erection when using latex condoms; and they can be used by people sensitive to latex. However they break more often than latex condoms.[2] Natural "skin" condoms (made of lamb membrane) protect against pregnancy but contain pores (microscopic holes) that are large enough to let viruses pass through (but not large enough to let sperm pass through). Therefore, skin condoms do not protect against some STIs, including HIV.

Condoms are a good way for the man to share in birth control. In a shorter-term relationship, when you may not know whether you will be having intercourse, condoms can be very convenient. Although some men carry condoms, you should not expect the man to have a condom with him. Protect yourself by carrying condoms with you.

EFFECTIVENESS

Pregnancy Prevention

The contraceptive effectiveness of condoms varies from 87 percent to 98 percent depending on how well they are used. If used correctly *for every act of intercourse,* condoms are 98 percent effective at preventing pregnancy. This means that if a hundred couples use condoms correctly every time they have intercourse for a year, two women will become pregnant. When user error (such as not putting the condom on properly) is included, condoms have a contraceptive effectiveness closer to 87 percent. In cases of typical use, for a hundred women using condoms for a year, between four and fifteen women will become pregnant.

Some condoms (spermicidal condoms or spermicidally lubricated condoms) contain spermicide (a chemical that kills sperm). The concentration of spermicide is so low in these varieties, however, that they appear to be no more effective than condoms that don't contain spermicide (for more information on spermicide nonoxynol-9 and increased risk for HIV and other STIs, see p. 269). Combine condoms with a spermicidal foam, cream, or jelly in your vagina for close to 100 percent protection if the

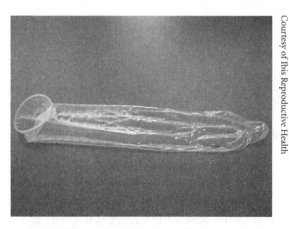

Male condom

condom is used correctly at every act of intercourse.

Sexually Transmitted Infection (STI) Prevention

The effectiveness of condoms in preventing STI transmission, including HIV, chlamydia, gonorrhea, and trichomonas, is similar to the effectiveness rate for pregnancy protection, or 98 percent with perfect use and 86 percent with typical use. For STIs that cause genital ulcers, such as syphilis, herpes, and chancroid, or for human papillomavirus (HPV)—genital warts—the protection is decreased because the condom may not cover all of the areas that could transmit the infection. Nevertheless, condoms provide the best protection currently available against these diseases.

ADVANTAGES

- Do not require advance planning, clinic visits, or a prescription
- Inexpensive and readily available
- Can be carried easily and discreetly by men and women
- Best means currently available of protection against STIs, including HIV
- By preventing STIs, condoms can protect fertility
- Allow men to participate in preventing pregnancy and infections
- May help prevent cervical cancer (see Chapter 15, "Sexually Transmitted Infections")
- May decrease premature ejaculation and prolong intercourse
- Catch the semen, so nothing drips from the vagina after intercourse
- Have minimal side effects
- Do not affect menstrual cycles

DISADVANTAGES

- May disrupt spontaneity during sex
- Can reduce sensitivity
- Some men cannot maintain an erection when using a condom
- Some men and women can develop an allergy or sensitivity to latex (in this case, polyurethane condoms may be used)

Though condoms do have disadvantages, many of them can be overcome with practice and experience or by switching to a different brand or type of condom.

HOW TO USE

Condom use can be fun for both partners when it is made part of sex. Discuss condom use *before* you have sex. Have more than one condom on hand in case one is torn or damaged before use or is put on incorrectly; if you have repeat intercourse; or if you change from anal to vaginal sex. Use a condom *before you have any genital contact*—long before ejaculation, the male may discharge a few drops of fluid. This preejaculatory fluid can contain sperm and may also expose you to HIV or other infectious organisms.

1. Carefully open the packet.

2. Unroll the condom onto the erect penis before the penis comes in contact with the partner's mouth, anus, or vagina. If the penis is uncircumcised, pull back the foreskin before putting on the condom.

3. Unroll the condom a short distance to be sure it is being unrolled in the right direction. Then squeeze the tip of the condom and unroll it down to the base of the erect penis. The loose end will hold the man's sperm. If you do not

leave space for the sperm, the condom is more likely to break.

4. Adequate lubrication is important. If you do not use a lubricated condom, use a water-based lubricant to prevent tearing, such as K-Y jelly or Astroglide. Never use Vaseline or other oil-based lubricants such as massage oils, suntan lotion, hand cream, or baby oil, which can weaken the rubber (though with polyurethane condoms, any type of lubricant can be used). Saliva is always an option, but it may increase your chances of developing a yeast infection. Apply the lubricant after the condom is on the penis.

5. Soon after ejaculation, the man must carefully withdraw his penis while it is still erect. Hold the condom firmly against the base of the penis to prevent leakage or slipping.

6. Check the condom for visible damage, such as holes or tears, then wrap it in tissue and discard. Do not flush condoms down the toilet, as this can cause plumbing problems.

7. **If the condom breaks, falls off, or was not used,** discuss the possibility of pregnancy or infection with your partner. Emergency contraception can be used to prevent pregnancy (see section on ECs, p. 374). To reduce the risk of STIs, gently wash the penis, vulva, anus, and adjacent area with soap and water immediately after intercourse. It should be stressed that washing *may* reduce the risk—it is *not a reliable method of preventing STIs.*

WHERE TO GET CONDOMS

You can find condoms in drugstores, supermarkets, on the Internet, at family planning agencies, in vending machines, and on many college campuses. Many family planning agencies, youth-serving organizations, and AIDS prevention programs make condoms available free of charge. The cost varies, depending on the brand and the store, so shop around. Polyurethane and skin condoms are more expensive than latex condoms.

MANAGING PROBLEMS

Allergic or Sensitive Reactions

If you or your partner have a reaction to using a condom, it may be a reaction to the lubricant, spermicide, or perfumes used on the condom. First try using a different brand, or a condom without lubrication. If you still have a reaction but it is not severe, try switching to polyurethane condoms; or if you need protection only against pregnancy, you can try natural skin condoms.

If you or your partner experience a severe reaction including severe swelling or wheezing, you should see a health care provider for follow-up.

Decreased Sensitivity

To enhance sensitivity, try different types of condoms, or add a water-based lubricant to the outside of the condom, or even a few drops to the inside tip of the condom.

FREQUENTLY ASKED QUESTIONS

• *Can the HIV/AIDS virus get through a condom?* No. Latex or polyurethane condoms, if used correctly, are the only way to effectively prevent the spread of HIV/AIDS. Condoms also protect against other STIs. Oil-based lubricants should not be used with latex condoms, as they can cause the latex to break down and could allow HIV/AIDS to pass through. Natural membrane condoms may also allow the HIV/AIDS virus to pass through.

Because heat is one of the causes of deterioration in condoms, do not store them over a month in a wallet or pocket.

- *Do condoms make sex less enjoyable?* This may vary from person to person. Condoms can have some positive effects. For instance, both partners may enjoy sex more if they don't have to worry about getting pregnant or contracting an STI. Using condoms also may prolong an erection.

  Some men believe that condoms are too small or tight for them. All condoms can stretch to accommodate various sizes.
- *Do condoms often break during sex?* A small percentage of condoms do break during sex. When they are used correctly, however, this rarely happens. Condoms are more likely to break if there is a lack of lubrication, so use a water-based lubricant to avoid this. Polyurethane condoms are more likely to break than latex ones.
- *Does a person need to use condoms to protect against STIs when having oral or anal sex?* Yes. STIs can pass from person to person during oral, vaginal, or anal sex. Condoms should be used during any of these sex acts. Anal sex is a particularly high-risk activity, even more than vaginal intercourse, because the tissue in the rectum tears easily. Using extra lubricant with a strong, preferably latex, condom is recommended.

THE FEMALE CONDOM

The female condom is a thin polyurethane sheath with a soft ring at each end. One ring, covered with polyurethane, fits over the cervix, acting as an anchor. The larger, open ring stays outside the vagina, covering part of the perineum and labia during intercourse.

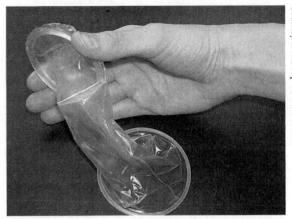

FC Female Condom

Presently there is only one female condom available, called FC Female Condom in the U.S. and Femidom in other countries (see photograph). It is available without a prescription as an over-the-counter barrier contraceptive that also protects against STIs. Because the condom is not made of latex, it will not deteriorate when used with oil-based lubricants. It can be inserted up to eight hours before intercourse but should be removed immediately after. The female condom is prelubricated but does not contain spermicide. It does not require precise placement over the cervix. Male and female condoms should *not* be used at the same time. Like the male condom, the female condom is intended for onetime use.

EFFECTIVENESS

The FC Female Condom was designed to protect women against both pregnancy and STIs. As a contraceptive, it is 95 percent effective when used consistently and correctly, similar to the diaphragm and cervical cap. With typical use, it is 79 percent effective.

STI PROTECTION

Consistent and correct use of the female condom gives more protection against STIs, including HIV infection, than the male condom, the diaphragm, or the cervical cap, because it covers the cervix, vagina, and the external labia.

ADVANTAGES

- Does not require advance planning, clinic visits, or a prescription
- Provides good protection against STIs, including HIV
- By preventing STIs, female condoms protect fertility
- You don't have to rely on a man to use a condom
- Provides broader coverage than the male condom, covering the labia, the perineal region, and the base of the penis
- Some women say the outer ring stimulates the clitoris and makes intercourse more enjoyable
- May help you know your body better
- No physical side effects
- Does not affect menstrual cycles

DISADVANTAGES

- Not as effective in preventing pregnancy as hormonal methods or male condom
- Expensive and not readily available
- May disrupt spontaneity
- Can be quite noisy, if there is not enough lubrication
- Can be difficult to use at first
- Some women find the outer ring causes discomfort

HOW TO USE

Female condom use can be fun for both partners when it is made part of sex. Discuss condom use *before* you have sex. Use a female condom *before you have any genital contact.* Long before ejaculation, the male may discharge a few drops of fluid. This pre-ejaculatory fluid can contain sperm and may also expose you to HIV or other

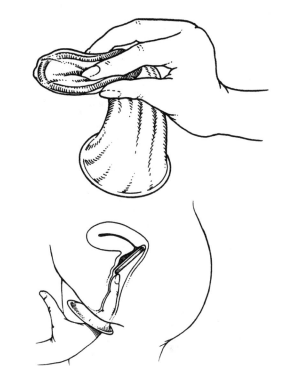

Insertion of FC Female Condom

infectious organisms. You can insert the female condom up to eight hours before intercourse.

1. Carefully open the packet.
2. Find the inner (smaller) ring, which is at the closed end of the condom.
3. Squeeze the inner ring together.
4. Put the inner ring in your vagina.
5. Push the inner ring up into your vagina with your finger. The outer ring stays outside the vagina.
6. When your partner's penis is hard, you will need to guide the penis through the outer ring, to make sure it is not pushed aside.
7. After sex, remove the female condom (if you are lying down, do this before you stand up). Squeeze and twist the outer ring to keep the man's sperm inside the pouch. Pull, and the condom should come out easily.

8. Wrap the condom in tissue and dispose of it. Do not flush it down the toilet.

If you find that the ring is being pulled into your vagina during intercourse, you need to add extra lubrication inside the condom. You can use any kind of lubricant with the female condom. A lubricant containing a spermicide provides the most effective protection against pregnancy, but it may not be the best protection against STIs.

HEALTH CONCERNS

Female condoms currently are the most effective women-controlled method for the prevention of STIs.

WHERE TO GET FEMALE CONDOMS

The female condom is available from the Internet, most drugstores, family planning clinics, and on many college campuses. The cost varies, so shop around.

FREQUENTLY ASKED QUESTIONS

- *Do female condoms come in different sizes; do they have to be fitted?* No, the female condom does not need to be fitted. It comes in one size that is designed to fit most women.
- *Can female condoms be used with male condoms?* No, female condoms should not be used at the same time as male condoms, because the added friction between the two condoms could cause them to tear.
- *Are female condoms more effective than male condoms?* Female condoms have similar efficacy to male condoms and other barrier methods.
- *Can spermicides or lubricants be used with female condoms?* Yes, it is perfectly safe and effective to use spermicides or lubricants with female condoms.

DIAPHRAGM

The diaphragm is a shallow, dome-shaped, soft rubber cup that fits securely in the vagina to cover the cervix. A spermicide is placed in the cup, facing the cervix, to kill or immobilize sperm and prevent them from entering the uterus and fertilizing an egg.

Diaphragms, correctly fitted and worn, prevent pregnancy and protect against some STIs, including gonorrhea and chlamydia, as well as pelvic inflammatory disease and cervical dysplasia. Though they are safer than the Pill or the IUD, they are not as effective in preventing unintended pregnancy. For many women, the diaphragm is an excellent method of contraception because it is woman-controlled and has few side effects, but it requires consistent and correct use. Many women find the device inconvenient, since it must be inserted prior to intercourse, and messy, because it must be used with a spermicide gel or cream.

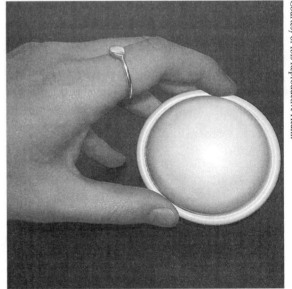

Courtesy of Ibis Reproductive Health

Diaphragm

EFFECTIVENESS

The diaphragm has an effectiveness rating of approximately 94 percent, if used properly, which means using it every time you have intercourse and adding additional spermicide if you have sex again before removal. With highly motivated consistent users, effectiveness can be as high as 98 percent. In typical use, however, the diaphragm is 80 percent effective.

ADVANTAGES

- Can be inserted up to six hours before sex
- May help you know your body better
- Does not affect menstrual cycles
- Provides some protection against most reproductive tract infections
- Can be used during menstruation to contain flow during intercourse
- Has minimal side effects
- Its use is controlled by you

DISADVANTAGES

- Does not provide as much protection against HIV as condoms
- May interrupt spontaneity
- Requires a fitting at a clinic
- Needs occasional refitting
- May increase risk of bladder infections
- Can be messy

HOW TO USE

Practice inserting and removing your diaphragm before sex play with a partner. It can be awkward at first, but it becomes easy with practice. You can put the diaphragm in any time within six hours before intercourse or vagina-to-penis contact. If more than six hours have passed, either insert an applicator full of spermi-

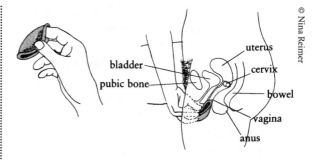

© Nina Reimer

Insertion of diaphragm

cide into your vagina, or remove the diaphragm, wash it out, and start again.

1. Put about 1 tablespoon of spermicidal cream or jelly (¾ inch from the tube) into the shallow cup.

2. Squeeze the diaphragm together by pressing the rim firmly between your thumb and third finger. If you have trouble, you can buy a plastic inserter (good only with a flat-spring diaphragm).

3. Squat, sit on the toilet bowl, stand with one foot raised, or lie down with your legs bent.

4. With your free hand, spread apart the lips of your vagina and push the diaphragm up to the upper third of your vagina with the cream or jelly facing up. Remember that your vagina angles toward the small of your back.

5. Push the lower rim with your finger until you feel the diaphragm fit into place.

6. You should then reach in to make sure you can feel the outline of your cervix through the soft rubber cup. When the diaphragm is in right and fits properly, you should not be able to feel it at all. Your partner probably won't, either, although some men notice that the tip of the penis

is touching soft rubber instead of cervical and vaginal tissue. (This is not painful.)

Leave the diaphragm in for at least six hours after intercourse. You can leave it in for up to twenty-four hours, but not longer. Douching is unnecessary, and routine douching—or douching with commercially prepared douches—can disrupt the natural environment of the vagina and promote infection. If you choose to douche, you must wait at least six hours after intercourse.

Subsequent Intercourse

If you have intercourse again, you must add more cream or jelly with an applicator. Put it into your vagina, leaving the diaphragm in place at least six hours after the last act of intercourse.

Removal

Remove the diaphragm by choosing a comfortable position, perhaps the same way you chose to insert it. If you have trouble reaching the diaphragm, try another position or bear down as if you were going to have a bowel movement. Slide a finger into your vagina and hook it under the lower rim of the diaphragm, either between the diaphragm and your vaginal wall or over the rubber dome. Pull the diaphragm forward and down. If you have long nails, take care not to rip the diaphragm.

Care

Wash the diaphragm with mild soap and warm water, rinse and dry it carefully, and put it into a container (away from light). Do not boil it. Occasionally check for holes by holding it up to the light or filling it with water and looking for leaks, especially around the rim. If you poke the dome with your finger, it will be easier to detect possible cracks along the rim. Oil-based creams, including some vaginal medications, can damage diaphragms, so avoid contact with those materials.

Get your diaphragm size rechecked after full-term pregnancy, after method failure, if you gain or lose more than ten pounds, or after any vaginal surgery. Diaphragms should be replaced every three years.

WHERE TO GET A DIAPHRAGM

Currently, getting a diaphragm requires a fitting in a clinic, though one-size-fits-all diaphragms are currently being developed. You can be fitted at most family planning clinics and at most women's health care providers. Ask in advance of your appointment. The person fitting the diaphragm can choose one of the three kinds of metal spring rim (arcing, coiled, or flat) to fit your particular anatomy. If one kind doesn't fit, try another kind.

Very important: When you have been measured and fitted, practice putting the diaphragm in and taking it out before you leave the practitioner's office, so she or he can tell you whether you are doing it right. (Or go home, practice, and come back in a few days with the diaphragm in place.) Reach in and see what it feels like when it is in correctly, and get help immediately if you have problems, so that when you actually use it, you won't be experimenting. The practitioner should have the diaphragm available right there or will give you a prescription for the proper size.

HEALTH CONCERNS

If you have a severely displaced uterus (e.g., severe prolapse), you may not be able to use a diaphragm. Because diaphragms require manual dexterity, women with some kinds of physical disabilities might not be able to use them effec-

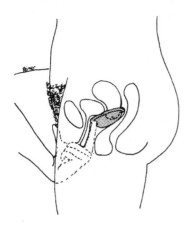
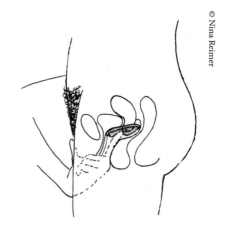

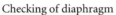

Checking of diaphragm

tively without assistance from their partners. Women with chronic urinary tract infections or a history of toxic shock syndrome should not use the diaphragm.

MANAGING PROBLEMS

Diaphragm use may cause some cramping as well as an increase in bladder infections (urethritis or recurrent cystitis—see p. 691 for more information). The diaphragm could also push backward on your rectum, which can be uncomfortable. Trying a different size or type of diaphragm (one that's less stiff, for example) could solve this problem. If you or your partner have discomfort when the diaphragm is in place, or if you experience genital itching or irritation, unusual vaginal discharge, or frequent bladder infections, call your provider for information and options. Bladder infections are a frequent side effect of the diaphragm, and you may need to be treated.

Some women may experience sensitivity or an allergic reaction to the rubber of the diaphragm or to the spermicide. If this happens and your spermicide has nonoxynol-9 or perfumes, try one without these chemicals.

FREQUENTLY ASKED QUESTIONS

- *If a woman uses the diaphragm without spermicide, will it work at all?* Yes, but using a diaphragm without spermicide will reduce its effectiveness. Studies are now under way to assess the effectiveness of using the diaphragm alone to prevent some STIs. If you do not have spermicide, it is advisable to use another method, such as condoms, or have emergency contraceptive pills on hand.
- *Is it okay to leave a diaphragm in all day?* It is not recommended that a woman leave a diaphragm in all day, but if a woman is unable to put it in before intercourse, this may be an option. You should remove and wash the diaphragm every day to avoid urinary tract infections and toxic shock syndrome.
- *Can a woman use lubricants with a diaphragm?* As with condoms, only water-based lubricants should be used, because oil-based lubricants can damage the latex rubber of the diaphragm.

CERVICAL CAP

The cervical cap is a thimble-shaped rubber or silicone cap that fits snugly over the cervix (the entrance to the uterus) and is held in place by suction. The cervical cap is used with a spermicidal cream or jelly to kill or immobilize sperm and prevent it from entering the uterus and fertilizing an egg.

There are currently at least four types of cervical cap available:

The Prentif cap is made of rubber and must be fitted by a practitioner. It can be left in place for up to twenty-four hours. Its main disadvantage is that it fits only about 80 percent of women properly. It must be fitted by a medical provider.

The Lea's Shield is made of silicone and has a one-way valve that allows for the release of cervical fluids. It comes in one size designed to surround the cervix and not rest on it, so it does not need to be fitted by a medical provider.

The FemCap is made of silicone. It comes in three sizes and must be fitted by a provider. It has a loop for easy removal.

The Ovès cap, another recent design, is made of silicone and is disposable after a single use. The Ovès cap gently adheres to the cervix like a film covering. It cannot be felt by either partner during intercourse. Ovès can be worn for three days, allowing for greater sexual spontaneity (as of August 2004, it had not yet been approved for use in the United States).

EFFECTIVENESS

For women who have never given birth, the Prentif cap is 91 percent effective with perfect use and 84 percent effective with typical use. For women who have given birth, the cap is 74 percent effective with perfect use and 68 percent effective with typical use. The cap is less effective for women in the first year after pregnancy. Cer-vical caps do not protect against sexually transmitted infections, including HIV/AIDS.

ADVANTAGES

- Can be inserted up to six hours before sex
- Comfortable
- May help you better know your body
- Does not affect your period
- No physical side effects
- Its use is controlled by you

DISADVANTAGES

- Does not protect against STIs, including HIV
- Relatively high failure rate
- May interrupt spontaneity
- Some types require a fitting at a clinic
- Some women cannot be fitted
- Can be difficult to insert or remove
- Can be dislodged during intercourse

HOW TO USE

Except for the Lea's Shield, the effectiveness of a cervical cap depends on its fit as well as consistent and correct usage. The Prentif, FemCap, and Ovès caps come in different sizes and need to be fitted by a medical practitioner, who will show you how to insert the cap. Each cap has different instructions, so it is important to read them carefully. If you have questions, ask your practitioner or go to the website for your product.

Inserting a cervical cap can be difficult at first, but becomes easier with practice. Try practicing inserting and removing it before any sexual activity. You can put the cap in any time within six hours before intercourse or vagina-to-penis contact, but it is not recommended during your period.

During the first few months of use, there is a higher risk of pregnancy. To increase effectiveness during this time and every time you have a new partner, use a condom and check the position of the cap before and after intercourse to make sure it stays in place. If the cap moved during intercourse, consider using emergency contraception.

Insertion

1. Prepare the cervical cap with spermicide according to the instructions. If you are having oral sex, wipe any excess spermicide off your vulva—spermicides can have a bad taste.

2. To insert the cap, find a comfortable position. Try standing with one foot raised on a chair, sitting with knees apart, or lying down with knees bent.

3. Use one hand to separate your labia (lips).

4. The other hand can squeeze the rim of the cap and insert it far inside your vagina. Use a finger to push it over your cervix.

5. Run your finger around the cap's rim to make sure the cervix is covered. Test the suction of your cap by gently pinching and pulling on it. You should feel some resistance.

Removal

After intercourse, wait at least six hours before removing your cervical cap so that the spermicide will kill any sperm that may have gotten around the barrier. If you have trouble reaching the cap, try squatting and bearing down as if you were going to have a bowel movement.

Care

Silicone cervical caps should be washed after use. They are not damaged by oil-based lubricants. However, do not use oil-based lubricants with the Prentif cervical cap in place; oil-based lubricants, like Vaseline or edible oils, may dam-

age the cap. After use, wash the cap with mild soap and warm water. You can prevent odors by soaking your cervical cap in diluted lemon juice and drying it between uses. To make sure the cap stays effective, regularly check its condition by holding it up to the light or filling it with water to check for holes.

Refitting

Giving birth or having an abortion can affect the way some cervical caps fit. Three months after a birth or two weeks after an abortion, if you have a Prentif cap or a FemCap, have your medical provider check its fit.

HEALTH CONCERNS

Cervical caps are not recommended for women who have had toxic shock syndrome.

Side Effects

Some women may experience an allergic reaction to the rubber of the cervical cap or the spermicide they use. If this happens and your spermicide has nonoxynol-9 or perfumes, try one without these chemicals.

WHERE TO GET A CERVICAL CAP

Cervical caps are available at many family planning clinics and from other health care providers. Remember, for some types you must be fitted by a trained provider.

SPERMICIDES

A spermicide destroys or disables sperm so that it cannot fertilize an egg to cause a pregnancy. The chemical nonoxynol-9 is the active ingredient in most spermicides, which are available in different forms: foam, jelly, cream, film, and suppositories. Spermicides provide lubrication and are most effective when used consistently and correctly with a barrier method of birth control, such as a condom. They also kill germs, offering some protection against reproductive tract infections, but they give no protection against HIV and can increase risk.

EFFECTIVENESS

When used perfectly, spermicides are 94 percent effective.[3] With typical use, however, they are only about 74 percent effective. As with all methods that depend on use with each sexual act, a spermicide's effectiveness varies widely depending on how correctly and consistently you use it. Spermicides are most effective when used with a barrier method such as a condom, diaphragm, or cervical cap.

ADVANTAGES

- Available without a prescription
- Lubrication may increase pleasure

DISADVANTAGES

- Nonoxynol-9 can increase risk of HIV transmission
- Must be applied before penetration
- Can be messy
- May make oral sex less pleasant
- May irritate vulva or vagina and increase risk of urinary tract infection
- Can interrupt spontaneity

HOW TO USE

Spermicides can be used alone or with other birth control methods to reduce the risk of pregnancy. The lubrication they provide can increase pleasure. Insert your spermicide within a half hour before intercourse. If it was inserted over one hour before intercourse, it will have lost much of its effectiveness. Add more spermicide for repeated intercourse. Leave spermicide in your vagina for six hours after the last act of intercourse. Avoid douching in general, but if you must douche, wait for at least six hours (douching weakens spermicide). Spermicide preparations are available in most drugstores and do not require a prescription. If you become pregnant while using spermicide, the pregnancy will not be affected.

Foam

Foam comes in a can and is the consistency of shaving cream.

1. Shake the can well.

2. Place the applicator on the top of the can and press down or to the side, depending on the package directions. The plunger will rise as the applicator fills.

3. Insert the applicator about two or three inches into your vagina and press the plunger to deposit the foam over your cervix.

4. To avoid sucking foam back into the applicator, don't withdraw the plunger. Foam is effective immediately.

Creams and Jellies

Creams and jellies can be used with a diaphragm, a cervical cap, or a condom. They are inserted into the vagina with an applicator and take effect immediately.

Vaginal Contraceptive Film (VCF)

VCF comes as paper-thin squares that dissolve over the cervix.

1. Fold the film in half and then place it on the tip of your finger.

2. Insert your finger into your vagina and put the VCF over your cervix.

3. A dry finger and quick insertion will help the VCF stay in place and not stick to your finger.

4. It will take about fifteen minutes for the VCF to melt and become effective.

Suppositories

Suppositories are inserted into the vagina like a tampon and pushed up toward the cervix. It takes about twenty minutes for the capsule to dissolve and the suppository to become effective.

SIDE EFFECTS

You or your partner may experience genital irritation, a rash, or itchiness if either of you is allergic to ingredients in a spermicide such as nonoxynol-9. If this happens, try a spermicide without nonoxynol-9 or perfumes.

WHERE TO GET SPERMICIDES

Spermicides are available over the counter in any drugstore or can be bought in family planning clinics or on the Internet.

HORMONAL METHODS

HORMONAL METHODS AND MENSTRUAL BLEEDING

Normal menstrual bleeding is a result of the interaction of the hormones estrogen and progesterone in our bodies. Estrogen causes the lining of the uterus to develop in preparation for pregnancy; progesterone holds the lining of the uterus (the endometrium) in place during pregnancy. If no pregnancy occurs in the cycle, the body signals a fall in progesterone, and the lining is shed. This lining is what is expelled during menstruation.

Hormonal contraceptives use synthetic forms of human hormones to suppress ovulation and prevent pregnancy. Most pills contain both estrogen and synthetic forms of progesterone called *progestins* (the estrogen stabilizes the uterine lining and encourages more regular bleeding patterns). Progestin-only methods such as Depo-Provera, Norplant implants, and some pills contain no estrogen and thus frequently lead to irregular or absent bleeding. Many women worry that not bleeding while taking the Pill or using other hormonal methods may be harmful; one concern is that unshed blood might build up inside the uterus. (Because progestin-only methods prevent the lining of the uterus from building up, there is no regular bleeding. Irregular bleeding occurs most frequently in the beginning of method use, when the uterine lining has not completely thinned. It is not harmful, but it can be very disruptive.)

THE PILL-ORAL CONTRACEPTIVES

The Pill is the most popular type of birth control used in the United States and one of the most commonly used methods worldwide. There are many different brands of the Pill, and they come in packs of twenty-eight pills (outside of the U.S., packs of twenty-one pills are also available). One pill is taken every day. The first twenty-one pills have a combination of synthetic estrogen and progestin hormones; the last seven pills have no hormones and are called spacer pills, sugar pills, or inactive pills. Monthly bleeding occurs during this week.

The Pill works by stopping ovulation, thus preventing the ovaries from releasing eggs. It also causes the cervical fluid to thicken, making it harder for sperm to enter the uterus and preventing fertilization. The Pill is a very effective method of birth control, although it does not protect against sexually transmitted infections, including HIV/AIDS.

EFFECTIVENESS

With perfect use, the Pill is considered 99 percent effective. Perfect use means that the woman takes a pill at about the same time every day and never misses a pill. With typical use, the Pill is about 95 percent effective. That means that one in every twenty women who use the Pill become pregnant in the first year of use.

ADVANTAGES

- May cause lighter or more regular periods
- May reduce painful periods
- Easy to use
- Does not interrupt spontaneity
- Reduces incidence of ovarian cysts and fibrocystic breast changes
- May relieve premenstrual syndrome (PMS)
- Protects against uterine and ovarian cancers
- Provides some protection against pelvic inflammatory disease
- May reduce acne
- Can be used for emergency contraception

DISADVANTAGES

- Does not protect against STIs, including HIV
- Must be taken every day; can be difficult to remember
- Can have unpleasant side effects
- Raises risk of heart attack and stroke for some women
- Requires a prescription
- May cause depression

HOW TO USE

If you begin taking the Pill within five days after your period starts or within five days after an abortion, it is effective immediately. If you begin at any other time, the Pill becomes effective after one week (so use another backup method during that week).* To lower your risk of STIs, use

---

* Some health care practitioners now recommend the "Quick Start" method, whereby a woman takes her first pill in the clinic or office following counseling and the decision to use an oral contraceptive.

SAFETY OF THE PILL

The birth control pill is considered the most intensely researched medication in history. Since its development over forty years ago, it has been used by millions of women worldwide.

Despite problems associated with early pill formulations, researchers now maintain that the low-dose birth control pills on the market today are safe for most women. Concerns about blood clots, heart attack, and stroke spurred exhaustive research on oral contraceptives beginning in the 1960s and '70s. Current research concludes that healthy, nonsmoking women have little if any greater risk of heart attack or stroke than women who do not use the Pill. Any woman of any age has a tripling of her risk of blood clots while on the Pill, although this risk is quite small, about half the risk of getting a blood clot during pregnancy. Some cardiovascular conditions, some chronic illnesses, and heavy smoking in women over the age of thirty-five rule out Pill use. Women who use birth control pills develop liver tumors in rare cases and may have a slightly higher chance of getting cervical cancer than women who don't use the Pill.[4] Some evidence suggests that recent oral contraceptive use slightly increases risk of breast cancer among women under 35 years old.[5]

The increased safety of the Pill can be attributed to the lower estrogen content. Today's pills contain about one eighth to one tenth as much estrogen as early pills.

In addition, we now know that long-term use of the Pill provides significant noncontraceptive health benefits. Long-term use protects against ovarian and endometrial (uterine) cancers, and research suggests that these protective effects may last up to fifteen years or more. Women who take the Pill have lighter, shorter periods (thus reducing the risk of anemia), are less likely to develop certain ovarian cysts, and have a decreased incidence of pelvic inflammatory disease (PID).

Though the information listed above is based on research on the Pill only, it is reasonable to infer that the same cautions and side effects apply to all methods that contain both estrogen and progestin.

condoms as well. Combining condom and Pill use also increases your protection from pregnancy.

Starting the Pill

A common way to start taking the Pill is to begin on the first day of your period or the day of an abortion. Some women prefer to start on the first Sunday after they begin their period or the first Sunday after an abortion. Starting pills on Sundays has the advantage of usually having your period begin on a Monday or Tuesday, thus not having periods on weekends.

Continuing

Take one pill every day until you finish an entire pack. If you take the Pill at the same time you brush your teeth, eat a meal, or perform another daily activity, it may be easier to remember. If you have a twenty-eight-day pack, start a new pack immediately after you finish the old one. If you have a twenty-one-day pack, take one pill every day for twenty-one days, no pills for seven days, then start the new pack immediately, regardless of whether you still have your period.

Skipping Your Period

Some women are now opting to use pills continuously for three months in order to skip having periods. For a discussion of this practice, see p. 255 in Chapter 13, "Sexual Anatomy, Reproduction, and the Menstrual Cycle."

Missed Pills

Try to avoid starting the next package of pills late, as this may lead to a pregnancy. Make up for a late start as follows.

Late Start:

- If one day late starting the next package, take two pills as soon as you remember and one pill each day after. Use a backup form of birth control for one week.
- If two days late starting the next package, take two pills as soon as you remember and one pill each day after. Use a backup form of birth control for one week.
- If three or more days late starting the next package, throw away the pills you missed and start the rest of the pills in the package right on schedule. Use a backup method of birth control until you have taken seven active (hormonal) pills in a row. If you had unprotected intercourse during the time you missed pills, consider using emergency contraception (see p. 374). If you have questions, call your health care provider.

Missed Pills During the Cycle:

- If one pill is missed, take the missed pill as soon as you remember and take your next pill at your usual time. This may require taking two pills in one day.
- If two pills in a row are missed in the first two weeks, take two pills on the day you remember and finish the rest of the pack as

If you are more than three days late in starting the Pill and had unprotected intercourse, consider using emergency contraception (see p. 374).

usual. Use a backup form of birth control for one week.
- If two pills in a row are missed in the third week, keep taking one pill every day until you have finished the active (hormonal) pills. Then set aside the rest of the pack, including the spacers (inactive pills), and start taking a new pack of pills. Use a backup form of birth control for one week.
- If three or more pills in a row are missed in the first two weeks, take one pill as soon as you remember, then keep taking one pill every day. Use a backup method of birth control until you have taken seven active (hormonal) pills.
- If three or more pills in a row are missed in the third week, take one pill as soon as you remember, then keep taking one pill every day until you have finished the active (hormonal) pills. Then set aside the rest of the pack and start taking a new pack of pills. Use a backup form of birth control for one week.

Missing any of the last seven pills of a twenty-eight-day combined pill package will not raise your risk of pregnancy. Skip the pills you missed and be sure you start your next pack on time. (This is not the case for the Mini-Pill; see p. 350.)

Missed Periods

Women taking the Pill often have shorter and lighter periods. A drop of blood or a brown smudge on your underwear during the week you are taking no hormonal pills is counted as a period when you are on the Pill.

If you miss one period and you took all of your pills correctly, and you don't have any signs of pregnancy, the chances of pregnancy are very low. It is not uncommon to miss a period while on the Pill. If you often miss periods and are taking the Pill correctly, talk to your provider about whether you should change to a different pill.

If you miss two periods in a row or feel worried, do a pregnancy test, but keep taking your pills until pregnancy is verified. Pregnancy is more likely in the first few months of Pill use, if you missed taking any Pills, or if you have been sick (vomiting and/or diarrhea).

If you forget one or more pills and do not have a period that month, have a pregnancy test done at a clinic. If you miss two periods in a row, it could be either normal or a sign of pregnancy. Pregnancy tests are recommended right away. If you become pregnant while on the Pill and give birth to a child, there is very little evidence that the Pill will increase the risks of your baby being born with a disability.

HEALTH CONCERNS

Risks

Women who are over thirty-five and smoke or who have any of the following conditions **should not** take the Pill:

- History of heart attack or stroke
- Blood clots
- Unexplained vaginal bleeding
- Known or suspected cancer of the uterus, ovaries, cervix, breast, or vagina
- Known or suspected pregnancy
- Liver disease

Women who are under thirty-five and who smoke or have migraines, gallbladder disease, hypertension, diabetes, epilepsy, sickle cell disease, elective surgery, a history of blood clots, or liver or heart disease *may not* be able to take the Pill. Your health care provider can advise you.

Because the prognosis of women with current or recent breast cancer may worsen with Pill use, many health care providers advise these women to avoid the Pill.[6]

Benefits

Women using hormonal contraception have a decreased risk of endometrial cancer, ovarian cancer, endometriosis, and pelvic inflammatory disease. You may have less menstrual cramping and pain, lighter periods, and less chance of anemia.

Side Effects

Side effects of the Pill include:

- Irregular bleeding or spotting
- Nausea and sometimes vomiting
- Breast tenderness
- Weight gain and/or water retention
- Spotty darkening of the skin
- Mild headaches
- Mood changes, including depression or decreased sex drive

Side effects usually go away after two to three cycles. If any side effects are bothersome after two to three cycles, or if heavy bleeding occurs, continue taking your pills and call your health care provider for an appointment. Though these side effects can make you uncomfortable, they are not dangerous. If you feel that you must stop the Pill immediately, be sure to abstain from sex or use another form of contraception. The contraceptive effects of the Pill—as well as the side effects—go away as soon as you stop taking it.

Danger Signs

If you experience any of the following symptoms while taking the Pill, you should call your health care provider or go to an emergency room immediately:

- Severe abdominal pains
- Chest pain or shortness of breath
- Severe headaches
- Severe leg or arm pain or numbness
- Eye problems, such as blurred vision

DRUG INTERACTIONS

Certain medications reduce the effectiveness of the Pill. These include anti-seizure medications (e.g., phenytoin, phenobarbitol, carbamazepine), Griseofulvin (anti-fungal medication), Rifampin (tuberculosis drug), and St. John's wort. If you are taking any medications, tell the provider who is prescribing the Pill. You may need to add a backup method of birth control.

There have been anecdotal reports of antibiotics interacting with oral contraceptive pills. None of these reports have been solidly proved. There is no definite evidence that antibiotics (other than Rifampin) interfere with oral contraceptives. Because of the controversy surrounding this issue, some women choose to use a backup method (such as condoms) while taking antibiotics and oral contraceptive pills.

GETTING PREGNANT LATER

Women who want to become pregnant may stop using the Pill at any time. Pregnancy may occur right away or after several months. The Pill does not affect your long-term fertility.

EMERGENCY CONTRACEPTION

Some brands of the Pill can be used for emergency contraception (EC). EC is taken within three to five days after unprotected intercourse to prevent pregnancy. (For more information, see "Emergency Contraception," p. 374.)

MINI-PILLS (PROGESTIN-ONLY ORAL CONTRACEPTIVES)

Mini-Pills are progestin-only birth control pills. Mini-Pills come in packs of twenty-eight pills, and one is taken every day. They have progestin and no estrogen. The Mini-Pill controls fertilization by affecting the fluid around the cervix and preventing sperm from entering the uterus. It also affects the transport of the egg through the fallopian tubes. It does not protect against sexually transmitted infections (STIs), including HIV/AIDS.

EFFECTIVENESS

Mini-Pills are 98 to 99 percent effective with perfect use and 95 percent effective with typical use, slightly less than regular birth control pills. For nursing women, they provide almost 100 percent protection from pregnancy and do not affect milk supply.

ADVANTAGES

- Avoid estrogen side effects of combination birth control pills
- Contain no estrogen so can be used by many women who cannot use combined pills
- Easy to use
- Do not interrupt spontaneity
- Periods can be lighter, less painful, and less frequent
- Reduce incidence of ovarian cysts and fibrocystic breast changes
- May relieve premenstrual syndrome (PMS)
- Protect against uterine and ovarian cancers
- Provide some protection against pelvic inflammatory disease (PID)
- May reduce acne

DISADVANTAGES

- Do not protect against sexually transmitted infections (STIs), including HIV
- Must be taken every day at the same time; missing one pill can result in pregnancy
- Increase the risk of functional ovarian cysts (not dangerous)
- May cause irregular bleeding
- Require a prescription

HOW TO USE

Mini-Pills packs have no spacer pills. Each pill contains hormones, *so it is important to take a pill every day,* preferably at the same time. Forgetting a Mini-Pill or taking it late increases the chance of pregnancy more than missing a combined pill does.

Using a backup method such as condoms or spermicide increases Mini-Pill effectiveness. To lower your risk of sexually transmitted infection, use condoms as well.

Starting Mini-Pills

Take the first pill on the first day of your period. Take one pill daily, at the same time of day, even during your period.

After the First Pack

As soon as you finish one pack, begin the next one. Start your next pack even if you are still bleeding or have not started your period. Continue taking one pill every day.

If you have problems with the Mini-Pill, call your health care provider. If you stop taking Mini-Pills, you must use another birth control method to avoid pregnancy.

Missed Pills

- Three or more hours late: If three or more hours late, take a pill as soon as you remember. Use a backup method for forty-eight hours.
- One pill missed: If one day late, take a pill as soon as you remember, and take the next one at the usual time. This may mean taking two pills in one day. If you miss only one pill and make it up, you probably will not get pregnant. Use a backup method for two weeks.
- Two pills missed: If two days late, take two pills each day for the next two days. Use a backup method for two weeks. You may have some spotting or bleeding, but if the bleeding is like a period, call your provider.
- Three or more pills missed: If three or more days late, use a backup method and call your provider for instructions.

If you missed one or more pills and you had unprotected sex, you might want to use emergency contraception (EC). Progestin-only ECs (called "Plan B") are higher doses of the Mini-Pill. (See section on EC, p. 374.)

GETTING PREGNANT LATER

Women who want to become pregnant may stop using Mini-Pills at any time. Pregnancy may occur right away or after several months.

HEALTH CONCERNS

You should not use the Mini-Pill if you are already pregnant or have unexplained vaginal bleeding until after it is diagnosed. See page 349 regarding breast cancer and combined oral contraceptives (concerns are similar for the Mini-Pill).[7]

Benefits

Women using progestin-only hormonal contraception have a decreased risk of endometrial cancer, ovarian cancer, and pelvic inflammatory disease. You may have less menstrual cramping and pain, lighter periods, and less chance of anemia.

Side Effects

The most common side effect for women using Mini-Pills is irregular bleeding or no bleeding at all. If you do not bleed for sixty days, call your provider to arrange for a pregnancy test, but continue taking your pills.

The Mini-Pill may also cause mood changes, headaches, and loss of sex drive.

DRUG INTERACTIONS

Mini-Pills are affected by the same medications as the Pill. See "Drug Interactions" (p. 350) for information on which medications can decrease effectiveness.

CONTRACEPTIVE PATCH

The contraceptive Patch—currently marketed under the name Ortho Evra—is a prescription method of birth control. The contraceptive Patch looks like a square Band-Aid and is applied to the abdomen, buttocks, upper arm, or upper torso. The Patch is changed every week for three weeks, left off for one week, then resumed. The contraceptive Patch works by slowly releasing a combination of estrogen and progestin hormones through the skin. It has the same hormones as those found in the combined birth control pill and therefore works the same way and has the same side effects (see p. 349).

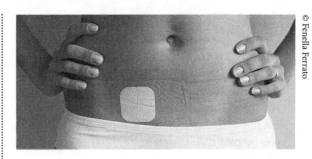

Birth control patch

EFFECTIVENESS

The Patch is a very effective reversible method of birth control. With typical use—although no comparative studies have yet been published—it is assumed that the Patch will be more effective than the Pill, since it should be easier to apply a Patch once a week rather than to remember to take a pill every day. With perfect use, the Patch is about 99 percent effective in women under 198 pounds (it is less reliable in women over 198 pounds).

The Patch works best when it is changed on the same day of the week for three weeks in a row. Pregnancy can happen if an error is made in using the Patch, especially if:

- It becomes loose or stays off for longer than twenty-four hours
- The same Patch is used—left on the skin—for longer than one week

If either of these things happens, follow the directions in your package insert, consider taking emergency contraception, and call your clinician.

ADVANTAGES

- These are the same as for the Pill (see p. 346), although some women find the Patch more convenient than the Pill.

DISADVANTAGES

- These are the same as for the Pill (see p. 346), except that you have to remember to use a new Patch once a week rather than to take a pill every day.

HOW TO USE

Apply the contraceptive Patch within five days of the first day of your period or within five days of a first-trimester abortion. One Patch per week is used for three weeks in a row. On the fourth week, no Patch should be worn, and your menstrual period should start. A new Patch is applied seven days after removal to start another month of birth control. If you start on the Sunday after an abortion or at the onset of menstruation after an abortion, you should use a backup method for seven days (for example: condom, spermicide, or diaphragm).

The day of the week you apply the Patch will be the same day you change it a week later. (After second-trimester abortion or having given birth, wait four weeks to apply your first Patch. If breast-feeding, consult your health care provider.) The Patch can be applied any place on the body that is clean and dry, except on the palms, on sores, and on the breasts. The Patch is effective immediately.

Health club studies have shown that the Patch can be worn swimming or in the shower but should be checked afterward. About 2 percent of the time, a Patch will completely fall off. If it partially or completely falls off, refer to the instructions.

HEALTH CONCERNS

As with all medications, there may be some side effects for some women taking combined hormone contraceptives. If you can use birth control pills, you can use the Patch. Women who cannot use the Pill for health reasons also cannot use the Patch. Also, drug interactions and danger signs are the same as for the Pill. (To learn more, see p. 349.)

Benefits

Women using hormonal contraception have a decreased risk of endometrial cancer, ovarian cancer, and pelvic inflammatory disease. You may have less menstrual cramping and pain, lighter periods, and less chance of anemia.

Side Effects

Side effects that usually clear up after two or three months of use include:

- Bleeding between periods
- Weight gain or loss
- Breast tenderness
- Nausea (rarely vomiting)
- Mood changes, including depression or decreased sex drive

Other possible side effects may include:

- Skin reaction at the site of application
- Problems with contact lens use—a change in vision or the inability to wear the lenses

WHERE TO GET THE PATCH

The Patch is available by prescription only, so you must see a health care provider. The clinician will discuss your medical history with you, check your blood pressure, and give you any other medical exam that may be needed. If the Patch is right for you, the clinician will give you a prescription. The Patch must be used as directed.

VAGINAL RING

A Vaginal Ring is a thin, transparent, flexible ring that you insert into the vagina to prevent pregnancy. The Vaginal Ring is left in place for three weeks and then removed for one week, providing one month of birth control. It slowly releases estrogen and progestin hormones into the body, stops ovulation, and thickens the cervical fluid, creating a barrier to prevent sperm from fertilizing an egg. The Vaginal Ring does not protect against sexually transmitted infections, including HIV/AIDS. Currently, the only type of Vaginal Ring available is NuvaRing.

EFFECTIVENESS

The Vaginal Ring is 99 percent effective as birth control when used perfectly. Because the Ring is inserted only once a month, the effectiveness with typical use should be about the same.

ADVANTAGES

- Easy to use, safe, and convenient
- Can be worn for three weeks
- Private—no visible patches or Pill packets
- Provides protection from pregnancy one month at a time
- Does not interrupt spontaneity

DISADVANTAGES

- Does not protect against STIs, including HIV
- Slightly raised risk of heart attack and stroke for some women (see "Health Concerns" under the Pill section on p. 349)
- Requires a prescription

HOW TO USE

The Vaginal Ring must be inserted within the first five days of beginning your period or within five days of a first-trimester abortion. (After second-trimester abortion or childbirth, wait four weeks to insert the Ring. If breast-feeding, consult your health care provider.) You may also choose to change the first Ring on the first day of the next month and use the calendar as your guide for when to replace each Ring. The Vaginal Ring is effective after seven days during its first use. After the first month, it is effective continuously, as long as you don't forget to insert a new Ring after the seven-day break. If it is out for longer than three additional hours, however, it is wise to wash and reinsert the Ring and use backup protection for a week.

If you're taking the Pill or using another form of hormonal birth control, you can switch to the Vaginal Ring without losing protection from pregnancy. (After an IUD or implant removal, backup is recommended for one week.)

- If you are taking the Pill, you should insert a Vaginal Ring within seven days after the last hormone-containing pill of your pack.
- If you are taking Mini-Pills, you should insert a Vaginal Ring on any day and discontinue Mini-Pills on that day.
- If you are using injectable contraceptives (Lunelle or Depo-Provera), then insert a Vaginal Ring on the day of your next scheduled injection.
- If you are using an IUD or implant, then insert a Vaginal Ring on the day of removal.

Inserting the Vaginal Ring is much like inserting a tampon or a diaphragm. The Vaginal Ring is not a barrier method, so incorrect insertion is usually not a problem. You may choose to squat; stand with one leg raised; or lie down. Squeeze the Ring between your thumb and index finger and gently push it into your vagina. Push the Ring far enough in so it feels comfortable. Sometimes you can't feel it at all.

The Vaginal Ring remains in the vagina for three weeks. It can be removed by inserting a finger into your vagina, hooking the side of the ring, and pulling it out. Carefully wrap it in its foil pouch and dispose of it in the trash, rather than the toilet, to prevent the hormones from being released into the environment. Your period should start within the next few days. For another month of birth control, insert a new Vaginal Ring seven days after removal of the last one, even if your period has not ended.

New Vaginal Rings should be stored until use in the refrigerator if possible, or at room temperature, but at no more than 77 degrees Fahrenheit, and away from direct sunlight.

If the Vaginal Ring slips out of your vagina and it has been out for less than three hours, you should still be protected from pregnancy. Rinse it with cold or lukewarm water (not hot) and reinsert it as soon as possible. If you lose the original Ring, insert a new one as soon as possible. If additional hours have passed, your protection is significantly reduced and you need another method of birth control until the Vaginal Ring has been back in place for seven days in a row. If more than three hours passed and then you had unprotected sex, consider using emergency contraception (see p. 374).

Missing a period while using the Vaginal Ring does not necessarily mean you are pregnant. However, if the Ring slips out of your vagina for more than three hours during the three weeks of use, you may want to get a pregnancy test. If you are pregnant, discontinue use of the Vaginal Ring.

Continuous Use

Some physicians recommend continuous use of the Vaginal Ring, which would prevent you from having a monthly period. Studies are being done about the safety of this approach. You would wear the Ring for three or four weeks, remove it, and insert a new one (a Ring may not protect against pregnancy after thirty days).

HEALTH CONCERNS

Women with an easily irritated vagina, dropped uterus, dropped bladder, rectal prolapse, severe constipation, or who are breast-feeding may not be able to use the Vaginal Ring. Your health care provider can help you decide.

The hormones found in the Vaginal Ring are similar to those found in the Pill. **Women who cannot use the Pill for health reasons also cannot use the Vaginal Ring.** Also, drug interactions and danger signs are the same as for the Pill. (To learn more, see p. 349.)

Male condoms can be used with the Vaginal Ring to provide protection against STIs.

Benefits

Women using hormonal contraception have a decreased risk of endometrial cancer, ovarian cancer, and pelvic inflammatory disease. You may have less menstrual cramping and pain, lighter periods, and less chance of anemia.

Side Effects

As your body adjusts to hormonal changes from the Vaginal Ring, you may experience some minor side effects, including:

- Vaginal discharge
- Vaginal irritation
- Headache
- Weight gain
- Nausea
- Irregular bleeding
- Breast tenderness

- Mood changes, including depression or decreased sex drive

INJECTABLE CONTRACEPTIVES

MONTHLY INJECTION (LUNELLE)

Lunelle is a monthly birth control injection (not available in the U.S. as of fall 2004). Lunelle can be injected into the arm, thigh, or hip. The shot has both synthetic estrogen and progestin hormones. Lunelle prevents ovulation and thickens the cervical fluid, creating a barrier to prevent sperm from fertilizing an egg. It also causes the uterine lining to become less prepared to support a fertilized egg. It requires monthly visits to a clinic or pharmacy. It does not protect against sexually transmitted infections, including HIV. For more information, see "Lunelle" (W43) on the companion website, www.ourbodiesour selves.org.

THREE-MONTH SHOT (DEPO-PROVERA)

Depo-Provera is an injection of the hormone progestin that prevents pregnancy for three months. It is usually given in the arm or buttock. The high level of progestin prevents fertilization by stopping the ovaries from releasing eggs, thickening the cervical fluid, and changing the uterine lining, making it harder for sperm to enter or survive in the uterus. You have to get a new shot every three months. Depo-Provera does not protect against sexually transmitted infections, including HIV.

The fact that Depo is a long-acting method is both its strength and its weakness. For women who like the shot, knowing that they are protected from pregnancy for at least three months is very important. But for those women who have side effects such as bleeding or depression, knowing that these effects may continue for another six or more months can be difficult. After the last shot of Depo-Provera, it can take over six months for the drug to leave the body. If you are considering using Depo, talk to your provider about what your options would be if you experience side effects.

Depo-Provera has long been a controversial method of birth control. Some women who feel that their lives have been negatively affected by the use of Depo are organizing to let other women know about their experiences. They are calling for further research on side effects and better disclosure of information to potential users.

EFFECTIVENESS

Depo-Provera is 99.7 percent effective as birth control.

ADVANTAGES

- Private
- Does not require regular supplies or attention
- Effective after twenty-four hours
- Does not interrupt sexual spontaneity
- Has no estrogen
- May decrease risk for ovarian and uterine cancers

DISADVANTAGES

- Does not protect against STIs, including HIV
- Requires injections every three months
- Delay of return to fertility
- Possible weight gain
- Possible irregular bleeding or no menstrual bleeding at all
- If side effects occur, they can last a long time

HOW TO USE

You will probably be given your first shot of Depo-Provera during—or within five days after—the start of your period. If there is no chance you are pregnant, it can first be given at any time during the cycle. After twenty-four hours, the shot provides effective birth control for the next thirteen weeks. You may find it useful to schedule your next injection slightly earlier than necessary to prevent a gap in birth control protection if you miss your appointment.

Depo can also be started six weeks after a birth or during the first seven days after an abortion, including immediately after an abortion.

If you are over a week late for your shot, use a backup method of birth control for the next two weeks. If your period is over two weeks late and you have had unprotected sex during that time, consider taking a pregnancy test before receiving the next dose.

If you have heavy or continuous bleeding after your first injection, you can have a second injection as early as four weeks after your first injection, which should stop your bleeding.

If you decide to switch from Depo-Provera to the birth control pill, the Vaginal Ring, or the contraceptive Patch, it is recommended that you start your new method on the date the next injection is due. If you decide to switch to an IUD, it can be inserted anytime during the three months following the last injection, but bleeding patterns may not normalize for six to twelve months.

GETTING PREGNANT LATER

If you want to become pregnant, you may stop using Depo-Provera at any time. Depo's contraceptive effect can last *an average of four to six months* after your last injection, and for some women, it will last up to eighteen months. This is not harmful and should be expected. If you

Though the contraceptive effects of Depo might last longer than three months, you should not expect it to last longer than thirteen weeks after your last shot.

think you might want to become pregnant in the next two years, Depo is probably not a good choice for you.

HEALTH CONCERNS

If you have any of the following conditions, you should not use Depo-Provera:

- Unexplained vaginal bleeding, until the condition has been investigated and found to be unrelated to a serious cause
- Known or suspected pregnancy

Depo-Provera may not be recommended if you are planning to get pregnant soon; are concerned about weight gain; or have liver disease, gallbladder disease, or a history of depression.

Risks

Depo-Provera causes some loss of bone density, though its long-term effects on bone strength remain unclear. Recent research indicates that bone density loss is worse with longer use of Depo-Provera and may not be completely reversible. Therefore, women should not use Depo for more than two years unless other birth control methods are inadequate. If you use Depo, it is advised to exercise regularly and take in calcium-rich foods (see Chapter 2, "Eating Well").

If you become pregnant while using Depo-Provera and continue your pregnancy, there may be a slight increased risk of premature birth. You can start Depo-Provera six weeks after giving birth.

The effects of Depo-Provera on breast cancer are still unknown.

Benefits

Women using Depo-Provera have a decreased risk of endometrial cancer and pelvic inflammatory disease. You may have less menstrual cramping and pain, fewer periods, and less chance of anemia.

Side Effects

All women who use Depo will experience changes in menstrual bleeding. This is not dangerous. Spotting, heavy bleeding, or no bleeding are common side effects. After a year of use, over half of all Depo users stop having periods; two thirds stop by the end of the second year. It is not possible to predict who will experience this amenorrhea. Many women like not having periods, while others find it unsettling. Irregular bleeding is the most common reason for discontinuing the use of Depo.

Seventy percent of women who use Depo-Provera will gain some weight due to increased appetite, usually gaining between five and ten pounds after one year of use.

Symptoms some women experience during use of Depo-Provera include headaches, nervousness, mood changes, bloating, hot flashes, decreased interest in sex, breast tenderness, acne, hair loss, and backache. After the last shot of Depo-Provera, it can take over six months for the drug to leave the body. Side effects may linger until the drug is completely gone.

DRUG INTERACTIONS

Few medications lower the effectiveness of Depo-Provera. If you are taking any medications, tell the provider who is giving you the shots. When taking medications that may interfere with Depo-Provera, add a backup method of birth control, such as condoms or spermicide.

IMPLANTS

Contraceptive implants are soft, hormone-filled capsules that are inserted under the skin in a woman's upper arm. They work in the same way as other hormonal methods, preventing ovulation and thickening the cervical fluid, thereby preventing sperm from entering the uterus. Contraceptive implants offer a safe, long-term, reversible contraceptive option. They do not protect against sexually transmitted infections, including HIV.

The first implant system available, called Norplant, consisted of six progestin-containing capsules and provided contraceptive protection for five years. Newer versions, including Norplant-2 (also known as Jadelle), a two-rod system that lasts for five years, and Implanon, a single-rod system that lasts for three years, are already being used in several countries outside the United States. Implanon will likely be approved for use in the United States during 2005. Several other implant systems are currently being developed as well.

Implant systems have come under criticism in many developing countries: While they are relatively easy to insert, removal can be difficult. Many women with implants who chose to discontinue the method were unable to find providers who could remove them. The newer implant systems have fewer problems with removal.

Implants have been implicated in rare cases of long-term problems, including damage to the optic nerve, causing sudden blindness. Some women who feel their lives have been negatively affected by Norplant have called for more thorough counseling about the potential problems associated with this method.

EFFECTIVENESS

Implants are 99 percent effective. They last three to five years, depending on the system.

ADVANTAGES

- Highly effective
- Do not interrupt spontaneity
- Provide protection from pregnancy for three to five years
- Fertility returns quickly once implants are removed
- Can be used by women who are breast-feeding
- You don't have to think about contraception for as long as the implants work
- If you change your mind, they can be removed

DISADVANTAGES

- Do not protect against STIs, including HIV
- Many women experience irregular bleeding and changes to periods
- Because they are long-acting, side effects can last a long time
- Can cause slight increase in ovarian cysts (which are not dangerous)
- Can be difficult to remove
- Require a trained medical provider to insert and remove
- Rarely, can cause an infection in the arm

HOW TO USE

Implant insertion needs to be done in a clinic or hospital. Implants are usually inserted during or a few days after your period to ensure that you are not pregnant. However, they can be inserted anytime, as long as you are sure you are not pregnant. The preference for insertion during menses should not be used to deny access to the method.

Insertion

A local anesthetic is used on the underside of the upper arm, and one small incision is made. Through this cut, the implants are placed under the skin. The arm may feel bruised or tender for several days. Implants are effective within twenty-four hours of insertion.

Removal

You can request to have implants removed on schedule (three or five years) or anytime before then. Removal can be more difficult than insertion. Local anesthetic is used on the arm, then a slightly larger incision is made and the clinician pulls out the implants. Fertility may return immediately or within a few months.

HEALTH CONCERNS

Women with the following conditions should not use implants:

- Unexplained abnormal vaginal bleeding, until after it is diagnosed
- Known or suspected pregnancy
- Known or suspected breast, cervical, or endometrial cancer

Implants are not recommended for women who have certain heart problems, intolerance to irregular bleeding, progestin allergies, or depression. It is recommended that breast-feeding women wait six weeks after giving birth to use implants. Cautions, side effects, and drug interactions are the same as with other long-acting progestin-only contraceptives. (For a complete discussion, see the section on Depo-Provera, p. 357.)

Risks

Irritation, scarring, or infection may occur where the implant is inserted. If your incision area becomes red, swollen, puffy, or painful, call your health care provider.

If you become pregnant while using implants, you have a higher risk of ectopic pregnancy (in which the fertilized egg implants outside the uterus) than someone who becomes pregnant while using no birth control. If you suspect that you might be pregnant, or if you have severe abdominal pain while using implants, seek medical help immediately.

Benefits

Women using Norplant may have a decreased risk of endometrial cancer, ovarian cancer, and pelvic inflammatory disease. You may have less menstrual cramping and pain, fewer periods, and less chance of anemia.

Side Effects

The most common complaint of women using implants is irregular bleeding, which occurs most often during the first months but can last up to a year. Bleeding patterns can be unpredictable, and some women have almost continuous spotting. Low-dose oral contraceptives or estrogen may help regulate cycles.

Some women may experience side effects such as weight gain, acne, and headaches. A small number of women have reported side effects such as mood swings, abdominal pain, painful periods, and hair loss. If you have negative side effects that are disrupting your life, you should be able to have your implants removed at any time.

IUD/STERILIZATION

IUD

IUDs are small plastic devices that contain copper or progestin and fit inside the uterus. One or more strings are attached to the IUD and extend downward through the cervix into the upper vagina, allowing you to check that the IUD is in place. The IUD is usually not noticeable during intercourse and is effective for ten years. It does not protect against sexually transmitted infections, including HIV/AIDS.

The presence of the IUD primarily affects the movement of eggs and sperm to prevent fertilization. It also creates a foreign-body reaction in the lining of the uterus, which prevents implantation. In addition, progestin-releasing IUDs cause changes in the thickness of the cervical fluid, which doesn't allow the sperm to advance

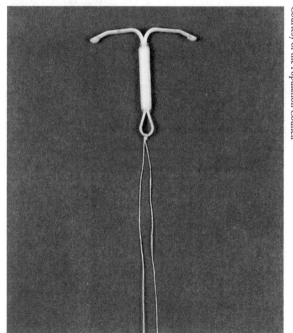

Courtesy of the Population Council

The Mirena IUD

from the vagina into the uterus. If sperm get through, they are less vigorous and less apt to fertilize an egg.

Currently, there are two types of IUDs available: ParaGard and Mirena. The ParaGard, also called the Copper T, has a tiny copper wire wrapped around the plastic body and should not be used by anyone who is allergic to copper. It is approved for use up to ten years. The Mirena releases small amounts of progestin, which decreases the bleeding and cramping that some women have with the copper-bearing IUD. It is approved for use up to five years.

The IUD is now used by more than 160 million women worldwide. It is one of the safest, best tolerated, and most effective methods of contraception available. It is not advised for women who are not in monogamous relationships or whose partners may have STIs.

EFFECTIVENESS

The IUD is 99 percent effective, as effective as tubal sterilization, but is reversible by simply removing the IUD. That means that for every one hundred women using an IUD, fewer than one will become pregnant in one year. IUDs are effective for five to ten years, depending on the type (the ParaGard is effective for twelve years, though approved only for ten years' use at the time of printing).

ADVANTAGES

- Immediately effective
- You don't have to think about contraception for as long as it is in place
- Effective for five to ten years, depending on type
- Does not interrupt sex play
- Does not interfere with breast-feeding
- The cost is very low over the life of the IUD

Though the IUD is the second most widely used method of birth control in the world, it is not popular in the U.S. This is largely due to the fact that in the 1970s, one type of IUD, the Dalkon Shield, was found to be unsafe, causing an increase in pelvic infections among users and resulting in the deaths of twenty women. Thousands of women filed lawsuits, and by 1985 the company had declared bankruptcy. All IUDs were pulled from the market at the time, and the reputation of IUDs was damaged. The IUDs now available are safer and have not been found to increase the risk of pelvic infections for women not at risk of STIs.

DISADVANTAGES

- Does not protect against STIs, including HIV
- Insertion and removal require clinic visits
- Can be expelled
- Can cause heavier than normal menstrual periods (more likely with ParaGard IUD)

HOW TO USE

The IUD needs to be inserted by a trained, skilled medical provider. Ask your provider about her or his experience inserting IUDs.

Providers should always insert the IUD gently. A good time to insert is during menses, when the cervix is dilated. However, IUDs can be inserted at any time in a woman's cycle, provided she has no chance of being pregnant (unless it is within three days of unprotected intercourse and is being used as emergency contraception; see p. 376). The preference for menstrual insertion should not be used to refuse access to the method. The insertion process takes only a few minutes and may cause strong cramping. It is recommended that you take a non-aspirin pain reliever (such as ibuprofen) before you have an IUD inserted. The cramping should go away in a few minutes or hours.

Six weeks after fitting, you should have a return visit with your provider to check the IUD strings and make sure there are no signs of infection. If you experience unusual vaginal bleeding, lower abdominal pain, abnormal discharge, or unexplained fever, you should see your provider as soon as possible.

The ParaGard can also be inserted by a trained provider immediately after childbirth (within forty-eight hours).

Checking IUD Strings

You should check your IUD strings before sex in the first month and then after each period to make sure the IUD has not been expelled. Expulsion is most common in the first three months after insertion. Check the strings by reaching a finger into your vagina and feeling for your cervix. You should be able to feel the strings against your cervix. If you cannot feel your IUD strings, or if you can feel the hard plastic of the IUD at the opening of your cervix, you should abstain from sex or use another contraceptive method until you see your provider to determine whether the IUD is still in place.

Missing Period

If you miss a period while using an IUD, you may want to take a pregnancy test. If you have any concerns about your IUD, call your health care provider.

HEALTH CONCERNS

Due to the risk of serious health problems, you should not use an IUD if you have any of the following conditions:

- Current, recent (in past three months), or repeated pelvic infection
- Known or suspected pregnancy
- Severe infection of the cervix
- Malignant lesions in the genital tract
- Unexplained vaginal bleeding
- HIV/AIDS
- Paralysis
- Physical inability to check IUD

IUDs are not recommended for women who are at risk for STIs, have lower immune response, or have had a recent abnormal Pap smear. Women with valvular heart disease or previous problems with an IUD should talk to a provider before considering an IUD. Women with anemia or a history of severe menstrual cramping and heavy flow should consider using the Mirena IUD to decrease menstrual flow.

Copper IUDs are not recommended for women with Wilson's disease or allergies to copper.

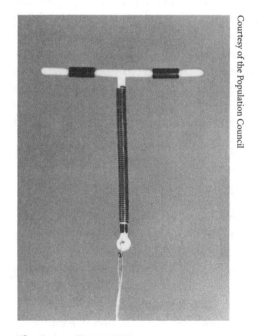

Courtesy of the Population Council

The Copper T 380A IUD

If you have a history of breast cancer, you cannot use the Mirena IUD. If you have diabetes, you should be monitored carefully if you use the Mirena. The Mirena is not recommended if you are breast-feeding, because the hormone will be in your breast milk.

Risks

The risk of pelvic infection from an IUD is very slight among women not at risk of STIs. However, if you have more than one partner, or if your partner has an STI or has sex with anyone else, the IUD may not be an appropriate contraceptive, because you are more likely to get an STI. STIs can lead to pelvic infection, which can cause infertility if untreated. If a pelvic infection does occur, it can be treated with antibiotics. There is no need to remove the IUD unless you choose to have it removed. Testing for STIs before IUD insertion and using condoms for protection against STIs are recommended.

Piercing or perforation of the uterine wall is a very rare event that can occur during IUD insertion (less than one time in a thousand insertions). In general, a partial perforation of the uterine wall heals quickly, and no treatment is required. Very rarely, it can cause more serious complications. More experienced medical providers have much lower rates of perforation.

Over time, an IUD may become imbedded in the uterine wall. An imbedded IUD is still effective, but it can be painful and may need to be removed. There is a risk of surgery and/or sterility if an IUD becomes imbedded, but this situation is rare.

If you become pregnant while using an IUD, have the IUD removed, whether or not you want to carry the pregnancy to term. An IUD in place increases the risk of miscarriage or premature birth.

Because the IUD is so effective in preventing pregnancy, women using IUDs are at lower risk of ectopic pregnancy (when a fertilized egg attaches and grows outside the uterus) than women using less effective contraception or no contraception at all. But if a woman does become pregnant while using an IUD, she is likelier to have an ectopic pregnancy than is a woman who gets pregnant using less effective contraception or no contraception. Ectopic pregnancy can be very dangerous and requires emergency medical attention.

Benefits

The IUD offers very effective protection from unintended pregnancy without systemic side effects. The Mirena IUD decreases menstrual bleeding and cramping. Studies report an 85 percent decrease in blood loss within the first three months of use and a 97 percent decrease by one year. Thirty percent of users stop having menstrual bleeding altogether.

Side Effects

Longer, heavier, and more painful menstrual periods are the most common complaint of ParaGard IUD users. Increased menstrual flow may cause anemia. Spotting between periods is common.

In the first three months of use, prolonged bleeding is also a common complaint with the Mirena. It takes about three months for the lining of the womb to thin down, and during this time, bleeding can be erratic or even heavy at times; it almost always settles down after three to six months. During the first month, 20 percent of users experience bleeding of over eight days in duration, but by the third month, only 3 percent have prolonged bleeding.

The side effects of the Mirena IUD are similar to those of other progestin-containing methods, but are generally less intense, because the effects are more local and the blood levels of progestins

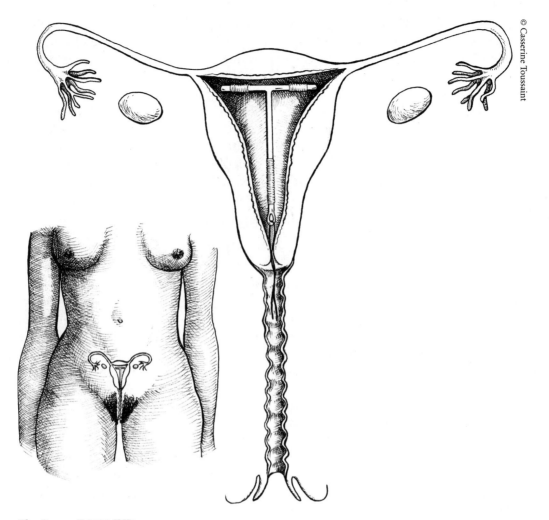

The Copper T 380A IUD

are much lower. The Mirena can cause a slight increase in ovarian cysts (from 0.4 percent to 1.2 percent). These cysts are benign and usually resolve in two to three months. Mirena can cause weight gain, headaches, acne, depression, and decrease in sex drive, but these symptoms are usually less intense than with other hormonal methods.

GETTING PREGNANT LATER

If you want to become pregnant, you may have the IUD removed at any time. Recent research has shown no connection between the use of an IUD and infertility, but for those women who get an STI while using an IUD, the STI may cause infertility. The hormone in Mirena is long-acting, so you may experience a delay in return to menstruation and fertility. Once the hormone is cleared from your body, your fertility returns. While most women who stop using IUDs are able to become pregnant, in very rare cases of perforation, imbedding, or pelvic infection, the uterus or tubes may become damaged and decrease the chance of future pregnancy.

EMERGENCY CONTRACEPTION

You can prevent pregnancy after unprotected intercourse by having a copper IUD inserted within five days of unprotected intercourse. They are 99 percent effective in preventing that pregnancy and can then be left in place as a method of birth control for up to ten years (see p. 376).

TUBAL LIGATION (FEMALE STERILIZATION)

I tried very hard after this last one to convince my husband to let me have my tubes tied, but he was adamant that this is just not happening. His way of thinking, for religious reasons—he is Church of Jesus Christ of the Latter-day Saints—he doesn't want it done. Because it's just not natural for a women to have her tubes tied. And you know, if God wants you to have babies, then you're going to have one. If He doesn't want you to have it, you weren't going to have it. Okay! Well, but it's me that has to carry it for the nine months, you know, with the morning sickness all day long through the whole nine months.

Tubal ligation, commonly known as "getting your tubes tied," is a surgical sterilization technique that closes the fallopian tubes. It stops the egg from traveling to the uterus from the ovary and also prevents sperm from reaching the fallopian tube to fertilize an egg. In this procedure, fallopian tubes are cut, burned, or blocked with rings, bands, or clips. The surgery is effective immediately. Tubal ligation does not protect against reproductive tract infections, including HIV/AIDS.

A tubal ligation is a surgical procedure performed under local or general anesthesia in a clinic, doctor's office, or hospital. Mini-laparotomies and laparoscopy are the two most common techniques. Other procedures include laparotomy, colpotomy, culdoscopy, hysteroscopy, and hysterectomy. Be sure to discuss the risks and benefits of different techniques with your health care provider before deciding which one to use.

In the laparoscopy procedure, the abdomen is filled with carbon dioxide gas so that the abdominal wall balloons away from the uterus and tubes. A laparoscope, a small telescopelike instrument, is inserted into a small cut just below the navel. Another instrument is inserted through an incision just above the pubic hairline to cut, sew, or burn the tubes.

After surgery, take two to three days off and perform only light activities for a week. You may have sex again when you feel comfortable, usually after a week. If you have surgery performed through your vagina, don't put anything into your vagina for two weeks to avoid infection.

EFFECTIVENESS

Tubal ligations are over 99 percent effective as birth control and should be considered permanent.[8]

Sterilization has a long history of abuse. Women with disabilities, poor women, and women of color have been disproportionately targeted for sterilization. Although U.S. federal guidelines now require that special informed consent procedures be followed, the problem of sterilization abuse remains in some places. (For a longer discussion of these abuses, see "Sterilization Abuse" [W44] on the companion website, www.ourbodiesourselves.org.)

A NEW FEMALE STERILIZATION TECHNIQUE

A new female sterilization technique considered to be a major advance over other surgical methods of sterilization involves the insertion into each fallopian tube of a soft, flexible device (Essure) that was approved in 2002 by the U.S. Food and Drug Administration (FDA). This sterilization technique poses fewer risks of complications than other female sterilization methods, according to the studies done so far.

A thin, flexible device is passed through the cervical canal into the uterus, and a doctor inserts a tiny device into each fallopian tube. Once placed in each of the fallopian tubes, the devices expand, and over the course of about three months, fibrous tissue grows into them to block the tubes.

Contraception becomes effective at three months (rather than immediately). In the U.S., the FDA requires a test three months after Essure insertion to confirm that both fallopian tubes are blocked and the devices are in the right place. Rarely, the devices are found to be in the wrong location or are found to have fallen out before fibrosis could occur.

Research has shown that the method blocked both fallopian tubes for 87 percent of 518 women who volunteered to use it. The most common reason for failure was that the doctor could not place the device in one or both fallopian tubes. Most women left the hospital about an hour after the procedure, returning to work the next day. Common side effects included mild uterine cramping or pain, nausea, and light bleeding. More serious complications included, in three women, a vasovagal response (slowing of the heart rate and dilation of the blood vessels, resulting in low blood pressure) and, in two women, fluid overload (the absorption of too much water in the body, which can, in rare instances, lead to serious breathing problems or other complications). However, all five women recovered quickly and did not need to stay overnight in the hospital.

The micro-insert method appears to be highly effective. As of 2003, there were no reports of pregnancy among women who had confirmed blockage of both fallopian tubes following placement of the device. Because of the metallic nature of the Essure device, women should always let doctors know about the device. Some procedures—such as electrocautery of the lining of the uterus—should not be done with a metallic object present. Although research to date has shown the method to be very safe, its relative newness means some risks may not have been identified yet.

ADVANTAGES

- Permanent birth control
- Immediately effective
- Does not interrupt sexual spontaneity
- Requires no daily attention
- Not messy
- Cost-effective in the long run

DISADVANTAGES

- Does not protect against STIs, including HIV
- Requires surgery
- Has risks associated with surgery
- Abnormal bleeding
- Bladder infections
- More complicated than male sterilization

- May not be reversible
- Possible regret

HEALTH CONCERNS

Women are fully able to enjoy sex after a tubal ligation. Usually, hormone levels and a woman's menstrual cycle are not noticeably changed by sterilization. Ovaries continue to release eggs, but the eggs stop in the tubes and are reabsorbed by the body. Some women experience improved sexual pleasure with the end of concerns about becoming pregnant.

Although pregnancy is unlikely after a tubal ligation, there is a slightly higher risk of ectopic pregnancy, compared with a pregnancy occurring in a nonsterilized woman. An ectopic pregnancy occurs when a fertilized egg attaches and grows outside the uterus. This can be very dangerous and requires immediate medical attention. Women who have surgery to reverse tubal ligation and become pregnant also have a higher chance of ectopic pregnancy.

Some women report irregular and painful periods or no periods, midcycle bleeding, lack of interest in sex, and other negative changes after having a tubal ligation.

GETTING PREGNANT LATER

Tubal ligation is considered a permanent method of birth control. Surgery to reverse a tubal ligation is not always effective. In addition, reversal is both difficult and expensive.

VASECTOMY

A vasectomy is a sterilization technique for men. It involves minor surgery to cut the *vasa deferentia,* the tubes that carry sperm from the testes to the penis. This operation keeps sperm from mixing into the semen when men ejaculate, so that sperm cannot fertilize an egg.

Male sterilization is a much more simple process than female sterilization. Usually done in a doctor's office or a clinic, the operation takes under fifteen minutes. The practitioner applies a local anesthetic (such as lidocaine), makes one or two small incisions in the scrotum, locates the two vasa deferentia (singular: vas deferens), removes a piece of each, and ties off the ends. Because sperm are already in the vasa deferentia, men are not sterile immediately. For this reason, it is important to use another method of birth control for two months or until the man has had two negative sperm counts. Since vasectomy does not protect against sexually transmitted infections, men should also continue to use condoms when needed to protect against STIs.

No-scalpel vasectomy is used increasingly throughout the world. It was developed in China, where it is now the standard technique used for vasectomies. In no-scalpel vasectomy, a practitioner uses an instrument to puncture a tiny hole in the scrotum, lifts the vas deferens out through the hole, removes a piece of it, and then ties off or seals the ends. No-scalpel vasectomy is as effective as the scalpel method but has a lower complication rate.[9]

Vasectomy does not affect a man's sexual function. It leaves the man's genital system basically unchanged. His sexual hormones remain operative, and there is no noticeable difference in his ejaculate, because sperm make up only a small part of the semen. Even if they know these facts, some men still worry that a vasectomy will affect their sexual performance. Talking with someone who has had a vasectomy can help relieve such anxieties.

Vasectomy has become increasingly popular over the past thirty years,[10] with about half a million American men having the surgery each year.[11] Men often choose vasectomy after the failure of another birth control method; when they want to spare their partner from more invasive surgery (female sterilization); or because they want to have complete control over their fertility.[12] Nearly 15 percent of U.S. married couples use vasectomy as their contraceptive,[13] and in some countries, such as New Zealand, almost half of the men over forty have opted for it.[14]

Recent advances have meant that some vasectomies can be reversed through an expensive microsurgical procedure. However, the longer a man has had his vasectomy, the lower the chance of success. Pregnancy rates after a vasectomy reversal vary widely; even a skilled surgeon may have only a 30 percent success rate.[15] Vasectomy should be considered permanent.

EFFECTIVENESS

Vasectomy should be considered permanent and is over 99 percent effective.

ADVANTAGES

- Permanent birth control
- Does not interrupt sexual spontaneity
- Requires no daily attention
- Does not affect pleasure
- Not messy
- Less complicated than female sterilization

DISADVANTAGES

- Does not protect against STIs, including HIV
- Not immediately effective
- Requires minor surgery
- Possible rejoining of the vas deferens
- May not be reversible
- Possible regret

EXPERIMENTAL MALE CONTRACEPTIVES

Since vasectomies are not reliably reversible, researchers are experimenting with new male contraceptives. The method closest to market in the U.S. is a male hormonal contraceptive (MHC), which probably will not be available until 2008. While it is often called the "male Pill," this contraceptive will be administered by injections or implants. Researchers are close to making an MHC as effective as the Pill, with a similar range of side effects.

Another method of male contraception close to market in India is called reversible inhibition of sperm under guidance, or RISUG. This involves injecting into the vas deferens a novel substance that makes sperm infertile. It is highly effective, begins acting immediately, has few reported side effects, and provides ten years of contraception. RISUG is very promising, but long-term reversibility rates in humans are still unknown.[16]

Several other promising methods of male contraception await further research and development. Both wet heat (a specific regimen of hot, shallow testicular baths) and miglustat (an oral compound) show promise. Since private industry stands to gain little profit from either of these contraceptive methods, the initiative for more research must come from public pressure.

ABSTINENCE

Some of us define abstinence as not having any sexual contact with another person. Others of us consider ourselves abstinent when we don't have intercourse, but engage in sexual practices such as hugging, caressing, or touching a partner's genitals. This section uses the terms *complete abstinence* and *lovemaking without intercourse* (sometimes called outercourse) to differentiate between these two kinds of abstinence.

EFFECTIVENESS

Complete, continuous abstinence is 100 percent effective.

Lovemaking without intercourse is 100 percent effective if no semen enters your vagina.

ADVANTAGES

Complete Abstinence

- The most effective form of birth control
- No physical side effects
- Protects against STIs
- Free

Lovemaking without Intercourse

- Highly effective form of birth control
- Free
- Allows you to experience sexual pleasure with a partner without risking pregnancy

DISADVANTAGES

Complete Abstinence

- Going without sex for long periods of time can be difficult for many of us.
- If our commitment wavers, we may become sexually active without protecting ourselves against pregnancy and STIs.

Lovemaking without Intercourse

- Slight risk of pregnancy if semen gets close to your vagina
- Risk of transmitting an STI

YOUR HEALTH

Women who abstain from intercourse are less likely to:

- Get a sexually transmitted infection
- Have an unplanned pregnancy
- Become infertile
- Develop cervical cancer[17]

Many of us who are abstinent will have intercourse at some time in our lives. If you're considering intercourse, take time to educate yourself about birth control options and safer sex, rather than making a spontaneous decision during a passionate moment.

FERTILITY AWARENESS METHOD (FAM) AND OTHER NATURAL METHODS

FAM is a scientifically validated method of natural birth control that involves charting fertility signs to determine whether or not you are fertile on any given day. Fertility awareness can also be used to achieve pregnancy or for greater body awareness in general. (For more information, see p. 245 in Chapter 13, "Sexual Anatomy, Reproduction, and the Menstrual Cycle.")

HOW NATURAL METHODS WORK

By charting one or more of your primary fertility signs (waking temperature, cervical fluid, and cervical position), you can determine which phase of the cycle you are currently in. Unlike the obsolete rhythm (or calendar) method, which relies on past cycles to predict future fertility, FAM effectively identifies your fertile phase, the time when ovulation is impending, and when it has occurred. You can then use your

THE DIFFERENCE AMONG NATURAL METHODS OF BIRTH CONTROL

	RHYTHM METHOD	STANDARD DAYS METHOD (SDM)	BILLINGS (OVULATION) METHOD	BBT (BASAL BODY TEMPERATURE) METHOD	FAM/NFP* (SYMPTO-THERMAL METHOD)
Fertility Signs That Are Observed	None	None	Cervical fluid	Waking temperature	Waking temperature, cervical fluid, and (optionally) cervical position
Comments	An obsolete method based on a mathematical formula using past cycle lengths to predict future fertile phases.	A variation of the rhythm method, in which unprotected intercourse is avoided on days 8 through 19 in women with consistent menstrual cycles between 26 to 32 days long. It is risky if a woman's cycle deviates from that range.	Because only cervical fluid is observed, you do not have the benefit of a thermal shift to confirm that ovulation has indeed occurred.	Because only temperature is observed, the first day of your cycle that you are considered safe is not until the third night after an obvious temperature shift.	Because the primary fertility signs are observed, as well as secondary signs (such as ovulatory pain or mid-cycle spotting), this method is considered the most comprehensive and reliable.

* Fertility awareness method (FAM) and natural family planning (NFP) are based on the same biological principles, but NFP is taught in a religious context, whereas FAM is nonsectarian. NFP rejects the use of any artificial contraception, including barrier methods, as well as nonprocreative sex and sex outside of heterosexual marriage. Those who practice FAM allow themselves to use a barrier method during fertile times.

daily fertility observations to know whether or not you are safe for unprotected intercourse on any given day.

Couples can choose to either abstain or use a barrier method during the woman's fertile phase. It should be understood, though, that if you choose to have intercourse using a barrier method during your fertile phase, FAM cannot be any more effective than the barrier itself.

It is beyond the scope of this chapter to explain the rules of FAM adequately. Refer to "Resources" for further information on how to use FAM as a method of birth control and to locate a qualified instructor in your area. (For more information on FAM, see p. 245.)

EFFECTIVENESS

If used perfectly by a motivated couple who abstain during the fertile phase (as is done with natural family planning), the effectiveness rate is approximately 98 percent over the course of a typical year for those couples who practice the symptothermal method (STM), which is the method that involves charting all three of the primary fertility signs. Various studies show that natural family planning effectiveness rates vary greatly, but 88 to 90 percent per year is about the average reported in the medical literature for STM. (The Billings method is not as effective as STM; while the BBT method is as effective as STM, that's only because women must consider themselves fertile, and thus abstain or use barriers, for the entire pre-ovulatory phase.) Ultimately, natural methods of contraception are most appropriate for strongly motivated women and couples who can commit to learning the method thoroughly and following the rules consistently.

ADVANTAGES

- No health risks or side effects
- Promotes healthful body awareness and information about gynecological health, hormonal balance, and fertility
- Promotes communication and responsibility between partners
- Allows for loving cooperation and male involvement
- Can increase a woman's awareness and understanding of her body
- After the cost of initial instruction, FAM and NFP cost nothing to practice

DISADVANTAGES

- To learn it correctly usually requires taking a class or reading a book, and it takes about two cycles to assimilate FAM's basic principles (the information presented here is not enough to effectively use FAM as a method of birth control)
- Does not protect against STIs, including HIV
- Requires considerable commitment, cooperation, and self-control, by both you and your partner
- Typical failure rate is higher than with other methods

- Can be challenging to practice while breast-feeding due to extended periods of potential fertility
- Takes a few minutes a day to take your temperature and chart your fertility signs

NEW TECHNOLOGIES

New technologies such as calculators, computer programs, saliva tests, and urine tests are becoming increasingly available to the public to help determine fertility. However, these high-tech methods are more appropriate for women who are trying to achieve pregnancy rather than avoid it. This is because most of these methods do not give you enough warning of impending ovulation to account for the possibility of sperm living up to five days beforehand.

BREAST-FEEDING AS BIRTH CONTROL

Breast-feeding can inhibit ovulation, and thus can work as a natural form of child spacing, but the *way* in which a woman breast-feeds is the primary factor in determining when fertility returns. You should never assume that you are infertile simply because you are breast-feeding. Frequency of feedings (not duration), the use of pacifiers, whether or not food or liquid other than breast milk is given to your baby, whether you sleep with your baby, and even the practice of a daily nap with your baby all influence your postpartum fertility.

A woman who wishes to practice a form of natural contraception following birth has several options.

- If you are breast-feeding, you may practice the lactational amenorrhea method (LAM), described briefly below, which applies to the first six months of breast-feeding.

- If you are breast-feeding, you may also practice fertility awareness, which, although more complicated than LAM, can be used throughout the return of your fertility, as well as afterward, if desired. The rules for practicing fertility awareness while breast-feeding differ from those used in other circumstances and are not described in this book but can be learned from a FAM or NFP instructor or from a very few books.
- If you are bottle feeding, you can still practice fertility awareness, but your fertility will return more quickly than it would if you were to breast-feed.

You can practice LAM if you meet the following three criteria:

- Your menses have not returned since childbirth.
- You are fully or nearly fully breast-feeding.
- Your baby is under six months old.

The first criterion of LAM is that you have not resumed menstruating. If you are breast-feeding, any vaginal bleeding before the fifty-sixth day after birth is almost always anovulatory (meaning no ovulation has taken place) and therefore can be ignored. Any bleeding after the fifty-sixth day should be considered a sign of resumed ovulation. However, if at any point you notice the return of cervical fluid; a wet vaginal sensation; or a high, soft, and open cervix, you should consider yourself fertile. If you do not know the rules for practicing fertility awareness while breast-feeding, you will need to use another method of birth control from this point forward.

Full breast-feeding means that you are not giving your baby any supplemental feeding. The contraceptive effectiveness of LAM is maintained if you are nearly fully breast-feeding, meaning that you supplement no more than 15

percent of all feedings. Full or nearly full breast-feeding means that intervals between feedings should not exceed four hours during the day or six hours at night. However, the shorter the intervals between feedings, and the closer you keep your baby to you, the more likely it is that you will remain infertile. Similarly, not giving your baby pacifiers, bottles, or foods and liquids other than breast milk will help you remain infertile.

To further increase the effectiveness of LAM, some instructors suggest that you nurse once or twice per hour during the day and several times at night during the baby's first few months. While that may seem excessive, it will usually create unambiguous infertility, meaning that you will have "dry cervical fluid" (essentially no wetness) and a dry vaginal sensation. Once you have established this dryness, you can usually nurse less frequently after the first few months and still maintain dryness indicative of infertility.

If you do not meet the LAM criteria, it is best to use another method of birth control.

ADVANTAGES

- Can be used immediately after childbirth
- Protects baby against allergies, asthma, and other ailments
- No cost

SUITABLE CONTRACEPTIVE METHODS TO USE WHILE BREAST-FEEDING

- Barrier methods
- Copper T IUD
- Depo-Provera injection
- FAM/LAM
- Mini-Pills (progesterone-only pills)

DISADVANTAGES

- No protection against STIs, including HIV
- Sexual pleasure may be affected negatively if breasts become tender

WITHDRAWAL (PULLING OUT)

Withdrawal involves removing the penis from the vagina just before ejaculation so that the sperm is deposited outside the vagina and away from the lips of the vagina. It is also called "pulling out." Pregnancy is possible if semen or pre-ejaculate is spilled on the vulva. Withdrawal offers no protection against sexually transmitted infections.

This method—while better than using nothing—is generally not recommended for couples unless they have been together for years and are willing to cope with an unintended pregnancy. Here are some of the reasons that withdrawal fails to work for many couples:

- Some men cannot tell when they are going to ejaculate.
- Some men ejaculate very quickly, before they realize it.
- Before ejaculation, almost all penises leak fluid containing sperm that can cause pregnancy.
- Some men lack the experience and self-control to pull out in time.
- Some men have been known to say they will pull out, but they get so excited and carried away that they don't.
- Some men have been known to say they will pull out, but they don't mean it.
- Women may have a harder time enjoying themselves because they worry about whether the partner will pull out in time.
- For both partners, the interruption of sexual pleasure is frustrating.

EFFECTIVENESS

Withdrawal is 81 to 96 percent effective as birth control, depending on how perfectly it is done. With typical use, nineteen of every hundred women whose partners use withdrawal will become pregnant during the first year. With perfect use, four of every hundred women whose partners use withdrawal will become pregnant during the first year. Pre-ejaculate can contain enough sperm to cause pregnancy. Pregnancy is also possible if semen or pre-ejaculate is spilled on the vulva.

ADVANTAGES

- Withdrawal can be used to prevent pregnancy when no other method is available.

DISADVANTAGES

- Does not protect against STIs, including HIV/AIDS
- Interrupts spontaneity
- Requires a great deal of self-control, experience, and trust
- May leave one or both partners very frustrated
- Not for men who ejaculate prematurely
- Not for men who don't know when to pull out
- Not recommended for sexually inexperienced men
- Not recommended for teens

HOW TO USE

The man withdraws his penis from the vagina before or when he feels he has reached the point when ejaculation can no longer be stopped or postponed. He ejaculates outside the vagina, being careful that semen does not spill onto his partner's vulva. Couples who have established great self-control, experience, and trust may use withdrawal if necessary. The men who use withdrawal must be able to know when they are reaching ejaculatory inevitability—the point in sexual excitement when ejaculation can no longer be stopped or postponed.

EMERGENCY CONTRACEPTION

- "The condom broke."
- "I didn't think we were going to have sex."
- "I didn't realize I had forgotten to take my pill."
- "I was raped."

It is always best to plan ahead and prevent an unintended pregnancy, but when we find ourselves at risk of a pregnancy that is unwanted, sometimes we need another option. Fortunately, we are no longer limited to waiting and worrying. There are now at least three safe and effective methods available to prevent an unplanned pregnancy even after sex has taken place. *Combined birth control pills, progestin-only pills, and IUDs can all be used for emergency contraception.*

WHAT IS EMERGENCY CONTRACEPTION (EC)?

Unlike regular methods of birth control that must be used before sex takes place, emergency contraception prevents pregnancy after sex has occurred. EC does not work if a woman is already pregnant. It does not cause abortion.[18] EC does not protect against sexually transmitted infections.

Emergency contraception pills (ECPs) have been used for several decades, yet most women and many providers still do not know that they are available and effective. In 1997 the FDA concluded that ordinary birth control pills were safe and effective for emergency contraception, paving the way for manufacturers to market

Anti-choice groups oppose EC and claim it is abortion, which ends a pregnancy, instead of contraception, which prevents one. However, EC works either by preventing ovulation or by preventing implantation of a fertilized egg in the uterus. The international medical community has said that pregnancy begins with implantation, so EC acts before pregnancy even occurs.

them as morning-after pills. It is estimated that if more women knew about and were able to get emergency contraception when needed, we could prevent 1.7 million unintended pregnancies and 800,000 abortions annually.

ECPs are available in some nations, such as France and Canada, without prescription. At the time of this writing, ECPs are available over the counter in a few states in the U.S., and several states have legislation pending to mandate that hospitals provide ECPs to victims of sexual assault. In 2004 the FDA rejected its medical board's recommendation to make ECPs available over the counter for all women. To learn more, see the ACLU Reproductive Rights web page: www.aclu.org/Reproductive Rights/ ReproductiveRightsMain.cfm.

EMERGENCY CONTRACEPTIVE PILLS (ECPS)

ECPs (also known as "post-coital contraception" or the "morning-after pill") work by changing a woman's hormone levels. They give the body a short, high burst of synthetic hormones that disrupt hormone patterns needed for pregnancy. This prevents pregnancy by inhibiting ovulation or by disrupting egg and sperm transport, fertilization, or implantation. Most women can safely use emergency contraceptive pills even if we cannot use birth control pills as our regular method of birth control. ECPs can be used within five days of unprotected sexual intercourse. The sooner after unprotected intercourse they are taken, the more effective they are.

It is not advisable to use ECPs as your only protection against pregnancy if you are sexually active or planning to be, because they are not as effective as other contraceptive methods. Using ECPs frequently won't hurt you, but it will get expensive (see the chart on p. 378 for a comparison of costs associated with methods of birth control).

There are currently two types of emergency contraceptive pills: pills that contain only progestin, and pills that contain both progestin and estrogen. (Mifepristone, or RU-486, can also be used for postcoital contraception. It is more effective—it has a lower pregnancy rate and fewer side effects than currently available pills— but has not been approved in the U.S. for this use.)[19]

Progestin-Only Pills

Progestin-only ECPs (Plan B, Mini-Pill) are slightly more effective than combination pills and cause few if any side effects. The brand Plan B is available through health care providers and, in some states, without a prescription in pharmacies.

Estrogen and Progestin

The second type of EC (combined ECPs, Preven) uses combination birth control pills in a higher dose. A few products have been studied and approved for this use, but it is likely that any available pill could be effective. This method often causes nausea and discomfort, but many women believe that the possible protection is worth it. One brand name specially packaged for use as emergency contraception is called Preven.

HEALTH CONCERNS

Even though the hormones used for emergency contraception are the same as those in some birth control pills, they are used for such a short time that most women can take them safely, and no long-term complications have been reported. If you have a serious health problem that prevents you from taking regular birth control pills, consult a health care provider. If you could be pregnant already, it is a good idea to have a pregnancy test before using emergency contraception. ECPs should not be used by women who are already pregnant—not because the pills are thought to be harmful, but because they are ineffective at terminating established pregnancies.

If after taking both doses of the pills, you become pregnant anyway, there is no evidence of potential danger to the fetus.

HOW TO USE

Some people call emergency contraceptive pills "morning-after pills." But you do not have to wait until the morning after. You can start the pills right away or up to five days after you have had unprotected sex—that is, sex during which you did not use birth control or your birth control may have failed. The sooner ECPs are started within the five-day (120-hour) window the more effective they are. Taken within twenty-four hours, EC is up to 95 percent effective.

HOW TO TAKE PROGESTIN-ONLY PILLS AS EC

Take both pills as soon after unprotected sex as possible. The packaging on Plan B may still advise you to take one pill and then wait twelve hours to take the second pill, but recent studies show that the pills are more effective when taken together.

EFFECTIVENESS

Plan B reduces the chance of pregnancy by 89 to 95 percent. (If a hundred women had unprotected intercourse once during the second or third week of their cycle, about eight would become pregnant; following treatment with Plan B, only one would become pregnant: an 89 percent reduction.) Plan B is 89 percent effective for all women who take the pills within the first three days. Taking the pill within the first twenty-four hours may increase effectiveness to as much as 95 percent.

HOW TO TAKE COMBINED ESTROGEN AND PROGESTIN PILLS AS EC

Directions for taking Preven are similar to Plan B (see package directions). There are currently at least twenty-one brands of birth control pills that can be used for emergency contraception. To determine which pills you can use and the proper dose for each, visit: http://ec.princeton.edu/questions/dose.html or www.not-2-late.com, or call the Emergency Contraception Hotline: 1-800-584-9911.

EFFECTIVENESS

Use of this type of EC reduces the chance of pregnancy by 75 percent (see "Effectiveness" for Plan B, above, for details).

Side Effects

Progestin-only pills and Plan B have few or no side effects. Nausea and vomiting are the most common negative effects when taking emergency pills that contain both estrogen and progestin; about half the women who take them feel nauseated, and about 20 percent vomit. For this reason, some practitioners advise taking the pills with food or with an anti-nausea medication such as an over-the-counter remedy for motion sickness. Other negative effects include breast tenderness, dizziness, abdominal pain, and headaches. Using combination pills for emergency contraception may also change the timing of your next menstrual period: It may begin a few days earlier or a few days later than usual.

HOW TO USE THE IUD AS EC

A copper IUD has proved very effective at preventing pregnancy if inserted within seven days after unprotected intercourse. The IUD probably works by preventing the implantation of a fertilized egg. Once inserted into the uterus, a copper IUD can be left in place and used as your regular method of birth control for up to ten years. Women who should not use the IUD for birth control (see p. 362) should not use it for emergency contraception, either.

EFFECTIVENESS

Using a Copper T IUD within seven days of unprotected sex reduces the risk of pregnancy by over 99 percent.

Risks

Many women can use IUDs as EC, but IUD use is not recommended for all women. In general, you should not use an IUD if you are pregnant; have an STI such as HIV, chlamydia, or gonorrhea; or have a recent history of pelvic inflammatory disease (PID). Your health care provider will discuss these issues with you before inserting an IUD.

WHERE TO GET EMERGENCY CONTRACEPTION

Emergency contraception is available in family planning clinics, health care providers' offices, and, in some states, at pharmacies. You can ask your provider to write you a prescription in advance so you have it on hand if you need it. The IUD must be inserted by a trained provider.

FREQUENTLY ASKED QUESTIONS

- *What is my risk of pregnancy from unprotected intercourse?* The likelihood of becoming pregnant after a single act of unprotected intercourse is low. Depending on where you are in your menstrual cycle and on your body's ability to conceive, the likelihood is between 0 and 20 percent. Yet almost any act of unprotected intercourse entails some risk of pregnancy, and EC reduces this risk substantially.

  With a single act of unprotected intercourse, the risk of either partner transmitting a bacterial STI—such as gonorrhea, chlamydia, or trichomoniasis—is much higher than the risk of the woman becoming pregnant. Emergency contraception does not reduce the risk of STIs.
- *What if I engage in unprotected sex but ejaculation does not occur? Is sperm present in pre-ejaculatory fluid?* The chance of pregnancy is probably extremely low. Two small studies found no motile sperm in pre-ejaculatory fluid, but that is the only evidence. However, HIV *can* be detected in pre-ejaculatory fluid. If you are worried about the possibility of pregnancy, or if you are not sure whether ejaculation did occur, ECPs should do no harm and may do some good.
- *When should my next period come after I take emergency contraceptive pills?* After taking ECPs, some women have a period early, and some women have irregular bleeding that is not really a period. The duration of the irregular bleeding is not predictable. You should have another, normal period within the next month. If not, you should get a pregnancy test just to make sure you're not pregnant.

- *What if I have sex after taking emergency contraceptive pills?* Emergency contraceptive pills will not protect against pregnancy from unprotected intercourse that occurs after the pills are taken.
- *Is there a limit to the number of times emergency contraceptive pills can be used?* There are no safety concerns with using ECPs repeatedly. However, ECPs are not as effective as many other methods of contraception. EC is also expensive to use repeatedly. Repeated use suggests that you need to find an ongoing method of contraception that you can use correctly and consistently.

For free information about preventing pregnancy after unprotected sex and to obtain names and telephone numbers of health care professionals in your area who can provide emergency contraception, call the Emergency Contraception Hotline: 1-800-584-9911.

When looking at effectiveness rates cited for each method listed here, keep in mind that there is a difference between the lowest expected failure rate—which is based on consistent and correct use of the method—and the higher typical failure rate, based on records of actual use of the method over time. Typical user failure rates include accidents such as forgetting a pill, failing to put on a condom early enough, and removing a diaphragm within six hours after intercourse. The typical failure rate will give you a more realistic idea of how effective the method is and will help you to consider the crucial question of how effectively you and your partner will use it.

COMPARING BIRTH CONTROL METHODS

METHOD	EFFECTIVENESS: NUMBER OF WOMEN IN 100 WHO WILL BECOME PREGNANT IN ONE YEAR WITH PERFECT USE*	EFFECTIVENESS: NUMBER OF WOMEN IN 100 WHO WILL BECOME PREGNANT IN ONE YEAR WITH TYPICAL USE**	STI PROTECTION	AVERAGE COST	COST PER YEAR
No Method	85	85	None		
Barrier Methods					
Male Latex Condom	3	14	Good	$.50–$3 each use	Dependent on use
Female Latex Condom	5	21	Good	$.50–$3 each use	Dependent on use
Diaphragm	6	20	Some	$100–$200 for method and fitting	$35–$65
Cervical Cap (no previous births)	9	20	Some	$100–$200 for method and fitting	$35–$65
Cervical Cap (previous births)	26	40	Some	$100–$200 for method and fitting	$35–$65
Spermicides (gel, foam, suppository, film)	6	26	Some	$.50–$3 each use	Dependent on use
Hormonal Methods					
Combined Pill	Fewer than 1	5	None	$20–$35 a month	$240–$420
Seasonale	Fewer than 1	n/a	None	$20–$35 a month	$240–$420
Progestin-only Pill	Fewer than 1	5	None	$20–$35 a month	$240–$420
Contraceptive Patch	Fewer than 1	n/a	None	$20–$35 a month	$240–$420
Vaginal Ring	Fewer than 1	n/a	None	$35–$40 a month	$420–$480
Injection (one month, Lunelle)	Fewer than 1	n/a	None	$20–$35 a month ($1,600 over 5 years)	$240–$420
Injection (three months, Depo-Provera)	Fewer than 1	Fewer than 1	None	$60–$75 for 3 months ($1,070 over 5 years)	$240–$300
Implant (Norplant)	Fewer than 1	Fewer than 1	None	$450–$750 over five years	$90–$150

(continued)

METHOD	EFFECTIVENESS: NUMBER OF WOMEN IN 100 WHO WILL BECOME PREGNANT IN ONE YEAR WITH PERFECT USE*	EFFECTIVENESS: NUMBER OF WOMEN IN 100 WHO WILL BECOME PREGNANT IN ONE YEAR WITH TYPICAL USE**	STI PROTECTION	AVERAGE COST	COST PER YEAR
Intrauterine Devices (IUDs)					
Copper T	Fewer than 1	Fewer than 1	None	$200-$300 over 10-12 years	$20-$30
Mirena– Progestin IUD	1.5	2	None	$395 over 5 years	$79
Female Sterilization					
Tubal Ligation	Fewer than 1	Fewer than 1	None	$2,500-5,000	n/a
Essure	Fewer than 1	Fewer than 1	None	$2,500-5,000	n/a
Sterilization					
Male Sterilization	Fewer than 1	Fewer than 1	None	$250-$400	n/a
Natural Methods					
Fertility Awareness	1-9	25	None	No cost	No cost
Breast-feeding	Within 6 months of birth, 1	Within 6 months of birth, 1	None	No cost	No cost
Withdrawal	4	19	None	No cost	No cost
Emergency Contraception					
Pills	Initiated within 72 hours of unprotected intercourse, reduces risk of pregnancy by 75-89 percent. Can be initiated within 120 hours of unprotected intercourse.		None	$15-$35	Dependent on use
IUD Insertion for Emergency Contraception	Inserted within seven days after unprotected intercourse, reduces the risk of pregnancy by over 99 percent.			$200-300 but can be used for up to 12 years	Dependent on use

* Perfect use refers to failure rates for women and men whose use is consistent and always correct.

** Typical use refers to failure rates for women and men whose use is neither consistent nor always correct.

NOTES

1. Linda Gordon, *The Moral Property of Women: A History of Birth Control Politics in America* (Chicago: University of Illinois Press, 2000).

2. M. F. Gallo, D. A. Grimes, K. F. Schulz, "Non-latex Versus Latex Male Condoms for Contraception," *Cochrane Review* 4 (2004).

3. The most recent data on spermicide effectiveness is available from a National Institutes of Health randomized trial of five N-9 spermicides. See E. G. Raymond, P. L. Chen, J. Luoto, "Contraceptive Effectiveness and Safety of Five Nonoxynol-9 Spermicides: A Randomized Trial," *Obstetrics and Gynecology* 103 (2004): 430–39.

4. This apparent increased risk of cervical cancer may be due to other reasons, such as having more sexual partners. U.S. Department of Health and Human Services, Food and Drug Administration, and Center for Drug Evaluation and Research, "Guidance for Industry: Labeling for Combined Oral Contraceptives," March 2004, Revision 1: 6, 19, accessed at www.fda.gov/cder/guidance/5197dft.doc on October 20, 2004.

5. M. D. Althuis, D. D. Brogan, R. J. Coates, et al., "Breast Cancers Among Very Young Premenopausal Women (United States)," *Cancer Causes and Control* 14, no. 2 (2003): 151–60.

6. World Health Organization, "Progestin-only Contraceptives," *Medical Eligibility Criteria for Contraceptive Use* (2004): 13, accessed at www.who.int/reproductive-health/publications/MEC_3/mec.pdf on October 25, 2004.

7. More detailed health concerns about the Mini-Pill may be found at World Health Organization, "Progestin-only Contraceptives," *Medical Eligibility Criteria for Contraceptive Use* (2004): 14, accessed at www.who.int/reproductive-health/publications/MEC_3/mec.pdf on October 25, 2004.

8. The Collaborative Review of Sterilization (CREST) study found that the failure rate for tubal ligation tends to increase with the time since the procedure was done (about 2 percent after ten years). See H. B. Peterson, G. Jeng, S. G. Folger, S. A. Hillis, P. A. Marchbanks, and L. S. Wilcox, U.S. Collaborative Review of Sterilization Working Group, "The Risk of Menstrual Abnormalities After Tubal Sterilization," *New England Journal of Medicine* 343, no. 23 (2000): 1681–87.

9. B. Xu and W. Huang, "No-scalpel Vasectomy Outside China," *Asian Journal of Andrology* 2 (2000): 21–24.

10. A. Chandra, "Surgical Sterilization in the United States: Prevalence and Characteristics, 1965–95." National Center for Health Statistics *Vital Health Statistics* 23, no. 20 (1998): 14.

11. J. M. Haws, G. T. Morgan, A. E. Pollack, L. M. Koonin, R. J. Magnani, P. M. Gargiullo, "Clinical Aspects of Vasectomies Performed in the United States in 1995," *Urology* 52, no. 4 (October 1998): 685–91.

12. P. J. Schwingl and H. A. Guess, "Safety and Effectiveness of Vasectomy," *Fertility and Sterility* 73, no. 5 (2000): 923–36.

13. J. M. Haws, et al.

14. M. J. Sneyd, B. Cox, C. Paul, D. C. Skegg, "High Prevalence of Vasectomy in New Zealand," *Contraception* 64, no. 3 (2001): 155–59.

15. I. Schroeder-Printzen, Th. Diemer, W. Weidner, "Vasovasostomy," *Urologia Internationalis* 70 (2003): 101–7.

16. K. M. J. Thompson, "Male Contraceptives Information Center: Experimental Methods." December 2003, accessed at www.malecontraceptives.org/methods/index.htm on October 25, 2004.

17. Planned Parenthood Federation of America, "Is Abstinence Right for You Now?" (2000), accessed at www.plannedparenthood.org/bc/abstinence.html on October 28, 2004.

18. World Health Organization, "Emergency Contraception," Fact Sheet 244 (2000), accessed at www.who.int/mediacentre/factsheets/fs244/en/print.html on October 20, 2004.

19. H. von Hertzen, G. Piaggio, J. Ding, J. Chen, S. Song, G. Bartfai, et al., "Low Dose Mifepristone and Two Regimens of Levonorgestrel for Emergency Contraception: A WHO Multicentre Randomised Trial," *Lancet* 360 (2002): 1807.

CHAPTER 19

Are you worried that you might be pregnant? You are among friends. At one time or another in our lives, almost half of all women become pregnant without planning.[1] Chances are that you just cannot believe you could be pregnant, whether you want a child or not.

If you think you are pregnant, the first step is to try to pinpoint the first day of your last period. The next step is to take a pregnancy test. While you may feel joyful and excited about the possibility of becoming a mother, you may also feel shocked, embarrassed, ashamed, or incompetent. You may not be sure if you want to be a parent right now. Early confirmation, especially within the first month, will provide you with the greatest number of options.

If you are afraid of the results, it is helpful to find someone equipped to give you the support you need. As you make your way through the process of finding out and deciding among your options, you have the right to receive whatever support and advice you want, and the right to make your own decisions.

If you *are* pregnant, you might know what you want to do immediately, or you might find it an agonizing decision. Many of us change our minds once we are faced with the reality of being pregnant, even if we thought we knew what we would do. Be gentle with yourself. Remember that there is help to guide you through this time, regardless of your circumstances.

SIGNS OF PREGNANCY

Early signs of pregnancy vary from woman to woman, and even from one pregnancy to the next in the same woman. Here are a few signs many women experience:

- A missed, lighter, or shorter menstrual period than usual
- Breast tenderness or enlargement
- Nipple sensitivity
- Frequent urination
- Feeling unusually tired
- Nausea and/or vomiting
- Feeling bloated
- Cramps
- Increased or decreased appetite
- Feeling more emotional than usual

There may be other reasons besides pregnancy that you are experiencing some of the above. If you do not want to be pregnant, do not assume that you are; use birth control until you take the test.

FINDING OUT

Any woman who has begun her period, has not experienced menopause, and who has vaginal intercourse with a man can become pregnant unexpectedly. Whether you are fourteen or forty-five, every method of birth control can fail, even tubal ligation. It is possible, though very rare, for you to become pregnant without intercourse if the man's sperm got near the entrance of your vagina. If you suspect you are pregnant now, try to take a test within the next twenty-four hours.

If it is under seventy-two hours from the time of intercourse or rape, you can prevent pregnancy by using emergency contraception. Call your health care provider or the Emergency Contraception Hotline: 1-800-584-9911.

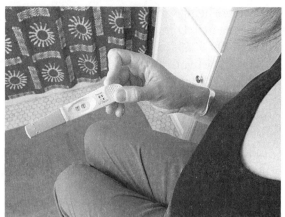

At age 45, I thought I knew my body well; you think you've got it covered. I was tired a lot, and my period was light, but I didn't even consider it. A colleague asked, "Could you be pregnant?" I bought a test and did it at lunch. I was so rattled I turned it upside down, and it said I wasn't pregnant. I did another the next day. It was positive. *

THE TEST

A simple way to find out is to take a home pregnancy test, which tests your first urination of the day. The test is easy to use, available in the family planning section of drugstores, and costs between $6 and $12. Follow the directions exactly. The test can detect pregnancy starting at the time of your missed period, about two weeks after ovulation.

Family planning clinics, women's health centers, and medical offices offer both urine and blood tests. A blood test can detect pregnancy six to eight days after ovulation.[6] Both tests, known as monoclonal antibody tests, detect human chorionic gonadotropin (hCG), a hormone present first in the bloodstream and then in urine during pregnancy. Be cautious about assuming that a negative urine result means you are not pregnant. Test results can be negative be-

cause the test wasn't performed correctly or because you tested too early in the pregnancy for the hCG levels to be detected.

Be aware that some clinics, sometimes called pregnancy crisis centers or abortion alternatives, offer free testing and counseling to frighten you away from considering abortion, or to convince you to choose adoption with their agency. When you seek testing, medical care, or counseling, it is normal to feel both greatly relieved and vulnerable. Professionals, consciously or not, may also treat you with some bias depending on how they perceive your age, marital status, race, disability, or other factors. No matter what your circumstance, you should receive advice that clarifies your needs and desires and does not presume anything about your life.

A SIGH OF RELIEF

If you suspected that you were pregnant but turn out not to be—and you don't want to become pregnant—here are some tips to avoid unwanted pregnancies:

- Find out if there are contraceptive methods more suited for you; there are continual improvements and choices. (See Chapter 18, "Birth Control.")

---

* To read additional personal stories of girls and women who had unexpected pregnancies, see "Unexpected Pregnancies" (W45) on the companion website, www.ourbodiesourselves.org.

- If you are being sexually abused, get help. Call the National Domestic Violence Hotline at 1-800-799-7233, or the Rape, Abuse & Incest National Network at 1-800-656-HOPE (4673), and see Chapter 8, "Violence and Abuse."
- Learn where to get emergency contraception. You may want to keep a package on hand as a backup.
- Talk with a counselor at a women's health or family planning clinic.

A SIGH OF REGRET

If you are not pregnant but realize that you wish you were, you now have time to prepare. To learn more about preconception care and conceiving a child, see Chapter 17, "Considering Parenting."

IT IS CONFIRMED: YOU ARE PREGNANT

If you learn that you are pregnant, you will need time to adjust to the news and the vast range of emotions that follow. Even if you are thrilled about being pregnant, you and/or your partner may feel emotionally, spiritually, or economically unprepared to become parents now. Trust yourself; you can discover what is best for you. Quiet reflection, talking with close friends or family, counseling, and writing can help you think through your possibilities.

TAKING A LONG TIME TO FIND OUT

It is not unusual to be more than two months into a pregnancy before we realize it. Our culture and family upbringing may influence how we interpret the changes in our body. Many of us think we have digestive problems, stress, or the flu. Some of us have taken so many risks without conceiving, or tried for so long without luck, that we think we are infertile. For some of us, it is unthinkable, and we just do not accept the signs. For others, we do not want to make decisions about the pregnancy, so we wait until we are so far along that our options are limited. Whatever the reasons that you might delay, it is important to seek medical care as soon as possible for your future and the health of a potential child.

I thought I was pregnant because I missed my period, but I tried not to think about it. My mother would never let me forget it, so I didn't want to tell her. I didn't want to tell my friends because I was afraid word would get around school. Finally, I told my boyfriend, and he found out where I could get a test, but I was scared. I'd make an appointment at the clinic, and then I wouldn't go. Weeks were going by, and finally, I talked to a counselor. She was great. She explained everything to me, and I got the test, but I was already five months pregnant.

DECIDING WHAT TO DO

Once you learn that you are pregnant, your next step is to decide whether to continue the pregnancy or to have an abortion. If you decide to

Insurance companies consider pregnancy a pre-existing condition. This means that if you do not already have insurance, they will not cover you. And if you do have insurance, it may not cover pregnancy or complications. Delivery costs about $6,000 and complications another $2,000 a day. If you have no or low income, you can receive insurance from the government (Medicaid) that covers all of pregnancy. And in an emergency, you cannot be turned away at a hospital. For more information, see "Care for Pregnant Women Without Health Insurance" on p. 427.

- A child will *not* automatically improve your relationship with your partner.
- Abortion is *not* more painful than labor.
- Abortion is *not* more expensive than having a child.
- Using drugs in the beginning of the pregnancy *does* hurt the fetus.
- Adoption does *not* necessarily cut you off completely from your child.
- Men *can* nurture and love a child the way a woman can.
- There *is* financial help for all of the options.

carry to term, you may choose to raise the child yourself, or have the child raised through closed or open adoption or foster care.

Many of us feel emotionally torn for a long time before we choose the next step. Your body will be going through hormonal changes that affect your feelings. Take time to listen to your instincts and needs. It is a *highly* responsible and moral act to clarify the right choice for you. If you let the pregnancy continue without medical care, you will limit your choices, and you may hurt the fetus. In addition, teens—whose bodies are still maturing and who tend to avoid getting medical care—are four times as likely to die from pregnancy-related causes as older women.[7] (For information and questions to help guide your research and reflection, see Chapter 17, "Considering Parenting.")

WHOM TO TURN TO

A partner who is loving and nurturing can offer wonderful support as you face an unexpected pregnancy. But even if you don't have such a person in your life, you deserve and need to be re-spected during all aspects of pregnancy and decision making.

FAMILY PRESSURE

Most of us have a relative who believes he or she knows what is best for everyone in the family. Some of us also have mothers or other relatives who always welcome a new child in their home and want us to carry to term and keep the child. This could be because of their religious beliefs, their mourning over the loss of another child, or their identity as a caretaker. Others of us have parents who are ashamed of us and concerned about the effects of a child on them.

A STRONG-WILLED PARTNER

Your partner may have reasons for wanting you to carry to term or to abort, but even his noble reasons might not consider what is best for you or a child. And sometimes his reasons are not so noble—for instance, he may fantasize that a child will suddenly change your tumultuous relationship into a beautiful partnership. Or he may use a child as another excuse to control your life.

If these situations are familiar, trust your instincts and seek support. If your loved ones have strong opinions about what you should do, you may need support to stand against their opinions, or to wait until you have made your decisions before telling them. Sometimes doing what

Poverty is the reality for many teen mothers and our children. Within five years after the birth of a first child, almost half of teen mothers and more than three quarters of unmarried teen mothers use welfare.[8] Teen women experiencing domestic violence (about one third of all teens in a relationship) are battered more after marriage.[9]

your heart says means going against what they want.

ABORTION

Abortion is safe and legal in the United States, although your financial situation, age (if you are under sixteen), and where you live can make it stressful. The safest, easiest, and most affordable time is within the first three months of pregnancy (calculated from the time of your last period). It is *very* difficult to have an abortion after twelve weeks (for more information, see Chapter 20, "Abortion").

I was using the pill with my long-term boyfriend. After we broke up, we had break-up sex, and the condom broke. One time was all it took! He did not want to be a father. I knew I could financially care for a child, but I did not feel it was moral to have a child who knew her/his father did not want her/him. I also did not feel emotionally secure [enough] to raise a child alone. I had an abortion and felt tremendously relieved.

CARRYING TO TERM

If you decide to carry your pregnancy to term, it is important to seek medical care *now*. Stop using alcohol and drugs, diet pills, herbal medicines, birth control, and over-the-counter medicines until you consult with a health care provider. If you are taking prescriptions, call your provider immediately (for more information, see Chapter 21, "Pregnancy").

PARENTING

Babies are remarkably resilient and adaptable when they have a consistent, emotionally nurturing caretaker and are comfortable, properly fed, and safe. As more children grow up with no father figure around, and women become empowered and economically independent, it is socially acceptable for us to parent on our own. We may also choose to parent with the father of our child.

I was in a stable, if long-distance, relationship, with a supportive guy who I knew would be behind me no matter what I chose. I spent a week thinking, wondering, agonizing, and writing. At the end, I realized that I wanted to be a parent. I told my significant other that he could leave now, or he could stay and be a father. I'm glad he decided to stay. I've told my daughter, who is three now, this story many times. It's one of her favorites. I want to make sure she knows that I wasn't forced into having her, that I chose to be her mother.

FOSTER CARE

Throughout history, shared child rearing in extended families and among friends has helped ensure that as many children as possible have a chance to thrive. This system is common throughout the United States and the world. The goal is to provide you time to resolve your situation. Obtain a lawyer for negotiations for either informal foster care or the government's formal foster care system. It is important to ensure that the guardian can make medical and educational decisions in your absence. You should also learn what process you must follow to regain custody.

Particularly with formal foster care, you put yourself at risk of losing your parental rights permanently. (For more information, see "Foster Care" [W46] on the companion website, www.ourbodiesourselves.org.)

ADOPTION

I started to take a real long look at my situation, and what kind of a parent I would be, and what I wanted my child's life to be like. It hit me like a ton of bricks: I was not ready, nor anywhere near ready, to be a mommy. I didn't have the financial resources to raise a child. Yes, there was state assistance . . . but I couldn't fathom raising my child on welfare. I know people who have done that, and it's not easy. I didn't want that stigma for my baby. I wanted my daughter to have a stable home, and I could barely pay the rent. There was no daddy around. I didn't want that life for my child. So I did a lot of thinking, a lot of crying, and a lot of soul searching, and I decided that the best option for me would be to place my child for adoption.

As recently as the 1970s, it was common for white middle-class families to hide the children of "unacceptable" relationships. Unwed women who became pregnant were sometimes sent away during pregnancy and coerced to surrender our babies for adoption. The secretive nature of closed adoptions is now considered psychologically unhealthy for you and your child. Today increasing numbers of birth mothers are choosing open adoptions, which allow us to have some level of ongoing contact with our children. If you choose closed adoption, consider picking an agency that will keep information about you to give to the child and adoptive family if they request it. Also be sure the agency will help you find out about how things are going later on, even if you feel now that you will never want to know.

Adoption can be a difficult choice. If you choose this route, you will be well served by creating a deliberate adoption plan with an adoption counselor and by using a reputable agency. A good agency pays for your legal and counseling services and does not offer you money. It treats you, not the adoptive family, as the client. To avoid a less desirable agency, call the National Adoption Information Clearinghouse, 1-888-251-0075, and ask how to contact the adoption specialist in your state. Most states require adoptive families to undergo an evaluation. If your state does not require one, consider what your own requirements would be for the family.

It is standard practice for you as the birth mother to choose the adoptive family from a pool of applicants in order to determine how comfortable you are having them raise your child. If you are not offered this opportunity, you may want to choose another agency. Many agencies require the adoptive families to provide yearly updates on the child's growth to the birth mother. It may be possible to write letters to the child and have them placed in a file for her or his future.

There have been many changes over the last twenty years in multiracial adoption. If they will affect you, be sure your agency is up to date on the issues. A good agency prioritizes matching the child's background with that of the adoptive parents. If it is not possible, look for a family with connections to a community with values similar to yours. If you or the birth father are of Native American descent, the Indian Child Welfare Act of 1978 may affect the adoption. (For more information, see the National Indian Child Welfare Association's website, www.nicwa.org.)

You can also find an adoptive family through a newspaper ad, an independent adoption facilitator, a medical practitioner, or a lawyer. In such circumstances, you create the adoption plan directly with the parents and/or their lawyer. Keep in mind that their lawyer will have the clients' best interest at heart, not yours. Whether you choose an agency or a private adoption, it is advisable to have your own lawyer and counselor. An adoption counselor can work with the birth father and both of your families as well.

NOW THAT YOU'VE MADE YOUR CHOICE

It is important to be gentle with yourself. Whatever route you decide to follow, you may grieve for the path you did not take. Grief is normal. It does not mean that you have made the wrong decision, but rather that you are feeling a loss. Remember that you need support during this time. The more informed you are about your options and feelings, the more power you will have to lead a satisfying life.

NOTES

1. Forty-eight percent of women between the ages of fifteen and forty-four have at least one unplanned pregnancy in their lives, not including miscarriages. Centers for Disease Control and Prevention, Vital and Health Statistics, 1995 National Survey of Family Growth, series 23, no. 19, 1997.
2. S. K. Henshaw, "Unintended Pregnancy in the United States," *Family Planning Perspectives* 1, no. 30 (1998): 24–29 and 46.
3. Alan Guttmacher Institute, *Fulfilling the Promise: Public Policy and U.S. Family Planning Clinics* (New York: AGI, 2000), 12.
4. Alan Guttmacher Institute, "Contraceptive Use: Facts in Brief," accessed at www.agi-usa.org/pubs/fb_contr_use.html on October 25, 2004.
5. Alan Guttmacher Institute, *Sharing Responsibility: Women Society & Abortion Worldwide* (New York: AGI, 1999), 30.
6. U.S. Department of Health and Human Services Office on Women's Health, "Pregnancy Tests," November 2002, accessed at www.4woman.gov/faq/pregtest.htm on October 21, 2004.
7. Marian Ringal, *Encyclopedia of Birth Control* (Phoenix, AZ: Oryx Press, 2000).
8. "What Docs Should Know About . . . the Impact of Teen Pregnancy on Young Children," accessed at www.teenpregnancy.org/resources/reading/pdf/tots.pdf on October 25, 2004.
9. Mayor's Office to Combat Domestic Violence, City of New York, 2004, U.S. Department of Justice.

Unless women can freely decide whether and when to have children, it is impossible for us to control our lives, to achieve sexual freedom, and to participate fully in society. Even though we have more contraceptive options now than ever before, no method is 100 percent effective, and access to reproductive health information and services is unevenly distributed, both in the U.S. and worldwide. Unintended pregnancies happen, and nobody should be forced to stay pregnant or to become a mother against her will. All women are entitled to safe, legal, and affordable abortion.

On the basis of current abortion rates, about one in three women in the United States—varying in age, race, religion, and class—will have an abortion by age forty-five.[1] A pregnancy may be terminated for all kinds of personal reasons, or because it could pose a health risk or is the result of rape or incest. Even a woman with a planned pregnancy may choose abortion if the fetus has a fatal condition or a severe disability (see Chapter 21, "Pregnancy").

Women must decide whether or not to continue a pregnancy based on what we believe is best for us (see Chapter 19, "Unexpected Pregnancy"). The government should not restrict our ability to make this personal decision. Unfortunately, abortion opponents in the U.S. have succeeded in placing many obstacles in the way of abortion access. (For the history and current status of abortion access in the U.S., please see p. 406.)

FINDING AN ABORTION PROVIDER

Abortion is legal in all U.S. states; however, accessibility depends on which state you live in, how far away you are from a provider, how much money you have or what your insurance will cover, and how far along the pregnancy is. Planned Parenthood (1-800-230-PLAN) has clinics in almost every state, and some of these clinics provide abortions. The National Abortion Federation hotline (1-800-772-9100) provides referrals and can help identify sources of funding. You can also check Abortion Clinics Online (www.gynpages.com) or under "Abortion Providers" or "Abortion Services" in the Yellow Pages. Gynecology clinics at non-Catholic hospitals, neighborhood health centers, and women's centers may also be good sources of information and referrals. You might also ask your primary care provider or obstetrician-gynecologist, if you have one.

Beware of "pregnancy crisis centers," often listed under "abortion alternatives" in the phone book. They are run by anti-choice groups and advertise themselves as counseling and referral agencies—often with the draw of free pregnancy testing—but actually try to dissuade women from having abortions by giving misleading and inaccurate information. For example, they may tell you the pregnancy is further along than it really is, or that abortions are dangerous. Such centers are often located close to clinics that do provide abortions and have similar names. One woman describes her experience at a crisis center:

They brought me into a room and did an ultrasound scan of my belly. They showed me the monitor and said, "There's your son." They told me that I was seventeen weeks pregnant, which shocked me because it seemed impossible based on when I had had sex. But they said that sometimes the way pregnancies are dated can be confusing. The ultrasound image on the monitor looked strange—like it was the same image playing over and over again, but they said it was because the baby didn't move very much at this age. Then they left me alone in the room with the ultrasound monitor. I eventually left feeling very confused. I called a hotline and got the number for another clinic. As it turned out, I was only six weeks pregnant, and I was able to have the abortion I wanted. Now that I look back on it, I think they didn't even do an ultrasound, and what they showed me was a videotape of another ultrasound from a woman who was much more pregnant than I was.

WHAT TO LOOK FOR IN A FACILITY

Most abortions are done in freestanding clinics that are not part of hospitals. Some specialize in abortion care exclusively, while others provide a range of reproductive health care services. Some are quite small, and others care for thousands of women a year. Abortions are also done in doctors' offices, hospital outpatient clinics, and hospitals.

It may be reassuring to know that most

WHAT YOU NEED TO KNOW

The following list includes some of the questions you may want to ask when you call for an appointment.

Medical Issues

1. What abortion methods are available to me? What are the differences in terms of numbers of visits, costs, and restrictions?
2. Is there anything in my medical history that would interfere with my getting an abortion at your facility?
3. What anesthesia and other medications are available? What is the difference in cost?
4. Will the clinic be responsible for routine follow-up care? For treating complications? What type of backup services are available in case of emergency?
5. I need my annual exam and Pap test. Can I get these done when I come in for the abortion?
6. Will birth control be available if I want it?
7. Will you perform an abortion if I'm HIV-positive?

Financial Issues

1. What does it cost? Must the fee be paid all at once? Is everything included, or will there be additional charges?
2. Will Medicaid or health insurance cover any of the cost?

State Laws

1. Are there age requirements? Do I have to tell my parents, get their consent, and/or bring proof of age? Will my parent or guardian need to visit the clinic?
2. Is there a mandatory waiting period between the counseling and when I can have my abortion?

Clinic Procedures

1. How long should I expect to be at the clinic? Will everything be done in one visit?
2. Can I bring someone else with me? Can she or he stay with me throughout the counseling and the procedure? If not, why?
3. Will there be a counselor or nurse with me before, during, and after the abortion?
4. How will my privacy be protected before, during, and after the procedure? Will my medical records be protected? Used for teaching purposes?
5. Will there be staff people who speak my native language? If not, will an interpreter be provided?
6. Can you accommodate any special needs I have (for example, wheelchair accessibility)?

The National Abortion Federation's brochure "Having an Abortion: Your Guide to Good Care," available online at www.prochoice.org, provides additional guidance about what you might want to ask.

women who have abortions in the U.S. are highly satisfied with the care.[2] When you call to make an appointment (and, of course, while you are at your appointment), ask about *anything* that concerns you. Trust your feelings about the way you are treated on the phone as well as in person. You should not have to defend your reasoning to anyone.

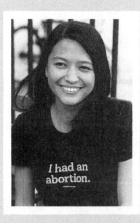

I had an
abortion.

"IF I HAD LISTENED"

A'YEN TRAN

If I had listened to the subway ads for post-abortion trauma counseling, or the men at the clinic brandishing rosaries and yelling racist pleas not to "kill your black/Hispanic/ Oriental baby," things would be different. I would not hold a degree, and I would not be building a career. My child's father would have been a man who sexually, emotionally, and mentally abused me. Worst of all, my child would not have the financial and emotional support necessary for a healthy life.

When I was nineteen, I got pregnant for the first time. On the recommendation of a friend, I opted for a medical abortion using methotrexate (a shot that detaches the products of conception from the uterus) and misoprostol (tablets that cause the uterus to shed its lining). I was left to go through the process alone, which made the experience difficult. While my side effects were unusually strong, I was grateful and relieved to have been able to have an abortion.

Several years later, in college, I got pregnant again. The pregnancy may have been from a condom breaking or from carelessness in not applying the condom before the first moment of penetration. This time I had a surgical abortion. The doctor was kind and caring, and her assistant held my hand and told me what was happening.

I told my friends that I was having an abortion, and they offered ample emotional support. I didn't feel alienated, because I was part of a vocally pro-choice community. Now I coordinate a group of abortion clinic escorts to deflect the harassment of anti- choice protesters.

If I had listened to the anti-choice protesters, I would not be able to pursue my life goals. Currently, about 80,000 women die every year due to lack of access to safe abortion services. I want to change that. The world I envision is filled with happy, healthy, nourished babies and parents.

A staff member at a feminist clinic describes how it should and can be:

At our clinic, counselors are trained to help each woman sort out her feelings. We do not invade anyone's privacy if she tells us that her decision is clear and not coerced, and that she does not want to discuss her reasons or feelings. At the same time, if she needs to talk through what she's feeling, we spend time working through those emotions with her. Women talk with each other, not just with the counselor. We provide very detailed and accurate information about the abortion procedure. A woman can have a friend stay with her during the abortion. When there is a decision to be made, the woman herself is an active participant.

PREPARING FOR YOUR ABORTION

It's natural to feel anxiety and anticipation before your appointment, as you might before any medical procedure. Planning ways to nurture yourself and preparing for your visit can help alleviate some of these feelings.

Try to go about your normal activities and get a good night's sleep. Meditation, deep breathing, or herbal teas may help you relax and sleep better. It's best to avoid excessive alcohol, street drugs, or strong sleeping pills.

If you are planning to have IV sedation or general anesthesia, then you will probably be advised to avoid food after midnight, though clear liquids may be allowed. This advice is important for your safety, so be sure you know and follow what the clinic recommends.

Prepare for variable temperatures in the clinic rooms by dressing in layers. If you enjoy music, bring a portable music player—you may even be able to listen to it during the procedure. Be sure you have documentation that the clinic requires, such as identification and your insurance card, or some other means of paying for the abortion.

Finally, give yourself positive messages. Like countless other women, you have made a decision that is the best one for your life right now. You are not alone, and you *can* do this!

WHAT TO EXPECT AT THE CLINIC

While doctors' offices and some clinics rarely attract protesters, at others they are not uncommon. If you are concerned, call ahead and ask what you might encounter. Abortion providers are well prepared—there may be escorts, who will meet you outside and accompany you into the clinic, and security personnel and procedures. Some women find it helpful to bring a friend, or to go by the clinic ahead of time to get familiar with the area.

Once inside the clinic, you will fill out a medical history form. A health worker will check your blood pressure, pulse, and temperature (vital signs); repeat a urine pregnancy test; and draw blood to check for anemia and the Rh factor.* You may have an ultrasound exam to confirm how many weeks pregnant you are.

A counselor or clinician will talk to you about your decision to have an abortion and tell you what to expect during and after the procedure. The counseling session is a time for you to ask questions and express any concerns. The clinic may also offer informational videos or group counseling sessions where you can talk with other women who are having abortions. Once you have the information you need and your questions have been answered, you will be asked to sign consent forms. The next steps in your visit depend on the type of abortion you are having.

ABORTION METHODS

Most abortions (88 percent) are performed during the first trimester, using one of two preferred methods: vacuum aspiration or medication abortion. In a medication abortion, the pregnancy is interrupted and expelled over the course of a few days using drugs; in vacuum aspiration, suction is used to terminate the pregnancy in one appointment. In the United States, most second-trimester abortions are done by dilation and evacuation (D&E), which involves dilation of the cervix and the use of instruments. Keep in mind that the length of a pregnancy is usually counted from the first day of the last normal menstrual period (LMP) and not from the day of conception (fertilization).† The chart on

the following page summarizes the various abortion methods and the stage of pregnancy at which they are used.

Which abortion method is used will depend on how pregnant you are; your medical history, including any medical conditions or drug allergies; the training of the person performing the abortion; the equipment and supplies available; the approaches favored by the local medical community; and your own preferences. If you have a choice of abortion procedures, some factors you may consider include:

- Effectiveness
- Duration and predictability
- Pain and pain-relief options
- Comfort, convenience, and privacy—will you be in a medical setting or at home when you expel the pregnancy?
- Whether or not you'll want genetic testing of the fetus
- Cost

MEDICATION ABORTION

A medication abortion (also called "medical abortion")‡ consists of a two-drug regimen that ends a pregnancy within the first nine weeks. In the United States, the most common is mifepristone (also known as Mifeprex, RU-486, or the "abortion pill"), which is taken orally, followed by misoprostol (brand name Cytotec), which is

---

* Blood is either Rh positive or Rh negative. If you are Rh negative and the fetus is Rh positive, you may form antibodies against the Rh factor in the fetal blood cells. In a subsequent pregnancy, these antibodies can react against an Rh-positive fetus, causing serious harm. To prevent you from forming these antibodies, your provider will give you an injection of a blood derivative (one brand name is RhoGAM) within seventy-two hours after the abortion.

† While the date of your last normal period can provide an estimate of how pregnant you are, LMP dating can be inaccurate, particularly for women with irregular menstrual cycles. A clinician will make the final assessment about how advanced the pregnancy is through a pelvic exam or an ultrasound.

‡ While "medical abortion" was originally chosen as the best way to describe this new option by those involved in advancing it, the term is a source of confusion. As stated in a recent editorial, "In popular use, the term 'medical' is often associated with medical necessity and with physician-based practices. To those outside the abortion field, all abortions are 'medical,' except for those performed illegally and/or unsafely." "Medication" abortion has been proposed as a clearer and more accurate term for this method, and it is used in this chapter, even though it may not be as familiar to some as "medical abortion." T. A. Weitz, A. Foster, C. Ellertson, D. Grossman, F. H. Stewart, " 'Medical' and 'Surgical' Abortion: Rethinking the Modifier," *Contraception* 69 (2004): 77–78.

Methods of Abortion*

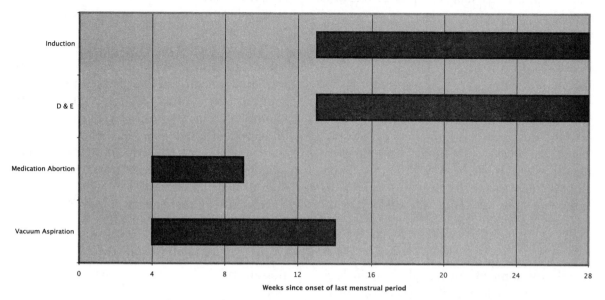

Induction

D & E

Medication Abortion

Vacuum Aspiration

| 0 | 4 | 8 | 12 | 16 | 20 | 24 | 28 |

Weeks since onset of last menstrual period

*Dates correspond to when each procedure is generally available. Individual providers may have some variation in what procedures they offer and when.

either swallowed or inserted into the vagina.* Mifepristone works by blocking progesterone, a hormone that is needed for the uterus to sustain a pregnancy. Without progesterone, the embryo detaches from the uterine lining. Another drug, called methotrexate, can also be used with misoprostol, but it works slightly differently, halting the ongoing process of implantation, and is usually administered via injection.

Misoprostol, a prostaglandin, is taken within two days after the mifepristone (or three to seven days after the methotrexate); it causes the cervix to become soft and the uterus to cramp. The embryo is then expelled in what seems like a heavy period. Medication abortion with mifepristone/misoprostol is very safe and about 95 to 98 percent effective. In 2 to 5 percent of cases, women will need a vacuum aspiration to complete the abortion. This may be because the drugs didn't

* Some researchers are studying whether putting the misoprostol between your cheek and gums or under your tongue is as effective as swallowing it or inserting it into the vagina.

work and the pregnancy continues (about 1 percent of the time) or because of heavy or prolonged bleeding. Between September 2000 (when the Food and Drug Administration approved mifepristone) and fall 2004, more than 350,000 women in the U.S. used mifepristone/misoprostol. Millions of women worldwide have safely used mifepristone since it first became available in France in the late 1980s.

The preliminaries of having a medication abortion are no different than for any other abortion method. After you complete your paperwork, lab work, examination, and counseling, you will swallow the mifepristone. Protocol and dosage may vary by clinic—you may have to return for the misoprostol, or your provider might send you home with the tablets and a prescription for any pain medications you might need. You may be directed either to swallow the misoprostol or to insert it into your vagina. Your provider may also give you a prescription for contraception that can be started as early as the day you use the misoprostol (see "Starting Contraception After an Abortion," p. 403). She or he should also give you a contact person to call if you have any questions or concerns.

After taking the mifepristone, you may experience bleeding, nausea, or fatigue. Even if you have had bleeding, it is very important to take the misoprostol as instructed, usually a day or two after taking the mifepristone. Most women take the misoprostol at home, or perhaps at a friend's or loved one's home. Cramping and bleeding will usually begin within a few hours, and they may be heavier than your normal period. The most common side effects include nausea, vomiting, diarrhea, chills, or fatigue. These symptoms should not last long and usually resolve on their own. It is normal to pass blood clots, some of which might be quite large. You may also see light pink or gray wispy tissue, which is the gestational sac. The embryo is under half a centimeter long at this stage and is often embedded in a blood clot. Severe lower abdominal cramps typically mean that pregnancy tissue is passing down the cervix. The cramping may occur in waves (see "Controlling Pain and Anxiety," following page, for coping ideas). Generally, cramping will subside after the tissue passes (about four hours). After a few days, the bleeding decreases to a light flow, then spotting, which may continue for several days or a few weeks.

You will need a follow-up visit to confirm that the abortion is complete. Do not try to make this determination yourself.* The clinician will do a physical examination, ultrasound, or blood pregnancy test. If the pregnancy is continuing, it is important to complete the abortion with a vacuum aspiration, since misoprostol can cause serious birth defects. If the embryo has stopped growing but some pregnancy tissue still remains in the uterus (sometimes called an *in-complete abortion*), the clinician may give you more misoprostol or may simply ask you to return for another visit.

Most women have our next period within about four to six weeks after using the misoprostol. Some women find that this first period after a medication abortion is heavier or has more clots than normal. A small percentage of us have an episode of extra-heavy bleeding about three to five weeks after the misoprostol. A good guideline for deciding whether you should call your provider about this bleeding is if you soak through two or more maxi pads per hour for two hours in a row (see "Aftercare," p. 402, and "Symptoms to Watch for After Any Abortion," p. 404, for general abortion aftercare information and other symptoms that may warrant a call to your provider).

EXPERIENCES OF WOMEN WHO HAVE HAD A MEDICATION ABORTION

In France, Sweden, and Scotland, where mifepristone has been available for over a decade, about half of women seeking an early abortion choose medication abortion.[3] In the U.S., the percentage of women who choose the method varies quite a bit from region to region and clinic to clinic. Some of the reasons women choose early medication abortion include a desire to avoid an invasive procedure; a perception that it is better, easier, or more "natural" ("like a miscarriage"); and that it feels more private. Most important, studies show that the overwhelming majority of women surveyed are satisfied with whatever method they choose.[4] Here are reflections of two women who each had a medication abortion:

The cramping was intense and almost unbearable for 6 hours. A hot water bottle helped, and afterward, it was worth it. I wish the cramping could have been lessened a bit, but otherwise, the proce-

---

* Clinicians are working to make the medication abortion process less complicated, but at this point, a follow-up appointment is necessary.

dure was as straightforward and simple as it could have been.

This was a very personal and private procedure, which enabled me to have some control over this difficult situation. This procedure is not for every woman. The bleeding and cramping last longer and are somewhat unpredictable. The hardest thing is the waiting between taking the medication and finishing the abortion. Aspiration would have been faster. However, for me it was better because I'm more private. I was comfortable being in my own home. Even though I did have side effects, this was easier than an invasive procedure, both emotionally and physically.

MEDICATION ABORTION THROUGHOUT THE WORLD

Medication abortion holds much promise to make abortion safer and more accessible in places where vacuum aspiration is not widely available, and misoprostol alone also holds great promise to expand access where abortion is illegal or severely restricted. Misoprostol is widely available, fairly effective for abortion, and very inexpensive. In Brazil, for example, where abortion is illegal, women have self-induced with misoprostol for years. This frequently results in an incomplete abortion (often because information on proper use is variable), but since misoprostol usually causes bleeding, women can get treatment at the hospital that completes the abortion. In essence, these women are able to have an abortion in a safe, hygienic setting. Unsupervised use of misoprostol has spread to other countries, notably in Latin America and Africa.

Because of its potential to offer a safe abortion option for millions of women who would otherwise be at risk of injury or death from unsafe methods, some activists are working to spread information about the safe use of miso-

CONTROLLING PAIN AND ANXIETY

Although it's natural to feel scared or anxious about experiencing pain during any abortion procedure, most women find the cramping tolerable. Deep rhythmic breathing, which you can do on your own or with a support person, is a powerful way to reduce pain and anxiety during any kind of abortion. Some women find that a hot water bottle or a heating pad can help. If you are having a medication abortion at home, your provider may offer you a prescription for pain medications or suggest over-the-counter pain relievers. For vacuum aspiration, local anesthesia injected into the cervix helps relieve pain that may occur during dilation (opening) of the cervix. In addition, the clinic may offer medications either orally or through an IV that will help you relax and feel less discomfort. Some facilities offer general anesthesia for women who want to be asleep during the abortion; however, general anesthesia carries its own risks. Many women find that local anesthesia is sufficient for the brief vacuum aspiration procedure even when general anesthesia is available. Because each of us has different ways of experiencing and coping with pain, it's important to talk with your provider about what the clinic offers, the difference in cost, and what will work best for you.

prostol. Research to date suggests that an 800 mcg dose of misoprostol inserted vaginally and followed twenty-four hours later by another 800 mcg dose is approximately 85 to 90 percent effective in terminating pregnancies up to sixty-three days since the last menstrual period.[5] Wetting the tablets with a few drops of water after insertion may increase efficacy. Most med-

TYPES OF ANESTHESIA USED FOR ABORTION

TYPE OF ANESTHESIA	POSSIBLE SIDE EFFECTS OR COMPLICATIONS
Local Anesthesia: Injection of medication into the cervix to numb the nerves around the cervix. Reduces pain associated with dilation (opening) of the cervix, but does not take away cramping.	Brief ringing in the ears or numbness of the lips and tongue. Seizures or serious allergic reactions rare.
Moderate Intravenous (IV) Sedation (sometimes called conscious sedation): Injection of pain medications or sedatives into a vein to reduce pain and anxiety without causing loss of consciousness. Usually combined with local anesthesia.	Nausea, vomiting. Serious allergic, breathing, or heart problems rare.
General Anesthesia: Administration of drugs (usually IV) to cause unconsciousness.	Nausea, vomiting, drowsiness. Because the costs and risks of serious complications may be somewhat higher, fewer facilities offer general anesthesia for abortion.

ical and public health experts agree that having access to medical supervision for any abortion is preferred. However, even without proper medical backup, the unsupervised use of misoprostol (and mifepristone, if available) at appropriate doses would eliminate infections caused by the use of unclean instruments. Unsupervised use of medication abortion, however, raises concerns about birth defects when these efforts fail and a pregnancy continues, and about the woman's health should she have excessive bleeding or another complication.

VACUUM ASPIRATION ABORTION

In the United States, vacuum aspiration (also called *suction curettage*) is the method used for most first-trimester abortions. In vacuum aspiration abortion, the uterine contents are removed by suction (aspiration), which is applied through a cannula, a thin tube that is inserted into the uterus and connected to a source of suc-

tion, either an electric pump or a handheld syringe. In countries where vacuum aspiration has not been introduced into training and practice, abortions may still be done by an older method called *dilation and curettage* (D&C).

The terms can be confusing, because D&C, surgical abortion, and suction curettage are often used interchangeably when describing vacuum aspiration. The distinction between vacuum aspiration and D&C, however, is important, because vacuum aspiration carries a lower risk of infection and injury. If a provider tells you about a D&C abortion, find out if she or he actually means vacuum aspiration.

Vacuum aspiration abortion is a safe medical procedure. Serious complications occur in fewer than 1 in 200 cases. The risk of dying from an early vacuum aspiration abortion is about 1 in 160,000, which is lower than the chance of dying from an injection of penicillin,[6] and much, much lower than the mortality risk involved in carrying a pregnancy to term.

Before starting the procedure, the clinician

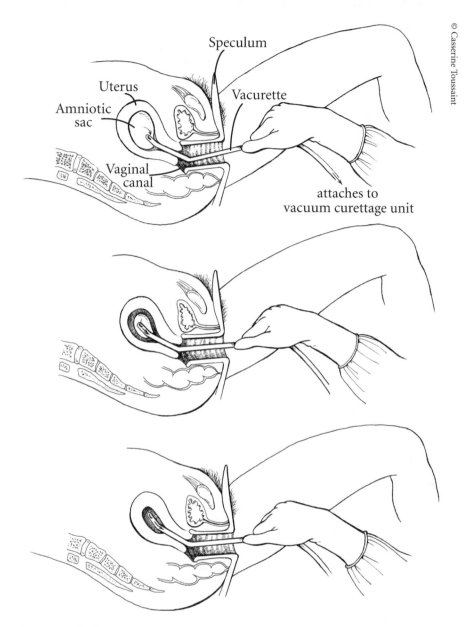

Speculum

Uterus

Amniotic
sac

Vaginal
canal

Vacurette

attaches to
vacuum curettage unit

© Casserine Toussaint

Vacuum aspiration

performs a pelvic exam to check the size and position of your uterus. Be sure to tell your provider if this is your first pelvic exam, and feel free to ask questions. Taking deep, slow breaths and staying as relaxed as possible will make the exam more comfortable.

Next, the clinician inserts a speculum into your vagina to separate the vaginal walls and bring your cervix into view. Although you may feel pressure, this should not hurt. Ask the practitioner to readjust the speculum if it pinches.

After washing the cervix with antiseptic solution, the clinician will place a tenaculum (a long-handled, slender instrument) on the cervix. This instrument allows the clinician to hold the cervix in the proper position during the abortion; you may feel a pinch or a cramp when it is applied. Next, the local anesthetic solution is injected around the cervix in two or more places. Although many women fear this step, injections into the cervix are usually less painful than injections in other parts of the body. You may feel pressure, a pinch, or nothing at all.

Once the cervix is numbed, the provider will gradually stretch the opening of the cervix by inserting and removing dilators (tapered rods) of increasing size. You will probably feel pressure and perhaps some cramps on and off. Dilating typically takes under two minutes.

Next, the cannula—a sterile strawlike tube—is inserted through the cervix into the uterus. The size of the cannula depends on how pregnant you are; it may range from the size of a small drinking straw to that of a large pen (half an inch). The clinician connects the cannula to a handheld vacuum device (manual vacuum aspiration) or an electric vacuum device and then moves the cannula back and forth to draw out the pregnancy tissue. If the clinician uses a vacuum machine (electric vacuum aspiration), then you may hear the humming of the machine and a whooshing noise when the cannula is removed. The aspiration usually takes only a few minutes.

You'll feel some cramping as the uterus contracts and empties. The contractions are important, because they squeeze the blood vessels of the uterus shut. The cramps may range from mild to intense, but they usually lessen immediately after the cannula is removed or within the next several minutes.

After wiping out your vagina and checking for bleeding, the practitioner will remove the speculum. She may examine the tissue to be sure the pregnancy tissue has been fully removed. A staff person will make sure you are feeling okay.

Then you can move into a more comfortable room to sit or lie down for a while. Sometimes women ask to see the pregnancy tissue. If you would like to, let the provider know.

I was really nervous about being awake during the abortion, especially because I'm afraid of needles. But the numbing part felt more like pressure than pain, and the cramps were bad for only a few minutes. I held my partner's hand, did some deep breathing, and I couldn't believe how fast it was over!

I experienced some pain with the procedure, but mostly, it was just a series of new sensations. I had never been so aware of my uterus. I spent an hour lying down to recover. I remember being elated—it was over! The only way to describe it was relief!

SECOND-TRIMESTER ABORTION

In the United States, about 12 percent of abortions take place at thirteen weeks of pregnancy or later. They occur for a number of reasons, most often because we do not realize that we are pregnant or do not know how far along we are, or because difficulty in raising money for an early abortion causes a delay. Teenagers who live in states that require parental notification or consent can be held up dealing with parents or trying to obtain a judicial bypass. And women who live in a state that requires a one- or two-day waiting period between counseling and the procedure may have to wait even longer. Women may also have later abortions because health problems develop or worsen during pregnancy, or because serious fetal impairments are detected.* Second-trimester abortions cost more,

---

* To read one woman's story of her late-term abortion, see "My Late-Term Abortion" (W47) on the companion website, www.ourbodiesourselves.org.

require more time off from work or school, and may require longer travel distances to find a provider.

The most common method of second-trimester abortion in the United States is *dilation and evacuation* (D&E), which involves removing the fetal and placental tissue with a combination of suction and instruments. About 4 percent of second-trimester abortions are done by inducing labor with drugs, a procedure called *induction abortion.*[7] Although second-trimester abortion carries greater risks than medication abortion or vacuum aspiration, the complications rates are still very low.[8]

The vast majority of women prefer D&E to induction because it is quicker and does not require hospitalization or going through the physical and emotional stresses of labor. However, because many doctors are not trained to do D&E abortions, labor induction may be the only method available in your area. Occasionally, women ending wanted pregnancies (because unexpected problems arise) decide to labor in order to hold the fetus and say goodbye. This may also be possible after some D&E procedures (called *intact D&E*).

DILATION AND EVACUATION

Having a dilation and evacuation (D&E) abortion is similar in many ways to having a vacuum aspiration procedure (see p. 398). Because your pregnancy is further along, however, your cervix needs to be opened wider to allow the pregnancy tissue to pass, which requires the clinician to soften and dilate your cervix ahead of time. This process of cervical preparation can take anywhere from a few hours in the early second trimester to a day or two for later procedures.

There are two main methods of cervical preparation: osmotic dilators and misoprostol, one of the drugs used in medication abortion. Osmotic dilators are short, thin rods made of seaweed (Laminaria) or synthetic material (Lamicel or Dilapan). After inserting a speculum, the clinician places one or more osmotic dilators in the cervical opening. The placement takes only a few minutes. The dilators absorb moisture and expand over the next several hours, gradually stretching the cervix open. You may feel pressure or intermittent cramping as your cervix dilates. If you are having a later second-trimester abortion, you may have more osmotic dilators placed on the following day. Once osmotic dilators are inserted, it is important to keep your appointment to complete the abortion; if you miss your appointment and the osmotic dilators are left in the cervix, you are at increased risk of infection, bleeding, and miscarriage.

Misoprostol is a prostaglandin that softens the cervix (for more information about misoprostol, see "Medication Abortion," p. 394). The small misoprostol tablets can be swallowed or placed between your cheeks and gums, under your tongue, or in the vagina a few hours before your abortion. Side effects with the doses used for cervical preparation are uncommon but may include cramping, nausea, mild diarrhea, or a transient fever. Sometimes osmotic dilators and misoprostol are used together, particularly for later abortions or intact D&Es.

The osmotic dilators are removed at the time of the abortion. Your provider may recommend stronger pain medication or sedatives than would be necessary for vacuum aspiration, in addition to local anesthesia in the cervix. If necessary, the provider uses dilator instruments to enlarge the cervical opening further. Then the clinician removes the fetal and placental tissue with vacuum aspiration, forceps, and a curette (a small, spoonlike instrument). This takes a few minutes, and you may feel a tugging sensation and some strong cramping as the uterus empties.

INDUCTION ABORTION

As the name implies, induction abortion involves medications that cause the uterus to contract and expel the pregnancy. Painful contractions may last for several hours or even a day or so. The procedure usually takes place in hospitals, where the quality of care and degree of personal attention vary. Although a few specialized facilities have dedicated space for induction abortion, most general hospitals don't. Therefore, you may find yourself on a ward with women who are delivering babies. If possible, bring a partner or friend to support you and to help assure that you get the compassionate treatment you deserve.

Preparation for an induction abortion is much the same as for dilation and evacuation, except that you need to plan for an overnight stay in the hospital. You will have blood tests and an ultrasound exam, and the clinician may use osmotic dilators to prepare your cervix (see p. 401).

Medications to induce abortion can be given in a number of ways. Most commonly, prostaglandin suppositories or misoprostol tablets are inserted into your vagina every few hours. Oxytocin (brand name Pitocin) may be given through an IV line. Occasionally, prostaglandins are injected into your arm, or medications (saline or urea) are injected through a needle in your abdomen into the amniotic sac (bag of water) surrounding the fetus. Although this may sound scary, the abdomen is numbed before the injection, and you will probably feel only a slight cramp when the needle enters your uterus.

Each woman's experience is different. The contractions will probably feel like mild cramps at first and then become more intense. When the amniotic sac breaks, you will feel a gushing of warm liquid from the vagina. Later, you may experience a lot of pressure in the rectal area as the fetus is expelled. If the placenta does not come out within an hour or two, your provider may use suction or a curette to remove it.

For pain, you may be given strong medications, sedatives, or epidural anesthesia (regional anesthesia commonly used in childbirth). Relaxation exercises, deep breathing, and the support of a friend can help make the contractions easier to tolerate. Medications are also available to control common side effects like nausea, vomiting, and fever. You should be as comfortable as possible during the abortion process, so be sure to ask for more pain medication or support if you need it.

AFTERCARE

After a vacuum aspiration or D&E abortion, you will go to a recovery area to rest. The staff will periodically check your vital signs and bleeding. It is normal to bleed moderately or even to pass small clots, and the intensity of the cramping usually lessens during the first half hour. Depending on the procedure, the type of anesthesia you had, and how you are feeling, you may stay in the recovery area from twenty minutes to an hour or more. If you had IV sedation or general anesthesia, you will need someone to drive or accompany you home.

Before you go home, the staff will provide information about what to expect over the next few days and what signs to look for that might indicate a complication (see "Symptoms to Watch for After Any Abortion," p. 404). Be sure you know the emergency number to call in case problems arise. You may also receive antibiotics to prevent infection, and a medication to help keep your bleeding to a minimum.

Because you can get pregnant shortly after an abortion, even before your first period, it's important to use reliable birth control if you don't want another pregnancy. Your provider will tell you about the different types of contraception

STARTING CONTRACEPTION AFTER AN ABORTION

METHOD	WHEN TO START AFTER VACUUM ASPIRATION OR D&E	WHEN TO START AFTER MEDICATION ABORTION
Birth Control Pills, Depo-Provera*	Day of abortion or within 7 days after	Day of misoprostol use or within 5 days after
Patch, Vaginal Ring*	Day of abortion or within 5 days after	Day of misoprostol insertion or within 5 days after
Intrauterine Device (IUD)	Immediately after abortion or at a follow-up visit. Expulsion rate may be higher if the IUD is inserted immediately after second-trimester abortion.	When passage of the pregnancy has been confirmed
Condoms	As soon as you resume vaginal intercourse	As soon as you resume vaginal intercourse
Diaphragm, Cervical Cap	As soon as you resume vaginal intercourse after first-trimester abortion. Wait 2 weeks to be fitted for diaphragm or cap after second-trimester abortion.	As soon as you resume vaginal intercourse

* Talk to your provider about how to prevent pregnancy if you plan to start one of these methods at a later time.

available and give you a method or prescription before you leave the clinic, if you so choose. Most contraceptive methods can be started immediately following the abortion (see table above). Remember that most forms of birth control will prevent pregnancy but not sexually transmitted infections. To protect yourself from HIV/AIDS and other diseases, use condoms even if you are using another form of birth control.

You will be given a follow-up appointment for two to three weeks after the abortion. At this visit, the clinician will check how you are doing physically and emotionally. Most of us feel fine and do not have any problems after an abortion, but it's also normal to feel tired or to have cramps for several days. Bleeding ranges from none at all to a light or moderate flow, which may stop and then start again. Some signs of pregnancy (such as nausea) usually get better in a day or two, while others (such as breast tenderness) may take a week or two. Emotionally, most women report feeling relief after an abortion, but it is also perfectly normal to have mixed or even negative feelings. The decision to terminate a pregnancy can be sad or stressful. It may be made more upsetting by the stigma perpetuated by the anti-abortion movement.

One woman describes such an experience when she became pregnant at age nineteen:

Nothing scarier had ever happened to me. I knew from the moment I found out that I didn't want to carry the pregnancy to term, but I was overwhelmed by images everywhere telling me that it was "wrong" to consider abortion. I felt more alone than ever before. When I searched for information on the Internet, I was bombarded by religious websites with brutal pictures of aborted fetuses. When I tried to go to my friends for help, I was told they were "so excited" and couldn't wait for me to have a baby. My boyfriend kept saying how much he wanted a son. No one asked me what I wanted. I felt robbed of choice, like my body was being controlled by everyone but me.

My dreams of going to college and moving out were over because of one mistake. Finally, some kind of switch went off in my head. I couldn't afford to care what other people thought. I wanted my life back. If that is selfish, then I was willing to be selfish. What kind of mother would I be, anyways? The next day I made an appointment, but it was hard. I cried a lot. But that was two years ago, and I will be graduating from college in a few months. Most importantly, I tell myself every day that I made the right choice, and I know in my heart that I did.

Another young woman says:

I am a 15-year-old Latina and couldn't tell my family. My pregnancy would be considered a disgrace and an insult. I would have to leave the house. My boyfriend thought I should have an abortion, so I did. I didn't really feel I had a choice. We did not have the time or money to bring a child into this world. I know what I did was right. I also know that after the abortion, I wept tears of sadness and tears of relief.

Clinics often give a list of dos and don'ts to follow after an abortion. We may be told to rest and to avoid heavy lifting, strenuous exercise, tub baths, swimming, tampons, and vaginal intercourse. While caring for ourselves is important, work, school, and family circumstances make some of these recommendations unrealistic. In addition, no studies have shown that these activities actually increase the risk of complications after abortion. The best guide is to listen to your body and use common sense. Important things to avoid are alcohol (which can increase bleeding) and douching (which can increase the risk of infection).

SYMPTOMS TO WATCH FOR AFTER ANY ABORTION

Your abortion provider is usually the best source of information or care if problems arise. If you require medical attention and cannot return to your abortion provider for care, ask for the best place to go in your area. You may not have a choice in emergency situations, but try to stay away from Catholic hospitals or practitioners who are against abortion, as they may not give you the most compassionate and appropriate care. If possible, bring a support person with you.

Abortion-related complications are rare in the United States, but they do happen. Below is a list of symptoms that may indicate a problem. If you have any of these symptoms or other concerns, call your provider immediately.

HEAVY BLEEDING

Heavy bleeding requiring treatment occurs in fewer than 1 in 100 cases, and fewer than 1 in 1,000 women bleed enough to need a blood transfusion.[9] The best way to tell if you are bleeding too much after an abortion is to keep track of the number of pads you are using and the number and size of any clots. Call your provider if you soak two maxi pads an hour for two hours in a row; if you pass large clots; or if you begin to feel light-headed.

The main way that your uterus controls

bleeding after an abortion is to contract, squeezing the blood vessels shut. Heavy bleeding can occur if your uterus relaxes too much (uterine atony) or if some fetal or placental tissue is left in the uterus (retained tissue or incomplete abortion). Very rarely, excessive bleeding can be due to a uterine injury that occurred during the abortion.

PAIN

Uterine cramping is normal after any kind of abortion, but persistent or severe pelvic pain may indicate an infection. Contact your provider if intense pain persists after you've used a heating pad and taken pain relievers, or if you have a fever. Infection of the uterus is uncommon after medication abortion because no instruments are inserted into the uterus, and the rate of infection after vacuum aspiration is under 2.5 percent.[10] Most infections are mild and can be treated at home with antibiotics prescribed by your provider.

Post-procedure pain may also be caused by retained fetal or placental tissue (incomplete abortion) or clots (hematometra). If the tissue or clots don't pass on their own, you may need medication or a vacuum aspiration to empty the uterus.

Pain may also indicate ectopic pregnancy, when an embryo is implanted outside of the uterus, most commonly in a fallopian tube. A growing pregnancy can stretch and burst the tube, causing severe pain and bleeding in your abdomen (see p. 500). An ectopic pregnancy is not removed by vacuum aspiration or medication abortion using mifepristone. It is usually treated with methotrexate or surgery. Although ectopic pregnancy is rare, it requires immediate medical attention.

FEVER

Fever means a sustained body temperature above 100.4 degrees Fahrenheit when taken with an oral thermometer; it can indicate an infection. Misoprostol can cause a short-term fever. However, if your temperature remains elevated for several hours, or if you have other symptoms of infection, call your provider.

CONTINUED SYMPTOMS OF PREGNANCY

Symptoms of pregnancy, such as nausea, bloating, or breast tenderness, typically resolve over the week or two following an abortion. If these symptoms persist, you may still be pregnant and should visit your provider. Taking a home pregnancy test is not useful, because you can continue to test positive for four to six weeks even after a complete abortion. Continuing pregnancy occurs in fewer than one in a hundred women who have vacuum aspiration or medication abortion.[11,12] Sometimes hormonal birth control methods (the Pill, Patch, or Vaginal Ring) can cause pregnancy-like symptoms, particularly during the first few months of use.

ABORTION OUTSIDE A MEDICAL CONTEXT

Some women claim that herbs, acupuncture, or acupressure can be effective in inducing abortion, especially within one to four weeks after conception. However, much of the information about these techniques is incomplete, vague, or inaccurate. Taking herbs like pennyroyal—known as an abortifacient—can be dangerous without expert guidance. Some medical professionals report that pennyroyal poisoning occurs regularly and is potentially deadly. They also say that it fails to induce abortion in most cases.[13]

FREQUENTLY ASKED QUESTIONS

Women, and the public in general, are exposed to a great deal of misinformation about abortion. In some cases, anti-choice activists have intentionally spread myths. What follows are the facts.

- **Will having an abortion affect my ability to bear children in the future?** Uncomplicated early abortion poses virtually no risk to a woman's future reproductive health, as shown by numerous studies. Very rarely, serious pelvic infection can cause damage to the fallopian tubes, which can increase the risk of ectopic pregnancy or fertility problems. You can decrease this risk by taking antibiotics at the time of the abortion and by seeking prompt treatment if symptoms of infection occur. Less research has been done on second-trimester D&E; however, studies thus far are reassuring.

- **Does having an abortion increase my risk of breast cancer?** No. In February 2003 the National Cancer Institute convened a workshop of more than a hundred experts from around the world to evaluate the research. These experts concluded "induced abortion is not associated with an increase in breast cancer risk."[14]

- **Do women who have had an abortion suffer from post-traumatic stress disorder or "post-abortion syndrome" (also called post-abortion stress syndrome)?** No. In spite of claims by anti-choice activists that women who have had an abortion are at risk for PAS or PASS, no such syndrome is recognized by any mainstream professional organization.[15] In fact, studies have shown that women most frequently report relief, positive emotions, and decreased stress after an abortion.[16] Some women also feel sadness and loss after an abortion, but abortion is not associated with long-term psychological distress. (For more information on feelings after an abortion, see the National Abortion Federation website, www.prochoice.org.)

Some women use a technique called menstrual extraction (ME), which was developed in the early 1970s by women's health activists and was practiced by "self-help" groups. A small plastic cannula and suction remove the lining of the uterus at the time of the expected menstrual period, controlling menstrual symptoms and regulating fertility. ME is not performed in clinics in the U.S. but exists in clinical settings worldwide.*

* In some countries, such as Bangladesh, where abortion is illegal but "menstrual regulation" is permitted up to at least ten weeks, this method is performed by paramedics in clinical settings.

HISTORY OF ABORTION IN THE U.S.

Abortion has been used to control fertility in every society we know about, regardless of its legality. It was practiced legally in the United States until about 1880, by which time most states had banned it except to save the life of the woman. Anti-abortion legislation was part of a backlash to the growing movements for suffrage and birth control—an effort to control women and confine them to their traditional childbearing role.[17] It was also a way for the medical profession to tighten its control over women's health care.[18] Midwives, who performed abortions, were a threat to the male medical establishment. Finally, with the declining birth rate among whites in the late 1800s, the U.S. government and the eugenics movement were concerned about "race suicide" and wanted white U.S.-born women to reproduce. More than most other medical procedures, abortion is linked to women's status and political power, as well as to the population objectives of the society.

WHEN ABORTION WAS A CRIME

I had an illegal abortion, which led to infection, and I was close to death. I ended up in a legal hospital with a real doctor who managed to pull me through. Thank god the pregnancy was terminated. All this rubbish about guilt feelings is just that. Ask me if I would do it again knowing the risks—YES—absolutely. Thank heaven it's legal now, so women don't have to endure life-threatening situations.

Abortion was widely practiced during the entire period when it was illegal. In the 1890s, there were an estimated 2 million abortions per year and 1 to 2 million annually during the 1920s and '30s (compared with 1.3 million today). Whether a woman could obtain an abortion at all, let alone one that was safe, depended upon her economic situation, her race, and where she lived. Women with money could leave the country or find pricey doctors. Poor women, for the most part, were at the mercy of incompetent practitioners with questionable motivations; or they tried dangerous self-abortions, such as inserting knitting needles or coat hangers into the vagina and uterus, douching with dangerous solutions like lye, or swallowing strong drugs or chemicals. All women were subject to the desperation, shame, and fear created by the criminalization of abortion.

When I was 15 and pregnant, abortion was illegal. I was denied any choice—I had a baby that I gave up for adoption. This experience has been a driving force in my life. I became an OB/GYN; I do abortions because I am totally committed to making sure that other women have the options that I didn't have.

Laws prohibiting abortion took a heavy toll on women's lives and health. Because many deaths were not officially attributed to unsafe, illegal abortion, we can never really know the exact number. However, scholars estimate that approximately five thousand women died annually in the U.S. because of unsafe abortions.[19] Several hundred thousand women a year were treated for health complications due to botched, unsanitary, or self-induced abortions; many were left infertile or with chronic illness and pain. Poor women and women of color were at the greatest risk. Nearly four times as many women of color as white women died as a result of illegal abortion.[20]

MAKING ILLEGAL ABORTION SAFER

Before abortion was legalized, some dedicated and well-trained physicians and other medical practitioners risked imprisonment, fines, and loss of their medical licenses to provide abortions. Through word of mouth, women found out how to obtain abortions. By the 1960s, the Clergy Consultation, a network of concerned pastors and rabbis, and feminist groups had set up referral services to help women find safer illegal abortions.

In Chicago, a group of trained laywomen called the Jane Collective went even further, creating an underground feminist abortion service. They provided safe, effective, inexpensive, and supportive illegal abortions. Over a four-year

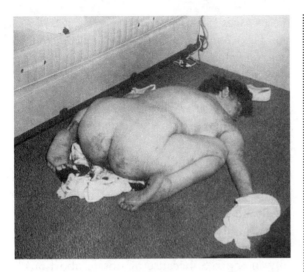

This controversial photograph first came to widespread notice when it appeared in *Ms.* magazine in the early 1970s. It was later included in *The New Our Bodies, Ourselves* as a depiction of an anonymous victim of an illegal abortion. We now know that the photo is of Geraldine Santoro. The story of her life and tragic death from an illegal abortion is told in the documentary film *Leona's Sister Gerri* (see "Resources"). (Files of Dr. Milton Halpern, former medical examiner, New York City.)

period, the Jane Collective provided more than eleven thousand first- and second-trimester abortions with a safety record comparable to that of today's legal medical facilities. Laura Kaplan, a former Jane member and author of *The Story of Jane*, describes the women involved:

We were ordinary women who, working together, accomplished something extraordinary. Our actions, which we saw as potentially transforming for other women, changed us, too. By taking responsibility, we became responsible. Most of us grew stronger, more self-assured, confident in our own abilities. In picking up the tools of our own liberation, in our case medical instruments, we broke a powerful taboo. That act was terrifying, but it was also exhilarating. We ourselves felt exactly the same powerfulness that we wanted other women to feel.[21]

Throughout the world, wherever abortion is illegal and unsafe, committed people take enormous risks to provide safe abortions clandestinely, to treat women who have complications, and to help women find safe providers.

ORGANIZING TO CHANGE THE LAW

In the 1960s, inspired by the civil rights and anti-war movements, women began to organize and took up the issue of abortion. Some of us marched, rallied, and lobbied for legislative reform. At speak-outs, women talked publicly for the first time about illegal abortion experiences. This activism led a few states to liberalize abortion laws, allowing women access to the procedure in certain circumstances, such as rape or incest. In 1970, New York became the first state to legalize abortion on demand through the twenty-fourth week of pregnancy. A few other states followed suit, and women who could afford it began flocking to the few places where abortions were legal. Feminist networks offered support, loans, and referrals and fought to keep prices down. But for every woman who managed to get to New York, many others with limited financial resources or mobility still sought illegal abortions.

Finally, on January 22, 1973, the U.S. Supreme Court struck down all existing criminal abortion laws in the landmark *Roe* v. *Wade* decision. The court found that a woman's decision whether or not to terminate a pregnancy in the first trimester was protected under the "right of privacy . . . founded in the Fourteenth Amendment's concept of personal liberty." The court allowed states to place restrictions in the second trimester to protect a woman's health, and in the third trimester to protect a viable fetus. However, the court held that if a pregnant woman's life or health were endangered, she would not be forced to continue the pregnancy at any stage.

While legal abortion was ultimately won in the courts, the political activism of the 1960s was critical to the judicial victory. The women's movement made visible the millions of women who were willing to break the law and risk health and life to obtain an abortion. The movement also connected abortion rights to gender equality.

LEGALITY AND ACCESSIBILITY

The positive impact of *Roe* v. *Wade* on women's health in the United States was enormous. Fatal infections and hemorrhaging due to abortion complications became things of the past. However, the court did not secure abortion access for all women. *Roe* and subsequent court decisions (see "Weakening the Constitutional Protection for Abortion," p. 410) left the door open for the hundreds of state restrictions that make it extremely difficult for many women to obtain abortions.

Roe v. *Wade* also galvanized abortion opponents, who label themselves "pro-life" or "right to life." Supporters of abortion rights, however, call them "anti-woman" and "anti-choice." Initially led by the Catholic Church and joined by fundamentalist Christian groups in the 1980s, the movement began an aggressive, often violent campaign to intimidate abortion providers, to block access to clinics, to stigmatize abortion, and to pass legal restrictions. Operation Rescue, which has since changed its name to Operation Save America, gained notoriety in the 1980s for blockading clinic entrances, which provoked tens of thousands of arrests nationwide.[22] Clinics have also been the targets of bombings, arson, anthrax threats, and acid attacks. As of July 2004, seven doctors and clinic workers had been murdered.

The massive protests and invasions of clinics decreased after Congress passed the Freedom of Access to Clinic Entrances Act (FACE) in 1994, but FACE has not stopped the strategy of harassing individual doctors and their families, picketing their homes, circulating wanted posters, or listing their names on the Web.

A health care provider speaks about the impact of the violence:

The fear of violence has become part of the life of every abortion provider in the country. As doctors, we are being warned not to open big envelopes with no return addresses in case a mail bomb is enclosed. I know colleagues who have had their homes picketed and their children threatened. Some wear bulletproof vests and have remote starters for their cars. Even going to work and facing the disapproving looks from coworkers— isolation and marginalization from colleagues is part of it.

The ultimate goal of the anti-choice movement is to outlaw abortion entirely, but its approach has been to erode access. And it has been quite successful. Harassment and violence against providers have led to a sharp decrease in services. Meanwhile, state restrictions have been devastating for the most vulnerable women: young women; women with low incomes, of whom a disproportionate number are women of color; women who live in rural areas; and any women who depend on the government for health care. Nowhere is this clearer than in the case of funding restrictions. After *Roe* v. *Wade*, federal Medicaid funds paid for about a third of all abortions. Even then it was estimated that one third of eligible women were unable to obtain a publicly funded abortion because services were not available or accessible, or because state policies prohibited coverage. In 1976, Congress passed the Hyde Amendment, which banned federal Medicaid funding for abortion unless the woman's life was in danger. Although Hyde has since been altered to include exceptions for rape and incest, it is conservatively estimated that one fifth of women who are eligible for Medicaid and need an abortion are unable to obtain one.

Following the lead of the federal government, many states stopped funding abortions, making an exception only if the pregnancy threatened the woman's life. (For more information, see "Medicaid Coverage of Abortion" [W48] on the companion website, www.ourbodiesourselves .org.) Without state funding, many poor women have been and are forced to have babies or to pay for abortions using money needed to sustain families, and some of us have sought and will seek cheaper illegal procedures or attempt to self-abort. In October 1977, Rosie Jiménez became the first woman known to have died from an illegal abortion because she could not afford a safe and legal one.

Parental consent or notification laws are enforced in thirty-three states, affecting many of the approximately eight hundred thousand teenage women who become pregnant each year. Seventy-four to 95 percent of these pregnancies are unintended, and one third end in abortion.[23] The abortion rate among teens has been steadily declining since the late 1980s. While in part this reflects a decline in pregnancy rates, it may also be due to restrictive laws that limit access.

Mandatory waiting periods—which require women to wait up to thirty-six hours between receiving state-imposed, often biased, counseling and having an abortion—frequently burden women with extra costs and stress. Women often have to travel to the clinic, stay overnight and pay for a hotel, take time off from school or work, or arrange for child care. As of March 2004, such restrictions had been passed in twenty-seven states.

Another strategy to erode abortion access is targeted regulation of abortion providers (TRAP) laws. These laws impose burdensome and medically unnecessary requirements, which are sometimes extremely expensive to implement. TRAP laws make abortion services more expensive and dangerous, and they force the closure of some clinics. Thirty-five states have at least one TRAP law.

Declining hospital services also decrease access. Over the past twenty years, the number of hospitals providing abortions has decreased— from 1,405 in 1982 to only 603 in 2000.[24] The impact is greatest on women in rural areas, low-income women who depend on hospitals for health care, and women whose health requires hospital services.

The "partial birth abortion" ban, signed by

WEAKENING THE CONSTITUTIONAL PROTECTION FOR ABORTION

In 1980 the Supreme Court began eroding the constitutional protection for abortion rights when it upheld the Hyde Amendment. Since then, there have been other severe blows. In *Webster* v. *Reproductive Health Services* (1989), the Court opened the door to new state restrictions on abortion. In *Hodgson* v. *Minnesota* (1990), the Court upheld one of the strictest parental notification laws in the country. In 1992 the *Planned Parenthood* v. *Casey* decision upheld a highly restrictive Pennsylvania law that included mandatory waiting periods, parental consent, and biased counseling. In *Casey*, the court abandoned the trimester framework of *Roe*. In its place, it sanctioned the regulation of abortion at any stage, so long as it does not place an "undue burden" on a woman's access to abortion. While the decision said that spousal consent was an undue burden, in the aftermath of *Casey*, hundreds of restrictions have been passed and not seen to be in violation of the new standard.

President George W. Bush in 2004 and immediately challenged in the courts, will hopefully be found unconstitutional. Nevertheless, it has succeeded in confusing the public and focusing attention on the fetus rather than on women. The term "partial birth abortion" is purely political: It does not refer to any one procedure or gestational period, and it is not recognized by any medical authority. If found constitutional, the ban would compromise women's access to the safest abortion procedures and would again turn physicians into criminals.

These campaigns are also part of a broader anti-choice effort to stigmatize abortion; to shame women who have abortions and those who provide them; and to convince the public that women who have abortions are selfish, sexually irresponsible, or victims of uncaring men and families. The effort may be succeeding. Polling data shows that younger women are more supportive of restrictive abortion legislation than women in midlife.

REPRODUCTIVE FREEDOM VS. POPULATION CONTROL

Reproductive freedom means the right to have children as well as the right not to. However, the pro-choice movement has not always been supportive of both aspects. Some people and organizations within the movement are pro-choice because they believe in population control, an ideology that blames overpopulation for social problems ranging from global poverty to ethnic conflict and environmental degradation. Historically, policies driven by population control objectives have focused on limiting the reproduction of women in developing countries—not empowering women—and this has often led to coercive policies and practices. Some women have been sterilized without knowing what was happening or giving consent, or have been offered only long-term hormonal

contraceptives, such as Depo-Provera and Norplant, rather than a range of choices, some of which can prevent the transmission of STIs. The pro-choice movement, historically focused only on gaining and protecting the right to abortion, has not always been careful to separate itself from those advocating population control.

Population control has been practiced in the U.S. as well, and poor women and women of color have been most affected. During the 1970s, women's health activists exposed and fought to eradicate sterilization abuses in the U.S. (See p. 365 in Chapter 18, "Birth Control"). Despite these efforts, women of color and low-income women continue to face coercive and unethical tactics. For example, HIV-positive women, overwhelmingly women of color, continue to be pressured to have abortions, and the federal gov-

ABORTION WORLDWIDE

Abortion is still illegal and unsafe in many countries. The World Health Organization estimates that sixty-seven thousand women die each year from unsafe abortions,[30] and many more women suffer lifelong injury. Decriminalizing abortion is a necessary step toward making access to safe abortion a reality for all women. The World Health Organization, the Alan Guttmacher Institute, and the Center for Reproductive Rights make the following estimates:

- An estimated 46 million abortions occur globally each year, and about half of them are unsafe.
- Ninety-five percent of unsafe abortions occur in developing countries.
- There are 20 million unsafe abortions annually.
- Over two thirds of countries in the Southern Hemisphere do not have safe, legal abortion.
- Approximately 13 percent of preventable maternal deaths are due to complications of unsafe abortion, and 99 percent of those deaths occur in developing countries.
- About 40 percent of the world's population has access to legal abortion (almost all in Europe, the former Soviet Union, Asia, and North America).
- Twenty-five percent of the world's population lives in countries where abortion is highly restricted, mostly in Latin America, Africa, and Asia.

For more information, see "Abortion Worldwide" (W49) on the companion website, www.ourbodiesourselves.org.

ernment refuses to pay for abortions for women on Medicaid but encourages sterilization by continuing to pay for it.

In order to secure abortion rights and to combat these ongoing reproductive abuses, the pro-choice movement needs to affirm every woman's right to make her own reproductive decisions. Increasingly, it is doing so. At the 2004 March for Women's Lives, many signs and speakers affirmed a broader agenda, calling for reproductive justice and linking it to human rights.

TAKING ACTION

Abortion opponents have created an atmosphere that is stigmatizing, threatening, and too often violent. Sometimes just identifying oneself as pro-choice can feel risky. But abortion rights

WHAT YOU CAN DO

- Be visible about your support for reproductive freedom—talk to your family, friends, and coworkers; write to your legislators; wear a button; put a bumper sticker on your car.
- Break your own silence—talk about your experiences with abortion, sterilization, contraception.
- Join a reproductive rights organization (see "Resources").
- Give financial support to organizations fighting for reproductive freedom.
- Ask your ob-gyn if he or she performs abortions.
- Learn more about the threats to reproductive freedom.
- Participate in or organize a demonstration.

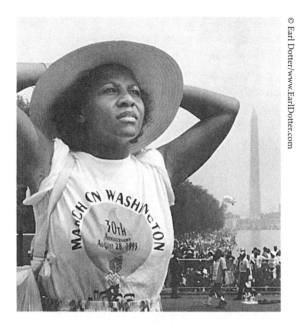

activists continue to stand up against these forces in all kinds of ways—by organizing large national demonstrations, clinic defense, public education campaigns, and support for abortion providers, and by giving direct financial assistance to women seeking abortions.

Women's health groups and organizations of women of color continue to push the mainstream pro-choice movement to promote a broader understanding of women's reproductive rights and health, placing abortion within a larger framework that includes maternal and infant health, economic justice, racial equality, and ending violence against women. Such groups prioritize the rights of the least privileged women and see reproductive freedom as part of the larger fight for human rights.

AFRICAN-AMERICAN WOMEN FOR REPRODUCTIVE FREEDOM

The following is an excerpt from a statement signed in 1989 by sixteen African-American leaders; in 1994 it was signed by twenty-nine others. (For the full statement and list of signatories, see "African-American Women for Reproductive Freedom" [W50] on the companion website, www.ourbodiesourselves.org.)

"Choice is the essence of freedom. It's what we African-Americans have struggled for all these years. The right to choose where we would sit on a bus. The right to vote. The right for each of us to select our own paths, to dream and reach for our dreams. The right to choose how we would or would not live our lives.

"This freedom—to choose and to exercise our choices—is what we've fought and died for. Brought here in chains, worked like mules, bred like beasts, whipped one day, sold the next: 244 years we were held in bondage. Somebody said that we were less than human and not fit for freedom. Somebody said we were like children and could not be trusted to think for ourselves. Somebody owned our flesh and decided if and when and with whom and how our bodies were to be used. Somebody said that black women could be raped, held in concubinage, forced to bear children year in and year out, but often not raise them. Oh, yes, we have known how painful it is to be without choice in this land. . . .

"Now once again, somebody is trying to say that we can't handle the freedom of choice. . . . Somebody's saying that we must have babies whether we choose to or not. Doesn't matter what we say, doesn't matter how we feel. Some say that abortion under any circumstance is wrong, others say that rape and incest and danger to the life of the woman are the only exceptions. Doesn't matter that nobody's saying who decides if it was rape or incest, if a woman's word is good enough, if she must go into court and prove it. Doesn't matter that she may not be able to take care of a baby, that the problem also affects girls barely out of adolescence, that our children are having children. Doesn't matter if you're poor and pregnant—go on welfare or walk away.

"What does matter is that we know abortions will still be done, legal or not. We know the consequences when women are forced to make choices without protection—the coat hangers and knitting needles that punctured the wombs of women forced to seek back-alley abortions on kitchen tables at the hands of butchers. The women who died screaming in agony, awash in their own blood. The women who were made sterile. All the women who endured the pain of makeshift surgery with no anesthetics and risked fatal infection. . . .

"We understand why African-American women risked their lives then and why they seek safe, legal abortion now. It's been a matter of survival. . . . African-American women once again will be among the first forced to risk their lives if abortion is made illegal.

"There have always been those who have stood in the way of our exercising our rights, who tried to restrict our choices. There probably always will be. But we who have been oppressed should not be swayed in our opposition to tyranny of any kind, especially attempts to take away our reproductive freedom. You may believe abortion is wrong. We respect your belief and we will do all in our power to protect that choice for you. You may decide that abortion is not an option you would choose. Reproductive freedom guarantees your right not to. All that we ask is that no one deny another human being the right to make her own choice. That no one condemn her to exercising her choices in ways that endanger her health, her life. And that no one prevent others from creating safe, affordable, legal conditions to accommodate women, whatever the choices they make. Reproductive freedom gives each of us the right to make our own choices and guarantees us a safe, legal, affordable support system. It's the right to choose. . . .

". . . Those somebodies who claim they're 'pro-life' aren't moved to help the living. They're not out there fighting to break the stranglehold of drugs and violence in our communities, trying to save our children or moving to provide infant and maternal nutrition and health programs. Eradicating poverty isn't on their agenda. No—somebody's too busy picketing, vandalizing, and sometimes bombing family planning clinics, harassing women and denying funds to poor women seeking abortions.

"So when somebody denouncing abortion claims that they're 'pro-life,' remind them of an old saying that our grandmothers often used: 'It's not important what people say, it's what they do.' And remember who we are, remember our history, our continuing struggle for freedom. Remember to tell them that we remember!"

NOTES

1. "State Facts About Abortion," Alan Guttmacher Institute, www.guttmacher.org/pubs/sfaa/pdf/alabama.pdf, accessed July 2004.

2. Picker Institute, *From the Patient's Perspective: Quality of Abortion Care* (Menlo Park, CA: The Kaiser Family Foundation, 1999).

3. R. K. Jones, S. Henshaw, "Mifepristone for Early Medical Abortion: Experiences in France, Great Britain, and Sweden," *Perspectives on Sexual and Reproductive Health* 34 (2002): 154–61.

4. S. M. Harvey, L. J. Beckman, S. J. Satre, "Choice of and Satisfaction with Methods of Medical and Surgical Abortion Among U.S. Clinic Patients," *Family Planning Perspectives* 33 (2001): 212–16.

5. "Consensus Statement—Instructions for Use: Abortion Induction with Misoprostol in Pregnancies up to 9 Weeks LMP," expert meeting on misoprostol, sponsored by Reproductive Health Technologies Project and Gynuity Health Projects, July 28, 2003, Washington, D.C.

6. L. Elam-Evans, L. T. Strauss, J. Herndon, W. Y. Parker, S. V. Bowens, S. Zane, C. J. Berg, "Abortion Surveillance—United States, 2000," *Morbidity and Mortality Weekly Report* 52, no. SS12 (2003): 1–32.

7. Ibid.

8. E. S. Lichtenberg, D. A. Grimes, M. Paul, "Abortion Complications: Prevention and Management," in M. Paul, E. S. Lichtenberg, L. Borgatta, D. A. Grimes, P. G. Stubblefield, eds., *A Clinician's Guide to Medical and Surgical Abortion* (New York: Churchill Livingstone, 1999), 197–216.

9. R. H. Allen, C. Westhoff, L. DeNonno, S. Fielding, E. A. Schaff, "Curettage After Mifepristone-Induced Abortion: Frequency, Timing, and Indications," *Obstetrics and Gynecology* 98 (2001): 101–6.

10. Lichtenberg, Grimes, Paul, "Abortion Complications."

11. Ibid.

12. Allen, Westhoff, DeNonno, Fielding, Schaff, "Curettage After Mifepristone-Induced Abortion."

13. Associated Press, "Herb Dangerous Alternative to Abortion, Experts Say," *American Medical News* (December 16, 1996): 44.

14. National Cancer Institute, "Summary Report: Early Reproductive Events and Breast Cancer Workshop," National Cancer Institute, 2003, accessed at www.cancer.gov/cancerinfo/ere-workshop-report on October 20, 2004.

15. N. L. Stotland, "The Myth of the Abortion Trauma Syndrome," *Journal of the American Medical Association* 268 (1992): 2078–79.

16. N. A. Adler, H. P. David, B. N. Major, S. H. Roth, N. F. Russo, G. E. Wyatt, "Psychological Responses After Abortion," *Science* 248 (1990): 41–44.

17. Leslie Reagan, *When Abortion Was a Crime: Women, Medicine and Law in the United States, 1897–1973* (Berkeley: University of California Press, 1997), 11–12.

18. For more on this, see Petchesky, *Abortion and Women's Choice: The State, Sexuality, and Reproductive Freedom* (Boston: Northeastern University Press, 1990), Chapter 2; and Kristin Luker, *Abortion and the Politics of Motherhood* (Berkeley: University of California Press, 1984), Chapter 2.

19. Zad Leavy and Jerome Kummer, "Criminal Abortion: Human Hardship and Unyielding Laws," *Southern California Law Review* 35 (1962): 126.

20. Reagan, *When Abortion Was a Crime*, 211–13.

21. "Jane," "Just Call Jane," in *From Abortion to Reproductive Freedom: Transforming a Movement* (Boston: South End Press, 1990), 100.

22. The National Abortion Federation (www.prochoice.org) and the Feminist Majority Foundation (www.feminist.org) keep annual statistics about anti-choice violence.

23. Tamarah Moss, "Adolescent Pregnancy and Childbearing in the United States," January 2003, Advocates for Youth. Accessed at www.advocatesforyouth.org/publications/factsheet/fsprechd.pdf on October 20, 2004.

24. L. B. Finer and S. K. Henshaw, "Abortion Incidence and Services in the United States, 2000," *Perspectives on Sexual and Reproductive Health* (January/February 2003), 6–15.

25. Ibid, 10–11.

26. S. K. Henshaw, "Abortion Incidence and Services in the United States, 1995–98," *Family Planning Perspectives* (November/December 1998), 269.

27. Kaiser Family Foundation Fact Sheet, "Abortion in the U.S.," January 2003.

28. "Legal but Out of Reach," fourth edition, Spring 2003, National Network of Abortion Funds.

29. R. Almeling, L. Tens, and S. Dudley, "Abortion Training in Obstetrics and Gynecology Residency Programs, 1998," *Family Planning Perspectives* 32, no. 6 (November/December 2000): 268–71, 320.

30. "Safe Abortion: Technical and Policy Guidance for Health Systems," World Health Organization, Geneva, 2003.

Childbearing

CHAPTER 21

CREATING A CLIMATE OF CONFIDENCE
FOR PREGNANCY AND BIRTH

Pregnancy and birth are as ordinary and extraordinary as breathing, thinking, or loving. Whether you are pregnant for the first time or are already a mother, each pregnancy will call on all your capacities for creativity, flexibility, determination, intuition, endurance, and humor.

When you are pregnant, you deserve high-quality prenatal care; a safe work and home environment; enough time for childbearing leave, with assured job continuation; and clear, accurate information about pregnancy and birth. You deserve nourishing food; time for rest and exercise; encouragement, love, and support from those close to you; and skilled and compassionate health care providers. When you are in labor, you deserve to be in the birth environment of your choice, attended by caregivers who sustain and guide you through the natural processes of birth. You deserve to be an active participant in your labor. You deserve to experience your pregnancy and birth within a *climate of confidence* that reinforces your strength and power and minimizes fear.

Some of the factors that contribute to such a climate can be achieved only through collective efforts to create a just maternity care system; others are more likely to be within your personal control. As you enter your pregnancy, seek out friends and family who can provide support; choose caregivers who listen to you and respect the birthing process; and select a birthing environment in which you feel comfortable.

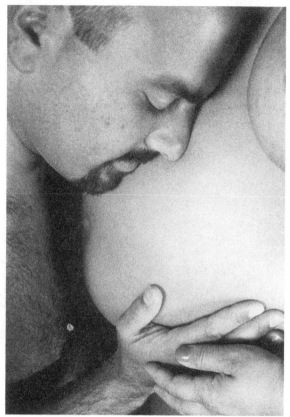

I planned to leave all my care and my decisions to my doctor. He seemed nice enough. I didn't know very much about childbirth. The big change happened after a few months. I told him that I wanted a doula (a trained birth attendant) with me during labor. "What book are you reading?" His tone of voice was so scornful and angry. "If it's not written by a doctor, I can't comment on it."

. . . So I decided to leave. Now my labor had become my own responsibility. I wasn't ready for that. So I began to learn about nutrition, everything! What is hard to express is the endurance—I spent five months of pregnancy asking questions. I found a wonderful nurse-midwife practicing in a hospital. . . . My beautiful labor and the birth of my daughter were the culmination of a lot of decisions I'm happy with. I experienced the strength I always knew I had.

Another woman describes her experience:

I transferred to a smaller hospital closer to home at around 32 weeks and told them I wanted my

two daughters, family, and friends to be there. The birthing center staff and my doctor were so accommodating, telling us, "Every family is different—we'll work with you, and make it work." They respected all of my wishes. I felt right at home.

The day arrived. I was 7 centimeters dilated, felt no contractions. My friends convinced me to go to the hospital around 7 P.M. ("We don't want you to give birth on Interstate 89," they joked.) There, I read and rested, everyone sent out for pizzas, the doctor did puzzles with my daughters. Around 10, I felt something happening. . . . I had back labor, [so] my husband massaged me and held my hips from behind to ease it. I was so much in my own space that I had no idea that anyone was there. At midnight I wanted to be on the bed, and was ready to push. Elan was born at 12:20. I had him all to myself, and nursed him . . . before he was examined and bathed nearby. It was all so calm and gentle.

Learning about childbearing will help you make good decisions throughout pregnancy and birth, so you can better handle the expected circumstances and unexpected incidents that occur. Respectful care will be key to supporting your health and the health of your baby.

Unfortunately, a climate of doubt prevails in thinking about pregnancy and childbirth in the U.S. today. Childbirth is seen as an unbearably painful, risky process to be "managed" in a hospital setting with a wide array of tests, drugs, and technologies. Routine medical practices regularly disregard and disrupt the natural rhythms of labor ("physiologic" labor) and often fail to support a woman's inherent capacity to give birth.

During my prenatal visits, my obstetrician encouraged me to have an epidural for labor. He told me there was no need to suffer as women had in the past. He assured me that epidurals were totally safe. I wasn't sure, but when he ended up inducing my labor with Pitocin because I was "late," I found the contractions unbearable. My husband and I were left in the room alone except when a nurse came in to look at the monitor and check my blood pressure. I couldn't push well, and my doctor used the "Mighty Vac" to pull my son out. [My son] had such a hard time getting on to my breast; it was days before he really sucked well. I was upset when I found out that many babies born to women with epidurals have this difficulty. I've wondered what [the doctor] meant by "safe."

Some medical interventions common to labor and childbirth are widely used despite World Health Organization recommendations that they not be,[1] and ample evidence that with appropriate maternity care, most mothers and babies do not need them.[2] A national survey of 1,583 childbearing women, "Listening to Mothers,"* revealed that the majority of women experienced each of the following procedures: continuous electronic fetal monitoring (EFM); intravenous (IV) drip; artificially ruptured membranes (deliberately breaking the amniotic fluid sac around the baby); epidural analgesia; intravenous Pitocin, or "Pit" (a synthetic oxytocin), to stimulate labor contractions; bladder catheter; and perineal stitches. Many women described these as disruptive, painful, and undermining.

The survey participants also experienced many restrictions that may do more harm than good. Most women were not allowed to drink or eat food, were completely immobile once admitted to the hospital and in "active" labor, and gave birth lying on their backs (a position that poses challenges for giving birth). Some felt "overwhelmed" (48 percent), "frightened" (39 percent), "weak" (41 percent), and "helpless" (25 percent). They also ended up with an array of self-described major and minor postpartum physical health concerns, and 19 percent scored as probably depressed in the week before taking the survey.† This is a troubling situation for a population of women who are overwhelmingly well and experiencing the normal life process of birth.

Finally, the cesarean section rate is at record levels in the U.S. and continues to climb rapidly. Cesarean sections can be lifesaving and health-enhancing in emergency situations, but unnecessary cesareans expose more mothers and babies to the risks of major surgery, without any clear gains for maternal and child health overall.

Why is all of this happening? Although most

* For the complete report of this first-ever national survey, see www.maternitywise.org/listeningtomothers/index.html.

† Based on the widely used and validated Edinburgh Postnatal Depression Scale.

caregivers are dedicated and well intentioned, they are working in a dysfunctional system and are influenced by many powerful forces that promote interests other than those of mothers and babies. The current maternity care system often:

- Standardizes and routinizes the management of labor so that birth is more predictable and convenient for health providers in hospitals. Often this care is not in accordance with the safe and effective practices now endorsed by a growing worldwide consensus among experts who have been studying evidence-based care for many years.
- Makes frequent use of procedures that can be billed for but may not be necessary. Tests and drugs that generate valued revenue for hospitals and health care providers often do not benefit mothers and babies. (We all pay a high price for these unnecessary expenses in terms of increased premiums that individuals and employers cannot afford, decreased access to insurance and care, and even jobs going abroad because employers can no longer afford to cover health benefits for their employees.)
- Makes providers fearful of legal claims, thus leading to more unnecessary interventions. To avoid lawsuits, many doctors and some midwives feel compelled to do "too much" rather than be accused of doing "too little." Obstetrical interventions play a valuable role under selective circumstances, but they are now vastly overused.

Moreover, insurers have largely ignored their responsibility to follow evidence-based research to determine which procedures are covered. Thus, they typically have not addressed questions of appropriate care, quality, and overuse, and this failure leads to higher premium costs and to practices often contrary to the best interests of childbearing women. Many providers who care for women lack adequate knowledge about physiologic birth; devalue such alternatives as birthing centers and access to midwives; or ignore the legal and ethical principles of informed consent. Malpractice insurance companies have also raised premiums for maternity care providers, thus leading to the closing of obstetric and midwifery practices as well as birth centers. This seriously limits valuable choices.

Several other factors contribute to a climate of doubt and make it harder for women to get accurate information about pregnancy and birth:

1. **The media.** When was the last time you saw a newspaper article titled "4 Million American Women Had Normal Labors and Healthy Babies This Year" or a TV episode that showed a healthy woman giving birth to a healthy newborn in the setting of her choice? TV portrays women in emergency situations and doctors rescuing babies. The message is: *Birth is unsafe.* Yet of the 4 million women who give birth each year in the United States, only a small percentage encounters the complications or problems reported daily in the media.

2. **Medical language.** Often-used medical terms define women as passive "patients," rather than as actively involved in demanding work. Physicians, and not women, "manage labors" and "deliver babies." Other medical terms imply that something is wrong with our bodies: An extended labor may be called "failure to progress" because of an "inadequate pelvis." Many of these outdated terms reflect a patriarchal system that influences how we see ourselves and how our care providers unconsciously see us.

3. **Doctors' training and practice.** Most women in the United States give birth in a hospital, attended by an obstetrician. Obstetricians are surgeons whose medical training emphasizes identifying and managing the complications of

pregnancy and childbirth. In contrast, the training of midwives and family practice physicians places importance on knowing what happens in typical births and learning the caring behaviors that support healthy pregnancy and birth. Obstetrical expertise can be lifesaving in times of crisis but is not needed in the vast majority of labors and births.

Direct-entry (independent) and nurse-midwives in the U.S. have attended women in homes, birthing centers, and hospitals for many decades. Numerous studies attest to their success, with outcomes as good as or better than those of obstetricians.[3] However, in hospitals, midwives may have a limited degree of autonomy and power or may not be available at all. Family practice doctors are also finding it more difficult to practice, partly because there are too many obstetricians for existing needs in the United States.

The history of childbirth and midwives in the U.S. offers many important lessons about how politics and power relations affect the choices of childbearing women (for a more complete discussion, see "The History of Childbirth" [W51] on the companion website, www.ourbodiesour selves.org). Despite all the evidence supporting the expansion of access to a midwifery model of care, including more freestanding birth centers, this is not the current trend. Reversing this situation will take active and dedicated childbirth activists—including mothers, fathers, family members, concerned practitioners, and the many organizations (see "Resources") that have long worked to recognize women's childbearing rights, respect the natural rhythms of labors, and humanize hospital routines.

Empower yourself with knowledge. Do your own research, and don't rely on your care provider for all the information you need. That's the most important thing I can think of for mothers to know.[4]

Two things about a birth center make it different from a hospital. One is that it is founded on the philosophy that pregnancy is a wellness event, not an illness. The second is that it is a maxi-home rather than a mini-hospital.[5]

Childbirth raises perfectly natural fears of pain and the unknown, and we can never be completely sure of the outcome, no matter where or how we give birth, or how much we've planned or prepared for it. Yet birth is intrinsically a healthy process, successful in most instances when understood, respected, and supported. Our own confidence can be enhanced when our providers—who may include doctors, midwives, nurses, and doulas—adopt approaches long characteristic of midwifery care: companionship, intelligent guidance, watchful waiting, patience, encouragement, and ways to support labor so that it unfolds on its own. Used in conjunction with appropriate medical interventions for managing complications, these practices help ensure that we give birth in a true climate of confidence.

YOUR PREGNANCY

You are pregnant! During the coming nine months, you will experience enormous physical and emotional changes as the embryo* grows from a single fertilized cell into a fully developed fetus.

You may sense that you are pregnant even before you know for sure. You can buy a pregnancy test at most drugstores or supermarkets to confirm whether or not you are pregnant. These tests detect a hormone (human chorionic gonadotropin, or hCG) that is present in your urine and blood during pregnancy. You can take

---

* In this chapter, we use the words "embryo" and "fetus" for the first trimester, and "baby" for the rest of pregnancy and birth.

a test as early as the first day that you miss your period, if you have regular periods. If the results are positive, you are pregnant. If they are negative and your period has still not arrived several days later, take the test again. Your hCG levels may be too low for the test to detect until seven days after a missed period. Blood testing is accurate at an earlier point but requires a visit to a health care provider.

Your approximate due date is 40 weeks after the first day of your last menstrual period. Pregnancies usually range from 37 weeks to 43 weeks, with most women giving birth between 39 weeks and 41 weeks. Your due date is merely the middle of that window.

YOUR FEELINGS

Your feelings can shift from delirious joy and contentment to melancholy, with a whole range of possibilities in between. You'll have questions: How will my pregnancy change me and my life, or our lives? How do I feel about my body changing shape? What supports do I have? Can I physically handle labor and birth? How long can I keep working? Will I be laid off? Do we have enough money? Will my baby be healthy? Will I be a good parent?

Many women report heightened perceptions, increased energy, and feelings of being in love, special, fertile, potent, and creative. You may also have surprisingly strong negative emotions and thoughts: I'm losing my individuality. I don't want to be a mother. I'm not ready to be a mother again. I'm ambivalent about this baby growing in me. I'm angry, scared, worried, tired, sick, in shock. I feel so alone.*

Sometimes it seemed like I had gotten pregnant on a whim—and it was a hell of a responsibility to

take on a whim. Sometimes I was overwhelmed by what I had done. A lot of that came from realizing that I had chosen to have the baby without the support of a man. I was scared up until the third trimester that I wasn't going to make it.

Negative or anxious feelings are natural. Most of us feel more positive as we get used to the fact of pregnancy, become attached to the growing baby, and prepare for labor and birth. Yet even during the most desired pregnancies, you may have moments, hours, or days of anxiety, confusion, and feeling blue. By talking with your partner or other loved ones, a counselor, or the practitioner you choose, you come to know yourself better. It can help to write down your concerns or keep a journal.

YOUR PARTNER'S FEELINGS

I am ecstatic about the birth, scared, happy, more emotions than I thought I could feel at any time. The personality, emotions, mind, life force of Ruth and I are in this growing child, a magical combination of the two of us that I can't wait to meet. . . .

If you have a partner, his or her feelings are probably as complex as your own. Like your own, they can be affected by family background, treatment when growing up, attitudes toward self, and ideas about beauty and slimness.

In the best of circumstances, your partner can reflect back to you the ways in which you are changing, and help you care for yourself and receive care from others. At times your partner may be feeling tired, left out, or neglected, or may find it hard to support you. Try to involve him or her in your pregnancy, so that the two of you can prepare, plan, and learn together. If your partner cannot provide the support you need, seek out a friend or family member who can.

---

* If your pregnancy was not planned, or if you are deeply ambivalent about whether you want to raise a child, see Chapter 19, "Unexpected Pregnancy."

CHOOSING A PRACTITIONER AND A PLACE FOR YOUR BIRTH

PROVIDERS

Choose your birth attendants and place of birth with care, because where you give birth and who attends you during birth will strongly affect the care you receive. Health care providers and place of birth are linked and you will need to find out who practices in the birth setting that best matches your personal circumstances and wishes. In all settings, you will find midwives and physicians attending births. In **hospitals,** most often the midwives are *certified nurse-midwives* (CNMs) and the physicians are *obstetricians.* In **birthing centers,** midwives may be *CNMs* or *direct-entry midwives* (certified professional midwives or CPMs, also called lay, independent, community, empirical, or traditional midwives) and *physicians* may be of various backgrounds. At **home,** midwives and physicians are overwhelmingly *direct-entry midwives* and *family physicians.* Increasingly, women giving birth in hospitals choose *doulas* (women skilled in attending labors) for care during labor and birth, in addition to a midwife or doctor.

While all practitioners perform many of the same tasks, they have distinct and different bodies of knowledge and often have substantial differences in their approach to pregnancy and childbirth. The profession of midwifery developed out of the support women have offered one another in times of need for millennia. The profession of obstetrics evolved from the profession of surgery; historically, surgeons were called upon to treat complications of pregnancy and childbirth. These two different origins contribute to the difference in philosophies often held by midwives and obstetricians.

MIDWIVES

In most countries, midwives attend the majority of births. In industrialized countries, this is often in collaboration with obstetricians, who provide backup care for complicated births. In the United States each year, midwives attend the births of approximately 10 percent of the women who have a baby. Midwives can provide all necessary health care services throughout the childbearing cycle for women who don't have medical complications. There are two broad categories of midwives practicing in the U.S.: certified nurse-midwives (CNMs) and direct-entry midwives.

Certified Nurse-Midwives (CNMs)

Most midwives practicing in the U.S. are CNMs. They attend births primarily in hospitals and in freestanding birth centers, and some offer home birth services. You will find CNMs in midwifery-owned practices, physicians' practices, or as employees of hospitals, health plans, or public agencies.

Certified nurse-midwives have offered prenatal and birthing services in the United States since 1925. They have helped create out-of-hospital birthing centers and woman-centered in-hospital maternity care programs. Some doctors appreciate and depend upon the high-quality care CNMs offer. Others consider them a challenge to their competence, as well as an economic threat. CNMs are licensed by a state board of nursing or medical board and are recognized practitioners in all fifty states.

Direct-Entry Midwives

Direct-entry midwives are also called *lay, independent, community, empirical,* or *traditional* midwives. They attend primarily women having home births. Direct-entry midwives learn midwifery through a combination of apprenticeship and/or attendance at one of several independent midwifery schools. Many have the certified professional midwife credential (CPM). Direct-entry midwives maintain communication with the medical community so that women will have adequate backup care if an emergency occurs, although the degree of cooperative backup for direct-entry midwives varies. Some direct-entry midwives use a local emergency room as backup rather than a specific physician. Licensure for

direct-entry midwives varies. Some states recognize the CPM certification; other states have no provision for recognizing home birth practitioners.

PHYSICIANS

Doctors assist at about 90 percent of births in the U.S. Physicians who provide care to pregnant women may be family physicians, obstetrician-gynecologists, or perinatologists.

Obstetrician-Gynecologists

Ob-gyns are surgeons who complete a four-year program of training in obstetrics and gynecology following medical school. They provide medical and surgical care for women during pregnancy and birth and for women of all ages with reproductive tract problems. *Perinatologists* are obstetrician-gynecologists who specialize in caring for women with medical or obstetrical complications during pregnancy or birth.

Family Practitioners

FPs are physicians trained in family medicine. Family practice physicians provide primary care for people of all ages. Some family practice physicians have specialized training and experience in obstetrics. With family practice physicians, general family care leads seamlessly to maternity care, and maternity care leads directly into women's postpartum health care, newborn, and baby care.

Since medical training focuses on identifying and managing health problems, physicians are optimal caregivers for women who have medical complications during pregnancy.

DOULAS

Research has shown that continuous emotional and physical support is an important component of care for women during labor. Yet doctors and midwives are often not able to provide one-on-one attention and care. Doulas—women trained to assist and provide continuous support to the mother before, during, and just after childbirth—are becoming more widely available. Studies demonstrate that women who give birth in a doula's presence need less medication, have lower cesarean section rates, and are more satisfied with their birth experiences. Doulas complement midwifery and medical care, offering a wide range of services, sometimes including home visits after the baby is born.[6]

Your health care organization may provide doula services or a list of local women you can hire privately. Doulas usually make an initial visit during pregnancy and then arrange to be with you during labor. If you have come to the U.S. from another country and find that hospital practitioners know little about your culture, it may be invaluable to have a doula who belongs to your community and speaks your language as well as English, acting as linguistic and cultural interpreter in addition to labor support.

While it is crucial to understand the differing philosophies and training among practitioners, it is also true that the letters after someone's name don't tell you much about her or him as an individual. There are some doctors whose styles and approaches are similar to the midwifery model, and some midwives whose practices incorporate the medical model more common to doctors. Find a practitioner you feel comfortable with—one who respects the birthing process, works in partnership with you, and offers appropriate guidance.

FINDING A PROVIDER

In some areas of the United States, women have more choices of types of practitioners and where to give birth than in others. Some institutions offer a full array of options, and others have

CARE FOR PREGNANT WOMEN WITHOUT HEALTH INSURANCE

Finding appropriate medical care and services can be difficult if you do not have health insurance. You may be eligible for Medicaid: Eligibility requirements in all states are expanded for pregnant women, and there is a special program called *presumptive eligibility* that pays for medical care for pregnant women whose applications have not yet been approved. To find out if you are eligible for Medicaid, contact your state office (see www.nasmd.org/members.htm for a list of all state Medicaid offices).

Many states have special health care insurance for pregnant women who do not have other insurance and are not eligible for Medicaid. Your local medical assistance, welfare, social services, or public health office can help you find a clinic that will offer you care or refer you to an insurance program that is available to you.

One program available everywhere in the United States is the Women, Infants, and Children (WIC) program, a federal supplemental food program.* WIC provides milk, fruit, cereal, juice, cheese, and eggs, and offers some prenatal and breast-feeding education. The program may be housed in the local health department, schools, or free clinics. It is available to everyone and is often the best place to start when you're looking for affordable prenatal care. People in the WIC office can refer you to health care providers and other programs and services that are available to you during pregnancy.

* Information about the Women, Infants, and Children Program is available at www.fns.usda.gov/wic/. The website lists toll-free phone numbers for WIC agencies in each state.

QUESTIONS TO CONSIDER ASKING MIDWIVES AND DOCTORS

- What is your philosophy of childbirth?
- How long have you been practicing?
- How many births have you attended as the primary attendant?
- Do you practice alone or with others?
- If with others, what is their experience? Do they share your beliefs and manner of practice?
- Who attends births for you when you are away?
- How can I reach you?
- How often will I see you during these next months?
- What kind of childbirth preparation do you recommend?
- What tests do you recommend for pregnant women? Why?
- Do you provide labor support and stay with women throughout labor?
- Do the nurses provide one-on-one nursing care for women during labor?
- How do you feel about doulas, labor assistants, or family and friends being present?
- Do you support moving around during labor, changing positions, and eating and drinking?
- Will I see you after the birth takes place?
- If I want to hold my baby right after birth, breast-feed, and not be separated, will that be supported?
- Under what circumstances do you recommend IVs, continuous electronic fetal monitoring, Pitocin, forceps or vacuum, or episiotomy?
- What is your protocol for the birth of twins and breech births?
- Do you attend vaginal births after cesareans (VBACs)?
- How much do you charge?
- Are your services covered by my insurance?

Additional Questions for Midwives Who Attend Birth at Home

- How do you define and handle complications?
- What drugs and equipment do you use in the home?
- Do you have a formal agreement with an obstetrician-gynecologist to provide care if complications occur?
- Do you recommend that I meet the physician who will assist me in case of a complication?
- Which hospital will I be transported to if a complication occurs during labor?
- Under what conditions would we go to the hospital?
- Would you stay with me if we transfer?
- Are you trained in newborn resuscitation?
- How many times do you visit after my baby is born?

Additional Questions for Nurse-Midwives and Physicians Practicing in Freestanding Birth Centers

- What do you require for admission?
- What are your backup arrangements if I have a complication that requires hospitalization?
- When and why do you advise women to go into the hospital?
- What percentage of your clients transfer to a hospital during labor?

more limited traditional practices or policies. Your health insurance coverage, personal income, geographic location, and medical history will affect what provider you choose for prenatal care and what setting you choose to give birth in. Keep in mind that even though you might not have a choice about provider or birth site, you can still make many decisions that will affect your experience.

To find a doctor, midwife, or doula, talk with other women about their experiences and ask them for the names of providers they like and trust. If you have health insurance, find out which providers and services it covers. The professional organizations that represent doulas, certified nurse-midwives, direct-entry midwives, family practice physicians, and obstetricians can often direct you to a practitioner in your community (see "Resources"). Once you have some names, make an initial appointment to talk with one or more of the providers.

If, at any point after choosing a provider, you are dissatisfied with the care you receive, consider changing to a different practitioner, if possible. You do not have to be loyal to someone who makes you uncomfortable.

BIRTH PLACES

GIVING BIRTH AT HOME

I had a homebirth, and choosing this was never a question for me. I knew in my bones and flesh that this was the way I needed to approach my pregnancy and birth. . . . I would have my baby in the warmth and familiarity of my home.

Giving birth at home is a proven safe choice unless specific risk factors are present before labor or develop during labor.[7] In familiar surroundings, labor usually unfolds harmoniously over a period of hours or sometimes days. Your birth attendants know you. You may want only your caregiver, partner, or close family members with you, or you may invite additional family and friends. A study of many home birth studies demonstrates that when healthy women have trained attendants with access to hospital backup, home births are as safe as hospital births, with fewer interventions, fewer infections, and less trauma.[8]

FREESTANDING BIRTH CENTERS

Freestanding birth centers are homelike centers with access to specialist consultation and hospital acute care services as needed. The birth center philosophy is simple—pregnancy and birth are normal until proved otherwise. Birth centers are guided by the wellness model of pregnancy and birth. Freestanding birth centers provide comprehensive family-centered care for women during pregnancy, birth, and the postpartum period. The National Association of Childbearing Centers (www.birthcenters.org) can tell you if there is a freestanding birth center in your community.

TRANSFERRING TO A HOSPITAL

Although figures vary, approximately 8 to 13 percent of women who labor at home or in a freestanding birth center will need to transfer to a hospital for assistance during labor. However, complications that require rapid emergency transfer are very rare. Midwives and other practitioners who attend women at home or at freestanding birth centers arrange for medical consultation and for hospital transport when necessary. Birth attendants have differing criteria for transferring a birth to the hospital. Their decisions may vary depending on the nature of the problem, their experience, the available equipment, their agreements with supporting physicians, and the nature and distance of the backup facility.

HOSPITAL LABOR AND BIRTHING ROOMS

I chose the hospital because I wanted the whole experience to be separate from the rest of my life, and I felt safest there.

Hospitals, the site of 99 percent of all U.S. births, care primarily for people who are ill and need medical treatment. Many of the routines in hospital settings are practices that facilitate emergency medical treatment, which is unlikely to be necessary for most women during labor. It is important to investigate hospital practices before you are in labor. Some of the common standard hospital routines, such as IVs, have not been scientifically proved to be helpful for healthy women in labor.*

Most hospitals offer labor, delivery, recovery, and postpartum rooms (LDRPs) where you can labor and give birth in the same room. In the best of these institutions, the philosophy will center on you and be family-oriented, flexible, respectful, and as noninterventionist as possible. However, the mere existence of these rooms does not always guarantee you an autonomous labor and delivery. If you plan to give birth in a hospital, or if you want to be assured about the care you will receive if you need to be hospitalized, learn about your options and rights as early as possible in pregnancy so that your informed decisions are respected when labor begins.

MAKING SURE YOUR DECISIONS ARE SUPPORTED

The Coalition for Improving Maternity Services (CIMS) (www.motherfriendly.org) promotes an evidence-based wellness model of maternity care to improve birth outcomes. CIMS has a Mother-Friendly Childbirth Initiative whereby a hospital, birth center, or home birth service that promotes philosophical principles related to the normalcy of birth—empowerment, autonomy, responsibility, and a commitment to do no harm—can be designated "mother-friendly." This designation is granted only to settings that fulfill the Ten Steps of Mother-Friendly Care,† a set of criteria CIMS has developed for women to use when evaluating birth settings and birth classes. These steps can be useful guides in your evaluation of possible birth sites.

THE FIRST TRIMESTER (WEEKS 1 TO 14)

You may experience nausea and fatigue during early pregnancy, but nausea usually disappears after the first three months. Even if you can't eat as much or the same foods as usual during this time, your fetus will be well nourished. Eat small amounts frequently throughout the day. Fruit juices or carbonated water can help, as can munching dry crackers or toast early in the morning. Ginger capsules, ginger or mint tea, and acupuncture may also help relieve nausea. If nausea continues or is severe, you can also take vitamin B_6, either alone or in combination with one Unisom tablet (available without a prescription in drugstores). Consult your midwife or doctor for information on how to use these medications. There are also prescription medications your caregiver can provide that may help and are considered safe for you and your fetus.

It takes a lot of energy to form a new human being, so make time to rest when you feel especially tired.

Hormonal changes cause you to urinate fre-

---

* See the Maternity Center Association's "Listening to Mothers" survey at www.maternitywise.org.

† For a complete description of the Ten Steps, see www.mother friendly.org/MFCI/steps.html.

RIGHTS OF WOMEN DURING PREGNANCY AND BIRTH

No matter what situations you face when you are pregnant and in labor, understanding your rights as a childbearing woman is key to making good decisions. In the United States today, essential health care is not guaranteed for all women and infants, nor are scientific data about best maternity care practices consistently applied in maternity care services. More important, women are not routinely given complete information about the benefits and risks of drugs, tests, or treatments. Often we are unaware of our legal right to make health care choices for ourselves and our babies.

The statement below, adapted from the Maternity Center Association, outlines a set of basic rights for childbearing women. It applies widely accepted human rights to the specific situation of maternity care. Most of these rights are granted to women in the United States by law, yet they are not always honored.*

Every Woman Has the Right to:

- Choose her birth setting from the full range of safe options available in her community, on the basis of complete objective information about the benefits, risks, and costs of these options.

- Receive information about the professional identity and qualifications of those involved in her care, and to know when any are trainees.

- Communicate with caregivers, receive all care in privacy (which may involve exclud-

* For the full text of this statement, see the Maternity Center Association's "Rights of Childbearing Women" at www.maternitywise.org/mw/rights.html.

ing nonessential personnel), and have all personal information treated according to standards of confidentiality.

- Accept or refuse procedures, drugs, tests, and treatments, and to have her choices honored. She has the right to change her mind.

- Leave her maternity caregiver and select another if she becomes dissatisfied with the care.

- Be informed if her caregivers wish to enroll her or her infant in a research study. She should receive full information about all known and possible benefits and risks of participation, and she has the right to decide whether to participate, free from coercion and without negative consequences.

- Have unrestricted access to all available records about her pregnancy, her labor, and her infant; to obtain a full copy of them, and to receive help in understanding them, if necessary.

- Receive maternity care that is appropriate to her cultural and religious background, and to receive information in a language in which she can communicate.

- Receive full advance information about risks and benefits of all reasonably available methods for relieving pain during labor and birth, including methods that do not require the use of drugs. She has the right to choose which methods will be used and to change her mind at any time.

- Enjoy freedom of movement during labor, unencumbered by tubes, wires, or other apparatuses. She also has the right to give birth in the position of her choosing.

quently, and the enlarging uterus begins to press on your bladder and bowel, which can cause constipation. To maintain bowel regularity, eat fresh fruits and vegetables and other foods high in fiber, and drink lots of water. Your breasts swell and become tender, the veins become more prominent, and your nipples and the area around them (the areola) may darken.

The hormones your body makes during pregnancy cause vaginal changes as well; clear, nonirritating vaginal secretions may increase. Check with a health care practitioner if the discharge is thick, itchy, or yellowish (see p. 651 for vaginal infection remedies).

Some women lose weight in the first trimester, while others begin to gain. A weight gain of up to ten pounds during the first three months is typical.

Some women have slight occasional vaginal bleeding (spotting) during the first weeks of pregnancy. Spotting can be normal, or it can be a sign of impending miscarriage. If you have spotting for several days, or period-like bleeding and cramping, you should contact your health care provider. If you experience pain with spotting for any length of time, contact your provider right away.

It's important to understand that pregnancy is a wonderful *possibility*. At least one in five pregnancies end early in miscarriage, usually in the first trimester. Most of the time, miscarriage is your body's way of responding when the fetus has a problem that will not support life. Most miscarriages occur for no known reason. If you have one or two miscarriages, you still have an excellent chance of getting pregnant and having a healthy baby the next time. (For more information, see "Miscarriage," p. 496.)

PRENATAL CARE IN THE FIRST TRIMESTER

Pregnant women have always been considered "special," the subject of special treatment and taboos. Historical writings suggest that pregnant women should gaze at beautiful things, get fresh air, keep their feet warm, and be surrounded by cheerful company to help their babies grow strong and healthy—good advice even today!

Although new tests and technologies have been added to basic prenatal care, it has remained strikingly unchanged for over half a century. The goal of prenatal care is to promote the health and well-being of the pregnant woman, the baby, and the family.

Prenatal care consists of three interrelated elements: (1) regular visits with your midwife or doctor; (2) the care you give yourself; and (3) the care you receive from friends, family, or other support people.

The effects of warmth and kindness on measurable outcomes of pregnancy may be difficult to demonstrate, but these qualities are simply good in themselves. Many things that really count cannot be counted.[9]

In the first trimester, prenatal visits to your health care provider are recommended every four to six weeks. The timing of your visits may vary depending on your individual needs. Each visit will include weight, blood pressure, and urine checks for you; listening to the baby's heartbeat (after ten to twelve weeks); and measuring his or her growth by placing a measuring tape on your abdomen. Ideally, you will have enough time to talk about any concerns, review test results if any tests were done, and discuss future plans.

First Visit

Come with questions (see p. 428). Bring your partner or a friend. At the first prenatal visit, you will be asked about your health history and your family's history, your background, occupation, and what support you have at home. You will talk about your diet, exercise, and drug and alcohol use. The purpose of this visit is to help you identify any problem areas, such as physical and psychological concerns. If you are experiencing physical or sexual abuse, your midwife or doctor can help by giving you referrals and scheduling more frequent visits if needed.

This is usually the only visit for which you get undressed. The exam usually includes a check of your heart and breasts and a pelvic exam to collect a Pap smear and to feel the size of your uterus. If you want to see your vagina and cervix, ask for a mirror. (For more information on understanding your reproductive system, see Chapter 13, "Sexual Anatomy, Reproduction, and the Menstrual Cycle.") If it is ten to twelve weeks after your last period, you may be able to hear the baby's heartbeat with an electronic Doppler (ultrasound wave device). Some doctors' offices and clinics have ultrasound machines and use them at this first visit to see the fetal heartbeat and confirm how far along you are. However, office ultrasounds are not routine in all settings or necessary for most pregnant women. The quality of the pictures produced frequently cannot provide relevant information about your baby's health.

Before leaving, ask when to return, what to expect from future visits, and where and when to call with problems and concerns. The practitioner should provide you with any other information you may need, such as written materials and referrals to classes and nearby resource centers. You should leave feeling listened to and well cared for—off to a good start. If you don't think this person is a good fit for you, seek a different provider, if possible.

TAKING CARE OF YOURSELF

Pregnancy is often a good time to improve or add healthy habits. It is especially important to eat nourishing foods, get plenty of rest, and avoid substances likely to be harmful. You may find that you naturally choose healthier options because they make you feel better. Women who smoke are sometimes able to stop smoking early in pregnancy because the smell of cigarettes is distasteful. If you normally eat very sweet foods first thing in the morning, you may find that healthier foods make you feel less nauseated. Pregnancy is an opportunity to make positive changes that will serve you well for a lifetime.

EATING WELL

By nourishing yourself and your baby, you enable all the systems that support pregnancy to function at their best. Many of your nutritional needs during pregnancy are the same as at other times in your life: Eat a well-balanced diet that includes plenty of whole grains, healthy proteins, and fruits and vegetables; and avoid highly processed foods (especially those with transfats) and excessive sugar. (For a full discussion of nutrition, see Chapter 2, "Eating Well.")

During your pregnancy, you have several unique nutritional needs, including the following:

- **Folic acid** is an essential component that your baby needs to grow. You can find folic acid in green leafy vegetables; citrus fruits and juice; dried peas, beans, and lentils; liver; and beef. In addition, many ready-to-eat breakfast cereals, breads, and pastas are fortified with folic acid. When you get enough folic acid just before pregnancy and during the first trimester of pregnancy, you reduce the already small possibility of neural tube defects (spina bifida). Some women do not get enough folic acid through food, so folic acid vitamins are generally recommended for all women trying to get pregnant and during early pregnancy.
- **Iron** is found in prune juice; dried fruits, beans, or peas; blackstrap molasses; lean meat; liver; egg yolk; and food cooked in iron pans. During your pregnancy, your baby absorbs all the iron she or he will get for the first six

months of life. Vitamins with iron in them can make some women more nauseated or constipated—you can get enough iron in a healthy diet without taking iron tablets.

- Women's bodies absorb **calcium** efficiently during pregnancy. Babies have mechanisms for getting all they need. Extra calcium in the form of more dairy products or other dietary sources is recommended only for women whose diets are significantly low in calcium.
- If you eat a variety of foods rich in **protein**— such as meat, soy products, beans and grains—you do not need to worry about getting enough protein in pregnancy. Vegetarian diets can supply adequate protein.

Eating well during pregnancy is vital. If money is scarce, the WIC food supplement program can provide extra food for you and your family during your pregnancy. (For more information, see "Care for Pregnant Women Without Health Insurance," p. 427.)

WEIGHT GAIN

Pregnancy is a time to gain weight, *not* a time to diet. Your weight takes care of itself when you eat a well-balanced diet of healthy foods. When you consume adequate calories during pregnancy you help your baby to achieve a healthy birth weight. Women who enter pregnancy at an average weight usually gain between twenty and thirty-five pounds. If you are underweight, you may gain more; if heavier, you may gain less. The pattern of weight gain also varies. Some women gain steadily; some lose weight in the beginning and then gain quickly later; some gain in the beginning and then don't gain as much later in pregnancy.

EXERCISE AND MOVEMENT

Physical activity and exercise are important for good health. Continue doing what makes you happy, gives you energy, and creates a sense of well-being. If you regularly exercise and you are too tired in the beginning of pregnancy, cut back to activities that don't tire you. You can add back running or more vigorous exercise after the first trimester, when the fatigue goes away. Check out the resources in your community, from swimming to yoga.

Throughout pregnancy, you can practice labor positions such as squatting, a position that opens your pelvis and facilitates labor. Perineal exercises (popularly known as *Kegels*) consist of contracting and releasing your pelvic floor muscles and are simple to do. They help you prepare for childbirth by increasing your muscle tone so you will be able to consciously let go of tension in your pelvic area during labor. (For instructions on how to do Kegel exercises, see p. 235 in Chapter 13, "Sexual Anatomy, Reproduction, and the Menstrual Cycle.")

MAKING LOVE DURING PREGNANCY

I remember feeling very sexy. We were trying all these different positions. Now that we were having a baby, I felt a lot looser. I used to feel uptight about sex for its own sake, but when I was pregnant, I felt a lot freer.

You may feel open, giving, and sensuous, or turn inward and feel less like making love during pregnancy. With each month, each trimester, you may feel differently. Pregnancy can be a time to experiment with different ways of loving, from massage and touching to exploring sexual positions. Certain positions may be more comfortable than others.

Be assured that intercourse and other forms of making love will not hurt the baby. You should not have sex if you are experiencing vaginal bleeding or abdominal pain; if your membranes have ruptured (waters have broken); or if you have had preterm labor contractions and are being treated for premature labor. Orgasms and/or semen in the vagina may cause light uterine contractions. If either you or your partner has herpes, do not have sex if the lesions are active.

SUBSTANCES TO AVOID

In addition to environmental and workplace concerns (see "Precautions for Pregnant Women," p. 105 in Chapter 7, "Environmental and Occupational Health"), certain substances are known to be harmful to you or your baby during pregnancy.

The following substances have predictable negative effects.

ALCOHOL

No safe limit has been established for alcohol consumption during pregnancy. Fetal alcohol syndrome (FAS) is a syndrome associated with frequent, heavy drinking that is exacerbated by malnutrition, poverty, and lack of education or access to health care.* Children with FAS often experience mental health problems, a disrupted school experience, inappropriate sexual behavior, trouble with the law, alcohol and drug problems, difficulty caring for themselves and their children, and homelessness.[10] FAS is one of the leading causes of mental retardation. The risk of fetal alcohol syndrome associated with one or two drinks daily has not been determined, so the surgeon general recommends that pregnant women do not consume alcohol.

SMOKING

Smoking during pregnancy is associated with abnormalities of the placenta (placental abrup-

tion, placenta previa), low-birth-weight (growth-restricted) babies, and premature birth. Tobacco use during pregnancy has also been implicated in sudden infant death syndrome, and children exposed to tobacco in the home have more respiratory diseases. Frequent use of marijuana is also associated with low birth weight. Children exposed prenatally to marijuana can experience mild withdrawal symptoms at birth and have long-term nervous system effects.

COCAINE, HEROIN, AND OTHER ILLEGAL DRUGS

These drugs have been associated with premature delivery and poor fetal growth, with additional concerns raised about organ formation and neurodevelopment in fetuses. When a pregnant woman uses addictive drugs, including heroin or methadone, her baby may be born addicted and may experience prolonged symptoms of drug withdrawal, including extreme irritability and poor feeding ability. Cocaine use has also been implicated in placental abruption (when the placenta separates from the uterus wall prematurely), which can be life-threatening for both mother and baby. Using several drugs at once increases the risk of negative effects. Additionally, impurities and dilutants such as herbicides, arsenic, Coumadin (a blood thinner), and many other substances can be present in illegal drugs, and may harm both mother and fetus.

PRESCRIPTION MEDICATIONS

A few prescription medications are known to cause fetal malformations. Isotretinoin (Accutane), a treatment for severe acne, is the most well known. It can cause malformations in as many as 23 percent of infants born to mothers using it. If you require medications, discuss their safety with your health care practitioner.

* For a full discussion of this question, see "Fetal Alcohol Syndrome" by David J. Hanson at www2.potsdam.edu/alcohol-info/FAS/FAS.html.

GETTING HELP IF YOU ARE USING HARMFUL SUBSTANCES

If you use illegal drugs, or if you have trouble avoiding alcohol, seek substance abuse counseling. Finding safe, affordable treatments that address the needs of pregnant women can be difficult, and many pregnant women are afraid to seek treatment, not knowing whom to trust. If you are having trouble finding an appropriate program, or if you don't feel safe in any that exist, attend a local Alcoholics Anonymous (A.A.), Narcotics Anonymous (N.A.), or Women for Sobriety meeting. All are free and guarantee anonymity, and you may find someone there who can advise you and provide trustworthy contacts. Women's health centers or health care providers you trust may give you more leads.

If you need help quitting smoking, look for a local hospital, clinic, HMO, or community group that sponsors free or low-cost smoking cessation workshops and clinics.

For more information on getting help if you are using harmful substances, see "Finding Help," p. 53 in Chapter 3, "Alcohol, Tobacco, and Other Mood-Altering Drugs." For information on the legal rights of pregnant woman who use drugs or alcohol, see "Reproductive Autonomy," p. 707 in Chapter 30, "Navigating the Health Care System."

OVER-THE-COUNTER MEDICATIONS

There are no firm conclusions about the safety of many over-the-counter medications. Acetaminophen (Tylenol) has no known harmful effects on you or your baby, but both ibuprofen (Advil) and aspirin can be harmful. Pharmacists, as well as drug package labels and inserts, can provide information regarding over-the-counter medications and possible dangers during specific times in pregnancy.

HERBAL SUPPLEMENTS AND VITAMINS

Very large doses of some vitamins may cause problems. Herbal preparations, classified as dietary supplements by the Food and Drug Administration, are not regulated like other drugs; however, they *are* drugs. Some herbal remedies are known to be helpful, such as ginger for morning sickness, but there has been little scientific research on the effects of most commercial herbal preparations.

DIAGNOSTIC PROCEDURES

It is best to avoid all elective procedures during pregnancy, including X rays. If certain procedures become medically necessary, make sure your health care provider and all technicians involved are aware of your pregnancy. Take all appropriate precautions, and obtain guidelines for follow-up care from your provider.

LEARNING ABOUT PREGNANCY

Many factors shape how you learn about childbearing and mothering.

THE WOMEN IN YOUR LIFE

Inspiration and positive information can come from mothers, grandmothers, sisters, cousins, and aunts, as well as friends. When their experiences have been good and their messages are positive, you absorb their confidence, which makes it easy to approach birth joyfully and positively.

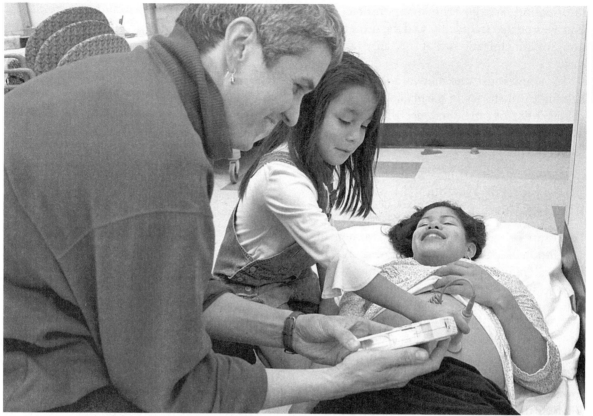

A girl listens to the heartbeat of her sibling-to-be during a session of Centering Pregnancy, or Embarazo Balanceado in Spanish, a group model of prenatal care.

If people close to you had negative experiences, you may feel scared as you progress through your pregnancy and approach labor and delivery. It can help to talk with your practitioner and to learn more about the birth process. Sometimes other women's unpleasant or difficult experiences may motivate you to seek new caregivers and/or places of birth.

BOOKS, WEBSITES, VIDEOS

Bookstore shelves are filled with childbearing advice books. Almost every book contains a bit of useful information. Some books are reissued year after year and serve as reliable, inspiring guides. But remarkably few books describe the childbearing year in a consistently realistic manner.[11] Some use excessive humor and thereby make light of situations that affect us deeply. Others quote risks of complications in a way that makes them seem highly likely and more dangerous than they really are. Most often these authors adopt medical language and undercut positive information with negative content.

Choose the ones that address your questions without instilling worry, doubt, confusion, or fear. Countless websites deal with childbearing. Keep in mind that books and websites vary widely in accuracy and often contain conflicting information. The best websites for pregnancy information are government-sponsored sites that are updated frequently, and the professional nonprofit organizations that specialize in health care.*

Sometimes just one or two books are most helpful; birth stories in particular can be compelling.† Videos can be an especially good way to learn about birth, teach relaxation, and dispel fears.‡

SUPPORT GROUPS AND BIRTH NETWORKS

Local support groups for expectant women and new mothers can be great sources of energy and practical information. Special swimming and yoga sessions for pregnant women may provide you with such a group. Birth Networks § are support groups dedicated to providing women with information about research supporting best birth practices, informed consent, informed refusal, and providers who will help you work toward the goal of a safe and satisfying birth. Most Birth Networks use the Internet to distribute information.

A local gay and lesbian health center helped us form a lesbian pregnancy group. We met every month, rotated houses, and ate dinner. None of us had known each other before, but we were all at just about the same place in our pregnancies. We talked about how pregnancy was changing our relationships, what it meant to our families, and issues like how the non-pregnant moms may have felt left out of the process at times. Now our babies are about one year old, and we are still meeting together.

If no support groups exist in your community, you may want to start one.

CHILDBIRTH CLASSES

In the past thirty years, childbirth education has evolved from the conditioned-response approach of Lamaze, through the husband-coached childbirth of the Bradley Method, to the more natural, relaxing orientation of Birth Works, and more recently, to hypno-birthing and mindfulness-based childbirth education classes. Childbirth classes teach you about the process of labor and offer techniques to help you relax and to go with the energy of labor.

Teach women how to breathe? Why, we know how to breathe, honey—we've been doing it all our lives!

Techniques that decrease stress or fear and exercises that improve confidence can help you cope with the pain of active labor contractions. Meditation techniques in particular can help you relax and cope with pain.|| Breathing techniques are another tool you might use to ride the waves of labor.

Hospital-sponsored classes tend to focus upon medical interventions and are less likely to

---

* For example, see the National Women's Health Information Center (www.4woman.gov); the March of Dimes (www.modimes.org); and the Maternity Center Association (www.maternitywise.org).

† Several books tell birth stories, including *Having Faith* by Sandra Steingraber; *Baby Catcher* by Peggy Vincent; *Operating Instructions* by Anne Lamott; and *Spiritual Midwifery and Guide to Childbirth* by Ina May Gaskin.

‡ For a list of videos, see "Resources" on the companion website (www.ourbodiesourselves.org). You might try *Relaxation, Rhythm, Ritual—The 3Rs of Childbirth, Gentle Birth Choices* or the audiotape *Journeying Through Pregnancy and Birth*.

§ Lamaze International houses a resource center for finding Birth Networks in your area, and their website includes information on starting Birth Networks: http://normalbirth.lamaze.org/institute/default.asp.

|| Mindfulness meditation techniques are an excellent preparation for parenting. Classes in mindfulness meditation can be found in stress reduction programs in many hospitals across the United States. They are often called "mindfulness-based stress reduction."

give you details about all of their risks and benefits or your rights. If a class you attend is less open to alternatives or more fear-oriented than you would like, find another or arrange a get-together with pregnant friends to explore childbirth information and stories together.

TESTS DURING PREGNANCY

In the thirty-five years since this book was first published, pregnancy and birth have become increasingly medicalized. The number of tests has multiplied, allowing increasing surveillance of both you and your fetus and more extensive monitoring during labor and birth. Some of these tests are routine tests recommended for all pregnant women, such as blood tests to find out if you are anemic or if you have immunity to rubella (German measles). These routine tests are important because they detect conditions in the woman that can often be treated. It is now recommended that all pregnant women be tested for HIV,* even if at low risk of having HIV, because detection and treatment during pregnancy can prevent transmission of the virus to your baby.

Other kinds of tests are performed to detect information about the fetus. Approximately one to three per hundred babies will be born with some condition classified under the traditional term "birth defect," though that term is misleading, since babies are not "defective." Many impairments are not disabling, and most occur for unknown reasons. No tests are available for most conditions, but a number have been developed to detect a few specific conditions that are genetic problems passed down in a family, or chromosomal problems that occur randomly. Your pro-

vider can refer you to a professional genetic counselor who can assist you in understanding genetic conditions and testing. (For more information on specific prenatal screening tests, see "Prenatal Care in the Second Semester," p. 441, and "Prenatal Care in the Third Trimester," p. 443.)

INFORMING YOURSELF ABOUT TESTS FOR FETAL IMPAIRMENTS

The number of tests available for birth impairments is expanding daily.† Although some are currently offered routinely, many are still experimental or are not available to everyone. Their names may vary. Testing, not testing, and what to do with any information the tests provide are extremely personal choices. Before choosing to have any test, it is important to know what the test is capable of telling you and what the advantages and disadvantages are.

To decide whether to have a specific test, ask:

- *What is the reason for the test?*
- *Is the test a screening test or a diagnostic test?* Screening tests such as ultrasounds and blood tests tell you if your baby's risk for a specific birth impairment or medical problem is "high" or "low." They do not give you a definitive diagnosis. Diagnostic tests such as chorionic villi sampling (CVS) or amniocentesis provide a definitive diagnosis of specific fetal impairments such as Down syndrome.
- *How accurate are the results?* The accuracy of screening tests varies. All screening tests have some chance of giving you a false positive result (the test result says that an impairment may exist when it doesn't) and a smaller chance of a false negative result (the test result says there is no problem when one actually exists). The results of diagnostic tests are accurate.

---

* If you refuse an HIV test, your practitioner may ask you to sign an informed refusal form that says the test has been offered and refused.

† For information on specific prenatal tests, see "Resources."

CARRIER TESTING OF PARENTS FOR GENETIC DISORDERS

Genetic (inherited) conditions are more common in certain families or people from specific ethnic groups. People who carry traits (genes) for these disorders usually do not have symptoms themselves. If both parents are carriers for the same genetic disorder, then that couple has a one-in-four chance of having a baby with the full disease and a one-in-two chance of having a baby who, like themselves, is a carrier without having symptoms. The risk is slightly different for each type of disorder. If you have a higher chance of carrying a gene for one of these disorders because of your family history or ethnic background, a blood test can determine whether or not you are a carrier. You can get tests performed before you are pregnant or during the first trimester of your pregnancy. Some of the more common genetic disorders and the groups associated with them are listed below:

GENETIC DISORDER	ETHNICITY/ANCESTRY AT HIGHER RISK
Tay-Sachs disease	Ashkenazi Jewish, French Canadian
Canavan disease	Ashkenazi Jewish
Cystic fibrosis	Caucasian people of Northern Europe
Sickle cell disease	African-American, African, Mediterranean, Hispanic
Thalassemia	Mediterranean, Southeast Asian

- *How might the information help me?* The result of a screening test can be reassuring. If the results indicate there is a higher risk that your baby has an impairment, and a diagnostic test is available for that condition, you can have the diagnostic test performed. If these results determine that a problem exists, you can choose to either terminate the pregnancy or prepare for a child who may have special needs. Disability advocates recommend that providers and genetic counselors arrange for women and couples to meet families with children who have the disability in question, to learn more about what it is like to raise a child with a particular condition and learn more about its real impact. (For more information, see "Prenatal Testing and Disability Rights" [W52] on the companion website, www.ourbodiesour selves.org.) Some programs offer this opportunity on a limited basis.

- *What are the advantages, disadvantages, and potential risks for me and my baby in having the test done?* Screening tests are of no known physical harm to you or your baby, although the long-term effects of ultrasound have never been sufficiently studied. The advantage of having a screening test is that a "good" test result, which is by far the most common kind, can be immensely comforting. However, a false positive may cause you needless anxiety and concern and can lead you to have further testing that was not in fact necessary. Diagnostic tests carry a small risk of miscarriage.

- *What type of preparation is necessary before having the test?*

It is important to note that none of the screening or diagnostic tests will give you a healthier baby; instead, they give you a certain amount of information.

SECOND TRIMESTER (WEEKS 14 TO 28)

The second trimester is usually the most physically comfortable time during pregnancy. Most of us have our normal energy and sleep well. You have made a lot of decisions, perhaps changed some daily habits, and can focus on enjoying the transition. At the beginning of the fourth month (16 to 20 weeks), many women notice occasional sharp pains in the abdomen at the level of the hip bone on one side. This pain is from a ligament (the round ligament) that is stretched by the growing uterus. It can hurt if you suddenly stretch it farther by standing up or swinging one of your legs out of bed. In some women, a dark line that extends down from the navel to the pubic region appears (the *linea negra*). The increased color around your nipples and in the line on your abdomen will fade after the baby is born. You may salivate or sweat more or notice that your gums bleed more often when you brush your teeth. Some women get cramps in their legs or thighs. If you experience this, pull your toes toward your knees to break the cramp. Regular exercise and good nutrition will minimize this occurrence and also prevent constipation.

Your baby will be big enough for you to feel his or her movements for the first time sometime between 18 and 22 weeks.

I was lying on my stomach and felt something, like someone lightly touching my deep insides. Then I just sat very still and for an alive moment felt the hugeness of having something living growing within me. Then I said, "No, it's not possible,
it's too early yet," and then I started to cry. . . . That one moment was my first body awareness of another living thing inside me.

The biggest day-to-day concern most of us grapple with during the second trimester is increasing weight, shifting body shape, and the need to keep changing the clothes we wear. Our culture celebrates women who are very slender, and it can be uncomfortable to feel "fat." Meet with other pregnant women. Sharing clothes, ideas, and support can help tremendously to counter the negative messages we get from the culture around us.

I was excited and delighted. I really got into eating well, caring for myself, getting enough sleep. I liked walking through the streets and having people notice me.

I don't like being pregnant. I feel like a big toad. I'm a dancer, used to being slim, and I can't believe what I look like from the side. I avoid mirrors.

PRENATAL CARE IN THE SECOND TRIMESTER

Visits with your midwife or doctor can be both a source of information tailored to your needs and a place to share the changes you feel happening. Some settings offer group prenatal care where you combine the prenatal visit with childbirth education and a support group.*

During the second trimester, your focus will probably shift to topics of labor, birth, and beyond. This is a good time to consider finding a

---

* Centering Pregnancy is one group prenatal care program that is an alternative to the traditional prenatal care model. In prenatal visit groups, you weigh and record measurements in your medical chart. The group session is moderated by your health care provider, but everyone in the group contributes to the discussion and learning.

childbirth class, touring the hospital, drafting a birth plan, choosing a pediatrician, and lining up help for after your baby has arrived.

PRENATAL SCREENING TESTS OFFERED DURING THE SECOND TRIMESTER

18 to 20 Weeks, Ultrasound

A screening sonogram or ultrasound, performed by a specialist, has become routine in many places. A sonogram can help confirm the due date, make sure twins or other multiples have not been missed by previous exams or testing, and take an overall look at the baby from head to toe as general reassurance. While the purpose of this test has nothing to do with identifying the sex of the baby, often the sex can be seen, and you can be told or not, as you choose.

Ultrasound is popular, but it is just a picture. The sonogram shows the shape and size of your baby and can confirm that the baby is growing normally, but it cannot identify problems that are not visible to ultrasound waves. It takes special training to interpret ultrasounds well. Most midwives and obstetricians can interpret basic features, but only specialized ultrasonographers can accurately interpret all the features of a sonogram.

Although there are commercial businesses that offer ultrasound pictures and keepsake videos to pregnant women, the FDA has issued a warning cautioning women not to expose babies to the high level of sound wave energy used to make these keepsake photos.[12] The long-term effects of the higher energies used by the newer ultrasound machines have not been determined, and frequently, the operators have not been trained adequately in interpreting the ultrasound results.

24 to 28 Weeks, Diabetes Test

In your fifth month, a blood test that screens for too much sugar in your blood is recommended. The blood is drawn one hour after you drink a measured amount of sugar (glucose). This test identifies women who are at higher risk of having a special form of diabetes called *gestational diabetes,* which develops in some women during pregnancy. If your blood sugar is higher than normal after you've drunk the sugar solution, you will be asked to do a second, three-hour test to determine if you have gestational diabetes. Gestational diabetes occurs in about 4 to 7 percent of women and is associated with higher rates of cesarean section and larger babies.

THIRD TRIMESTER (WEEK 28 TO BEGINNING OF LABOR)

Until 32 to 34 weeks, your baby changes positions frequently. Then she or he tends to settle in a head-down position. The sciatic nerve that runs from your lower spine across your buttocks and down your legs may get pinched and cause pain. Exercises, abdominal support bands, and chiropractic care may help. Pressure on your bladder may cause you to pee more often. You may experience occasional shortness of breath or heartburn. Your stomach is being squeezed. Once again, eat small amounts of food at a time, often, to forestall or relieve indigestion. Mild swelling (edema) of hands and feet is normal. However, if you have headaches, nausea, or dizziness, contact your practitioner right away.

Sometimes the increasing weight presses against the veins in your rectum, causing hemorrhoids. Over-the-counter treatments or herbal remedies may be soothing. You will naturally start sleeping on your side. Long body pillows can be comforting. Your uterus is becoming very large. It will contract more and more often,

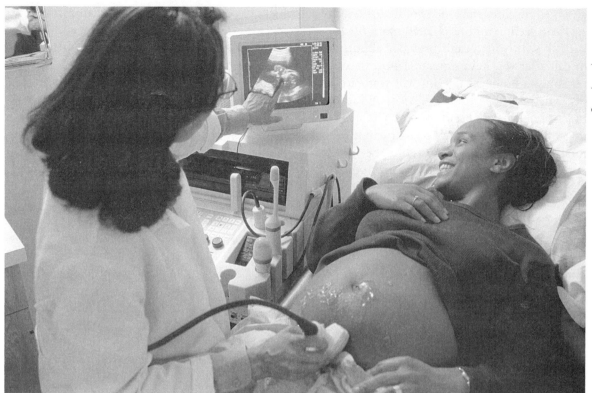

in practice contractions called Braxton-Hicks, preparing for eventual labor. These contractions do not come at regular intervals, nor do they cause your cervix to open. If you are experiencing contractions before 36 weeks that come regularly and cause low backache, cramps, or increased vaginal discharge, call your practitioner.

About two to four weeks before birth, and sometimes as early as the seventh month, your uterine muscles relax, and your baby's head may settle into your pelvis (called *lightening*), giving you more room to breathe and to eat.

I thought it would never end. I was enormous. I couldn't bend over and wash my feet. And it was incredibly hot. . . . I wonder what [my child] looks like. How fantastic that it only has to travel one and a half feet down to get born. . . . My kid is dancing under my heart.

(To learn how to recognize when labor begins, see "Signs of Labor," p. 452 in Chapter 22, "Childbirth.")

PRENATAL CARE IN THE THIRD TRIMESTER

You will have more frequent prenatal visits as you get close to the time of birth. You and your provider will continue to monitor your blood pressure, your weight gain, and the movements and position of your baby. If your baby is not in the head-down position in your uterus, you have what is called a *breech* presentation, and you should consider seeking help from a skilled doctor to turn the baby. This procedure, called an *external version,* is performed three to four weeks before your due date. It is often successful and especially important if you are planning to give birth in a hospital, many of which require a cesarean section for breech presentations.

Talk with your health provider about when to call after you have signs of labor. If you are planning a home birth, you will want to have necessary supplies gathered. Most home birth practitioners have a list of supplies you will need to get. If you are planning to give birth in a hospital or a freestanding birth center, be sure you are familiar with the physical surroundings as well as the institutional policies and procedures (most places offer booklets with this information). Consider a special class on breast-feeding and arrange for a doula, if you have decided to have one present. Choose a nurse-practitioner, family practice physician, or pediatrician who will become your baby's health care provider. Many pediatric providers welcome a prenatal visit from expectant parents.

PRENATAL SCREENING TESTS OFFERED DURING THE THIRD TRIMESTER

35 to 37 weeks, GBS Test

Ten to 30 percent of pregnant women normally have a bacterium called group B in the vagina or rectum. It is not a problem or infection for the women who carry it, but in rare cases, it results in a serious infection in the baby at birth. At 35 to 37 weeks, your practitioners or you will collect a culture from your vagina to test for GBS. If you have GBS as a normal inhabitant in your vagina, you will be offered antibiotics when you are in labor.

PREPARING FOR LABOR

During pregnancy, it is important to: (1) identify how strongly you want or do not want pain-relieving drugs; (2) learn about the benefits and risks of pain-relief methods available to you; (3) decide what options are best for you, with the awareness that you can never predict exactly how your labor will progress. The Pain Medications Preference Scale* is an excellent one-page list of statements that can help you clarify your feelings about pain and medications during labor. The chapter on childbirth reviews the advantages and disadvantages of the most common pain medications used in hospitals today.

BIRTH PLAN

Some women choose to create a birth plan. Writing a birth plan can allow you to express yourself clearly and firmly. The plan can specify the kind of care that you hope for and whom you want to attend you. If you plan to go to a hospital, you may want to send copies to your practitioner and his or her associates, the head of nursing, and the physician in charge of maternity care. Bring a copy with you when you are in labor and go to the hospital. If you choose to create a birth plan, remember that a plan is just that; it is not a guarantee that everything will happen as you would like.

PREPARATION FOR BREAST-FEEDING

Breast milk is the best food for babies; it provides all the nutrients your baby needs to grow, as well as antibodies that protect against infection. Nursing also provides numerous health benefits to mothers. Whether you are undecided about breastfeeding or committed to trying it, take time to talk with midwives, childbirth educators, and other mothers and to read available books. Having good support and plans in place before you give birth can help smooth the way. (For

---

* The Pain Medications Preference Scale is available at www.maternitywise.org.

more information, see "Breast-feeding Your Baby," p. 478.)

SPECIAL CONSIDERATIONS

WHAT IS A HIGH-RISK PREGNANCY?

A pre-existing medical condition such as diabetes or high blood pressure, clotting or immune disorders, or kidney disease may increase your chances (risk) for certain complications during pregnancy. You may need to consult with obstetricians or relevant specialists, and make more frequent prenatal visits or adjustments in your daily activities. But even though your risk for complications during pregnancy is higher if you have a pre-existing disease, you may not actually develop any worrisome complications.

If someone labels you high-risk, do some research to understand what's happening. If your pregnancy requires attention from a specialist, a midwife or family practice doctor can still give you the general care you need.

IN YOUR TEENS AND PREGNANT

Becoming pregnant as a teenager can present many challenges. Because of our society's negative attitudes toward teen pregnancy, we forget that in earlier times, and presently in many countries around the world, women often have several children before the age of twenty. Be assured that with support you can have a healthy pregnancy and birth, although very young teens (thirteen to fifteen years old) do have a higher rate of complicated births.

If you're a teenager, you are still growing yourself, and you need to eat a lot of healthy, nutritious food. You may have many changes to negotiate and plans to make as you prepare to give birth. You will need to know where you and the baby will live, and you may need to figure out how to stay in school or at your job, arrange health insurance, and ensure that you will have enough money. It can seem overwhelming. Take advantage of any support systems available to you; the more helpful people (family, friends, the baby's father, school counselors, public health nurses) you can surround yourself with, the better. They can encourage you to be and to stay healthy and feel positive about pregnancy and birth, and to plan for and make decisions about your and your baby's future. (If you are unsure whether you want to raise a child, see "Deciding What to Do," p. 384 in Chapter 19, "Unexpected Pregnancy.")

IF YOU ARE IN YOUR LATE THIRTIES OR EARLY FORTIES

Many more of us are becoming pregnant for the first time in our late thirties and early, middle, and sometimes even late forties. At this point, you may be in excellent health, knowledgeable about life, and sure of what you want. Unfortunately, the medical establishment, by virtue of your age alone, may label you as an "elderly primigravida," consider you high-risk, and view your baby as a "premium baby" requiring extensive, unnecessary interventions.

In reality, elevated risks associated with becoming a mother after the age of thirty-five are limited. There is an increased chance that you will have a baby with Down syndrome, and you have a higher chance of developing age-related conditions such as diabetes and high blood pressure. But many older women stay healthy throughout pregnancy and childbirth.

DRUG AND ALCOHOL TREATMENT: PROTECTING YOUR RIGHTS DURING PREGNANCY

District attorneys in several states have used existing laws about child abuse to argue that substance abuse is a criminal act against the fetus. Pregnant women who test positive for alcohol or drugs have been charged with civil or criminal child abuse or with delivering illegal substances to minors. Mandatory drug screening of pregnant women has been highly controversial.

The number of women prosecuted has increased despite unanimous opposition from medical professional organizations. The current status of fetal versus maternal rights varies in each state. In March 2001, the U.S. Supreme Court ruled that a woman must give consent before health care provi ders can test her for drugs. A positive test may result in a referral to the criminal justice system. (For more information on the legal rights of pregnant women seeking treatment, see "Reproductive Autonomy," p. 707 in Chapter 30, "Navigating the Health Care System.")

IF YOU HAVE EXPERIENCED SEXUAL ABUSE

The effects of previous sexual abuse may surface during your childbearing year. For example, you may feel invaded or violated during prenatal checkups, extraordinarily vulnerable in the midst of labor, or have unsettling flashbacks while nursing or bathing your baby. Try to find a health care practitioner who listens carefully to you, with whom you feel comfortable enough to tell at least part of your story. A therapist can help. After working with a therapist, many women who have feared vaginal births and had planned cesareans go on to have vaginal births. Find a family member or friend to talk with, if possible. Though having a history of sexual abuse may raise difficult issues, pregnancy, birth, and motherhood can be empowering and healing, physically and emotionally.[13]

IF YOU ARE EXPERIENCING ABUSE OR VIOLENCE

If you are being hurt verbally, emotionally, or physically, and you trust your health care practitioner enough to talk about it, prenatal visits can provide you with an opportunity to seek help. Some studies find that one in fifteen women are battered during pregnancy. Unfortunately, this figure may be misleadingly low. Many women experience abuse for the first time during pregnancy.

Violence can cause miscarriage and put you and your baby at risk during labor and birth. Many health care providers do not notice or recognize the marks of abuse (bruises, depression, drinking to cope), or they fail to address it. Current or former partners, or parents and other family members, are the usual assailants. If your partner's remarks change from loving to degrading, take notice. If you are isolated, do everything you can to end your isolation. Find other women to talk with. Exchange experiences, insights, and solutions. Try to get out of your situation, to protect yourself and your baby. Look in the phone book and/or call a local women's center to locate battered women's shelters offering refuge and help (see Chapter 8, "Violence and Abuse"). Ask your provider to help you find resources. There is never any justification for violence or abuse.*

IF YOU HAVE A DISABILITY OR CHRONIC DISEASE

Women with chronic diseases or physical, emotional, or cognitive disabilities have the right to the same choices as women without disabilities.

* Also see the Family Violence Prevention Fund: http://endabuse .org/resources/gethelp.

© Tanit Sakakini

"I LOVED BEING PREGNANT"

CINDY PURCELL

After a car accident left me paralyzed from the chest down, I had been fearful and wondered what kind of mom I could be. I had a pretty uneventful pregnancy except for a few urinary tract infections, which in my case could have been really dangerous. I loved being pregnant. I could feel all the changes going on inside me and used to watch him move, especially at nighttime.

Since Tanner was breech and my care providers thought turning the baby would have presented unnecessary risk because of my spinal cord injury, I was scheduled for a C-section on June 13. I had been working throughout the pregnancy, and I even worked on June 12, the day before the birth.

Now I think you can't let fear get in the way. If I had, I would have never had Tanner, and he is the best thing ever in my life.

However, you may encounter inaccessible facilities, insensitive practitioners, ignorance, and discrimination when attempting to get adequate care. There has been limited research, data, and training about disability and pregnancy. Be prepared to advocate for yourself and to educate your health practitioner, or to find someone who can help.

People may try to talk you out of having a baby, unable to imagine how you could cope. Don't let their ignorance affect your decision. Asking yourself questions beforehand can help clarify your thoughts and wishes: Will pregnancy and birth put my health at risk? If so, how? Are there ways to lessen the risk? Do I want to have a baby despite the risk? If my disability is genetic, how do I feel about the possibility of passing my disability on to the baby? Contact organizations that deal with your specific concerns.

Carefully choose the people who know you and your needs best to help you decide where you want to have your baby and to be with you during childbirth. If your health plan doesn't allow you to make these decisions, try to meet all of the members of the health "team" who might care for you. You may want to tour the hospital or birth center in advance. You also may want to write a brief statement about yourself and include a paragraph describing how you want to be treated (for example, "Don't talk to me through my attendant/interpreter; talk to me directly"). Hand out copies to everyone so that you won't have to answer the same questions over and over.

Being in the hospital and experiencing the intense physical changes of labor may trigger feelings of vulnerability or helplessness. Remember that you are the expert about your own needs. Trust yourself to handle difficult situations and people, and ask for help. Make sure someone accompanies you to act as your advocate.

YOU ARE READY FOR BIRTH

The transition to motherhood can be challenging, both physically and emotionally. Learning as much as you can and listening to other women's stories will give you information and inspiration to face the challenges of pregnancy and childbirth with greater confidence.

One woman describes her experience:

I found Kathy online, the one doula in our area. . . . We met once, were going to meet again, then, in the hospital, I started going into labor. Soon I was having serious contractions, a bit out of control, thrashing around wildly. Finally, I
called Kathy. She arrived and sat me on a chair. I immediately calmed down and spent a long time seated, barely noticing contractions, as we joked and talked. At some point she must have noticed a change and advised me to use the birthing ball. I did; it kept me feeling open. Her saying "That pain is bringing your baby closer to you" changed my whole perspective, made me feel so good.

A woman planning a home birth said:

My mother gave birth to me at home. Her mother had given birth to five children and had considered her labors her finest, strongest moments. I know I can give birth, and it is hard work, but I trust my body. At night I sit still, close my eyes, breathe deeply, and picture myself opening up. . . . My birth will be unique.

That woman's midwife recalls that when labor began, the expectant mother was too excited and was experiencing too many contractions to sleep, so she got up at two A.M. and baked bread, muffins, and a pie:

In the morning she called me and continued to work and walk in between contractions. By late afternoon her whole focus was on contractions. She changed positions often, and during a rest time, lying on her side, her cat draped himself across her rising and falling uterus. The purring, she said, gave her comfort. At one point, she opened her eyes, asking, "Ohhh, how long?" Late in the evening she gave birth while squatting on her bathroom floor, reaching down to welcome her son.

NOTES

1. Technical Working Group World Health Organization, "Care in Normal Births: Report of a Technical Working Group," 1997, accessed at www.who.int/reproductive-

health/publications/MSM_96_24/MSM_96_24_Chapter6.en.html on October 27, 2004.

2. Murray Enkin, *A Guide to Effective Care in Pregnancy and Childbirth*, 2nd ed. (Oxford: Oxford University Press, 1995), and text available in entirety from www.maternitywise.org; Henci Goer, *Obstetric Myths vs. Research Realities: A Guide to Medical Literature* (Westport, CT: Bergin & Garvey, 1995); and Marjorie Tew, *Safer Childbirth? A Critical History of Maternity Care*, 2nd ed. (London: Chapman & Hall, 1995).

3. J. P. Rooks, N. L. Weatherby, E.K.M. Ernst, S. Stapleton, D. Rosen, A. Rosenfield, "Outcomes of Care in Birth Centers," *New England Journal of Medicine* 321(1989): 1804–11. See also M. F. MacDorman, G. K. Singh, "Midwifery Care, Social and Medical Risk Factors, and Birth Outcomes in the U.S.A.," *Journal of Epidemiology and Community Health* 52 (1998): 310–17.

4. A "Listening to Mothers" survey participant, accessed at www.maternitywise.org on October 27, 2004.

5. Kate Bauer, executive director of the National Association of Childbearing Centers, personal correspondence, November 15, 2003.

6. E. D. Hodnett, S. Gates, G. J. Hofmeyr, C. Sakala, "Continuous Support for Women During Childbirth," *Cochrane Review*, in *The Cochrane Library*, Issue 4, 2003. (Chichester, UK: John Wiley & Sons, Ltd.)

7. MacDorman, Singh, "Midwifery Care, Social and Medical Risk Factors."

8. O. Olsen, "Meta-Analysis of the Safety of Home Birth," *Birth: Issues in Perinatal Care* 1 (March 24, 1997): 4–13. Results from the combined experiences of twenty-five thousand women in five countries.

9. Ellen S. Lazarus, quoting Enkin and Chalmers, "Poor Women, Poor Outcomes: Social Class and Reproductive Health," in Karen L. Michaelson, ed., *Childbirth in America: Anthropological Perspectives* (South Hadley, MA: Bergin & Garvey, 1988), 53.

10. A. Streissguth and J. Kanter, eds., *The Challenge of Fetal Alcohol Syndrome* (Seattle: University of Washington, 1997).

11. Jane Pincus, "A Consumer Viewpoint: Childbirth Advice Literature as It Relates to Two Childbirth Ideologies," *Birth* 27 (2000): 209–13.

12. Carol Rados, "FDA Cautions Against Ultrasound 'Keepsake' Images, *FDA Consumer Magazine* 38, no. 1 (January–February 2004), accessed at www.fda.gov/fdac/features/2004/104_images.html on October 27, 2004.

13. Penny Simkin and Phyllis Klaus, *When Survivors Give Birth: Understanding and Healing the Effects of Early Sexual Abuse on Childbearing Women* (Seattle: Classic Day Publishing, 2004).

CHAPTER 22

We bring to childbirth our histories, our relationships, our rituals, our needs and values that relate to intimacy, our sexuality, the quality and style of family life and community, and our deepest beliefs about life, birth and death.[1]

LABOR AND BIRTH*

Labor continues the process begun at conception. The finely tuned biological system that nurtures developing babies guides labor as well.

Your labor will be unique, influenced and shaped by many

* This section describes labor and birth as they can occur naturally without interruption or intervention. Given the present health care system, women in the U.S. don't always have such an experience, yet it is important to know what is possible when women give birth in supportive surroundings.

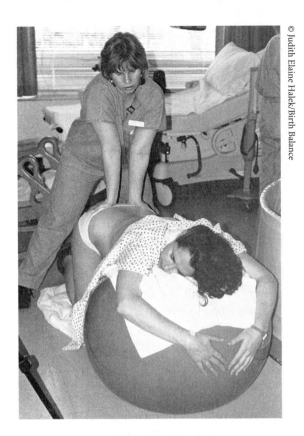

factors: your physiology, the size and position of your baby, your health and medical history, your expectations and feelings, the people who surround and support you, your professional attendants, and the place you labor and give birth. The experience of labor varies from woman to woman, in different phases of labor, and from one labor to another.

A woman tells the story of her home birth:

I had a long, drawn-out labor. Labor was painful. Pain isn't an adequate word. I was bowled over by the intensity of the physical experience. I remember thinking as labor got heavy, women are fantastic, they get pregnant over and over again and are strong enough, people go through this all the time. Nobody could have prepared me for it in words. But because everyone was saying, "Everything is fine," it was easy to keep going.

Then came the best time of all. Mary was holding the mirror; each time I pushed, I could see the effects. Laura: "Try breathing—blow out from really deep inside you. Let your cheeks puff out." It worked. I started squatting, then sitting up with Lewis behind me. My final delivery position was on my side, one leg up on Laura's shoulder. With every single push, I could see Emma coming out, bigger and bigger. After every push, Laura would massage my perineum. The little—no, the big!— head came out. Laura said to Lewis and me, "Reach down and lift up your baby." It was a big surprise to us! We did! I birthed her into our hands. I brought her to my breast. We were enthralled. The afterbirth came out with no problem. Laura showed it to us.

The whole experience changed my life. It taught me how deeply physical life is, and connected me much more with my body.

A woman who gave birth in a hospital birthing center says:

The baby was in breech position. We waited to have her turned (by external version) until around 3 weeks before she was due, to lessen the chance of becoming breech again. (If she had been breech, Lucy, our midwife, wouldn't have been

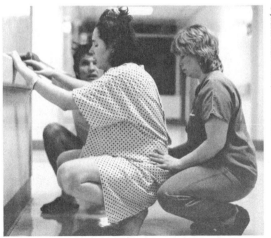

able to attend us, as it was a first-time breech—hospital rules.) The doctor at the hospital repositioned her, mainly by feel, using his hands. He was very still and quiet; it was like a massage. I said, "You just turned her, didn't you?" He said, "Yup." So simple and positive.

The day before she was born, I'd done everything: cooked, mopped, even put up a new mailbox in the bitter cold weather outside.

At 3 A.M. my waters broke. We didn't sleep much after that. We had an already scheduled appointment with Lucy at 10. Since I was only 1 centimeter dilated, she said, "Go on home." . . . Off we went, and all of a sudden, there I was in hard labor, doubled over. Back we drove to the hospital birth center. No one was expecting us; the place was empty. We got a room. I took a shower and curled into the yoga "child's position," letting hot water run down my back, relatively comfortable. Lucy finally arrived, saw I was completely dilated, and said, "Impressive! Good show!"

I pushed for two hours. I never doubted that I could do it, but it took so long, I was exhausted. Finally, Rosa crowned. Margaret caught her; I remember she put her on my belly. Since she didn't cry, they worried, took her to another room, but Marg said, "That's ridiculous: Bring her back!" And so they did. We stayed 2 nights. It was an amazing moment finally to bring her home.

APPROACHING LABOR

Just before labor begins, your body readies itself. The joints in your hips and pelvis relax and open, ligaments soften, and the baby may drop deeper in your pelvis in readiness. Toward the end of pregnancy—for some women, even earlier—you may occasionally feel a painless tightening of your uterus, called *Braxton-Hicks contractions*. These normal "practice contractions" do not come at regular intervals, nor do they cause your cervix to open. You will also feel increased pressure in your pelvis and on your bladder as the baby drops lower.

During the last few days before labor starts, your cervix changes from firm to very soft and then becomes very thin (it effaces). A degree of dilation (opening of the cervix) may occur before you feel regular contractions. Sometimes the cervical softening and thinning does not occur until active labor begins.

WHAT CAUSES LABOR AND WHEN IT BEGINS

We don't know all the biological mechanisms that cause labor to begin, or the best gestational length for a particular baby. Thus, we cannot predict or determine exactly when labor will start. Changes in hormonal levels in both you and your baby influence the timing of labor: Natural hormones called *prostaglandins* ripen or soften your cervix, while *oxytocin* causes regular rhythmic contractions that dilate your cervix. The baby's size and maturity, as well as placental changes, also play a role.

Normal-term pregnancies range from about 37 to 42 weeks; a due date marks the midpoint in this window of time.* Though artificial inductions are increasingly common, as long as mother and baby are healthy, there is no physiological reason or benefit to forcing or rushing the process.

SIGNS OF LABOR

As your cervix softens and opens, the mucus seal may begin to come out, tinged pink or streaked

---

* For information on labor that begins before 37 weeks, see "Premature Labor and Birth" (W53) on the companion website, www.ourbodiesourselves.org.

with blood ("bloody show"). Other signs of approaching labor may include loose stools, mucus discharge, crampiness, more frequent contractions, leaking of fluid, or rupture of membranes. Many women have a strong burst of energy, a nesting impulse that compels them to cook, clean house, or become more organized. If you are tired, go to bed early and nap during the day, if possible, since you will need to be well rested.

The sac containing the amniotic fluid that surrounds your baby may rupture (waters breaking), causing the fluid to gush or trickle out before contractions begin. A leak high up in the sac may trickle and seal up; sometimes fluid leaks out for a few days before labor starts. Call your practitioner when your bag of waters breaks or when you think you are leaking fluid. Your practitioner may want to check the baby's position and heartbeat and discuss the options of inducing labor or waiting until labor starts on its own. Notice the color of the fluid and tell your practitioner if there's any brown or green staining, a sign that meconium, the first stool in your baby's bowels, has been squeezed out. This can occasionally be a sign of fetal distress.

If there is no medical reason why your labor should be induced once the bag of waters is broken, waiting for labor to start spontaneously is best. You will be less likely to receive unnecessary interventions or to develop the complications that can occur from inducing labor. **To reduce the chance of infection, do not take baths until labor is clearly established; do not have intercourse; and *do not have* vaginal exams. Rest and drink often. Take your temperature twice a day.**

There is controversy about how long women should wait for labor to start after the bag of waters has broken. Some evidence supports a period of watchful waiting up to 72 hours for labor to begin on its own, while observing the above precautions. There is no clear justification for routine induction after 12 to 24 hours, as many doctors believe. After 48 hours, some practitioners will suggest various ways to stimulate labor, with castor oil, herbs, or nipple stimulation. Eight out of ten women begin labor naturally within 24 hours once membranes have clearly ruptured.

MYTH OR REALITY?

• *My doctor should cut the umbilical cord immediately after my baby is born.*

Myth. It has been routine medical practice to cut the cord as soon as the baby breathes, but there is no evidence that this is better than waiting. If you wait until the cord stops pulsating before cutting it, your baby receives additional blood and iron to support healthy red blood cell production.

• *Cesarean section rates in the United States are abnormally high compared to other countries.*

Reality. Today, 26 percent of all U.S. babies are born by cesarean section, a rate that is much higher than in other industrialized countries. In the 1960s, the U.S. cesarean rate was 5 percent. There are many reasons for today's high cesarean rate, including the underuse of care that enhances the natural progress of labor and birth, the tendency by doctors to practice "defensive medicine" because they fear being sued, and the wide use of medical interventions, such as induction of labor and epidurals, which might necessitate a cesarean.

LABOR BEGINS AND EARLY LABOR

Contractions gradually shorten uterine muscles and pull up on your cervix, moving your baby down. This pressure can feel like gas pains, menstrual cramps, backache, or painful throbbing in your thighs or pelvis. Early on, contractions may vary, occurring regularly or irregularly. They may be inconsistent, widely spaced, or short-lived. Frequently, they will come regularly for a few hours and then stop—sometimes even for a few days. You can still go about your normal routine during this time.

A little before 6 in the morning, I had what was probably my first contraction. The pressure I felt in my back signaled to me that this was different from the Braxton-Hicks contractions I'd had so many of throughout the latter half of my pregnancy. Since the pain wasn't that bad, the contractions were irregular, and I wasn't convinced I was in labor, I decided to go to work. In hindsight, I think this was a very wise decision, because spending the next twelve hours going about my everyday routine helped to minimize my attention to the pain and allowed my body to naturally prepare itself for the birth of my son.

When my husband came home from work, I told him I had a bad backache, probably from the cleaning and vacuuming I had been doing in preparation for the baby. Then I realized that my "backache" became more intense every few minutes, lasting for nearly a minute each time. I had always envisioned labor would feel like menstrual cramps—I'd been in early labor for hours and hadn't known it!

Some labors build up gradually, starting with any of the signs mentioned above, with crampiness evolving into stronger contractions that grow closer together over a long period of time, even over a period of days. At the other extreme, labor can begin abruptly, with strong regular contractions no more than five minutes apart, causing you to stop everything you are doing and requiring you to breathe and concentrate.

Labor frequently begins at night. Sometimes a hot bath or shower will slow things down, enabling you to sleep. If you feel contractions during the day, go about your usual routine if you can, but take time to eat and rest. Drink frequently.

Everyone responds differently to this phase of labor. Early on, walking, showering, taking long baths, or cuddling with loved ones can relax you and help labor progress.

When we went for a walk, we ran into friends. "What are you doing up? I thought you were in labor." It was fun changing people's image of a woman in labor.

These early hours may be sweet as you lie with your partner or sit alone, the baby still within you in the quiet of your home. Some women are too excited or apprehensive to sleep. You might want family and friends to come early on. Save your energy for active labor. Don't worry if contractions slow down when you lie down to rest.

ACTIVE LABOR

The body is malleable and birth is dynamic. . . . We have three forces, which interplay: the power of contractions, the baby's body, and the expandable passage. None of these can be considered separately; they form and re-form in relationship to each other; they touch, intertwine, converse, accommodate, embrace. It may be most appropriate to think of the process as dance.[2]

Some women are already effaced and dilated to 3 or 4 centimeters when active labor begins. Others have a "latent" phase that lasts for many hours, up to two days, with regular strong contractions that slowly efface and open the cervix to 4 centimeters.

When you feel strong, wavelike, regular, rhythmic contractions at least five minutes apart that last 45 to 60 seconds and are so intense that you can't talk while you are having one, you are most likely in active labor. The contractions may begin in your back, or you may feel them only in the front. Your uterus becomes hard. This is the time to gather your support people, to call your practitioner if you are having a home birth, or to prepare to go to the birth center or hospital.

In between contractions, rest, sleep, walk, or talk. If you are in a hospital, ask for intermittent monitoring by Doptone. (Many hospitals use continuous electronic fetal monitoring that prevents you from moving around—see section below.) Relaxing deeply between contractions renews your energy, allows contractions to work effectively, and helps reduce the intensity and pain. Pee as often as you can.

GIVING BIRTH

More rapid, intense contractions; a powerful "opening up" feeling; and rectal pressure are several signs that indicate you are completely dilated and ready to move your baby down through your vagina (birth canal) and give birth. Breathing deeply and focusing your energy can help you relax. Some women become quiet and focus inward. Others moan, hum, chant, or sing to match the new intensity.

Rocking, breathing, groaning, mouthing circles of distress, laughing, whistling, pounding, waving, digging, pulling, pushing—labor is the most involuntary work we do. My body gallops to these rhythms. Labor is a drama in which the body stars.[3]

Lying flat on the back is a painful position for many laboring women. Experiment with other positions that use the force of gravity until you find one that is comfortable for you. Kneel, squat, rock on your hands and knees, stand under running water in a shower, or submerge yourself in a tub or pool, if one is available.

Contractions may come so close together that they seem to merge into one long one with an overwhelming urge to push. Do whatever makes you feel more comfortable and helps you handle the intensity of labor. You may be irritable, nauseated, shaky, with trembly thighs and knees. Take comfort in knowing that this part of labor is almost complete. Often just before you feel like pushing or bearing down, contractions space out to provide a plateau that can last for a brief time, allowing you to rest, even to doze.

Pushing can be a great relief because it requires you to become an active participant, in contrast to the yielding and letting go necessary for opening the cervix. Pushing your baby out works best when you do just what your body wants, without external direction. Let others know which way of pushing feels best to you. Bear down only when you feel the urge and the feeling is overwhelming.

Pushing has a rhythm of its own. At the beginning, your baby's head moves down with a contraction, then retreats a little; down again during the next one, and back again. This to-and-fro gently molds the baby's flexible head bones to fit between your pelvic bones.

Depending on the baby's position, pushing can sometimes be very painful and very hard work, which may shock and disappoint you if you thought that it would be pain-free and exhilarating. Change positions to find the most comfortable one. Being upright (leaning, squatting, hanging from something or someone) helps you and your baby and often lessens pain and backache.

I told them I wanted to push, and the nurses decided to move me directly into the delivery room. I kept pausing to hold on to my doula, sounding more like an injured bear every moment. The whole time the nurses were telling me not to push, not to push, we'd get in the room and the doctor would arrive and then I could get started. What they didn't know is that I was secretly pushing. It felt so good to push, so necessary, and since I couldn't tell them about it, I just kept it to myself.

By the time I got up on the bed, the nurses got wise to me and told me to stop pushing, *and instead take little huffy breaths that at the time seemed impossible to master. The doctor finally arrived, slipped out of his jacket and into some surgical gloves. I screamed at him, "I have to push!" He said with a smile, "Well, why don't you just give me a little push, and we'll see what happens." I pushed once, and my daughter's head appeared; on the second push, she was out. I went from 3 to 10 centimeters and pushed her out all within twenty minutes.*

Another woman says of her experience:

To me, one of the more surprising things about giving birth was how little I had to actually think about what I was doing. I wrote a birth plan, read books, and generally prepared. But when I went into labor, logic and research became irrelevant—it wasn't an out-of-control feeling, more that my body was following some kind of preset plan. When it came time to push the baby out, my body's instincts took over and really pushed. It was shocking. I used muscles I didn't even know I had. And sure enough, my daughter came right out.

Shorter, spontaneous pushing is better for you and your baby than extended breath-holding. Between pushes, breathe deeply and rest. You might even fall asleep for a few minutes. Remember that—just as with earlier phases of labor—your uterus is designed to work involuntarily to move the baby down and out. Work with it, and give it time. Your labor may not progress as quickly as you had imagined, or as others around you expect.

Direct your energy downward and outward. Some women make deep, loud sounds as they push, while others simply "breathe" their babies out, concentrating intensely and making no sound at all.

It may take only one or two pushes, or a few hours of pushing, to birth your baby. As long as both you and your baby are doing fine and the baby is moving forward, there's no good reason to limit this phase of labor.

Women give birth in all sorts of ways: squatting, sitting on the toilet, side-lying with one leg supported, reclining in a tub for a water birth, on hands and knees. Some birth centers have stools or squatting bars to hold on to. In hospitals, your choice of positions may be more limited.

When the baby moves under your pubic arch, your perineum stretches slowly to accommodate the head. When you feel a burning sensation, breathe lightly so as not to push too rapidly and risk tearing. Your attendant may use oil to soften your tissues, and hot compresses for comfort and to promote circulation. Reaching down to touch your baby's head for the first time often produces an "Ahhhhhh" that opens you up even more.

Normally, your baby's head emerges first, then the body follows, sometimes slowly, inch by inch. Some babies are born in one continuous motion. Your attendant may check to see whether the umbilical cord is loosely around the baby's neck. This is usually not a problem. Breathe your baby out.

YOUR BABY IS BORN

Some babies breathe as they are being born, and look pink immediately. Others are still and may respond well if you rub their backs until they breathe in a regular, sustained way. Healthy babies are able to clear their own airways of fluid and mucus and do not need to be suctioned. If a baby's breathing is a little difficult at birth, or there is a lot of mucus, gentle suctioning may be helpful. Not all newborns cry. Some do for a moment, then stop. Often they breathe, blink, and look around, or cough, sneeze, and snuffle. Your baby's head may appear oddly shaped, having been temporarily molded by coming through the birth canal.

Mothers and babies belong together during this precious time. When you feel ready, hold your baby naked against your belly and breasts, near the familiar sound of your heart, so that she or he can touch your skin, smell, hear, and see you. Both of you need continuous peace and quiet. At home, it may be easy. In some hospitals, you may find it harder to preserve this important time.

I was in awe as I gazed into my baby's face for the first time. He wasn't crying, just looking intently at me. He was so tiny and new, but those eyes—they were so luminous and wise. He seemed regal; he had so much presence.

Practitioners can unobtrusively evaluate your baby's well-being and examine your baby in your arms. It is usually not necessary to have tests done right away. If there is a medical reason to take your baby away from you for a short time, your partner or support person can accompany the baby. If your baby needs special care, you will still have many ways of becoming attached to each other. You have been together for nine months, and bonding in humans is an ongoing process.*

* See *Your Amazing Newborn* by Marshall H. Klaus and Phyllis Klaus (Cambridge, MA and New York: Perseus Book Group, 2000).

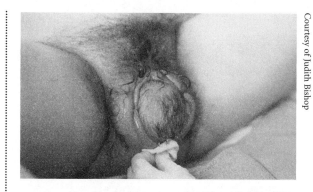

Courtesy of Judith Bishop

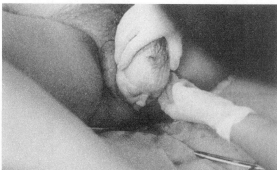

Courtesy of Judith Bishop

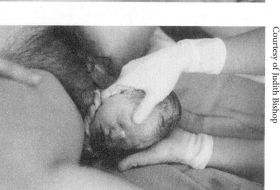

Courtesy of Judith Bishop

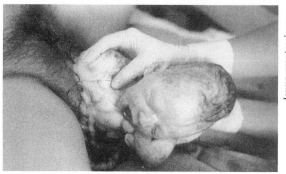

Courtesy of Judith Bishop

SUCKLING

Labor stimulates babies. Their first few hours of life are a time of heightened awareness that enhances their ability to focus and learn. Breast-feeding will be easier to establish if your baby nurses within the first hour or two after birth. Babies have an instinctive sucking reflex but show varying degrees of interest and take different amounts of time to nurse. Some latch on to the breast immediately, others more gradually over a period of hours. Smelling, licking, and exploring your breasts are part of the process. Allowing your baby to suckle, even if you don't plan to breast-feed, will give him or her the benefit of antibodies and nutrients from colostrum, the first "milk."

Nursing is important for you, too, since it stimulates oxytocin, which causes your uterus to contract to expel the placenta and to stay contracted afterward, slowing down any bleeding. *If you are planning to breast-feed, insist that the baby not be given any water or formula.* (For more on breast-feeding, see "Breast-feeding Your Baby," p. 478 in Chapter 23, "The First Year of Parenting.")

CUTTING THE CORD

After birth, your baby is still attached by the umbilical cord to the placenta inside you. There's no medical reason to cut it immediately. In hospitals, many practitioners cut the cord as soon as the baby breathes. Let your practitioners know what you want. If you wait until the cord stops pulsating, the baby receives up to 50 milligrams of iron to add to his or her reserves. The cord is clamped or tied off a short distance from the baby's navel. You may want your partner or family member to cut it. The bit of cord left on the navel will dry up and usually falls off within ten to fourteen days.

DELIVERY OF THE PLACENTA

Delivering the placenta completes the birthing process. After an interval that lasts from five to thirty minutes or so, the umbilical cord lengthens, a contraction occurs, and the placenta is expelled, often in a rush of blood. It's important not to pull on the placenta before it is separating from the uterine wall. It is extremely important that no fragments of the placenta remain in your uterus, as these fragments may allow blood vessels to remain open, causing hemorrhage. Retained fragments can also put you at risk for infection in the uterus. Contractions come sooner when you are sitting up or squatting and when your baby is suckling. Breast-feeding stimulates this process.

Once the placenta comes out, blood vessels close off. Your uterus contracts and begins to shrink. After the placenta is out, your baby's suckling helps keep your uterus firm and contracted.

Some view the placenta as a beautiful organ, with its pattern of blood vessels resembling a tree of life. Many cultures have rituals surrounding the afterbirth, including planting trees or flowering bushes above it. Let the staff know if you want to see and/or keep the placenta.

THE FIRST HOURS AND DAYS AFTER THE BABY IS BORN

At home and in birthing centers, it is usually easy for you both to be together, sleeping and waking together, getting to know each other, the baby nursing whenever she or he desires. In the hospital, specifically request that your baby remain with you. If a practitioner thinks that separation is needed, ask for an explanation. Even if medical observation or treatment becomes necessary, it is usually possible for you or your partner to stay with your baby.

If you have your baby in a hospital, the time you will stay will vary, from just a few hours to a few days if you have had a cesarean birth.

SITUATIONS THAT REQUIRE MEDICAL RESOURCES

Modern medicine has lifesaving and health-enhancing resources and tools to support women who have medically complicated pregnancies and births. Medical conditions that require special attention include insulin-dependent diabetes, high blood pressure, pre-eclampsia, multiple births, placenta previa, intrauterine growth restriction, and malpresentation—all relatively rare. Even when you find yourself in a hospital situation and interventions have been deemed necessary, your baby's birth can remain an emotionally and physically empowering event, and you can experience a positive transition to motherhood.

MEETING THE CHALLENGES OF LABOR AND BIRTH

Often, when you're in labor, it is almost impossible to connect with the fact that you are going to have a baby—it's really going to happen! Many aspects of labor and birth can be overwhelming: the intensity of contractions, the experience of pain, the uncertainty and unpredictability, the need to live in the moment, the newness of the experience for first-time mothers, the awareness

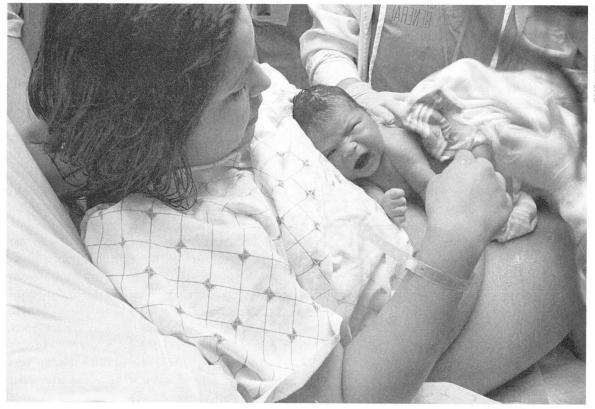

Chris T. Anderson © 2002

of impending parenthood. It helps to acknowledge and prepare as early as possible, as any or all of these elements can cause fear and panic.

Fear is a normal response to feeling overwhelmed or to not knowing what will come next. However, sustained fear can interfere with the effective functioning of labor, causing the secretion of adrenaline, which in turn may slow the labor process, which can lead to more uncertainty and more fear. When we are in labor, our bodies produce endorphins, the body's natural narcotic. These hormones reduce pain, help you ride out the contractions, and can create a euphoric "high" feeling that enables you to feel calm and peaceful in between pains.*

Women have described labor sensations in many ways: shocking, powerful, intense, painful, uncontrollable, difficult but doable, overwhelming. All are *making it happen,* moving toward a goal—the birth of your baby. Labor is an event of health. It need not be a cause for anxiety nor involve extreme distress. You do not have to be Superwoman to go through labor.

At first I was really scared of labor. I knew I wanted a birth as free of interventions as possible, but I thought this meant I had to be some kind of Amazon who squatted in the field, grunted out her baby, then stood up to pick the crops. Or else a super-fit marathon runner who had endless endurance and tolerance for pain. But the more I learned, the more I talked to other women, and the more support I got from my midwife, the more confident I felt. I took great comfort in the fact that women have been giving birth forever— every one of us had a mother who managed to birth us!

* See "Hormones Driving Labor and Birth" at www.maternitywise .org/mw/aboutmw/index.html?hormones.

STRATEGIES TO EASE LABOR

There are many different ways to deal with the intensity of labor and birth. A quiet environment with dim light is often most relaxing.

If you are having your baby in a hospital and you want to labor spontaneously, without interruption, you may have to be firm in insisting on having your wishes met at the very time when you should be focusing on your labor. Hospitals are not usually peaceful places. Most of them have or impose medical interventions that can deplete your sense of competence, your optimism, and your strength.

You can most successfully create your own pool of calm and determination in the midst of a busy atmosphere when supportive birth attendants inspire and sustain you; when they take responsibility for creating a safe cocoon or protected space around you; when they support your capacity to labor naturally; and when you have the freedom to incorporate into your experience some of the elements mentioned below.

The Presence of Others

Up until the twentieth century, when hospital births became the norm, female relatives, friends, and midwives attended women in labor. The continuous presence of people who love you and believe in you (your midwife or doula, a supportive physician and/or nurse, your husband, partner, or a family member or friend) can provide comfort and strength. The presence of a support person who stays with you continuously through labor makes labor shorter and more efficient; women who have support people have fewer medical interventions and are less likely to have a cesarean birth.[4] Choose people who understand your wishes and can focus on your needs. Even if you want to be left to yourself at times, nearby support is reassuring.

Listen to Yourself

Whatever you want or don't want during labor is fine. Don't be surprised if what you thought you *might* want differs from what you actually *do* want. Listen to your body's messages. Feel free to surrender yourself to each moment.

Surroundings

You may feel most comfortable at home, where you can create the atmosphere you want. In free-standing birth centers, you can cook, use the living room, walk outside, and spend time with children and friends. In hospitals, bring home along with you, in the form of clothes, personal objects, and recordings of music that you love. Most women need privacy, dim lights, and calm, all of which enable labor to flow efficiently and naturally.

Nourishment

Eat and drink what you want. Juices, teas, energy drinks, or light soups during labor keep you hydrated and give you energy. You are doing very hard work, after all, and need sustenance. Pee often.

Activity and Positions of Comfort

Moving around, being upright, walking, changing positions, dancing, rolling your hips, rocking on hands and knees if you are in back labor, squatting: All work with the forces of gravity and can help your uterus to work effectively. Many women find sitting or lying on large rubber birth balls useful.* Some women focus best, relax, and labor effectively lying on their side once active labor is established. **Lying flat on your back is not an ideal position.**

* See Janet Balaskas, *Active Birth* (Boston, MA: Harvard Common Press, 1992).

The Solace of Water

Water can be wonderfully soothing. It can help start contractions or pick them up into a new rhythm. Some women stay in the shower for hours. The flow of hot water on your back can ease discomfort, especially if you experience contractions and intense pressure mostly in your lower back (back labor). Immersion in a tub of deep water can help you feel lighter.

Touch

Sometimes you may seek support, touch, and massage, and sometimes not. Many midwives and doulas give wonderful massages. Ask others to help you when you stand, squat, or kneel, to let you hang from them, or to hold you however you want to be held. Application of cold or heat may be soothing. If anything feels wrong, say so.

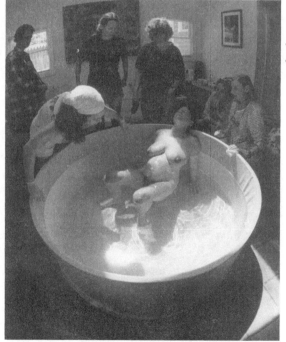

© Melissa Springer

Stillness

Sometimes being very still, being quiet and focusing inward, or sleeping between contractions leads to deep relaxation. You may want to draw upon skills learned in yoga, meditation practice, mindfulness-based childbirth preparation classes, or hypno-birthing classes.

Breathing

There really is no special way to breathe that works best during labor. Breathing takes care of itself. Focusing on natural rhythm can center you and help you work with your labor. You can pay attention to your breath, letting it anchor you to the moment as your contractions begin, become stronger, peak, and subside. Focusing on breathing out slowly between contractions can help you relax muscles and get rid of tension. Each breath brings you closer to when your baby will be born.

Imagery and Mantras

Some women focus on images that evoke peacefulness, relaxation, and openness or that serve as a mirror for what is happening in the body, such as blooming flowers, ever widening circles, or mandalas. Some cultures have special rituals to help women open. You may want to think of a phrase to repeat over and over, one that gives you strength and joy. Words and images might just come to you, but don't force the process.

During the most intense phase of labor, as each contraction geared up, I got on my hands and knees. While our doula pressed my hips together, my partner made me look into his eyes. He chanted to me. One time, out of nowhere, he said, "Think of Zachary's feet. Little feet in socks." "Little feet in socks" became the sustaining visualization of Zac's birth.

A midwife says:

I was with a mother who sang all during her labor. Her voice crescendoed with a lilting "Come" during each contraction. I sat across the room and observed her in the room dimly lit with candles as she began to push. With each "Come," her body seemed to close. After a while, I walked over and gently suggested that for this new phase of labor, she might try singing "Go." With each "Gooooo," her body opened, and she said she could feel her baby move through her pelvis.

Vocalizing

Women run the gamut of emotions during labor. You may feel exaltation, anger, fear, pain, or wonder. You may sing, laugh, giggle, or make low, open sounds, "ohhhhs" and "ahhhhs" and "oms." You may fear that making sounds means that you are losing control or being undignified. In fact, it means that you are present and aware, working with the descending, opening process as it is happening.[5] Feel the vibrations in your body.

Rhythm

In active labor, you turn inward, and a rhythm develops. You might rock back and forth, moan, curl around a partner's hand during each contraction, and then want massage or total silence in between. You might experience a cycle consisting of three parts: relaxation between contractions; rhythm during contraction; and a ritual that helps repeat and maintain the rhythm. Such a cycle is universal, yet the pattern that works for you will be uniquely yours.*

---

* In her book *Pregnancy, Childbirth, and the Newborn* (see "Resources"), Penny Simkin describes these helpful labor strategies as the 3 Rs: relaxation, rhythm, and ritual.

My doula told me there's nothing in life you can't do for one minute at a time. These words sustained me through an intense labor that lasted 20 hours. It was the rhythm of work, then rest; work, then rest, that made it possible to go on.

WHAT PARTNERS, FAMILY, AND FRIENDS CAN DO*

Be calm, strong, quiet, relaxed, caring, positive, and encouraging. See the rhythm in active labor that works for the woman you're supporting, and help her maintain it. Believe in her ability to get through labor, even if she doesn't believe it herself. Say, "You're doing it." Help her go from moment to moment. Suggest a walk, a shower, a bath, a change of position. Hold her. Sing, chant, moan, dance, rock with her, if that feels good to her. Breathe with her. Provide hot compresses, cool cloths, a fan, and liquids. Let her lean against you. She may not want you to touch her, or she may not want you to stop. She may just want you nearby. If she says, "I can't do this," tell her she *can* and she *is:* "You're doing really well." If she tells you to go away, don't take it personally.

ROUTINE MEDICAL PROCEDURES AND INTERVENTIONS DURING CHILDBIRTH†

Like a snowball rolling down the hill, as one unphysiological practice is employed . . . another frequently becomes necessary to counteract some of the disadvantages, large or small, inherent in the previous procedure.[6]

* For additional suggestions, see Penny Simkin, *The Birth Partner,* 2nd ed. (Boston: Harvard Common Press, 2001).

† For references on each procedure and intervention, and for help in making informed decisions guided by the best available research on safe and effective care, see the Maternity Center Association's website at www.maternitywise.org/home.html.

In some instances, medical interventions in labor are necessary and helpful. But many common hospital practices and interventions can interrupt, hinder, or accelerate the labor process unnecessarily. A 2002 U.S. national survey of birth practices showed that 93 percent of women had electronic fetal monitoring, 86 percent had IVs, 55 percent had artificially ruptured membranes, 53 percent had oxytocin, and 63 percent had epidurals.[7] These rates are higher than in any other country in the world. Many interventions have never been sufficiently evaluated for safety and effectiveness. None should be used routinely for women in normal labor.

Many women accept these interventions because hospital pressures are strong, and we don't know about alternatives to common medical practices. Nor do we learn about the negative effects of interventions.

In order to avoid unnecessary interventions, carefully choose your midwife or doctor and the place you give birth. Learn what you can, so you recognize when an intervention or practice is appropriate and when it may be unnecessary or potentially harmful.

On the following pages you'll find alternatives to routine medical practices in boldface type.

INTRAVENOUS INFUSION OF SALINE OR FLUIDS (IV)

Many hospitals routinely insert IVs in laboring women, just in case of emergency and for delivery of pain relief medication. Intravenous fluids are not necessary in normal labor. **Instead, it is important to eat and drink to keep up your energy.** Bring tea, juices, and other nourishment that you find appealing. Many hospitals have policies that limit food and drink intake, so discuss the situation with your practitioner ahead of time.

An IV restricts your freedom and ability to move about. **If you agree to have an IV to ac-**

commodate a routine recommendation, ask for a *heparin lock,* taped to your wrist but not attached to a pole, so that the IV line from the bag of saline can be attached only if you need the fluids. An IV will be used continuously if you are induced or have epidural anesthesia. It may be one of the first steps in a possible cascade of interventions.

ELECTRONIC FETAL MONITORING (EFM)

In most hospitals, thirty minutes of external ultrasound fetal monitoring to obtain a baseline reading of your baby's heart rate and response to contractions has become routine. After the baseline reading, your baby's heartbeat will be periodically monitored. In many hospitals, continuous (or nearly continuous) monitoring has become routine. Monitoring usually requires you to lie on your back, but some hospitals have fetal heart rate monitors that allow for wireless monitoring and more mobility.

Continuous monitoring has *not* been shown to improve outcomes in low-risk pregnancies, and it may lead to an inaccurate diagnosis of fetal distress and unnecessary cesarean sections. **Intermittent monitoring of the baby's heart has been shown to be as effective as continuous monitoring in women with low-risk pregnancies.**

IMMOBILITY AND LYING ON YOUR BACK

Lying flat on your back and immobility work against gravity and may make labor less effective and more painful. **Change position, walk and move around, take a shower or bath; let gravity work for you. When you want to rest, lie on your side.**

ARTIFICIAL RUPTURE OF MEMBRANES (AMNIOTOMY)

Rupturing the amniotic sac, while not painful, can have consequences. Early amniotomy, as it's called, carries risks: cord compression causing decelerations in the fetal heart rate; increased head pressure; malpositioning of the baby's head; and, rarely, cord prolapse (when the umbilical cord precedes the baby's head). Occasionally, when a woman is in active labor with a bulging sac of water in front of a well-descended head, her practitioner may rupture the membranes to facilitate contractions or to speed up a prolonged labor. This can provide relief. **Amniotomy does not need to be done routinely if your labor is progressing normally.** Eighty percent of membranes rupture spontaneously during pushing, if they haven't ruptured earlier in labor.

INDUCTION AND AUGMENTATION

Induction starts labor; augmentation strengthens contractions. If induction of your labor is required, prostaglandins inserted into the vagina as a tablet or gel may be used to soften the cervix and may be enough to initiate labor. Pitocin (synthetic oxytocin) given through an IV may also be used. Pitocin induction requires an IV and continuous fetal heart rate monitoring.

When labor contractions are weak or ineffective, Pitocin accelerates labor, making contractions more frequent and forceful. Augmentation of labor may be necessary if you have an epidural, and it can prevent cesarean birth if your contractions are not forceful enough on their own. Negative consequences to having labor augmented include being hooked up to an IV so you can't move around, and strong, prolonged contractions that reach a peak rapidly and may be more painful. Risks to the baby include fetal distress and prematurity (if the induction was mistimed).

Induction may be medically needed if a woman has pre-eclampsia, hemolytic disease (Rh factor), maternal diabetes, kidney disease, or a decrease in the amniotic fluid, or if she has not yet gone into labor past a point in time considered safe for the baby (check with your practitioner for her or his opinion on inducing women post-due dates).

In the absence of clear and compelling medical reasons for causing labor to start, wait patiently for it to unfold in its own time. When it is important to start labor within a few days, herbs, acupuncture, and castor oil have been helpful for some women, and walking can also help get things going.

PUSHING

Once you are completely dilated, attendants might ask you to hold your breath and push down as hard as you can for a count of ten. Breath-holding and sustained, directed bearing down can be exhausting and frequently are counterproductive. They are less effective than instinctive pushing. There is no justifiable reason to hold your breath during any part of labor.

ROUTINE EPISIOTOMY

Episiotomy is a cut made through perineal skin and muscles, between the vagina and the anus, to enlarge the vaginal opening. Doctors originally performed episiotomy to assist birth during difficult deliveries. For decades, episiotomy has been a routine practice, despite extensive, well-documented evidence that it does more harm than good. Episiotomies increase the chance you will have a more severe tear that extends into the rectum; evidence shows that naturally occurring tears are less extensive and not as deep. Episiotomy can speed delivery by a few

minutes, but normally, there is no need to hurry the process. Occasionally, it is necessary in rare cases of fetal distress.

Since episiotomy is a surgical procedure, practitioners should obtain consent from the woman involved. Too often it is done routinely, sometimes without consent.

When I was ready to give birth, I had to look my doctor in the eye and say to him as strongly as I could: "Don't cut me!" to avoid an episiotomy. He had to listen to me!

Avoid routine episiotomy. Your perineum is designed to stretch and expand to accommodate your baby. Hormones cause your tissues to stretch and soften. The baby's head slowly stretches these tissues as it moves back and forth. Techniques such as gentle guidance, touch, hot compresses and warm oils for comfort, encouraging favorable positions, and helping you breathe your baby out all work with this process and may prevent or minimize tearing.

PAIN AND PHARMACOLOGICAL METHODS OF PAIN RELIEF*

Many women equate labor with pain and anticipate using medication for pain relief. Many hospitals offer medication and anesthesia more readily than emotional support and encouragement. Yet all pain medications and anesthesia carry some risks.

Pain during labor is not a sign of danger. It is a signal that your cervix is opening. Good support during labor, including nondrug techniques, can help you cope better with the pain and reduce the need for medication. If you are

* For additional information on the effectiveness, benefits, and risks of various methods of pharmacological pain relief, see the Maternity Center Association's website, www.maternitywise.org.

alone, afraid, or exhausted, or if you feel helpless or overwhelmed or are treated disrespectfully, you are more likely to want medication for pain relief. Pain medication can ease complicated or unusually difficult labors and can make labor safer for women with heart disease and very high blood pressure.

MEDICATION GIVEN BY INJECTION

Opioids, also called narcotics, are the most commonly used medications given to relieve pain during labor. They include morphine, Demerol (meperidine), Nubain, Stadol, Fentanyl, and Nisentil. Each works for only a certain length of time and can be safely given only at certain times during labor. Though they "take the edge off," they do not take away the sensations. **Many women find tubs, showers, and birth balls more effective for relieving pain.*** Narcotics make you sleepy and may make you nauseated or dizzy. They cross the placenta, and they can depress your baby's breathing, muscle tone, and ability to suck if given too close to the time of birth, which can interfere with the initiation of breast-feeding.

EPIDURAL ANALGESIA

An *epidural*—a form of regional anesthesia—has become the most popular method of lessening labor pain in the U.S. Epidurals can be given as a onetime injection; as patient-controlled analgesia (on demand with a button you press to administer more as needed); or continuously. All epidurals require constant monitoring.

·An anesthesiologist or nurse-anesthetist numbs the skin on your back and introduces an anesthetic similar to Novocain into a tiny

* See the "Listening to Mothers" survey at www.maternitywise.org/listeningtomothers.

catheter placed through a needle. The needle is removed, and the catheter remains in place in the space just outside the spinal column. A specially designed pump keeps the anesthetic dripping in measured doses. Epidurals significantly diminish labor sensations in most cases and give adequate relief about 80 percent of the time. To limit the interference of epidurals with labor progress, some practitioners prefer to wait to administer the medication until contractions are well established.

When you choose to have an epidural, a number of interlocking procedures may follow, most of which increase the chance that you will need more interventions. You will need a blood pressure cuff attached to your arm, and an IV to deliver fluids into your bloodstream to keep your blood pressure normal. Your baby's heart rate will be measured, by either an external fetal monitor; an ultrasound plate belted around your abdomen; or, if there are problems, an internal fetal monitor attached directly to your baby's scalp. You will be unable to move the lower half of your body easily or to get out of bed. Unless you give birth within a few hours, you will need a urinary catheter placed to drain urine (although this can be done intermittently rather than continuously), since you lose the sensation of having to pee, and a full bladder can interfere with labor progress. You may have to be given Pitocin (oxytocin) to stimulate your uterus, because the fluids necessary to sustain blood pressure can dilute the natural hormones that stimulate contractions. Or your practitioner might break the bag of waters, if it has not already broken.

Because you don't feel your contractions, the epidural often lengthens the time it takes to push your baby out. This in turn can increase your chance of needing forceps or a vacuum extractor, either of which increases the risk that your vagina will tear more extensively, that you will need an episiotomy, or that your baby will suffer trauma to the face and head. There is a greater incidence of malpresentations, such as posterior or transverse position of the baby's head, and a reduced likelihood of spontaneous vaginal birth.

Epidurals can also cause your temperature to rise. Since it isn't possible to find out immediately whether this is the result of the epidural or of an infection, your baby may be treated as if she or he has an infection or is at risk for one. In rarer cases, she or he may be subjected to repeated cultures and blood tests; antibiotics administered by injection for forty-eight hours, until culture results come back from the lab; and possibly a spinal tap, a painful procedure that involves its own risks.

When I was pregnant with my first child, no one ever suggested to me that I could give birth without anesthesia. On my first visit to the obstetrician, I was assured that I could have an epidural. If anyone had ever told me that it [c]ould cause me to develop a fever, and that therefore my baby would be subjected to a spinal tap, repeated blood tests, and surveillance, I would never have had an epidural.

Epidural anesthesia is helpful during unusually difficult or complicated births. It enables you to remain awake and is much safer than general anesthesia if you need to give birth by cesarean.

WALKING EPIDURAL

The term "walking epidural" is used to refer to both a onetime injection of morphine into the spinal fluid and a newer epidural technique that offers women a lighter dose of anesthesia. The spinal injection of morphine does not cause your legs to be numb, and women who want to can walk. It can cause intense itching, nausea, and sometimes urinary retention that requires a catheter. The newer combined spinal epidural

consists of a mixture of anesthesia and morphine. Women are less numb following this technique than after a traditional epidural but may or may not have the ability to walk safely.

Although it certainly is better to be upright and walking, moving around becomes much less likely when you are hooked up to an IV or fetal monitor or when you have no one to assist you. Some practitioners do not allow walking because even a small amount of anesthesia in the epidural space can make walking unsafe.

TWO MECHANICAL WAYS TO ASSIST BIRTH

VACUUM EXTRACTOR AND FORCEPS

These devices can help mothers and babies when babies need to be born quickly. They are important tools in skilled hands. The *vacuum extractor* is a small suction cup that fits on the baby's emerging head when he or she is still in the vagina. A vacuum is created within the cup so it stays attached to the baby's scalp when the practitioner pulls upon it. It can cause a blood-filled swelling (cephalohematoma) on the baby's head. *Forceps* resemble hinged salad tongs with long spoons curved to fit the shape of a baby's head. They can cause serious damage to babies and mothers when used inappropriately or by unskilled practitioners.

The use of vacuum cup extraction has increased. Three factors account for this: (1) the increase in the use of epidural anesthesia, which lengthens the pushing stage; (2) a maximum time limit for pushing allotted to women in some hospitals; and (3) hospital efforts to lower the cesarean section rate. Vacuum cup extraction is often used with epidurals because the anesthetic blocks pushing sensations. If you have had an epidural, be patient after you are fully dilated. You can increase your chance of avoiding a difficult vacuum or forceps delivery or a cesarean by not pushing immediately when your cervix is completely dilated. If you wait until you feel the urge to push, or your baby's head is descended further, you will have more energy and can push more effectively.

Before using an extraction delivery method, if there is no immediate emergency, **move into different positions that open your pelvis. Try squatting or nipple stimulation to increase the strength of contractions and keep up your energy.**

BIRTH BY CESAREAN SECTION

In the United States, a woman is likely to have a cesarean:

. . . if she's too big or too small; too early or too late; too old or too fearful; too tired of being pregnant or too tired of being in labor; if she's having twins, if she's breech, if she's previously had a cesarean; or if she's due and so is the weekend, Christmas, Thanksgiving, or New Year's Eve. Then again, she's also at risk if her doctor is in doubt, scared of a lawsuit, too busy, going out of town, or convinced that a cesarean is always safer . . . the reasons go on.[8]

Surgical deliveries have increased alarmingly over the past thirty years. The 2002 cesarean rate in the U.S. was 26.1 percent, the highest ever in this country (in the 1960s, the national average was 5 percent). The rate varies from practice to practice and hospital to hospital.

A cesarean is major abdominal surgery. It must be done in a hospital, where anesthesia, antibiotics, and blood transfusions are available. Cesarean sections are lifesaving operations when performed on women who have certain problems during labor, including umbilical cord pro-

lapse (the umbilical cord precedes the baby's head); placenta previa (the placenta covers the cervix); placental dysfunction producing fetal distress; or failure of the baby to descend through the area between your pelvic bones.

I'd always dreamed of having a home birth, and if that wasn't possible, to give birth in a birth center with a midwife. At 32 weeks, I had some bright red spotting. My midwife came to the hospital with me for an ultrasound, which showed that my placenta was partially covering my cervical opening. The obstetrician held out the possibility that the placenta might still move away from the cervix, although he was doubtful. I returned home with directions to call immediately if there was any more bleeding. At 35 weeks, I woke to find blood pouring. With a towel between my legs, I called my midwife, jumped in the car, and headed to the hospital, where my lovely five-pound daughter Chiara was delivered by cesarean section.

If you need to give birth by cesarean section, you will be moved to an operating room, where you will receive a spinal or an epidural to make your abdomen and legs completely numb. A urinary catheter will be inserted to keep your bladder empty. You will remain awake. In the rare instance when a cesarean section needs to be performed very quickly, you may be given general anesthesia and put to sleep because it is faster than making you numb with a spinal or epidural.

When the anesthesia has taken effect, the physician will make a horizontal cut in the abdominal wall low down near the pubis (vertical cuts are reserved for rare emergencies), make another cut through the uterine muscle, and ease your baby out. She or he will suction your baby's nose and mouth, clamp and cut the umbilical cord, and assess the baby's breathing. Once all is well, you or your partner can hold your baby as the doctor removes the placenta and sews up the incision. The whole procedure takes about an hour.

Cesarean sections can be lifesaving and health-enhancing in emergency situations, but they are not simply another way of being born. While safer than they were fifty years ago, cesarean sections are still major operations that carry considerable risks to mother and baby that don't exist in vaginal birth. Although the overall incidence of death during childbirth is extremely small in the U.S.* (9.9 deaths per 100,000 live births in 2001),[9] cesarean sections are associated with a greater risk of death to the mother than vaginal deliveries. In addition, women who have a cesarean birth are more likely to experience an infection, be rehospitalized, and experience ongoing postpartum pain. A rare long-term risk to the mother, often unacknowledged, is death from bowel obstruction. This can happen up to twenty years after the surgery if the membrane that wraps around the uterus and bowels develops scarring and adhesions. Cesarean delivery is a special concern for women who have repeated pregnancies or plan large families, as it increases risks for subsequent infertility and serious placental problems for mothers and babies in future pregnancies. Babies born via cesarean section are more likely to have respiratory distress than babies born vaginally; are less likely to breast-feed; and are more likely to experience asthma in childhood and adulthood.† Why, then, despite the evidence, is the cesarean rate soaring in the U.S.?

- Caregivers are underusing the kind of care that can enhance the natural progress of labor and birth.

* This number may be too small, as it is generally agreed that maternal mortality is underreported in this country.

† For a complete list of the risks of cesarean sections to mother and baby, see *What Every Pregnant Woman Needs to Know About Cesarean Section* (www.maternitywise.org/cesareanbooklet).

- The side effects of widely used medical interventions (induction of labor, electronic fetal monitoring, and epidurals) lead to the "necessity" of cesareans.
- Physician training may favor operative deliveries—especially forceps and vacuum—over other approaches to problems, and concerns about liability often constrain a physician's willingness to adopt nonoperative approaches.
- Obstetricians are sometimes pressured to practice defensive medicine to avoid being sued or losing lawsuits. Thus, they may not offer women who have had previous cesareans the choice of a vaginal birth after cesarean (VBAC), or they may practice in a hospital where VBACs are no longer allowed. Some haven't learned the skills they need to deliver breech babies or twins vaginally.
- Elective cesareans (the term used for cesarean sections done without a medical need) are increasingly presented by doctors and the media as an option for healthy pregnant women. Women who fear labor or don't want to go through the stress of childbirth are being allowed to choose cesareans. So far, elective cesareans make up a tiny portion of all cesarean sections, but the numbers are growing. The latest "reasons" for the recent increase in elective cesareans include the concern that vaginal delivery leads to pelvic floor damage and urinary and fecal incontinence. There is limited evidence to support this concern, and more important, the absolute risk and magnitude of these problems are not sufficient for most obstetricians ever to recommend an elective cesarean, or for most women to choose an elective cesarean.

When considering a cesarean section, ask for a list of benefits and risks to you and your baby, both short-term and long-term. The information you are given should be based on the best evidence available as it applies to your pregnancy and situation.

IF YOU HAVE A CESAREAN SECTION

Women who have complicated labors and obstetric emergencies appreciate the necessity of cesarean sections. Others experience cesarean sections as a relief, even while wondering whether or not they were truly necessary. Some of us experience the surgery as intrusive, a violation of our bodies. Too many of us fault ourselves, feeling guilty or defensive that we didn't do "everything possible" to have a natural birth. In fact, we do the best we can, given our physical circumstances and the information and support available.

A midwife says:

I tell women who begin labor at home and end up in a hospital, "Who you are never changes. Your planning, ideals, beliefs, and principles never change just because you end up . . . with a cesarean. You are stronger than you would have been, because you've gone through all these decisions and made the choices you did."

VAGINAL BIRTH AFTER CESAREAN BIRTH (VBAC)

Women who give birth by cesarean section must decide whether to have a vaginal or cesarean birth with the next baby. In 1982 a large group of concerned parents and professionals founded the International Cesarean Awareness Network (ICAN, first called Cesarean Prevention Movement [CPM]). Its mission: to prevent unnecessary cesareans, to provide support for cesarean recovery, and to promote VBAC. Immediately, chapters blossomed in many communities, as people increasingly realized that many cesareans are medically unnecessary and are caused by a chain of obstetrical interventions, and that most women can labor naturally and deliver vaginally after having a cesarean. To do so, we need accurate information and encouragement.

Most often the condition that makes a cesarean necessary in one birth will not exist in the next. The most serious, and rarest, complication that can occur during a VBAC is a symptomatic separation of a previous uterine scar (a *rupture*).

In most cases, a VBAC is safer than a scheduled repeat cesarean. However, the physical and emotional toll of laboring and experiencing various labor interventions and then having cesarean surgery is likely to be worse than the toll of a planned repeat cesarean. Because the majority of women who plan a VBAC with supportive caregivers will go on to have one, it is worth doing some research to find a hospital and provider who can offer this option. You need to know the individual chances of harm to you and your baby, not the general fear-based risks you may hear about from the media or other sources.

If you had a cesarean and want a VBAC, it is essential to find out: (1) your chance of having a successful VBAC, which is dependent upon the events that occurred during your previous labor and the reason you had the surgery; (2) your risk for uterine rupture; (3) your practitioner's philosophy regarding VBAC; and (4) the birth center's or hospital's guidelines and practices regarding VBACs. Can a midwife care for you? Are there times or situations where VBAC would not be an option? How comfortable are nurses and physicians in caring for women having VBACs? What is the provider's/hospital's VBAC success rate? Explore these questions early in pregnancy and review your history so you have a good idea of whether or not you can plan to attempt a VBAC.* Depending on the an-

---

* See the International Cesarean Awareness Network (ICAN) website at www.ican-online.org.

Although everyone hopes for a healthy baby, in rare cases, some babies are born with serious medical problems. You may face challenges that you never anticipated. Very rarely, even the unthinkable happens: Babies die at birth. At these times, grief may feel unbearable. For more about childbearing loss, see Chapter 23.

swer, you may want to change practitioners or, if possible, find another hospital.

I really believe that childbirth is a normal, natural event in a woman's life that also serves as a rite of passage. Therefore, I was absolutely devastated when my planned homebirth with my first baby turned c-section. I eventually came to peace with the fact that the two week over-due pregnancy, the very, very long labor, the over 10-lb baby had a lot to do with it.

We had moved to the opposite coast when I became pregnant again. I had made sure to find a doctor who would support my choice for a VBAC, even if it meant having the baby at the big teaching hospital vs. the nice birthing center. I was so afraid of all the things that I was told "could" happen. But I also knew that I had to trust that my body could do the job. Not only did I not go overdue, did not have to be induced, or have such a terribly long labor, but I delivered a healthy, (much smaller) baby, rather quickly, into the hands of a former home-birth midwife turned labor nurse. How perfect it seemed! I felt so empowered by this vaginal birth. I had renewed trust in my body's ability and power. I was amazed at the sheer miracle of this process undisturbed. It was so incredible, and yet so normal all at the same time.

AFTERWORD

We relive the births of our children many times during the days, weeks, months, and years afterwards. Looking back upon your birth experience may call up a wide range of emotions. You may feel fulfilled, ecstatic, and immensely close to your loved ones and your baby, especially if you felt supported and respected throughout the process. You may feel joy, wonder, and a great sense of accomplishment.

On the other hand, if unexpected complications or medical interventions dominated your birth experience, you may feel a bewildering mix of joy and disappointment. You may feel distant from your baby. It is not uncommon to apologize for having wanted more ("It doesn't matter—after all, my baby is healthy and that's all that counts") or to feel sad or guilty about not having had the "natural" birth you prepared for. Worst of all, you may blame yourself—"my body just didn't work right"—instead of recognizing that you did not get the support that might have resulted in a different outcome or that birth is, after all, unpredictable.

It is normal to have doubts, regret, grief, or anger rising to the surface over time. Talk with your partner, good friends, or a counselor for comfort, understanding, and support. Women's groups and Internet chat rooms may also be helpful.

If you are dissatisfied and want to learn more about what happened, ask to see your birth records. Check them against your memories. Talk to the practitioner and others who attended your labor. Write letters to those who you feel did not meet your needs; it may help them to become more responsive and respectful in the future. Going through some of these processes may make it possible for you to feel more at peace.

The transformation from nonmother to mother is profound; the demands, huge. With a

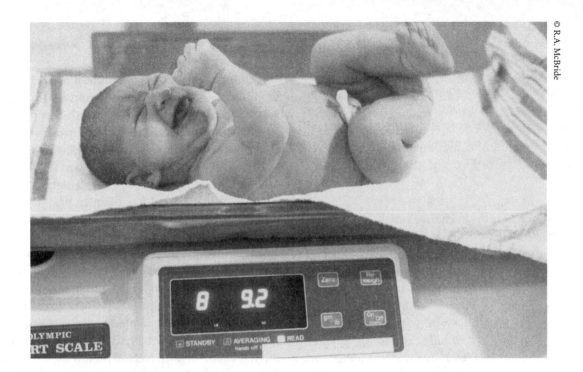
© R.A. McBride

new baby you experience a new identity and responsibilities, a connection with someone who, having been part of yourself for nine months, now becomes an individual outside of yourself. Our society provides mothers with few if any rituals, resources, or social supports for this transition. Most other Western industrialized societies offer generous paid maternity and paternity leave; flexible working conditions; quality state-run day care programs; and well-organized midwifery services. While there is little government support for new parents in the U.S., many communities have active doula groups, birth networks, or parents' organizations. These groups offer much-needed help with the joyful, difficult, passionate, challenging work of being a mother.

Even now, 24 years after my daughter's birth, I am still learning how powerful that event was. It is amazing how the experience of pregnancy, labor and birth keeps reaching across the years of my life to open doors in my heart.

NOTES

1. Judith Dickson Luce, "Birthing Women and Midwife," in Helen B. Holmes, Betty Hoskins, and Michael Gross, eds., *Birth Control and Controlling Birth* (Clifton, NJ: Humana Press, 1980), 240.
2. Penny Armstrong and Sheryl Feldman, *A Wise Birth* (New York: William Morrow, 1990), 30.
3. Louise Erdrich, *The Blue Jay's Dance: A Birth Year* (New York: HarperCollins, 1995), 42.
4. E. D. Hodnett, S. Gates, G. J. Hofmeyr, C. Sakala, "Continuous Support for Women During Childbirth," *Cochrane Review* 4 (2003).
5. Penny Simkin, *Pregnancy, Childbirth and the Newborn* (New York: Meadowbrook Press, 2001).
6. Doris Haire, *The Cultural Warping of Childbirth* (Minnesota: International Childbirth Education Association Publications, 1985), 32.
7. The Maternity Center Association, "Listening to Moth-

ers Study," accessed at www.maternitywise.org/listen ingtomothers/index.html on October 28, 2004.

8. Diony Young, "The Push Against Vaginal Birth," *Birth: Issues in Perinatal Care* 3 (September 2003): 151.

9. National Center for Health Statistics, "Mortality for Complications of Pregnancy, Childbirth, and the Puerperium, According to Race, Hispanic Origin, and Age: United States, Selected Years 1950–2001," accessed at www.cdc.gov/nchs/data/hus/tables/2003/03hus043.pdf on October 28, 2004.

CHAPTER 23 ■ ■ ■ ■ ■ ■ ■ ■ ■ ■ ■ ■ ■ ■ ■ ■ ■

BECOMING A MOTHER

You have a new baby! Whether you gave birth or adopted a child, whether you are a first-time mother or have other children, your identity, your relationships, and your perspectives all change from this moment on. Regardless of socioeconomic status, where or how you live, relationships, age, career, sexual orientation, or cultural and religious background, no woman is immune to feeling unsettled in the course of this transformation.

The period after a new baby arrives is a time of enormous change physically and emotionally. Those of us who gave birth are recovering from pregnancy and birth. Those of us who adopted are not going through the same physical changes, yet we, too, are experiencing many transitions. Our feelings range from exhilaration to exhaustion, joy to sadness, and confidence to uncertainty. Many factors affect how we experience this time in our lives: our health and the health of the baby, our feelings about the birth or adoption experience, whether feeding the baby is going well, our readiness to be mothers, and the amount and kind of support we receive from partners, families, friends, and other resources.

During those early weeks, sometimes I wasn't sure where the baby ended and I began. I felt that I had lost my old self and was too tired, physically and emotionally, to find her again. But I was also discovering a new part of myself that I hadn't known about before: unexpectedly intense feelings for my new baby, a resurgence of love for my mother, connection with other women. I went from despair to overwhelming feelings of tenderness, all within the space of an hour.

Many of us are encouraged to plan only for birth or adoption and are not adequately prepared for the many life changes that come with a new baby. Perhaps the most important thing you can do to prepare for your needs is to build up your support network in advance. This could include calling upon your partner, family members, old and new friends, neighbors, coworkers, professional care providers, and lactation consultants. Discuss with them what you will need and ways they can help you. Talk to other pregnant women and new mothers and their partners about their experiences. If possible, assign others some of the day-to-day tasks (making food, cleaning the house, caring for other children if you have them), so that you can devote your energy to caring for yourself and your baby.

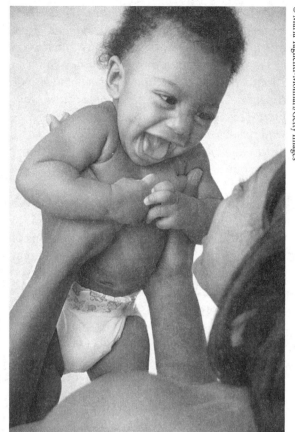

FOR WOMEN WHO HAVE GIVEN BIRTH

FEELINGS ABOUT THE BIRTH

The birth experience holds different meanings for different women. Some of us approach it as a means to an end, the end being a healthy baby. Others hope that the birth experience itself will be a transformative and spiritual experience. If the birth has gone well and your baby is healthy, you may feel incredibly happy, tremendously relieved, and proud of what you have just accomplished.

Even though I'd had a long and difficult labor, I felt ecstatic after the baby was born. I wanted to

*leap out of bed and run around the room to cele-
brate. Then, after a couple of hours, fatigue
caught up with me, and I began to feel utterly
exhausted. Every muscle and bone ached. Still,
I didn't mind somehow. It was a good kind of
tiredness—the kind that comes when you've been
pushed to the limits of your capabilities. Along
with the weariness came new, quieter feelings of
peace, happiness, tenderness for my baby, and a
connection to all womankind!*

But you may have other feelings, too, especially if
the birth did not live up to your expectations or
if you encountered unexpected interventions or
complications. If you are disappointed, you may
feel guilty and question how this happened; you
may feel angry at your providers; or you may become depressed.

*New motherhood for me consisted of an emer-
gency C-section followed by long hours sitting
bedside in a NICU [neonatal intensive care unit],
rushing between medical consults to pump breast
milk for my infant son's nasogastric feeding tube,
sleeping in snatches on a foldout cot for weeks,
eating if I had time or remembered, and enduring
round-the-clock interruptions of nurses, doctors,
medical students, interns, social workers, visitors,
and even cleaning people. Three years later, he is
whole and happy . . . while I am still grieving the
irretrievable loss of all his precious newborn firsts
and the anticipated joy of coming into my own as
a new mother.*

If your baby has health problems, you will
probably spend your time collaborating with
medical providers and making difficult decisions, forced to set aside, for the time being, your
own physical and emotional needs. Support
from others is especially important, be it from
social workers in the hospital, parent-support
organizations (see "Resources"), friends, family,
or other new parents. Trust your intuition in
terms of who is helpful and supportive, and
avoid those people who are not.

PHYSICAL CHANGES AFTER BIRTH

The course of pregnancy and giving birth is a
tremendous physical experience. No matter how
you gave birth, your body worked hard and
needs and deserves rest. Typically, it takes about
three months (sometimes called the "fourth trimester") for your body to recover fully.

The bleeding that happens after the birth is
called *lochia*. This bleeding happens whether the
birth is vaginal or cesarean. Lochia is blood combined with tissues no longer needed in the
uterus. It is red for a few days, then pink, then
brownish, then white before it stops, typically
after two to eight weeks. If bleeding is unusually
heavy or suddenly resumes after stopping, or if
the lochia smells bad or you develop a fever, this
may be a sign of infection, and you should check
with your midwife or physician.

Afterbirth pains are caused by the uterus
contracting to control bleeding. Often these
pains are worse with second and third births.
One way to relieve these cramps is to lie on your
stomach with a pillow right under the lower abdomen. Breast-feeding causes afterbirth pains
due to the hormones stimulated by suckling,
which make the uterus contract. This is why
women who breast-feed have a return to pre-
pregnant uterine size more quickly than women
who do not.

Nearly all women experience mild or moderate discomforts after birth. For instance, if you
had stitches (episiotomy), you will probably
have soreness in your genital area; if you had an
epidural, you may have a backache off and on.
Some women find that after birth, the pelvic
floor and abdominal walls feel weak and lax;
others experience painful intercourse, leaking
urine (incontinence), and other genital pain.
Though it can be embarrassing to talk about

these problems, it is important to tell your midwife or physician about them. Kegel exercises (see p. 235 in Chapter 13, "Sexual Anatomy, Reproduction, and the Menstrual Cycle") immediately after birth, followed by gentle abdominal exercises and leg lifts, will help restore your muscle tone. If you feel very tired or weak, you may be anemic. Be sure to eat enough iron-rich foods, and check with your health care provider about the advisability of iron and vitamin supplements if you are breast-feeding.

For me, physical recovery was no big deal. Because I had an easy birth and no episiotomy, I healed very fast and felt back to normal within a few days. The only things that bothered me were sore nipples (for the first couple of days) and night sweats, which lasted about a week. Otherwise, I felt terrific. Maybe I was just high from the birth, but I seemed to have a lot more energy then than I do now, several months later.

Every woman's body begins to make milk right after the afterbirth (placenta) comes out. If you are not breast-feeding, the milk backs up in the breast, causing feedback to the body, telling it to stop making milk. The second or third day, the breasts get hard and hot and may hurt (engorgement). If you have placed your baby for adoption or your baby has died, this may be an especially difficult time for you emotionally. Be sure to get support.

HELPFUL HINTS AFTER A VAGINAL BIRTH

During the first twenty-four hours after birth, apply ice packs to the genital area to reduce swelling. After twenty-four hours, try warm or cool sitz baths (sitting in a couple inches of water in the bathtub or in a toilet insert you can get at the hospital). Another recommendation for per-ineal care is to apply witch hazel directly to the perineum for pain relief.

After a vaginal birth, you will probably be up and about within a few hours. Getting on your feet soon after birth means fewer bladder and bowel problems and a quicker recovery of energy. This doesn't mean, however, that you should resume normal activities right away. Get as much help as you can, and rest when you're able.

RECOVERY AFTER A CESAREAN BIRTH

A cesarean birth is major abdominal surgery. You may feel sick and weak, and sore around the incision. It may be difficult to change positions, to get in and out of bed, or to position your baby for nursing. You may have an intravenous feeding tube (IV) and a catheter (to drain the bladder) for 24 to 48 hours. If the catheter is uncomfortable, ask if it can be removed earlier. Also ask that the IV be placed so that it doesn't interfere with nursing your baby. Do not do abdominal exercises until the midwife or physician says the incision is healed enough.

After a cesarean, you should be on your feet within a day. Walking will be painful, but it helps to get your digestive system going and to avoid blood clots in your legs (thrombosis). You should avoid heavy lifting and strenuous activity. You may have gas pains or a constipated feeling as your bowels begin to work again.

During your hospital stay, ask for whatever makes you feel better, whether it's frequent visits from your family and friends, food from home, or a massage when you're feeling tired and sore. Some hospitals allow partners to stay overnight.

Recovery from my C-section was completely different from recovery from my vaginal birth. The pain was much greater. There was an incision with stitches. After a C-section, you are recovering from something that was done to you, not some-thing your body was supposed to do. Bonding with the baby took longer because I was trying to take care of myself physically and get myself better before I could dedicate 100% to the baby.

FOR WOMEN WHO HAVE ADOPTED

The women in the new mothers' circle eyed me warily. I'd sat silently and politely listening, as they discussed their C-section scars, cracked nipples, and night-time feedings, and now, apparently, it was my turn. I had suffered insom-nia, jet lag and a radical life change, but I didn't feel I had a right to complain; after all, I'd been reminded more times than I could count, "You're lucky, you did it the easy way."

While many of the issues of adoptive mothers—exhaustion, isolation, adapting to a new baby—are the same as those of women who gave birth, women who adopt also face different logistical, emotional, and financial challenges. (For a more thorough discussion of these issues, see "Adoption," p. 317 in Chapter 17, "Consider-ing Parenting.")

BREAST-FEEDING YOUR BABY

I didn't breast-feed my first daughter. I was a new immigrant, I wanted to be like the Americans. Do I feel bad about it? Yes. Do I keep beating up on myself? No!! We have to get beyond our personal issues. I go up to women in the street who are breast-feeding and I say, "Great job!" And when women aren't breast-feeding, I say "What went wrong? Call me next time!" We need to help each other out on this one.

Breast milk is the best food for babies.[1] It pro-vides exactly the right balance of nutrients, adapting to your baby's changing requirements. Breast milk helps strengthen the infant's resis-tance to infection and disease. Not breast-feeding is associated with a higher risk of the child developing many short-term health prob-lems and chronic conditions, including ear and lower respiratory tract infections, gastrointesti-nal problems, Type 1 diabetes, leukemia, and other childhood cancers.[2] Breast-feeding also has health benefits for the mother, the most im-pressive of which is a greatly reduced incidence of breast cancer.[3] Some studies show that women who breast-feed two years or more have half the rate of breast cancer than women who do not breast-feed.[4] For premature infants, or infants with conditions such as Down syn-drome, the anti-infective properties of breast milk are especially beneficial.

Studies show that most women in the United States want to breast-feed but that practical barriers, early difficulties, and misinformation often jeopardize our success. In countries such as Sweden and Norway–where about 98 percent of mothers begin breast-feeding and 70 percent are still breast-feeding after six months—social acceptance, supportive hospital practices, and extended maternity leave all contribute to help-ing women achieve their breast-feeding goals. Unfortunately, in other developed nations, in-cluding the U.S., society's influences are differ-ent, and breast-feeding rates are low, especially among poor and minority women.[5] In the early 1970s, only 22 percent of women in the U.S. began breast-feeding their infants. By 2001 rates had risen to 70 percent, but only 46 percent of all babies received exclusively breast milk in the hospital setting.[6] Worldwide, over eighteen thousand hospitals have earned the WHO/ UNICEF "Baby-Friendly" designation for sup-portive breast-feeding practices, but in 2004 only forty-two of those were located in the U.S.

In developed countries in particular, where formula feeding is common, many of us do not have the wisdom and support of other women to help guide us in breast-feeding our child. The American Academy of Pediatrics recommends exclusive breast-feeding for approximately six months, then adding solids at six months, with continued breast-feeding to a year or beyond.[7] The WHO recommends that children be exclusively breast-fed for six months, with breast-feeding continued two or more years.

A GOOD START: ROOMING-IN

Infants who breast-feed in the first hour of life are more successful long-term breast-feeders.[8] Those who are placed on the mother's abdomen after birth will instinctively try to crawl to the breast and (especially if the birth was unmedicated) will usually find the breast and suckle within the first hour of life.[9]

Keeping your baby with you twenty-four hours a day also helps promote successful breast-feeding. Many mothers actually sleep better with their baby in the room. If you give birth in a hospital and want to room-in (as the practice is called), be clear with your caregiver and the nursing staff. It's a good idea to let them know before birth so that your newborn is not taken to the nursery. Remember: It's your right to be making decisions about your baby from the very beginning.

I am the nurse manager of a maternity unit at an inner-city hospital. I encourage the moms and babies under my care to room-in together. When my own daughter was born 20 years ago, hospital policy dictated that she was "not allowed" to stay with me at night. My breasts were engorged, I was in pain and longing to see my new child. I remember walking down the long hall to the nursery, crying, just so that I could glimpse her through the window. I am committed to my job because I never want another woman to go through such an experience.

The advantages to having your baby nearby in your hospital room include bonding; the chance to observe early feeding cues; and the opportunity to begin learning about your baby's care with skilled nurses to assist you.

I have no support. It's just me and my baby. I want him with me at all times, because that's where he's gonna be for a whole lot of years, and that's where I want him to be.

WHAT TO EXPECT IN THE FIRST FEW DAYS

Colostrum

Colostrum, the liquid in a mother's breasts before the milk actually comes in, is especially high in antibodies that protect the newborn against infections. Most women make about three tablespoons of milk in the first twenty-four hours after birth, and thirteen tablespoons on day two: just the right amount for your baby, whose stomach is only the size of her or his fist. Mothers who need to pump for medical reasons, such as the baby being in the intensive care unit, may find these first three days discouraging because the volume is so small. However, by day three or four, most mothers are pumping more milk.

Supply and Demand

The drop in progesterone levels after your baby is born starts milk production, which continues on the principle of supply meeting demand. When your baby suckles, nerves in the nipple and areola are stimulated and signal the pituitary gland to release oxytocin and prolactin. Oxytocin is responsible for the "letdown," or milk ejection reflex. It moves the milk from the glands toward and out of the nipple. Prolactin is responsible for milk production. As your breast is emptied, the milk glands respond to the prolactin, and more milk is made. The more frequently your breasts are emptied, the more milk you will make. This is why women who nurse twins make enough milk for both babies.

Latch and Positioning

The key to avoiding pain and ensuring milk transfer is for the baby to latch on well, taking as much breast as possible into her or his mouth, rather than pinching the nipple between the gums at the front of the mouth. To latch a newborn, support your breast with your fingers away from the nipple, making sure your fingers do not get in the infant's way. Stroke the center of your baby's lower lip with your nipple to elicit the rooting reflex. When your baby opens her or his mouth widely, hug the baby to your breast, so your nipple can get deep in his or her mouth and milk can flow easily.

Most of us naturally use the cradle hold to breast-feed our baby, with the infant in our arms on his or her side, facing us, tummy to tummy, nipple to nose. To prevent backache, use support under the baby and bring the baby to you, rather than leaning over. The football hold, with the baby at your side, feet tucked under your arm, is especially useful if you had a cesarean birth, as this position avoids pressure on abdominal sutures; and if you have large breasts, as it is easier to see the baby's mouth. You can also lie on your side next to your baby, tummy to tummy, with the baby nursing on his or her side and facing you.

BREAST-FEEDING CHALLENGES

Baby Cannot Latch

Some infants, especially those born early, have trouble latching, or are sleepy beyond the expected sleepiness of the first twelve to fourteen hours. If this happens, continue to offer the breast, and watch carefully for feeding cues. To

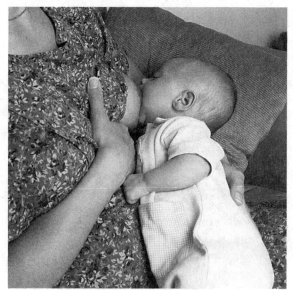

help rouse your infant, try tickling her or his feet, giving a full-body massage, undressing the baby or changing diapers, or laying the baby down in an open space away from you. Other infants are wide awake but fuss and cannot latch easily. Calming techniques—such as putting the infant skin to skin with you, offering a finger to suck before switching to the breast, and expressing colostrum onto the nipple—may calm the baby enough so he or she will begin eating. You may also need to test different holds on your breast, as one might work better than another. Some mothers need to stimulate the nipple to make it erect and firm enough for the baby to latch.

If your baby still cannot latch, you should begin to pump every three hours for about ten to fifteen minutes, with a high-quality double-pumping electric breast pump. The pump will give your body the message to make milk until your baby is sucking effectively. You can also use a small syringe to drip the milk in the baby's mouth as your volume increases.

If you leave the hospital before your baby is breast-feeding effectively, arrange for follow-up with someone who is knowledgeable about breast-feeding, such as an international board-certified lactation consultant (IBCLC).

My first baby refused to take the breast—it felt like he was rejecting me. It took hours to latch him on, and then after 10 minutes, I would have to "change sides" like the nurse said. My family all urged me to quit. After a week, I decided to pump and bottle-feed. With my next baby, I listened only to my friend who had breast-fed successfully. I breast-fed him for 13 months and my third baby for three years! If my first had been my third, I would have felt more confident and coped better. He probably would have latched on eventually.

Inverted Nipples

Some women's nipples evert (stick out or become erect) when rubbed or stimulated, while other women's nipples retract (invert) when pressure is put on the areola, making it difficult for most babies to latch. Other nipples have a slit or crease across the middle that can become painfully abraded. If your nipples are flat or mildly inverted, feeding the baby in the first hour of life and avoiding bottles may help. If the baby continues to be unable to latch, you may need to pump your milk and feed your baby with a bottle, cup, or syringe.

Engorgement

When your milk comes in, or transitions from colostrum to mature milk, the breasts may become so full and firm that your baby cannot latch easily. In this instance, you can either manually express milk or use an electric breast pump just long enough to soften the breast around the nipple so your baby can latch on (pumping for too long increases stimulation and leads to even more milk production). Ice packs or warm compresses can be used; whatever feels comfortable. Putting your baby to the breast as often as he or she will eat will ease engorgement more quickly.

Engorgement is temporary, and with careful management, most women are more comfortable within twenty-four to forty-eight hours. However, untreated engorgement can be a serious problem, because it decreases milk production by setting up the biofeedback mechanism for inhibiting prolactin. If you notice that your breasts are not softening significantly when your baby nurses, it is important to seek professional help from a lactation consultant or another knowledgeable health care professional, because breast softening is the first sign that the baby is getting milk.

Sore Nipples

Nipple pain in the early days usually results from poor latch, not from length of time at the breast. If your nipples hurt, work on positioning (see above). Breast milk on the nipples is healing; pure lanolin to rub into the chafed skin is also available over the counter. Hydrogels that were developed to treat burns can safely be used to protect the nipples between feedings and allow the skin to heal once the baby is latching on correctly. Limiting nursing time will *not* prevent sore nipples. Tolerating the pain will only lead to damage, and if the baby is not well latched, he or she will not get milk effectively.

Sore Breasts

Swelling, redness, or a painful lump in one area of your breast may signal a plugged duct. Warm compresses on the swollen area (or ice, if that feels better); massaging behind the area as the baby nurses or you pump; and increased nursing will usually ease the discomfort. If the swelling is accompanied by fever and/or a tired, run-down, achy, flu-like feeling, you probably have a breast infection (mastitis). In that case, your health care practitioner will probably recommend an antibiotic covering staph and strep bacteria, which means you can still continue to breast-feed.

Rarely, a breast infection will develop into an abscess that may have to be surgically drained.

Breast-feeding in Public

Some states have laws protecting a woman's right to breast-feed in public, and others are currently introducing them. If you encounter problems when breast-feeding in public, contact your local breast-feeding support organization (such as La Leche League) for supportive information regarding the laws in your area.

Returning to Work

Those of us who decide to continue breast-feeding after returning to work can hand-express breast milk or use an electric breast pump to produce a supply for our baby. An effective breast pump should have adequate pressure and mimic the infant's suck/swallow rhythm. Pumps may be either single or double pumping. It should take you ten to fifteen minutes to "empty" each breast. Contact your local La Leche League or the maternity unit of your hospital to obtain the names of good manufacturers.

BREAST-FEEDING UNDER SPECIAL CIRCUMSTANCES

If you have had breast surgery, successful breast-feeding may still be possible. Breast reduction surgery for cosmetic reasons or a lumpectomy (breast cancer treatment) can cause problems with milk supply. Breast augmentation surgery is usually less problematic. If you have had a mastectomy (breast removed), you can probably

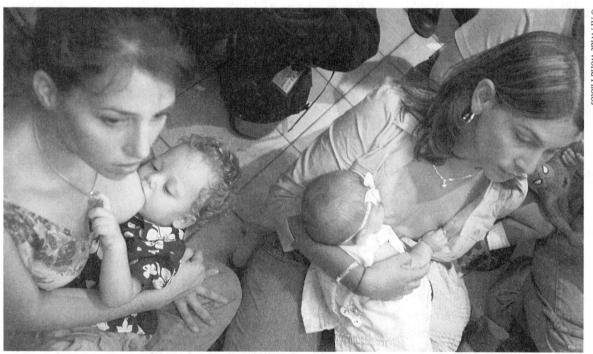

© AP/Wide World Photos

Dozens of mothers nurse their babies in protest on the floor of the Plaza las Americas Mall in San Juan, Puerto Rico, in July 2003. The women rallied after a mother was asked to leave a store for nursing her baby.

nurse with the remaining breast. Tell health care providers about your surgery, and be sure to monitor your baby's weight carefully. Even if you do not have sufficient glandular tissue to produce a full milk supply, you can usually breast-feed if you choose to, and supplement with formula.

Some of us who adopt a child also wish to breast-feed. It may be possible to create a milk supply even without giving birth, by frequently putting the baby to the breast. (Nipple stimulation can affect hormone levels that control milk supply.) It's a good idea to make enjoyment of the nursing relationship the main goal, and to regard milk supply as a bonus rather than a necessity, as the supply may not be copious. Pumping and medication may help to increase a supply, though little research exists on this in the Western world. If you decide to try to breast-feed your adopted baby, contact a lactation consultant for expert advice.

REASONS NOT TO BREAST-FEED

In specific situations, breast-feeding is not safe for the baby. The American Academy of Pediatrics cites the five following reasons not to breast-feed:

- HIV-positive status in the mother
- Active, untreated maternal tuberculosis
- Some maternal medications
- Illegal drug use by the mother
- Infant with galactosemia (a metabolic deficiency) [10]

Other medical reasons breast-feeding may not be possible or advisable for a mother include previous breast surgery (see above), nondevelopment of breast tissue, and certain rare hormonal conditions. There are also instances when pumped breast milk or formula supplementation may be temporarily advisable for the infant's health. These include: weight loss over 7 percent, low blood sugar, and unusually high levels of bilirubin (causing jaundice). For more information on formula, see p. 484.

THE HEALTH AND WELL-BEING OF MOTHERS

While caring for a new baby often takes all our physical and emotional energy, each of us, for our own sake and the sake of our children, should do our best to attend to our own basic needs. These include nutritious food, exercise, rest and sleep, and contact with others. Despite the preparations we may have made, after the baby comes, these basic aspects of life are changed in ways we never could have imagined.

One day when I was leaning over to put Ben in the crib, I realized I had no idea what clothes I had on. I stayed there with my eyes half closed, not looking, trying to figure it out. I couldn't. I tried to remember brushing my teeth, and I couldn't. I knew what shoes I had on, only because I only wore one pair—ever!

Nutrition and eating well are especially important. Continue to eat frequent small meals during the day to keep your energy level constant. When shopping, pick up easy foods to eat on the run, such as fruit, crackers, and cheese. Don't diet! This will stress your body and send it into a mode of conserving energy by slowing down.

LEARNING HOW TO MOTHER YOUR BABY

As I felt life begin and grow within me, my fear mounted. I felt totally inadequate to care for another human being. I enlisted the help of my

FORMULA AS AN ALTERNATIVE TO BREAST MILK

Some of us are unable to breast-feed, some of us prefer not to breast-feed, and some of us would like to but cannot due to situations in our lives beyond our control. In earlier times, the only option for a new mother not breast-feeding was to find a wet nurse for her infant. Today we have formula as an alternative. Depending upon the situation, some women use formula in combination with breast-feeding, and others exclusively formula-feed.

All formulas imitate human breast milk, but they are not a perfect substitute. Human breast milk contains living cells and proteins that provide immunity from disease, which formula does not have. Therefore, formula supplies the basic nutrients needed for normal growth and development, but it cannot supply the protection against disease that human milk provides.

Infant formula is made from either cow's milk or soy products. Both have additional nutrients added so the final product imitates human milk. The two types of formula have similar amounts of many nutrients, but the types of protein and sugar differ from those found in human milk. Some new formulas on the market modify either the type of protein or type of sugar (lactose or sucrose). These formulas are designed to feed babies with special needs, such as prema-ture babies or infants sensitive to lactose, which is the sugar in cow's milk formulas.[11] In recent years, formula manufacturers have introduced additional nutrients based on growing knowledge of the composition of human milk.[12]

Soy formula gained popularity in the 1990s, in response to concerns about allergies to cow's milk protein. Infants are particularly susceptible to developing allergies to the proteins in food, and about three of every hundred infants develop allergies to cow's milk protein.[13] It was thought that soy formula would prevent allergies. However, babies can be allergic to soy protein as well, so this hope was unfounded.[14] More recently, concerns have been raised about soy formula causing reproductive or thyroid problems because it contains isoflavones that are similar to female hormones. To date, research has found no short-term or long-term differences in growth or in the frequency of illness in babies who are fed cow's milk formula when compared with those who are fed soy formula.[15]

The inappropriate promotion of infant formula by corporations continues to undermine informed choices about breast-feeding among women worldwide. This is one reason that the U.S. government in June 2004 launched a national campaign to promote exclusive breast-feeding for the first six months of life.

---

therapist, a volunteer visiting mom, and new moms' groups. There was also a lot of trial and error. I can't say it's been easy, but when I look at my little girl, I marvel at the transformation that she and I have experienced together. She has brought passion and creativity into my life. I have so much more spontaneity and joy. And I am learning that I actually have it within me to be a mother.

Many of us grew up believing that because we are women, we will instinctively know how to love and care for a baby. But mothering is a learned skill in many ways. It may not feel natural. We may feel clumsy and worry that we are not doing a good job. Yet we can grow into the role of being a mother, learning as we go, just as we have learned many other skills in life. Talking with other mothers and making use of services such as home visitors and support groups can give us the confidence to try different things.

FATIGUE

Sleep deprivation is one of the most difficult aspects of having an infant. Some babies are up a lot at night and sleep a lot during the day for the first few weeks. You will get very little sleep if you try to keep up with your other activities while the baby is asleep, then care for the baby while she or he is awake. Exhaustion and sleep deprivation can lead to depression. It is very important to sleep **whenever** the baby sleeps.

For the first week after the birth, I was flying. I seemed to have plenty of energy for everything—my new baby, my husband, even the constant stream of visitors who filled the house. Then, one day, it just caught up with me. Suddenly, I could hardly get through the day [even] with two or three naps. By 9 A.M. I was exhausted. In addition, my perineum, which was nearly healed, suddenly began to ache and feel sore again. My body was clearly sending me a message. When I slowed down and began to take care of myself, I felt better, but I never did recapture that initial high of those days after the birth.

Some of us find it helpful to have a family member or friend help feed the baby, so that we can get some sleep. If you are breast-feeding and your sleep pattern has been severely disrupted, consider having your partner or other support person give the baby a middle-of-the-night bottle of pumped breast milk. (For more information, see "Breast-feeding Your Baby," p. 478.)

STRESS

Caring for infants and young children is rewarding but hard work. The experience can lead to stress, fatigue, loss of concentration and appetite, and even loss of self-esteem. It is almost inevitable that there will be times when you begin to feel that you have exhausted your resources and need a break. This is especially true for those of us who are on our own.

Continuous stress is not good for us—it puts us at risk for physical illness and psychological difficulties such as depression. Think about ways you can get help or support. For example, you might ask a trusted friend or family member to take care of your baby for a short time while you rest, exercise, read, take a relaxing bath or a walk, and/or enjoy social contacts. If there's no one around who can help in this way, you might take your baby along while visiting a neighbor or taking a walk.

PARTNERSHIP

When I think back on it, adding a baby was like sending our relationship through a wringer and planting a garden smack in its middle—both at once.

Throughout the first year, adult intimacy or conversations often lose out to a cry from the baby. If you have a partner, he or she becomes less a lover or companion and more "the other parent." This is not an easy transition. One of the most difficult issues for couples can be jealousy or competition for affection. Often there just doesn't seem to be enough energy, time, and affection for everyone.

As you become a parent, your role in your relationship may become uncertain. What may have been a smoothly functioning system, with each person comfortably taking certain responsibilities, may no longer work. Changes in the partner relationship are frequently experienced as highly stressful. Often it helps to communicate about these changes as soon as possible, so that they don't have a negative effect on your relationship and on your child(ren).

It's one of those "grass is greener" things—I envied, sometimes even hated, Sam when he went out to work. I don't know what I was imagining— that he hung around talking, went out to lunch, did interesting things. One time he was watching me bathe Annie in the sink. He asked if he could do it—he stood there, soaping her back over and over like he couldn't get enough of it, and he talked about how he hated to leave us in the morning, and how he worried he would be closed out, left looking in at what she and I had together.

(For more information on the impact of parenting on partnership, see *Becoming Parents* in "Resources.")

SEXUALITY

Some of us have little or no interest in sex after a child arrives. Others resume sexual activity fairly quickly.

It took a long time before sex was even on the radar screen for both of us. The sleep deprivation and exhaustion usurp that whole part of life. Desire never crossed my mind until the exhaustion thing got better.

Low sexual interest can result from having your life shaken up, feeling exhausted, or taking care of a new baby and possibly also other children. Some women discover that breast-feeding and physical contact with the baby fulfill a desire for physical closeness to some degree. Many of us

who are nursing find that sexual desire does not fully return until we wean our child.

Low sexual interest can have other physical causes. If you had an episiotomy or tear in the perineum during birth, the area may still be sore. Your vagina may feel dry, lacking its normal lubrication because of lowered estrogen levels (more common in nursing mothers). Penetration may hurt, although other kinds of lovemaking may be comfortable (see Chapter 12, "Sexuality," and "Resources").

If you gave birth, you should avoid intercourse or any vaginal penetration until all vaginal discharge has stopped. If you feel physically and psychologically ready, and the bleeding has stopped, there is no risk in lovemaking that includes penetration. If penetration is uncomfortable, you may want to use an unscented lubricant such as K-Y jelly. If you are having intercourse and do not want to conceive, ask your midwife or physician to recommend a stable method of birth control, because the body can make an egg in the ovary about four to five weeks after birth, and pregnancy can occur. Some women come to a six-week checkup pregnant, due to not taking precautions. While many women who are breast-feeding do not menstruate for many months, you cannot depend on breast-feeding for birth control (unless you use it in conjunction with fertility awareness methods), since your first ovulation will occur before your first period. (For more information on birth control, see Chapter 18 and for more information on sexuality and motherhood, see *The Mother's Guide to Sex* in "Resources.")

LIFESTYLE CHANGES

For many of us, life with a new baby can feel monotonous and lonely. Days may go by without adult company. Making contact with other mothers is important. Local parks, playgrounds, churches, community centers, and new-mother or adoption support groups are good places to connect with other parents.

When Willie was just a few months old, I joined a playgroup with several other mothers in the area. While the group was formed to get the babies together, its real function was as a support group for the mothers. It was reassuring to hear that someone else's baby was colicky and had been up all night, and to trade information and suggestions as to what we could do. It was also a help to share some of my ambivalent feelings about motherhood and discover that I wasn't the only one. I came to look on the playgroup as an oasis in what was otherwise a somewhat lonely existence.

As new mothers, we are on twenty-four-hour call. Some of us are resentful about giving up activities we used to take for granted; others are happy if we can stay at home for a while. Within a few months, when the baby is older and on a more predictable schedule, there will be more flexibility.

Your network of friends may begin to change when you have children. You may find you have more in common with friends who have children, and less connection to those without. Friends who do not have children may not want to spend as much time with you now that your life centers on your baby—or, on the other hand, they may be a great source of help and support.

RETURNING TO WORK

At some point during the first year, most women and families have to deal with the issues of who will be financially supporting the family and how. Some of us will have no choice but to return to work outside the home; others will prefer to work outside the home; and some of us will decide to stay home. Many factors contribute to the solution each family creates. Each solution has its benefits and disadvantages.

All mothers have feelings—frequently mixed—about spending time away from our babies. If we need to return to work (or school) soon after the baby's birth, we may feel relieved, or grief-stricken, or a combination of both.

As it got closer to the time when I had to return to work, I kept wondering why no one had told me how hard it would be to leave my baby. I asked someone I thought of as wise, "Why didn't you tell me I would fall in love with my baby?" The wise person just shrugged and said, "I thought you knew how you wanted to do things." There was no choice but to go back to work; I was earning most of the family income. But I just wasn't prepared for how wrenching it would be.

THOUGHTS AND FEELINGS

FOR THOSE OF US WHO GAVE BIRTH

I was so emotional that I could hardly watch TV. I was set off immediately by anything the least bit sentimental, like stories about children or animals or even the news, especially if there were any problems that concerned a child. When my son was only days old, I watched a made-for-TV movie about babies who were switched at birth. I was weeping through the whole thing. I was so vulnerable to those feelings—like, Is this baby really mine? If my husband came home from work and didn't pay attention to me right away, I would cry. A friend told me that after you have a baby, you wear your heart on the outside, and it's so true.

Almost all of us (up to 80 percent) will experience some ups and downs in our moods within the first few weeks after giving birth.[16] This is often referred to as "the baby blues" or "the blues." Quite a few of us (about 10 to 15 percent)

POST-ADOPTION DEPRESSION

As an adoptive mother, I sometimes seemed to have little in common with other new moms. My baby was ten months old, not a few weeks. She didn't look like me. I hadn't given birth to her. And I had other different issues—insensitive comments, for example, or fears about a shortened parental leave (which at that time was seventeen weeks instead of the six months' maternity leave for biological mothers), not bonding with her, or she with me. There was only one thing that I was certain I shared with some biological mothers: I was extremely depressed.

Is it possible to get postpartum depression without having given birth? While few studies have been done, post-adoption depression clearly exists. Physical exhaustion, isolation, financial worries, and stress from the adoption process have all been cited as causes of post-adoption depression. Sometimes unresolved feelings about infertility arise. Some adoptive parents see the adoption as bittersweet, dwelling on the loss experienced by the child's birth mother. There is also a huge disconnect between outsiders' assumptions about adoptive parents and the real stresses that any new parent experiences. Adoptive mothers often hesitate to ask for help, because we get comments like "Don't be silly, you had it easy, you didn't have to give birth or breastfeed." Or "Isn't this what you wanted for so long?"

Strategies for coping with post-adoption depression are similar to those for coping with postpartum depression: Acknowledge that this sort of depression exists; seek out support, especially from other mothers; ask for help; take care of yourself.

will have problems with our feelings and moods that last longer and do not seem to go away. This is often referred to as *postpartum depression* or *postpartum anxiety.** A few women (one or two per thousand) experience such severe problems with mood and thinking that we feel disconnected from reality and from the people around us. This is referred to as *postpartum psychosis.* A discussion of treatment options follows, along with a description and ideas about what to do in the table on pp. 490–91.

* To read a story about a woman's struggle with postpartum difficulties, see "I Knew I Was in Trouble" (W54) on the companion website, www.ourbodiesourselves.org.

PHYSICAL, PSYCHOLOGICAL, AND SOCIAL RISK FACTORS

Certain factors make it more likely that some of us will have more difficulties in the postpartum period:

- History of PMS or difficult menstrual cycles
- History of physical, sexual, or emotional abuse
- History of depression, anxiety, or bipolar illness
- Previous history of postpartum problems, such as depression or anxiety
- History of infertility, abortion, miscarriage, or stillbirth
- Recent loss through death or moving
- Negative or traumatic birth experience
- Relationship problems

- Ill partner or family member
- Housing problems
- Current domestic violence
- Financial problems
- Postpartum pain
- Fatigue
- Lack of support
- Social isolation and loneliness
- Thyroid problems*
- Premature or sick baby
- Challenging baby
- Breast-feeding problems
- Poor nutrition

Postpartum difficulties can sometimes be prevented and often minimized, and are definitely treatable. If you are experiencing difficult thoughts and feelings, regardless of whether you are awaiting giving birth or are already home with your baby, seek out support from a social worker, psychiatrist, psychologist, psychiatric nurse, mental health counselor, or established organizations such as Postpartum Support International, www.postpartum.net or 805-967-7636; or Depression After Delivery, www.depressionafterdelivery.com or 1-800-944-4773.

COMMON POSTPARTUM EMOTIONAL PROBLEMS

While there are no official diagnostic categories or criteria for postpartum difficulties, the information in the chart on p. 491 is widely agreed upon among experienced professionals.

This chart is a guideline, but categories of emotional problems are not always so clear-cut. Additional recommendations include:

- Trust your intuition about how you are feeling.

* Thyroid problems are often overlooked, especially in postpartum women, and can be confused with postpartum depression.

- One woman's blues may be another woman's depression.
- Err on the side of caution if you are concerned about how you are feeling.
- If someone tries to brush you aside, find someone who will take you seriously.
- Be persistent in seeking experienced professional care.
- You may feel ashamed, but remember these are medical problems that are common, treatable, and not your fault.
- You deserve to feel the best you can.

If you believe you may be at risk for postpartum depression, discuss it with your health care provider, and ask for help in finding suitable supportive resources, such as a knowledgeable counselor who can help you assess your specific needs and find ways to meet them.

TREATMENT

An experienced professional will listen carefully to how you are feeling, ask some questions, and work with you to create a treatment plan, which might include counseling, medication, support groups, and/or home visitors. It might include some discussions with you and your partner together, or alternatives such as acupuncture and homeopathy. If you do not feel that the person you see is responsive to your preferences, or if you are not comfortable with what he or she is recommending, seek a second opinion. New information on research about treatment options is constantly becoming available, but many health care providers have inadequate or outdated knowledge.

Research has shown that some medications are safe to take while breast-feeding. If a practitioner says you must wean your baby in order to take medication, ask if there is an alternative medication that is safe to take while nursing. If the answer is no, get a second opinion.

	BLUES	DEPRESSION	ANXIETY	PSYCHOSIS
Symptoms	Tearfulness, restlessness, sudden mood changes, irritability, not feeling like yourself, asking questions such as "What did I get myself into?"	Sadness, hopelessness, low self-esteem, guilt, suicidal ideas, sleep disturbances, eating disturbances, inability to be comforted, exhaustion, emptiness, inability to enjoy anything, social withdrawal, low energy. Easily frustrated, not feeling like you can take care of the baby. These symptoms can range from mild to severe and can feel quite frightening and overwhelming.	Scary thoughts about the baby getting hurt or about you hurting the baby, even though you have no urge to actually hurt your baby and you realize these are odd thoughts. Repetitive images of things that can hurt the baby. Difficulty getting rid of these thoughts. Feeling wound up, with rapid heartbeat, rapid breathing.	You may feel that you are being ordered by God or a power outside yourself to do things you normally wouldn't, such as harm yourself or your baby; you may feel confused or agitated; you may see or hear things that others don't; you may have extreme highs or lows of energy or mood; you may not be able to take care of your baby; you may experience your thoughts and feelings as being out of your control. This is a rare but very serious condition.
When can it start?	A few days after birth; often appears just as your milk comes in. Hormonal changes may be at least partly responsible.	May be what is happening if the blues are not going away. Can occur anytime in the first year. Can occur with and without anxiety.	Anytime in the first year. Can occur with or without depression.	Usually within 2–4 weeks postpartum.
How long will it last?	A few days; it will end by itself.	Treatment can reduce the severity and length. Depression can last a few weeks to several months. Untreated, it may or may not go away.	Same as depression.	Treatment is essential in order for it to go away.

What can I do about it?	Take good care of yourself. Talk to people around you, especially other mothers. Be patient with yourself.	Take yourself seriously. Ask for help and support from an experienced professional. (Refer to the organizations Postpartum Support International, and Depression After Delivery, in "Resources.") See the section preceding this chart for more information on treatment.	Same as for depression.	Ask someone to take you to a knowledgeable health care provider or to an emergency room and explain that you believe you are having a serious postpartum reaction and you need help from a provider who specializes in this condition. Be assured that it can be successfully treated.*
Common Treatment	Supportive professional counseling, support groups, home visitors.	Supportive professional counseling, support groups, home visitors, medication.	Supportive professional counseling, support groups, home visitors, medication.	Immediate professional attention and psychiatric treatment, including medication, supportive professional counseling, support groups, home visitors.

* This condition is thought by many to be connected in some way to the massive hormonal changes that occur after childbirth, although no one yet knows why some mothers are more vulnerable to postpartum psychosis than others.

Chart adapted from original chart created by Kathleen Kendall-Tackett. Original at www.granitescientific.com/. Click on "Depression in Mothers," then "Conference Handouts," then "Depression in New Mothers: Causes and Consequences." Accessed October 2004.

Many practitioners believe that medication and hospitalization are necessary in the treatment of postpartum psychosis and severe postpartum depression. Unfortunately, temporary weaning and separation of mother from baby may be necessitated in this case, because few units in the U.S. accept mothers and babies together. Depending on the medications used and the type of treatment, a breast-feeding mother could pump while hospitalized and send frozen milk home for the baby. You may be able to negotiate frequent, regular visits with your baby, with assistance and oversight by caregivers, during the short time when hospitalization is needed.

Some innovative, determined, energetic families, with considerable community support, may be able to arrange alternative forms of care for individual mothers. This should not be undertaken lightly, however. Ongoing therapy, monitoring, and consultation by experienced and knowledgeable caregivers are a necessary part of such an alternative plan.*

MOTHERING AGAIN: THE SECOND TIME AROUND

If you had a difficult time following the birth of your first child because of postpartum depression or other distress, you may find yourself worrying about whether it will happen again. There is no way to predict this. The arrival of a second child can be a very different experience. Some aspects may be much easier; having been through it all before, you know what to expect and are comfortable with many of the practical issues of child care and parenthood. However, there are still unknowns that can make the arrival of second and subsequent children diffi-

* We know of only one mother-baby unit in the U.S. that offers a day treatment program in which mothers and babies can be together: Women and Infants Hospital in Providence, Rhode Island.

cult. For example, your new baby may have a different temperament than the first. Your relationship with your partner may be different. In addition, you now have two or more children and must find ways to balance their needs. You also have changed.

I had a really hard time emotionally after the birth of my first child. He had lots of problems right after birth, and we didn't know if he would make it. I remember crying constantly. We almost lost this child that we wanted so desperately. How could I give my heart to him, when I was afraid I'd lose him? It took me a long time to let myself love him, but then I loved him so much. With my second child, it was very different. I had such an easy birth, and my daughter was a wonderful baby. I felt like a traitor to my son.

Taking preventive measures, such as lining up help and support before the baby is born, will increase your chances of an easier time after the birth.

CONCLUSION

Becoming a mother for the first time happens only once. This life transition is unique, sensitive, and all-consuming. It requires support, care, community, and patience. Yet our society in the United States does not automatically supply these ingredients for new mothers and families. As a result, we must rely on ourselves to create the support systems we need for a successful transition to parenthood. Sometimes unexpected challenges, such as housing and financial problems, health or relationship problems, and emotional problems, create extra stress and increase the need for support.

Most communities have some resources for new mothers, though they are not always well coordinated or easy to find. Check with libraries, synagogues and churches, social service agencies, YMCAs, your city or town hall, preschools, public schools, WIC, and online. The Internet offers information, chat rooms, and e-mail listservs (see "Resources"). If you do not have a computer at home, see if your local library or community center has one you can use.

Having a new baby is the beginning of an awesome journey. Your competence as a parent grows, along with your baby, during this first year. Like all journeys, it's a balance of challenges, pleasures, and the satisfactions of success.

NOTES

1. Work Group on Breastfeeding, American Academy of Pediatrics, "Breastfeeding and the Use of Human Milk," *Pediatrics* 100, no. 6 (1997): 1035–39.
2. B. Duncan, J. Ey, C. J. Holberg, A. L. Wright, F. D. Martinez, L. M. Taussig, "Exclusive Breast-feeding for at Least 4 Months Protects Against Otitis Media," *Pediatrics* 91, no. 5 (1993): 867–72. See also Work Group on Breastfeeding, "Breastfeeding and the Use of Human Milk"; E. J. Mayer, R. F. Hamman, E. C. Gay, D. C. Lezotte, D. A. Savitz, G. J. Klingensmith, "Reduced Risk of IDDM Among Breast-fed Children: The Colorado IDDM Registry," *Diabetes* 37, no. 12 (1988): 1625–32; S. M. Virtanen, L. Rasanen, K. Ylonen, et al., "Early Introduction of Dairy Products Associated with Increased Risk of IDDM in Finnish Children: The Childhood Diabetes in Finland Study Group," *Diabetes* 42, no. 12 (1993): 1786–90; X. O. Shu, M. S. Linet, M. Steinbuch, et al., "Breast-feeding and Risk of Childhood Acute Leukemia," *Journal of the National Cancer Institute* 91, no. 20 (1999): 1765–72; F. Perrillat, J. Clavel, M. F. Auclerc, et al., "Day-care, Early Common Infections and Childhood Acute Leukemia: A Multicentre French Case-Control Study," *British Journal of Cancer* 86, no. 7 (2002): 1064–69; V. B. Smulevich, L. G. Solionova, S. V. Belyakova, "Parental Occupation and Other Factors and Cancer Risk in Children: I. Study Methodology and Non-occupational Factors," *International Journal of Cancer* 83, no. 6 (1999): 712–17; M. K. Davis, D. A. Savitz, B. I. Graubard, "Infant Feeding and Childhood Cancer," *Lancet* 2, no. 8607 (1988): 365–89; L. Tryggvadottir, H. Tulinius, J. E. Eyfjord, T. Sigurvinsson, "Breastfeeding and Reduced Risk of Breast Cancer in an Icelandic Cohort Study," *American Journal of Epidemiology* 154, no. 1 (2001): 37–42; V. Tovar-Guzman, C. Hernandez-Giron, E. Lazcano-Ponce, I. Romieu, Avila M. Hernandez, "Breast Cancer in Mexican Women: An Epidemiological Study with Cervical Cancer Control," *Revista de Salude Publica* 34, no. 2 (2000): 113–19; M. McCredie, C. Paul, D. C. Skegg, S. Williams, "Breast Cancer in Maori and Non-Maori Women," *International Journal of Epidemiology* 28, no. 2 (1999): 189–95; T. Zheng, L. Duan, Y. Liu, et al., "Lactation Reduces Breast Cancer Risk in Shandong Province, China," *American Journal of Epidemiology* 152, no. 12 (2000): 1129–35; T. Zheng, T. R. Holford, S. T. Mayne, et al., "Lactation and Breast Cancer Risk: A Case-Control Study in Connecticut," *British Journal of Cancer* 84, no. 11 (2001): 1472–76; R. Ing, N. L. Petrakis, J. H. Ho, "Unilateral Breast-feeding and Breast Cancer," *Lancet* 2, no. 8029 (1977): 124–27; and Collaborative Group on Hormonal Factors in Breast Cancer, "Breast Cancer and Breastfeeding: Collaborative Reanalysis of Individual Data from 47 Epidemiological Studies in 30 Countries, Including 50,302 Women with Breast Cancer and 96,973 Women Without the Disease," *Lancet* 360, no. 9328 (2002): 187–95.
3. Tryggvadottir et al., "Breastfeeding and Reduced Risk of Breast Cancer." See also Tovar-Guzman et al., "Breast Cancer in Mexican Women"; McCredie et al., "Breast Cancer in Maori and Non-Maori Women"; Zheng et al., "Lactation Reduces Breast Cancer Risk in Shandong Province, China"; Zheng et al., "Lactation and Breast Cancer Risk"; Ing et al., "Unilateral Breast-feeding and Breast Cancer"; and Collaborative Group on Hormonal Factors in Breast Cancer, "Breast Cancer and Breastfeeding."
4. Zheng et al., "Lactation Reduces Breast Cancer Risk in Shandong Province, China."
5. Office on Women's Health, U.S. Department of Health and Human Services, "Health and Human Services Blueprint for Action on Breastfeeding," Washington, D.C., 2000.
6. A. S. Ryan, Z. Wenjun, A. Acosta, "Breastfeeding Continues to Increase into the New Millennium," *Pediatrics* 110, no. 6 (2002): 1103–9.
7. Work Group on Breastfeeding, "Breastfeeding and the Use of Human Milk."
8. L. Righard, M. O. Alade, "Effect of Delivery Room Routines on Success of First Breast-feed," *Lancet* 336, no. 8723 (1990): 1105–7. See also L. Righard, M. O. Alade, "Sucking Technique and Its Effect on Success of Breastfeeding," *Birth* 19, no. 4 (1992): 185–89; L. Righard,

"How Do Newborns Find Their Mother's Breast?," *Birth* 22, no. 3 (1995): 174–75; and L. Righard, "Early Enhancement of Successful Breast-feeding," *World Health Forum* 17, no. 1 (1996): 92–7.

9. Righard, "How Do Newborns Find Their Mother's Breast?"

10. Work Group on Breastfeeding, "Breastfeeding and the Use of Human Milk."

11. A. L. Morrow, "Choosing an Infant or Pediatric Formula," *Journal of Pediatric Health Care* 18 (2004): 49–52.

12. A. Donnelly, H. M. Snowden, M. J. Renfrew, M. W. Woolridge, "Commercial Hospital Discharge Packs for Breastfeeding Women," *Cochrane Review,* in *The Cochrane Library* 2 (Chichester, UK: John Wiley & Sons, Ltd.).

13. S. L. Bahna, "Cow's Milk Allergy Versus Cow Milk Intolerance," *Annals of Allergy, Asthma and Immunology* 89, no. 6 (2002): 546–60.

14. C. W. Low, et al., "Infant Formula, Past and Future: Opportunities for Improvement," *American Journal of Clinical Nutrition* 63 (1996): 636S–50S.

15. B. L. Strom, et al., "Exposure to Soy-Based Formula in Infancy and Endocrinological and Reproductive Outcomes in Young Adulthood," *Journal of the American Medical Association* 286 (2001): 807–14.

16. A. LoCicero, D. Weiss, and D. Issokson, "Postpartum Depression: Proposal for Prevention Through an Integrated Care and Support Network," *Applied and Preventive Psychology* 6 (1997): 169–78.

■ ■ ■ ■ ■ ■ ■ ■ ■ ■ ■ ■ ■ ■ ■ ■ ■ ■ ■ ■**CHAPTER 24**

Childbearing loss occurs in many different ways. Miscarriage, stillbirth, early infant death, loss in a multiple gestation, ectopic or molar pregnancies, and the decision not to carry to term a baby with impairments are all childbearing losses. In each of these cases, the impact of the loss on a woman who wishes to become a mother can be devastating. While a miscarriage may come as a welcome relief to some women, even those who have chosen to terminate an unwanted pregnancy may experience sadness and grief. Loss of a pregnancy or a newborn infant challenges us physically, psychologically, and spiritually and can cut to the core of our identity as women.

Women experiencing childbearing loss need and deserve the

same emotional support and quality health care as women who have experienced viable pregnancies. Those of us experiencing loss are often too devastated to make decisions readily or face our emotional challenges alone. It is important to have a trusted partner, relative, friend, or counselor to provide needed support and help you choose the best options.

Unfortunately, childbearing loss is a common experience, one that has become even more common in recent years.[1] It becomes more likely as women and men age and is also more common in very young women. Certain types of reproductive technologies, such as in vitro fertilization, result in higher rates of pregnancy loss (see Chapter 25, "Infertility and Assisted Reproduction"). Women who conceive two or more embryos are also more likely to experience loss. Home pregnancy tests and early ultrasounds mean that what was once considered a heavy, late period may now be experienced as a pregnancy loss.

Those of us who are African-American are nearly twice as likely to suffer pregnancy loss and about three times as likely to give birth to very low-birth-weight babies, who account for up to half of the deaths of newborns. African-American women also have a higher incidence of ectopic pregnancy, which occurs when the fertilized egg starts developing outside the uterus.[2]

Community expectations and cultural background can add to the emotional struggles surrounding loss.

As a Cuban Jewish immigrant to the United States, I deeply transgressed my own family-based expectations that we would have our children in our early twenties, when I chose a professional path. Remarried at forty, I have since experienced five miscarriages. . . . As part of my search both for fertility treatment and for a way of understanding the texture of my grief, I have explored the interwoven threads of emotional loss and of

unyielding, accusing inner voices which tell me that, without my own baby, I will never prove that I am a "good woman" after all. This hard-won knowledge based on a profound sense of loss is a gift that has expanded my capacity to love and to give in the many relationships with children, students, and other loved ones, which I cherish now more than ever.

Women are rarely prepared for the experience of childbearing loss. Despite its frequency, it is often shrouded in secrecy. Whereas in some cultures, women speak openly about reproductive hardships, in the United States, many women do not readily share pregnancy loss stories, or do so only with others who have had a similar experience. Some health care providers do not inform women of the possibility of loss or give us information about medical options until the crisis is upon us.

Some of us have been so disturbed by the way we were treated during pregnancy loss that we have become activists working to improve the experience for others. You may be the beneficiary of such work; or, if you lose a pregnancy, you may feel moved to use your experience to help others. In the last twenty years, activists have improved the support women receive, especially for losses that occur later in the pregnancy. Many hospitals now have bereavement teams ready to help.

MISCARRIAGE

Miscarriage is the premature ending of a pregnancy before the fetus can live outside the womb (that is, during the first five months). Miscarriage is also called "spontaneous abortion." It is by far the most common type of pregnancy loss, occurring in approximately one in every five pregnancies. Most miscarriages take place within the first twelve weeks of pregnancy.

Miscarriage often comes as a cruel shock.

When I found out I was pregnant, I danced around the house. My pregnancy was an easy one. My body was slowly and pleasantly changing. Because it was a conscious and well-thought-out decision to have a child, I felt free to revel in my pregnancy and motherhood. It was a special time. I mention all of this because it is partially by understanding the depth of the joy that one can understand the depth of the loss.

The first symptoms are usually spotting or bleeding, followed by cramps. Sometimes these signs will disappear and nothing more will happen. If you are having symptoms, your health care provider may want to order blood tests to check your hormone levels. If they are declining, then a miscarriage is presumed. If you are miscarrying, bleeding becomes heavy, cramps increase, and the cervix dilates. In losses that occur after nine to ten weeks, you may feel painful contractions.

My husband held me and we cried together. The deepest and most obvious feeling was the sense of loss. Almost as strong was the fear. We did not understand what was happening and why it was happening to us. We were also frightened by the look of what was pouring out of me. It was bad enough that we were losing our baby, but in the midst of all that pain, we had to stay strong enough to deal with all that blood. Why hadn't anyone given us any preparation?

Sometimes pregnancy losses are discovered at a routine prenatal visit. Often families anticipate visits with pleasure, bringing along loved ones with the expectation of hearing the heartbeat or seeing the baby on ultrasound, only to learn that there is no detectable embryo or that the fetus has died. In some cases, you may see and/or hear a heartbeat at one prenatal visit, and then at the next, find the screen deadly still. In the room that had been filled with the galloping sound of the fast-paced fetal heartbeat, there is thundering silence.

If a blood test or sonogram indicates that you are about to have a miscarriage, you have a number of options, which may be affected by how far your pregnancy has developed. Some women choose to allow the miscarriage to occur naturally, while others find that scheduling a medication or aspiration abortion provides a sense of control and closure. Medication abortions involve taking a drug such as misoprostol, which will bring on the miscarriage. An aspiration abortion may be performed on an outpatient basis in a hospital, abortion clinic, obstetrical office, or emergency room (for a description of this procedure, see p. 398 in Chapter 20, "Abortion"). Sometimes a woman may schedule an abortion but then miscarry at home before it takes place. If you are worried this might happen, supplemental progesterone can be given to prolong the pregnancy until the abortion can be done.

I had three miscarriages, all in different settings. I found having a D&C in my doctor's office far superior to the first one, which took place in the emergency room, although it was hard to sit in the waiting room with all those pregnant bellies and hard to face walking past them afterward with my newly emptied womb. The D&C I had in the abortion clinic was the most positive experience because not ending up with a baby to take home was not seen as a failure.

If you choose to miscarry naturally or to induce it with medication, you will probably have your miscarriage at home. Once the miscarriage begins, it may be over quickly or take several days. The fetus, amniotic sac, and placenta, along with a lot of blood, will be expelled. If you have reached eight to ten weeks, try to arrange for a trusted, knowledgeable person to be with you throughout the process, realizing that this

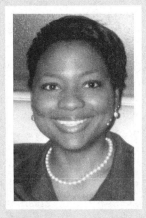

"I FELT COMPLETELY DISMISSED"

MARY HINTON

I had two pregnancy losses in one year—the first at about eight and half weeks, the second at eleven weeks. I was devastated. My emotions cascaded from guilt and shame to depression and anger. I had spent my entire college career working with pregnant teenagers and had seen fourteen-year-olds who could successfully carry a pregnancy, yet I couldn't. I'd done all the "right things" and still couldn't seem to get this right. I got tired of people saying to me, "Oh, don't worry, you'll have a baby." I wanted to shout back, "I don't want a baby! I want the baby I was just carrying!" I searched for services that could help me, but couldn't find any. One doctor told me that I was "just being too upset about the whole thing." I felt completely dismissed.

I decided to deal with my grief by helping others, and came up with the idea of the Glimmer Fund, a nonprofit that raises funds to help organizations support women who have suffered pregnancy loss. So far we have made grants to RTS Bereavement for scholarships to train lay people and medical personnel as bereavement counselors. We also made a grant to SHARE to help publish material about miscarriage in Spanish. We are currently raising funds for projects in underserved communities and also hope to support a Spanish-language project here in New York.

Pregnancy loss touches a million women a year. I hope we can get some momentum going and eventually achieve the same kind of progress for this women's health problem as breast cancer activists have.

may well involve staying through the night. Think about where you will be most comfortable and what you will need. Hot water bottles and massage may comfort and help with cramping. Bed liners and sanitary pads may be helpful. You may want to think about and discuss with others what you would like to do with the remains. There will be some blood clots, and you may notice some tissue that is firmer or lumpy-looking, which is placental or afterbirth tissue. You may or may not see tissue that looks like a fetus.

Once everything in your uterus has been expelled, you may still feel pregnant for a while. Bleeding will continue, but it will lessen over several days. If bleeding increases or stays bright red, or if you have odd or foul-smelling discharge or a fever, contact your health care practitioner. Sometimes bleeding continues because fetal tissue remains in your uterus. At that point, your practitioner must perform a D&C to remove the tissue and prevent infection. After the bleeding has stopped and the cervix is closed, you can make love (including penetration) with no risk of infection. You should have a repeat pregnancy test to make sure your hormone levels are normal a few weeks later. If you feel dizzy or tired, ask for a test to check for anemia. If you do not know your blood type, get a blood test within a few days of miscarrying to determine what it is. If you are RH negative, it's important to get a shot within 72 hours after the miscarriage to protect you from making dangerous antibodies.

At present, it is not common for women to miscarry naturally in hospitals. But just as consumer demand and the women's health movement led to more comfortable, homey birthing environments in hospitals, if women begin to ask for more nurturing health care environments in which to have our losses, such facilities may become available.

After a miscarriage, it can be helpful, although emotionally painful, to try to learn why the miscarriage occurred. If you are at home when you miscarry and there is fetal or afterbirth tissue that you can collect, you might want to bring it in a clean container to a hospital-based laboratory for examination. You may request tests, such as cultures for infection, genetic studies of the tissue, and blood tests to determine whether there is an immunologic cause for your pregnancy loss. Be sure to see the pathology report and ask for a full explanation of all terminology. If the explanations don't satisfy you, find someone else to help you, or see if further tests can be done.

In most instances, the exact cause cannot be known. Early losses often occur without a detectable embryo (sometimes there is just an empty sac, or what doctors call a blighted ovum). In cases with embryos, 50 percent test as normal. Chromosomal anomalies can be detected in about 30 percent of miscarriages that occur after eight weeks. Other known reasons for miscarriage include infection, hormonal imbalances, structural problems of the uterus, and autoimmune problems. Environmental and industrial toxins can be responsible, as can physical trauma, including domestic violence. In rare cases, a woman will miscarry after certain tests during pregnancy, such as chorionic villi sampling (CVS) or amniocentesis. Most miscarriages that occur during the second trimester

MYTH OR REALITY?

- *If I have a miscarriage, I won't be able to have healthy babies in the future.*

Myth. The vast majority of women are able to have a baby after a miscarriage. If you have two miscarriages in a row, you may want to ask your health care provider about investigating the causes.

involve a normal fetus and are caused by weak cervical muscles.

ECTOPIC AND MOLAR PREGNANCIES

Ectopic pregnancy is a form of pregnancy loss in which the fertilized egg starts developing outside the uterus, usually in the fallopian tube. An ectopic pregnancy can be a life-threatening condition and requires immediate treatment. It can happen to anyone, but the risk is higher for women who have had previous tubal surgery, including surgery for a previous ectopic pregnancy and tubal reversal surgery; women who have pelvic inflammatory disease (PID) or who used IUDs; women whose mothers were given DES; and African-American women. Approximately one in every fifty pregnancies is ectopic.[3]

Molar pregnancies happen in the initial cell division, when the cells that are supposed to develop into the placenta instead develop into a tumor. Molar pregnancies are rare in the U.S. (one in fifteen hundred live births), but rates go up with age and are much higher among Asian women.

(For more information on these two types of pregnancy loss, see "Ectopic and Molar Pregnancies" [W55] on the companion website, www.ourbodiesourselves.org.)

MULTIPLE GESTATION PREGNANCIES

The number of women conceiving multiples has increased dramatically in recent years. One reason is that more women are undergoing infertility treatments such as in vitro fertilization and ovulation-stimulating medications. These increase the chance of a multiple gestation pregnancy. In addition, older women are more likely to conceive multiples. Unfortunately, pregnancy loss is much more likely in pregnancies involving more than one embryo or fetus.

LOSS AFTER PRENATAL DIAGNOSIS

Some of us choose to end a pregnancy after discovering that we are carrying a fetus with severe impairments. Loss from terminating a pregnancy is different from other childbearing losses because it arises out of our own decision. Facing such a loss is often painful and difficult. Many of us find that we are best able to come to peace with our decision if we feel supported by those around us and if we have received accurate and adequate information about the diagnosed disability and its potential impact.

Religions, subcultures, communities, and individuals have a wide range of beliefs about the ethics of ending a pregnancy because of a diagnosed impairment. Often those of us who experience this kind of loss do not speak openly about it because we fear being judged. If you face such a loss, it may be helpful to seek the support of others who have suffered similar losses.

STILLBIRTH

Stillbirth refers to pregnancy loss that occurs after twenty weeks' gestation. Although stillbirth is much less common than miscarriage, twenty-six thousand stillbirths occur each year in the U.S. Until recently there has been very little research on the causes of stillbirths, despite these numbers. However, in 2003 the National Institutes of Health allocated close to $3 million to fund research on stillbirth, or SADS *(sudden antenatal death syndrome)*. Unlike earlier losses, stillbirths often involve apparently healthy fetuses. Some causes of stillbirth are known, such as diabetes, high blood pressure, or umbilical

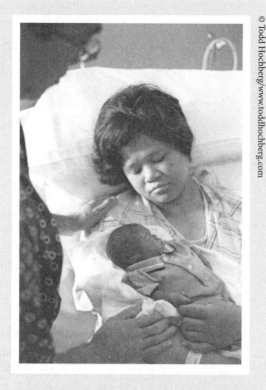

"WE WANTED SOMETHING TO REMEMBER NICHOLAS'S LIFE"

STELLA NG

As I held Nicholas, I was happy that he was born alive, even though I knew he was dying slowly in my arms. There were no cries, no eyes opening, just a faint heartbeat. He looked just like my daughter when she was born. Even though he was slightly smaller, his toes and fingers were perfectly formed. He was a fighter until I could no longer support his life inside me. When Todd arrived to take pictures, I was glad that Nicholas was dressed and ready.

His birth was another step in our grieving process, which had started more than two months earlier. Tests had shown that there was no chance for Nicholas to live, because his blood lacked the components that carry oxygen to the rest of the body. When the hospital's bereavement program gave us the option of having a photographer document our time with Nicholas, we were very interested. We wanted something to remember Nicholas's life and not to just let time pass and forget about what had happened. We also wanted something tangible to show our three-year-old daughter when she could understand. We wanted her to know she had a brother and not to hide the fact that he died.

Our family has since moved back to the East Coast, but we visit the garden where Nicholas's ashes are buried once a year. My daughter wishes her brother were alive and makes sure she gets flowers to put in his garden. From time to time, we remember Nicholas by looking at the album Todd created, which the hospital's bereavement program gave us at no charge. My daughter feels she knows her brother through his pictures and our words.

cord accidents. However, the cause of over half of all stillbirths is unknown.[4]

If you know in advance that you are going to have a stillbirth, choose the location and birth attendants you think will be able to help you best.

Once the baby has been delivered, birth attendants should handle her or him in a reverent manner. You will decide whether you want to see her or him, either immediately or later on. You may want to hold your dead baby, name him or her if you haven't already done so, and take photos. You will also have to decide whether or not you want an autopsy to try to find the cause of death. Most likely, the loss was totally beyond your control or the doctor's. If you do suspect malpractice by your doctor, seek legal counsel and have the facts analyzed.

SUDDEN INFANT DEATH SYNDROME (SIDS)

Every year in the United States, about twenty-five hundred apparently healthy infants die in their sleep. These deaths are called SIDS: *sudden infant death syndrome.* The cause of SIDS is unknown. Between 1994 and 2000, SIDS deaths were reduced by over half, likely because of the discovery that it is safer to have babies sleep on their backs rather than their stomachs. African-

American and Native American women are more than twice as likely to suffer this devastating loss.[5]

COPING WITH LOSS

We went home from the hospital dazed and tired. I was weak and enormously sad. I don't know that I've ever experienced such deep emotional pain. The loss was so great and so complete in a way that only death is. For the first few days I couldn't talk to anyone, but at the same time, it was painful to be alone. I would just cry and cry without stopping. One of the clearest reminders that I was no longer pregnant was all the speedy changes my body went through. Within two days, my breasts, which had grown quite swollen, were back to their normal size. My stomach, which had grown hard, was now soft again. My body was no longer preparing for the birth of a child. It was simple and blatant. Tiredness was replaced with weakness. And then there was the bleeding. My body would not let me forget. I knew things would improve once we could make love again and would be even better when we were full of hope. But it seemed so far away.

Childbearing loss evokes many emotions. You and your partner, if you have one, may feel buffeted and torn by confusion, relief, shame, anger, sorrow, fear, powerlessness, or despair. You might need to withdraw at first and you might feel numb about a reality that may be too much to bear. You may want those around you to comfort you physically and listen empathetically. Platitudes such as "You'll have another baby before you know it" or "Think of your wonderful children at home" are usually not comforting. Thoughtful compassion from family, friends, and health care practitioners is crucial.

A tremendous void and sense of loneliness often follow childbearing loss. You may find that your feelings differ from your partner's in strength or content. Grief may be mixed with guilt; both can cause tension between you. You may wonder if either of you did something "wrong" (too much activity, too much sex, not enough good food, etc.). Acknowledge and talk out your feelings as much as you can.

Most people didn't know how to give me support, and perhaps I didn't really know how to ask for it. People were more comfortable talking about the physical, and not the emotional, side of miscarriage. I needed to talk about both. It was also difficult for my husband, because people could at least ask how my body was doing. Unfortunately, he would sometimes be completely bypassed when someone called to talk with us, despite the fact that he, too, was in deep emotional pain.

In addition to emotional responses to loss, you have experienced a pregnancy, and your body will be going through changes (see Chapter 23, "The First Year of Parenting"). You may find it difficult to be around pregnant women or events like Mother's Day or baby showers. Obstetricians' waiting rooms can be especially hard.

When I went back for my post-birth checkup for myself at the doctor's nobody had bothered to tell

the nurse that I had lost my baby. I went in there and I sat down. The nurse came in and went through this long list of probably twenty or more questions, all about the birth, and ended with the last question, "Are you breast-feeding or bottle-feeding?" I completely lost it. I started shrieking. I ran out of the room. I was shrieking to all these ladies in the waiting room.

You may feel a strong resurgence of grief on the date when your baby would have been born, or when you see children the same age as your child would have been. The depth of grief is not simply related to the duration of the pregnancy.

The first time I got pregnant, I miscarried after six weeks. Although I was told that the fetus was only the size of a grain of rice, I deeply grieved the loss. I remember nine months later, feeling a deep sadness wash over me, and finally, I connected it with the fact that if I hadn't miscarried, I would have been giving birth that month.

Our society has few formal ways of dealing with pregnancy loss. Some kind of ceremony may help. Giving to a favorite charity or planting a tree has offered solace to some. During the weeks, months, and even years to come, you may feel alone in your grief. Talking to others who have experienced the loss of a child can help. If you do not know anyone to whom this has happened, and if no support groups exist in your area, there are websites and books that can help you. (For more information, see "Resources.")

SUBSEQUENT PREGNANCY

Pregnancy loss does not mean that you cannot have a normal subsequent pregnancy. The vast majority of women are able to have a baby after a miscarriage. If you have two miscarriages in a row, you may want to begin investigating possible causes and preventive treatments with your current health care practitioner, or see an infertility specialist.

Pregnancy after a loss can feel scary. Depending on your experience, you may choose to remain with your health care provider, or you may want to find a new caregiver. If you're choosing a new provider, ask in advance what his or her policy is for dealing with pregnancy loss and monitoring a woman who has had a prior loss.

During subsequent pregnancies, we sometimes cherish each moment of the pregnancy, knowing that the pregnancy itself may be the only opportunity for mothering the child we hope to have. We may embrace the use of technologies such as home pregnancy tests and ultrasounds that help us feel more connected. More often, however, we try to protect ourselves emotionally by not becoming too attached. During a subsequent pregnancy, we may try to avoid learning the sex, buying things, or choosing a name. Then we may worry that we aren't being fair, or that we may somehow be harming the fetus by these actions. Be gentle with yourself and give yourself permission to cope in ways that work for you. If the pregnancy results in a baby to bring home, there will be plenty of time for love.

You are likely to feel most anxious around the time in the pregnancy that the previous loss occurred.

I remember the impact of all those losses on the pregnancy I did manage to carry; how I shifted my conviction that things could and would go wrong, from one source of anxiety to the next, throughout the course of the pregnancy. First I was certain that I would lose it between the eighth and tenth week, as was my pattern. Once I made it past that critical point, I was so worried that the amnio would cause a miscarriage, I made myself physically ill. Then I worried about the amnio results, and once that was behind me, about

whether I would make it to twenty-four weeks gestation, after which fetuses have a chance of making it outside the womb.

The anxiety isn't necessarily alleviated once one has had a successful subsequent pregnancy.

Two and a half years later, I became pregnant again, and I was an emotional wreck. I worried a lot, but tried to focus on the fact that everything in the pregnancy was going very well. At first I was reluctant to tell anyone that I was pregnant, then realized that if no one knew and I miscarried again, I would have no support; we then told everyone. Everything turned out fine.

You will be better able to deal with the anxiety and tension if you have compassionate caregivers and supportive partners and friends. Sometimes psychotherapists or support groups specifically for women who become pregnant after a loss can be helpful. If possible, talk with women who have had the same experience to learn how they managed the tension and fear and then found the courage and optimism to try again. You may be able to use your energy, sorrow, anger, and determination to learn about what happened, to heal yourself further, gain wisdom, and possibly to learn from it, to work to make the experience of childbearing loss less painful for those who come after.

NOTES

1. Stephanie J. Ventura, William D. Mosher, Sally C. Curtin, and Joyce C. Abma, "Trends in Pregnancy Rates for the United States, 1976–97: An Update," *National Vital Statistics Reports* 49, no. 4 (2001): 5–8.
2. Stephanie J. Ventura et al., "Trends in Pregnancies and Pregnancy Rates: Estimates for the United States, 1980–92," *Monthly Vital Statistics Report* 43, no. 11 (May 25, 1995), Centers for Disease Control and Prevention/National Center for Health Statistics. See also U.S. Dept. of Health and Human Services, *Child Health*

USA 1999, Washington, D.C.: U.S. Government Printing Office, 1999; F. Gary Cunningham, Norman F. Gant, Kenneth J. Leveno, Larry C. Gilstrap III, John C. Hauth, Katharine D. Wenstrom, *Williams Obstetrics 21st Edition.* (New York: McGraw-Hill, 2001).

3. Stephen J. Fleischman, M.D., "Ectopic Pregnancy," in *Parenthood Lost,* Michael R. Berman, ed. (Westport, CT: Borgin and Garvey, 2001), 141–44.

4. U.S. Department of Health and Human Services, National Institutes of Health, www.nichd.nih.gov; see press release, November 19, 2003, "NICHD Funds Major Effort to Determine Extent and Causes of Stillbirth."

5. First Candle. www.firstcandle.org, accessed July 2004.

CHAPTER 25 ■ ■ ■ ■ ■ ■ ■ ■ ■ ■ ■ ■ ■ ■ ■ ■ ■ ■ ■

I have always had regular periods. In fact, I used to worry about getting pregnant. I can't believe we have been trying for 10 months to get pregnant, and now we can't. I am 39 years old; finally, my life is settled enough to start having a family. Imagine my horror when the doctor did a blood test and told me that even though I had regular menstrual periods, my ovarian function was poor, that I was premenopausal, and that my chances of getting pregnant and not miscarrying were low.

I've been working through my feelings over my failed procedure, over the probability that I will never be pregnant. . . . I am feeling really sad, very discouraged . . . angry, [and] frustrated at the fact that we did the best we could but hit another brick wall. . . . I am really uncertain how to proceed. . . . Does it make sense to put more money into a procedure with no guaranteed outcome? How will we feel if we do this one more time and [fail again]? Maybe I should cut my losses and proceed with adoption. On the other hand, I have been pursuing the dream of raising a birth child for a decade. . . . I still deeply want to raise a child I give birth to. I may always wonder if I could have been successful on my second try.

Many of us grow up dreaming of, playing at, and planning for the day when we will have and hold our own baby. The inner and outer forces that contribute to these dreams and desires are complex and powerful. For many women, wanting children feels like a primal need, and being unable to conceive or to carry a child to term is devastating. The inability to bear a child can challenge our assumptions about the course of our lives and our ability to control events, and make us question our capacities and worth.

Societal pressures can intensify the pain of infertility. U.S. society, like so many others, often measures our worth as women by our fertility. Some of us are seen as irresponsible for having "too many" children (especially if we are poor or black), while others of us are pitied or seen as not truly fulfilled if we don't have children. Community expectations and our particular cultural background can make the pain of not being able to bear a child even more difficult. For example, in some Latino communities, infertility—seen as only the woman's problem—is considered grounds for divorce.

When you're faced with infertility, initial reactions of shock and denial are normal. It may be difficult to spend time with your friends' children. Feelings of envy, jealousy, and "Why them and not me?" are common. Because holidays are so child-centered, they can become stressful, lonely, depressing times. You may feel isolated

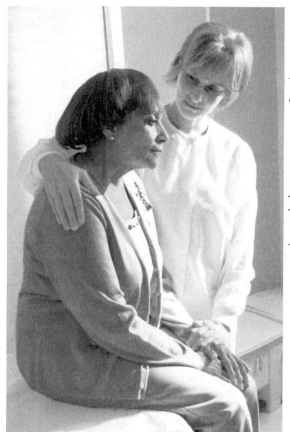

from friends and your partner, if you have one. You and a partner may each react differently to infertility.

Anger, too, is natural—but where and toward whom to direct it? We want to find reasons. You may feel that something you or your partner did in the past caused your present inability to conceive or to stay pregnant. Could past abortions (even though properly performed), drug or alcohol use, masturbation, or unusual sex practices be "responsible"? Though these experiences do *not* cause infertility, we want explanations for the unexpected and latch on to all kinds of culprits.

I . . . always believed that I would have children without any problems—as many as I wished and

THE ETHICS OF THE INFERTILITY BUSINESS

Treating infertility in the United States has become a highly technical, competitive business in which the physician providing the treatment is often the business owner trying to make a profit. In this context, some assisted reproductive technologies (ARTs) raise complicated ethical questions. On one hand, these technologies offer reproductive alternatives to infertile couples, single people, lesbian and gay couples, postmenopausal women, women who have had chemotherapy, and fertile couples at risk of passing on a genetic disorder. But at the same time, these high-cost, invasive procedures have low success rates and are not well studied for their long-term risks to both women and children.

Moreover, the increasing pressures on women to pursue ever more experimental procedures when treatments fail may lead to the use of paid "donors" of eggs, sperm, and embryos. Such practices raise concerns about the potential for social or economic pressures to coerce low-income women to enter into contract ("surrogate") pregnancies or "donate" (sell) eggs. Furthermore, new practical and ethical dilemmas are posed by the creation and storage of embryos outside women's bodies, and by procedures that can separate women's genetic ties to children from gestational ties. These procedures also open the way to further stigmatization of people with disabilities, especially when we envision a future in which parents could choose the characteristics of children. (See Chapter 31, "The Politics of Women's Health," p. 732.)

Those of us considering the use of these technologies to manage infertility or genetic risk need to be sure we understand all the issues—medical, social, psychological, and financial—involved before making any decisions.

---

when I decided it was the right time. Unfortunately, after four years of trial and error, tests, operations, et cetera, my husband and I are realizing that life does not always happen the way we plan it. I have found it quite hard dealing not only with our infertility problem but also with the reactions of people around me. I'm sick of people telling me to "relax," "stop thinking it out," "adopt and you'll get pregnant," and all the other wonderful clichés that, although said to be comforting, ring of insensitivity.

WHAT IS INFERTILITY?

Physicians define infertility as the inability to get pregnant after a year or more of well-timed, unprotected vaginal intercourse or sperm insemination. Women are also considered infertile if we are unable to carry a pregnancy to term. Overall, about 10 percent of Americans of reproductive age experience some kind of infertility.[1] An average woman experiences peak fertility in her twenties with a 20 to 30 percent chance of conceiving each menstrual cycle. Fertility begins to drop slowly in the early thirties, and more steeply in the late thirties. By age forty, a woman's chance of getting pregnant without medical assistance is approximately 5 percent each cycle.[2] Women over forty who undergo assisted reproduction using our own eggs have pregnancy rates from 5 to 15 percent per cycle depending on the type of technology used.[3,4]

Infertility may be a temporary or a permanent condition; this depends on the cause, the available treatments, and the fertility of the partner at any particular point in time. About 15 percent of women in the childbearing years have received some kind of infertility service, with the proportions much greater among high- than low-income women.[5] Many insurers do not cover advanced infertility treatments, or they offer only a limited benefit, making infertility treatments too expensive for the average person.

DEBUNKING MYTHS ABOUT INFERTILITY

Infertility is often considered "the woman's problem," but that is just not so. Both the man and the woman should be evaluated, and treated if necessary, to improve the couple's chances of conceiving a child together. In straight couples who underwent an infertility evaluation in 2001, female factors contributed to nearly 50 percent of cases, and male factors were involved in 34 percent; in the remaining 16 percent, infertility was either unexplained or due to other factors.[6]

Approximately 50 percent of couples who are treated for infertility become pregnant. Even after giving up fertility treatments, many couples may still become pregnant, sometimes even years after treatment ends.

The use of birth control pills does not kill a woman's eggs, nor has it caused an infertility epidemic. But it may give women an illusion of control over *fertility,* whereas birth control is really only some measure of control over *unplanned pregnancy.* There are concerns that increasing numbers and kinds of chemicals and toxins in the environment may be interfering with men's and women's fertility.[7]

Even though age-specific infertility rates in the United States do not seem to be changing markedly, the number of infertility visits has skyrocketed due to women delaying childbearing for economic, professional, or personal reasons, as well as the broader social acceptance of infertility treatments and the increasing number of technologies available.

GETTING STARTED WHEN YOU HAVE CONCERNS ABOUT (IN)FERTILITY

INFORMING YOURSELF

You may want to begin learning about infertility, especially from women who have already experienced diagnoses and treatments. They can supplement the information you receive from your physician with firsthand knowledge about feelings and resources. You may also want to join an infertility support group to have a regularly scheduled place to talk with people going through similar experiences, as well as to explore nontechnological ways to deal with infertility.

It may also be helpful to talk with friends and other women who have used assisted reproductive technologies, and those who have chosen not to. Be on the lookout for knowledgeable and compassionate support and the kind of people and material that will help you make decisions that will serve you best in the long run.

FERTILITY AWARENESS

Before you begin any kind of fertility testing or treatment, it is important to be sure that you are timing intercourse or inseminations properly. Charting your menstrual cycle and observing your body's fertility signals can tell you if and when you are ovulating and can help you maximize your chances of conceiving. (To learn more, see Chapter 13, "Sexual Anatomy, Reproduction, and the Menstrual Cycle," p. 227.)

For many women, the Internet has become a major source of health information and advice about treatment and coping. However, be wary of sites that are strictly commercial profit-making ventures. Three national organizations provide information about infertility, its treatments, and ways of coping: RESOLVE, the American Fertility Association, and the Inter-National Council on Infertility Information Dissemination (INCIID). Each receives financial support from pharmaceutical companies and private, for-profit fertility clinics, and accepts commercial advertising.

FINDING A PHYSICIAN WHO SPECIALIZES IN INFERTILITY

Your current practitioner, partner, close friends, or an infertility support group can help you find physicians. The most highly trained specialists are reproductive endocrinologists, obstetrician-gynecologists who have trained for two additional years in the field of infertility.

It is crucial to have a good relationship with your physician, and important for all of your caregivers to respect your mind and body and to make themselves available when you need them. Clinicians vary greatly in their approach to problems, so ask your physician for her or his track record and expectations. Select a physician with whom you feel comfortable, one who will take the time to listen to all your hopes and fears and answer all your questions. You may also want to look for a clinic that provides counseling for you and, if you have one, your partner.

Discuss with your health care practitioner the time frame in which you will be trying to become pregnant: how long you want to undergo treatments and, if they aren't working, how you will decide when it's right for you to stop. Also discuss this with your partner or supportive friends before beginning a process that can take on a momentum of its own.

All of your caregivers should explain words and procedures clearly and patiently so that you fully understand them. It can be helpful to bring a list of questions to each appointment and to ask a partner or friend to accompany you for support. If you don't like your doctor's methods or attitudes, go elsewhere. Confer with a second, even a third clinician—though this may be more difficult in certain health care plans. (For a complete discussion of questions to ask and lists of clinics, see the websites of RESOLVE, www.resolve.org, the American Fertility Association, www.theafa.org, or INCIID, www.inciid.org.)

In choosing a clinic, be aware that it is in a clinic's interest to promise high success rates. Also be aware that comparing clinics' success rates may be difficult, since some take on cases and/or age groups that others refuse, and this can greatly influence results.

CAUSES OF INFERTILITY

Fertility is based on several physiological events and their timing. For pregnancy to occur, there must be a sufficient quantity of healthy sperm and the presence of a mature egg. Sperm must be deposited in your vagina and move upward through cervical mucus and the fluids of the uterus (womb) to meet the ovum (egg) while it is still in the tube (oviduct). Timing of intercourse or insemination is important, since an ovum generally lives only twenty-four hours. (Sperm, on the other hand, can live up to five days inside a woman's vagina.) Once the sperm and ovum join, this single cell begins to divide to become an embryo, and this new organism must implant properly in the uterine lining and proceed to grow. A couple's infertility can be caused when there is a malfunction in any one or more of these steps.

Some of the common causes for a couple's

infertility (not in any particular order) are noted below.

A MAN MAY EXPERIENCE INFERTILITY BECAUSE OF:

1. *Problems of production and maturation of the sperm.* These can be caused by previous infections, such as mumps after puberty; undescended testicles; chemical and environmental factors; drugs (including cancer treatments); occupational hazards; and sports injuries. Sperm are sensitive to temperature, so hot saunas and baths, hot work environments, extended times in overheated vehicles, or high fevers that cause overly high temperatures in the scrotal sac can affect sperm production for up to a few months. Even wearing tight underwear can raise scrotal temperature in the same way. The most common source of male infertility (15 to 25 percent of cases) is a varicocele (a varicose vein in the scrotum), which can raise scrotal temperature and affect sperm production.

2. *Problems with the movement (motility) of the sperm.* This may be due to chronic prostatitis (inflammation of the prostate gland) and abnormally thick seminal fluid. In addition, certain drugs used to treat depression, emotional stress, stomach ulcers, and hypertension can affect sperm production and motility.

3. *Problems of transport resulting from scar tissue* in the delicate passageways through which the sperm travel. These may be caused by infections or untreated STIs; intentional blockage is created by vasectomy. Some men are missing their vas deferens; this may warrant genetic testing, because it usually indicates that the man is a carrier for cystic fibrosis.

4. *Inability to deposit the sperm into the cervix.* This may be the result of sexual dysfunction, such as impotence or premature ejaculation, as well as of structural problems in the penis (for example, when the opening is on either the top or the underside of the penis instead of at the tip). Spinal cord injuries and various neurological diseases can also interfere with erection and ejaculation. Retrograde ejaculation occurs when the semen gets pushed back into the bladder rather than into the penis; it can be caused by blood pressure medications.

5. *Other factors affecting male fertility* may include poor nutrition and poor general health. Increasing attention is being given to various chemicals present in the environment that may affect sperm, but definitive links are not yet established. If taken in excess, marijuana, tobacco, and alcohol can affect sperm quality, as can the use of anabolic steroids (testosterone-like drugs). Some researchers recommend that men seeking to improve their fertility eat well and take zinc, vitamin C, and vitamin E.

A WOMAN MAY EXPERIENCE INFERTILITY BECAUSE OF:

1. *Mechanical barriers preventing the union of the sperm and ovum,* caused by scarring in the tubes or around the ovaries. Scarring can result from previous pelvic inflammatory disease (PID) or pelvic surgery (especially an appendectomy); from infection caused by certain IUDs; or from an abortion that was not properly performed or followed up on. An untreated STI, such as gonorrhea or chlamydia, can also cause scarring and tubal blockage.

2. *Endometriosis* (see p. 628 in Chapter 28, "Unique to Women"), which can cause scarring, tubal blockage, and possibly immune responses.

3. *Endocrine problems.* A malfunction of the ovaries, pituitary, hypothalamus, thyroid, or ad-

renal glands may lead to failure to ovulate regularly or to irregular menstrual periods. These organs secrete several hormones at specific times in the normal menstrual cycle, and if any one of them is over- or underproduced, the whole cycle can be thrown off. Irregular cycles can decrease the chances of conception, as ovulation occurs less often and less predictably. Women often develop amenorrhea (absence of menstrual periods) following significant weight loss, strenuous exercise, or episodes of high stress. Rarely, a woman who uses Depo-Provera as a contraceptive will find that it continues to suppress ovulation even eighteen months after the last shot. (For more on the hormones of the menstrual cycle, see Chapter 13, "Sexual Anatomy, Reproduction, and the Menstrual Cycle.")

4. *Structural problems in the uterus or cervix* due to congenital problems or DES exposure in utero.

5. *Polycystic ovarian syndrome (PCOS),* a complex set of poorly understood symptoms usually characterized by ovaries with multiple cysts, irregular menstrual cycles and ovulations, and excess production of both estrogen and androgens (male hormones). Elevated male hormones may result in increased body hair (hirsutism), facial hair, and acne. Women with PCOS may experience elevated body weight and blood sugar levels and be at increased risk of heart disease and diabetes. (For more information on PCOS, see p. 632 in Chapter 28, "Unique to Women.")

6. *Cervical mucus that is too thick or too acidic* (due to vaginal infections). This acts as a barrier to the normal movement of the sperm up into the uterus. Mucus can be too thick under the influence of progesterone (higher levels in birth control pills, or during the days of the menstrual cycle after ovulation) or if estrogen levels are too low. Infections in the reproductive tract, such as T-mycoplasma (a virus-like microorganism that can cause miscarriage) can be diagnosed from a cervical smear.

7. *Immunological response.* You or your partner or donor may have sperm antibodies that tend to destroy the sperm's action by immobilizing sperm or causing them to clump. Women with certain autoimmune disorders, such as Hashimoto's thyroiditis, Raynaud's disease, lupus, or rheumatoid arthritis may have higher miscarriage rates. Blood tests can check for this possibility. In other cases, very early miscarriages in healthy women may be the result of as yet unknown immunological responses against the embryo that disrupt implantation. Such miscarriages may also occur when changes in the chromosomes of the fetus lead to its early death.

8. *Age-related factors.* Beginning around age thirty, most women experience a gradual decline in the number and function of the eggs in the ovaries (the medical term is *ovarian reserve*). This reduces both our ability to ovulate and the eggs' ability to become fertilized, and grow into embryos.[8] This decline occurs more rapidly as women approach age thirty-five, and is even more dramatic after age forty.[9]

9. *Other factors,* such as genetic abnormalities, extreme weight loss or weight gain, excessive exercise, poor nutrition, cancer treatments, and environmental and industrial toxins. Breastfeeding after childbirth also slows the return of regular ovulation, though it should not be counted on for birth control. In many cases, the difficulties conceiving may be temporary and resolve when the underlying cause (breastfeeding, weight change, etc.) is removed.

DOUCHING

Douching destroys the normal vaginal bacteria–the lactobacilli, or the "good" bacteria–that produce hydrogen peroxide, a natural disinfectant that keeps the vaginal tract clean and in the proper acid range of pH (around 4). It is possible that women who douche have more vaginal tract infections, which can lead to increased risk of pelvic inflammatory disease, ectopic pregnancy (a fertilized egg developing outside the uterus), or preterm delivery.

CHANGING DIAGNOSES AND TREATMENTS

The field of infertility diagnosis and treatment is evolving rapidly. As drug companies, hospitals, and physicians introduce new technologies and drugs into medical practice and the marketplace, diagnoses and treatments of infertility continue to change. New causes of infertility will probably be revealed as we learn more about environmental toxins, and about how our genes interact with the changing environment. New techniques and treatments appear regularly, but these are rarely studied in controlled, randomized trials that could establish their safety and effectiveness. Some procedures used today are tried and true; many others are experimental. Practitioners will agree about the efficacy of some drugs and procedures and differ about others. You have a right to know whether your treatment is new or experimental, and whether and how it has been studied scientifically. You also have the right to know about the possible risks and side effects of each, and about the amount of time and money that will be required by diagnosis and treatment. Try to learn about

the latest, safest, and least taxing treatments. Whenever possible, develop with your doctor a written course of treatment—including when to stop—that is tailored to your needs. And always be sure you understand all you need to know to give truly informed consent to diagnostic and treatment approaches.

DIAGNOSIS

THE INFERTILITY WORKUP

An infertility workup tests all the links in the chain of events from ovulation to an established pregnancy in an orderly way. It can take as long as six to twelve months, because many tests have to be scheduled at specific times in your cycle and can't be combined. Some of these tests for women are invasive, painful, and emotionally exhausting. Workups are expensive, and unfortunately, medical insurance coverage can be limited, even for infertility diagnosis. Though the sequence of diagnostic tests may vary with different doctors or clinics, it can include some or all of the following:

1. *A general and medical history of you and your male partner, if you have one.* This will in-

Perhaps more than any other field, infertility medicine is filled with negative medical terms borrowed from the military or agricultural industry that often are insensitive and appear to blame the woman for her condition. Examples include: hostile cervical mucus; habitual abortion; incompetent cervix; elderly primipara; dominant follicle; blighted ovum; vaginal probe; ovarian failure; harvesting eggs.

clude a review of your menstrual history and the nature of your menstrual periods, as well as details about any previous pregnancies, episodes of STI, or abortions; your use of birth control; DES exposure; sexual relations (frequency and position); where you live and whether your job has exposed you to any toxins that may have affected your reproductive system; and behavioral factors, such as stress, nutrition, smoking, drinking, and use of drugs (both prescribed and "recreational"). Before starting your infertility workup, have toxoplasmosis screening done and get tests to determine if you've been exposed to chicken pox (varicella), German measles (rubella), and HIV.

2. *A gynecologic examination,* primarily to check your uterus, ovaries, breasts, and general pelvic area.

3. *Monitoring ovulation.* A thorough practitioner will make sure you understand your menstrual cycle, and will help you track your ovulation, usually by taking your basal temperature every morning or by using a urine test kit. (See "Fertility Awareness," p. 509.)

4. *Hormonal profile.* You will need blood tests to check levels of all hormones that relate to your menstrual cycles, ovulation, and fertility, as well as the levels of your thyroid hormones.

5. *Ovarian reserve.* This term refers to the capacity of the ovaries to grow healthy eggs that can ovulate and be fertilized. Doctors can evaluate ovarian reserve in two ways: by checking blood levels of the hormones inhibin B and FSH on cycle day three; and by using daily ultrasound scans to observe the number and size of the growing follicles (balls of cells in the ovary containing eggs).

6. *Semen analysis.* The man will be asked to ejaculate semen into a clean container, and the specimen will be examined under a microscope to assess sperm count, shape, and motility.

If either the motility or the shape of the sperm is abnormal, additional tests may be done. The American Society for Reproductive Medicine website (www.asrm.org) provides patient fact sheets describing these tests and the expected range of results for them. Because a man's sperm can fluctuate in count and motility for many reasons, he may be asked to repeat the semen analysis at least every six months. If the result is abnormal, your male partner or sperm donor should pursue his own diagnosis before you have further tests done.

My husband's sperm count was very low; we were both crushed. I don't think my husband believed it was actually happening. In fact, he often talked in the third person, not truly accepting the results. I love him and therefore hurt for him. I didn't know what to say. I couldn't say the typical, "Oh, it's all right," because we both knew it really wasn't all right.

If all male factors are normal, and none of the above exams reveal a specific problem that can be treated, you can choose whether or not to continue with the following tests or procedures. Some must be done in hospitals with radiology facilities, while others take place in physicians' offices or clinics. Remember: You can always say no to a specific test or treatment.

- A *uterotubogram or hysterosalpingogram (hsg).* This test determines if there are any blockages in the fallopian tubes. A radio-opaque dye is injected into the vagina and uterus, and a series of X rays is taken. This test can be very painful, as the dye produces cramping. You can have local cervical anesthesia or an oral medication to help you relax before this test. Taking ibuprofen thirty minutes in advance can help reduce the pain, as can deep breathing and relaxation techniques. Pregnancy rates are slightly increased in the cycle immediately following this test, perhaps because the dye "cleans out" any mucus plugs in the fallopian tubes.

- *An endometrial biopsy.* This test determines whether you are ovulating and whether your uterine lining is thick enough for embryo implantation. It is not done if you might be pregnant, since it could cause a miscarriage. For this biopsy, the doctor inserts a small instrument into your uterus after partially dilating your cervix (this will cause painful cramping); scrapes a tiny piece of tissue from the lining of the uterus (endometrium); and has it examined under a microscope for signs of ovulation.

- *Laparoscopy.* One of the most invasive infertility tests, *laparoscopy* allows a practitioner to view the tubes, the ovaries, the exterior of the uterus, and the surrounding tissue of the pelvic cavity. It is the only test that can confirm endometriosis. Performed under spinal or general anesthesia, usually on an outpatient basis, laparoscopy involves making a tiny incision near your navel (belly button). Carbon dioxide gas is used to inflate the abdomen and allow the practitioner to view the pelvic organs. Sometimes a dye is flushed through the fallopian tubes to see whether they are open. If endometriosis or scar tissue is found, it can often be removed during the procedure. A *hysteroscopy* (the insertion of a small fiber-optic instrument through the cervix to view the uterus) may be done at the same time or as a separate office procedure. If scar tissue or polyps are present, they can sometimes be removed with the hysteroscope.

In addition to the stress of going for tests and treatments during an infertility workup, you may be subject to other pressures at home and at work. Relatives may ask you, "Well, has it happened yet?" Perhaps worse is when they don't say anything but look at you and sigh a lot. People you hardly know may comment on your problem. Trying to work and find time to schedule these tests is difficult. Many women don't want bosses to know, so this adds yet another pressure: secrecy. When you are going through these tests, your sex life once again comes under scientific scrutiny.

We were supposed to make love at seven o'clock in the morning, and then I had to run to my doctor's for the postcoital test. Who feels like making love at seven in the morning during a busy week anyway?

The demands of your infertility workup and treatments can affect your sexual life. Spontaneity in lovemaking decreases. Men may experience performance anxiety and be unable to get an erection. You have to plan your sex life around your menstrual cycle and days of fertility; it becomes less an act of loving and pleasure and more a pass-fail clinical procedure. Recording the time of your sexual relations on a temperature chart may make you feel as if nothing is private or sacred in your life anymore.

Hopefully, during these hard times, you and your partner can support each other and try to maintain a fulfilling, intimate sex life despite the need to time sex according to your fertile intervals. Many of us find that a sense of humor helps, as does taking a vacation from trying.

In more than four out of five cases, a reason can be found for infertility. Furthermore, diagnostic procedures themselves sometimes result in success—as when, for example, the hysterosalpingogram clears your tubes. Once a diagnosis is made, you and your doctor should outline a treatment plan, and revisit it to consider alternative options, including stopping, as you reach each milestone.

About 10 percent of women and couples are eventually given the diagnosis of *unexplained infertility*. This simply means that even after an extensive diagnostic workup, doctors cannot find a clear-cut medical cause for your infertility. Such a diagnosis can give you hope—or it can be difficult to cope with. Since new medical treatments are proliferating, it is tempting to hope that the next intervention will be the one to work; it can be hard to decide when to stop. Science has not yet identified all the possible causes of infertility. It is helpful to know that many couples with unexplained infertility eventually conceive without treatment.[10]

TREATMENT

TREATMENT FOR FEMALE INFERTILITY

In general, treatment may involve the use of drugs or some surgical intervention, or both.

Drugs

Doctors use a variety of drugs to correct hormonal imbalances in women, to help induce ovulation, and to correct problems after ovulation (the luteal phase). It is important to understand how these drugs work, how they affect you, and how long you should use them. (To find out more about the informed use of drugs in general, see "Informed Consent and Informed Decision Making," p. 702 in Chapter 30, "Navigating the Health Care System.") The long-term safety of many of these drugs has not been adequately studied, though some good national studies are now under way. And some of the drugs used may not (yet) be approved for infertility treatment, though they might have FDA approval to treat other conditions. Be aware, too, that trade names for drugs may change as new drugs come on the market.

The drugs used to *induce ovulation* include both natural hormones (extracted from the human placenta or the urine of postmenopausal women), and synthetic drugs designed to mimic *(agonists)* or block *(antagonists)* the action of natural hormones. Some are taken orally, while others require injections. Women often have a combination of problems, and treatment can involve combining several medications.

Taking fertility drugs is stressful. The drugs are expensive (although many may be covered by insurance) and can cause unpleasant, possibly dangerous side effects. While some early research suggested an increased risk for ovarian cancer among women treated for many cycles with some infertility drugs, more recent studies do not find more cancers than among untreated, *infertile* women. As a result, researchers are not sure whether it is the drugs or the infertility (especially if a woman never becomes pregnant after treatment) that puts infertile women at higher risk.

Surgery

Surgical techniques can sometimes correct structural problems of the cervix, uterus, and tubes. *Microsurgery* may repair tubes and remove adhesions. *Balloon-catheter techniques* have also been successful, in outpatient settings, to unblock tubes. *Laser surgery* using the carbon dioxide or argon laser, often in combination with microsurgery, may remove scar tissue or endometrial adhesions. If there is significant tubal damage, *in vitro fertilization* (IVF) may offer a higher chance of a successful pregnancy than surgical repair of the tubes, but IVF does not have high success rates in general (see p. 520 and following). Surgery and medications are often used together to treat endometriosis (see "Endometriosis," p. 628 in Chapter 28, "Unique to Women"). Unless fibroids are causing blockages, distortion of the uterus, or heavy bleeding, they are not usually removed surgically and do not seem to hinder fertility.

Other Treatments

Complementary treatments such as acupuncture, herbal medicine, and relaxation techniques may help you feel and cope better and may also improve your chances of becoming pregnant. Some infertility clinics now include an acupuncturist on the treatment team. If you want to try any herbal remedies (teas, pills, creams), first find out about evidence supporting their safe use, as some involve serious risks for you or your baby.

TREATMENT FOR MALE INFERTILITY

If infection is causing a decrease in sperm motility, it can be corrected by treatment with antibiotics. A varicocele (a varicose vein in the scrotum) can be corrected surgically or in a nonsurgical procedure using a tiny balloon to block off the vein; a rise in sperm count and motility is usually seen three months after surgery. If your partner's sperm count is low, or if the sperm have poor motility or morphology, his semen may be inseminated into your cervix or uterus (intrauterine insemination) (see "Donor Insemination," below). If the tubes that bring the sperm from the testicle are blocked, sperm can be extracted with a needle, joined with your egg in a petri dish, and replaced in your tube or uterus. (This technique is called *intracytoplasmic sperm injection* [ICSI]; see discussion on p. 521.)

Different types of doctors usually treat male and female infertility problems. Men see a urologist or an andrologist (a urologist specializing in male infertility). Women see a gynecologist, an infertility specialist, or a reproductive endocrinologist. *Your doctors must communicate with each other.* This is especially important since, as treatments begin, you may start to feel that you have lost control and become overly enticed by the succession of available procedures. As one woman said, "If there's always something more that you can do, it becomes a situation where you don't even have control over when is enough."

Some women end up conceiving without any medical or surgical treatment, often after many years of trying, or after adopting a child. How these pregnancies come about is a mystery and a great joy. But other women do go on to consider further assisted reproductive options.

DONOR INSEMINATION

Donor insemination (DI) involves attempting to conceive using the sperm of a man who is not your partner. DI is used by single women, lesbian couples, and straight couples with male infertility. Straight couples may also opt to use donor sperm if the man has a hereditary disease or disorder that would put the baby at risk. DI is a simple, widely used assisted reproductive technology that has increased in popularity in recent years. It is estimated that between thirty thousand and fifty thousand babies are conceived this way each year in the U.S.

CHOOSING A SPERM DONOR

You will first need to decide whether you want to use the sperm of someone you know (a known donor) or someone who has donated to a sperm bank on either an anonymous or an identity-release basis. (Some donors agree to have their identity released to their offspring at the age of eighteen, or sometimes sooner if a serious medical or psychological need arises.) Each approach has pros and cons; the option you choose depends on your individual situation, the kind of family you want, and what you believe will be in the best interest of the child you hope to have.

If you choose to use an *unknown* donor, you will most likely be working with a sperm bank

IS DI RIGHT FOR ME?

DI isn't right for everybody. It raises different questions for different people. Some married women have said they felt as though they were committing adultery. (Some religious institutions, including the Roman Catholic Church, do consider DI adultery.) A partner may not feel as involved in the pregnancy or parenting as you had hoped, because the baby isn't his or her biological child. If genetic continuity and family resemblances are very important to you, then DI may not be for you. Think about what you will tell close friends and family, and—most important—what you will tell your child. In the past, many parents kept DI a secret, perhaps thinking this would protect the man from the embarrassment of having

people know he was infertile. (Fertility and sexual potency—particularly in the sense of the ability to achieve erection and ejaculation—are often mistakenly linked.) Today many believe such secrecy can be damaging, and increasing numbers of people are recognizing that children born through donor insemination, like children who are adopted, have a right to know of their origins and genetic histories. Several organizations (such as the Donor Conception Network, www.dcnetwork.org; the Donor Conception Support Group, members.optushome.com.au/dcsg; and the Infertility Network, www.infertilitynetwork.org) offer excellent books, newsletters, video documentaries, support groups, and seminars (live and on tape) to help families deal with the issue of disclosure.

and using frozen sperm. Your health care provider might work with a particular sperm bank, or you can research different banks on your own. (The Human Rights Campaign [www.hrc.org] maintains a list of accredited sperm banks, including lesbian-friendly banks and banks that allow the family to have contact with the donor.)

If you use fresh sperm from a *known* donor, it's important to know his medical and sexual history and to decide whether you trust him. Inseminating with a man's semen exposes you to the same risks as having unprotected intercourse. Many clinics can screen a potential donor for a range of illnesses and sexually transmitted infections, including HIV, hepatitis B, chlamydia, and gonorrhea. Clinics routinely screen for unknown donors.

Legal issues related to access, parenting roles, and financial support also must be addressed in order to protect the interests of all parties, including the child.

INSEMINATING

One of the humorous aspects of becoming a single mom was getting pregnant. In the absence of a significant other to do the inseminating, I asked various friends to do the honors. I inserted the speculum while three of them crowded between my legs, squinting through the flashlight and ogling my textbook-perfect cervix. As if being initiated into a revered secret society, each one enthusiastically took her turn drawing the specimen into the syringe and dribbling it into my mucus-covered os. We just laughed and laughed at this insemination by committee.

There are several ways to inseminate using donor sperm. The most low-tech way is to inseminate at home, using a syringe without a needle to put the sperm into your vagina.

The other types of insemination are generally performed in a practitioner's office (although

If you are using fresh sperm—which can live in a woman's body for up to five days—it is best to inseminate every day to every other day for the five days before you ovulate, as well as on the day of ovulation. If you are using frozen sperm—which, once thawed, can live inside a woman's body for under twenty-four hours—it is best to inseminate the day before and the day of ovulation.

When inseminating at home, use the sperm as quickly as possible, within thirty minutes after ejaculation or thawing. The sperm should be at body temperature. You can insert it by yourself, or you may choose to have a partner or friend do it. Some fertility experts recommend that a woman remain on her back with her hips elevated for twenty minutes or so following the insemination; others say doing so is unnecessary.

There is some evidence that when a woman has an orgasm after the man during intercourse, her cervix dips down into the pool of semen, increasing the chances that sperm will swim through the cervix into the uterus. Some women inseminating at home try to have an orgasm afterward in hopes of facilitating conception.

some midwives will perform them in your home). *Intracervical inseminations* (ICI) and *intrauterine inseminations* (IUI) both appear to have slightly higher pregnancy rates than home inseminations, particularly if you are using frozen sperm. In ICI inseminations, the sperm is injected through a tiny, strawlike tube into the opening of the cervix. During IUI inseminations, a thin catheter is threaded all the way through the cervix, allowing the sperm to be injected directly into the uterus. ICI is a very quick procedure, usually lasting only about five min-

utes. IUI, which is a slightly more invasive and more expensive procedure—and which may also cause some cramping—appears to have higher success rates than ICI.

The Cost of Donor Insemination

The cost of DI is variable, depending on where you live, whether you use fresh or frozen sperm, how many inseminations you do, and whether you inseminate at home or in a practitioner's office. If you choose to use a sperm bank, you will probably need to pay a registration fee (perhaps $50 to $200) as well as the cost of each vial of frozen sperm (between $175 and $275). If you inseminate in a practitioner's office, you will also have office fees, which may or may not be covered by your health insurance. Health insurance generally will not pay for inseminations unless a woman has a diagnosis of infertility; and the cost of sperm, as a rule, is not covered unless there is an infertile man involved. Check with your health care practitioner or insurance plan for more information about medical fees.

HIGH-TECH ASSISTED REPRODUCTIVE TECHNOLOGIES

For those who decide to pursue the more high-tech assisted reproductive technologies (ARTs)—in which both eggs and sperm are handled—it is important to become fully informed of the physical, emotional, and financial burdens involved. You will also want to gather the support you will need for what is frequently an arduous path, and to ensure that you stay as much in charge as possible.

Making the decision to do IVF was a difficult one. Everything felt so clinical. I had to carry my husband's sperm to the lab, and have my eggs taken from me and my embryos put back into me

IVF PROCEDURE

IVF involves the woman taking drugs to trigger the development of multiple ripe (egg) follicles in the next menstrual cycle. If this happens, the eggs are retrieved from the ovary using ultrasound-guided needle aspiration (suction). Eggs that pass visual inspection are then placed into an incubator to mature for about 2 to 36 hours, and then they are mixed with sperm and incubated for a further 12 to 18 hours for fertilization to occur. If fertilization takes place, the embryos are transferred to your uterus when they are at a 4- to 8-cell stage. A pregnancy test is then done about 12 to 14 days after the transfer. If the results are positive, you will get progesterone suppositories or shots for as long as 10 to 12 weeks to maintain the pregnancy until the placenta is fully functioning. In any attempt, *only about 10 to 15 percent of women undergoing IVF reach this point*. For women who enter into more than one IVF process, the cycle may start in subsequent tries at the embryo transfer stage, using embryos that were kept frozen after their production in previous attempts.

in a treatment room in a clinic. It was a far cry from making our baby at home. When the clinic called to say that my eggs had fertilized, I started to feel bonded to them. When they didn't implant and I got my period, I really grieved for what we almost had.

Pressures to use more and more technological options sometimes arise because of the commercialization of ARTs, our culture's fascination with technologies, our own determination to have one of these procedures succeed, and a persistent desire for a biologically related child.

However, it is important to remember that *you* can decide to stop when you want to, despite the pressures to "succeed" and to bear children of "your own."

I always felt in control of my life and body. Now nothing feels in control. I live month to month, period to period. I can't stop medical treatment, because after all this effort, how can I walk away empty-handed, defeated?

Assisted reproductive technologies now account for about 1 percent of all births in the United States each year. Some estimates put the revenues of the assisted reproductive industry at about $4 billion per year. The basis for many of these ARTs is *in vitro fertilization* (IVF).

"In vitro" is Latin for "in glass." IVF involves extracting ripe eggs from your ovary, fertilizing them with sperm in a glass dish, and placing the embryo back in your—or another woman's—womb (uterus). Though IVF has been around for a quarter century, and a million babies have been conceived through the procedure worldwide, there is still insufficient research about the risks it poses to women and to the children conceived.

IVF was intended originally for women with normal ovaries and uteruses who had blocked fallopian tubes that prevented fertilization and implantation. Today it is used for both male and female infertility. However, it still requires that the woman undergo the associated risks and pressures. And it is expensive, approximately $10,000 to $15,000 per cycle in addition to the medical expenses associated with pregnancy and birth.[11]

It is important to know the risks involved with IVF, but our information about the potential adverse effects for women and children is still, unfortunately, very inadequate. Some of the risks are associated with the drugs, and some with the procedure itself. In general, the risks associated with the egg retrieval and embryo transfer involved in IVF include infection, needle injuries, adverse reactions to anesthesia, and reduced uterine receptivity because of a thinner endometrium. With IVF, ectopic pregnancy (pregnancy in the fallopian tube) still occurs in about 4 percent of pregnancies, due to underlying tubal problems that don't get corrected. Miscarriage rates are as high as 20 to 24 percent.

Most important, you have a much greater chance of multiple-birth pregnancies, which carry significant risks for long-term health problems for the babies. In the United States in 2001, over half of IVF infants were born in multiple-birth deliveries: 46 percent were twins, and 8 percent were triplets or higher-order multiples.[12] That compares with a twin birth rate of 3.1 percent, and a triplet or higher-order birth rate of 0.2 percent, for women who become pregnant naturally.[13]

EMERGING RISKS TO THE CHILDREN BORN OF IVF

Few studies have been done in the United States on babies conceived through assisted reproductive technologies, though about 250 studies have been published in other countries where clinics are required to keep more complete birth records. Most earlier studies suggested that singleton babies conceived with ARTs are not different from other babies, with rates of physical and mental development about the same. But more recent research suggests caution. Studies have begun to show an association between assisted reproductive technology and a higher risk of cancer, birth defects, and genetic diseases.[14] These associations may depend on the procedures used during IVF (e.g., fresh or frozen embryos; multiple or single sperm; etc.).

TECHNIQUES RELATED TO IVF

Intracytoplasmic Sperm Injection

ICSI is a procedure in which a single sperm is injected into an egg in an attempt to achieve fertilization outside the body. The sperm may be surgically removed from the epididymis (the male reproductive duct that houses immature sperm) and matured in vitro before it is injected. This technique, developed for men with very few or even no sperm in their semen, may also be used to inject processed sperm from men who are HIV-positive to remove all the viral particles and produce healthy, HIV-free babies.

ICSI is an expensive procedure, costing an additional $2,000 to $4,000 above the $10,000 to $15,000 per cycle for IVF. The experimental process requires that healthy and fertile women undergo stressful hormone treatment to make egg cells available in vitro. Moreover, using sperm cells that have not been able to fertilize an egg on their own, or sperm from men with very few or no sperm in their semen, might lead to as yet unknown problems in the children born. We do not yet know whether genetic factors that might underlie the man's infertility may be transferred by ICSI to subsequent generations, but there are some data suggesting a higher than expected rate of health problems or genetic anomalies in these children. As well, men who congenitally lack at least one vas deferens may be carriers of cystic fibrosis, and prospective parents may want this to be determined. For these and other reasons, ICSI should be used only after the most careful consideration of the possible risks and then with great caution.

Micromanipulation

Micromanipulation, or zona "drilling" of the egg (making a small opening in the outer membrane of the egg wall with either a glass needle or laser) is another technique used to increase fertilization rates.

Donor Egg IVF

This technique has become an option for women with early menopause (premature ovarian failure), age-related infertility, or disorders that may be transmitted in the genes. In these instances, either a woman or a clinic finds another woman willing to "donate" her eggs, often in exchange for money. This donor will undergo the same hormone treatment to induce ovulation as do the women undergoing IVF, but once her eggs have been retrieved and fertilized, any resulting embryos will be placed in the uterus of the woman who is trying to become pregnant.

Any woman considering being a donor must discuss carefully with professionals and others the possible risks—physical, emotional, and social—she may face. These risks may be weighed differently if the woman will, or will not, be seeking her own pregnancy. (For more information, see "Being or Using an Egg Donor" [W56] on the companion website, ourbodiesour selves.org.)

Moreover, it is important to learn how donors are recruited and compensated, if at all. Concerns have been raised about the potential for commercialization and commodification when women are paid to "donate," or if we are undergoing IVF ourselves, when we are offered reduced rates for IVF if we agree to "share" our eggs and embryos.

Donor egg IVF has been used by some lesbian couples. When one member of a couple donates the egg and the other is the birth mother, both have a biological connection to the child.

As with sperm donors, egg donors may be anonymous or known to a woman. Many of the same questions about disclosure and medical, social, and psychological issues for the parents and children involved need to be considered.

Contract (or "Surrogate") Motherhood

Contract motherhood is another activity made possible through the use of either of two ARTs: donor insemination or embryo transfer after IVF. In both cases, a woman goes through a pregnancy and gives birth to a baby destined for another person or couple. This is highly controversial.

Various terms are used for this practice: artificial insemination (AI); surrogacy; surrogate motherhood; and contract motherhood. (From time to time, this book will use the word "surrogate" in quotes, because the term implies that the woman who carries the baby is not its mother.) In the most common form of surrogacy in the U.S., one woman—the "surrogate" mother—contracts with a man, or with a couple, to be inseminated with his sperm via donor insemination and to bear a child that she will turn over to him or them at birth. Typically, the man is married, and his wife adopts the baby. They pay the "surrogate" mother her expenses and a fee, usually about $15,000. (In 2004 the Canadian government passed a bill prohibiting payment for surrogacy services.) A mediating agency and/or a lawyer may require substantial additional fees. The Organization of Parents Through Surrogacy estimates that almost ten thousand surrogate births have occurred in the United States since the mid-1970s.[15]

In gestational surrogacy (sometimes called being a gestational carrier), the egg used to create the embryo is not that of the woman who carries (gestates) and gives birth to the baby. Thus, the woman who is the gestational carrier has no genetic relationship to the child. Rather, the eggs and sperm (the donated gametes) of the contracting couple, or of others who provided them, are brought together using IVF techniques. The resulting embryo is implanted in the gestational surrogate.

Surrogacy can be a problematic venture, with many pitfalls and considerations that need exploration. (For more information about the social, psychological, legal, and financial questions raised, see "Surrogacy" [W57] on the companion website, www.ourbodiesourselves.org.)

Preimplantation Genetic Diagnosis

Preimplantation genetic diagnosis (PGD) IVF is sometimes used when no infertility is involved, to allow screening of the embryo for people who want to avoid passing severe genetic conditions to the next generation. PGD begins with the creation of an embryo using IVF and then involves obtaining and examining DNA from one of the early cells for the presence of certain transmissible characteristics before the embryo is placed in the uterus to develop. (By contrast, prenatal diagnosis [PND] tests for the same characteristics but uses cells from the 8- to 12-week fetus of an already-started pregnancy.) Only the embryos that pass this screen—that do not have the characteristic being tested for—are implanted. This procedure does not guarantee a healthy baby, only one that will not develop the condition(s) for which the embryos have been tested.

This technology is also being marketed as a way to choose the sex of future children. Some IVF centers are offering it routinely to women over age thirty-five as a check for Down syndrome.

DRAWING THE LINE

By this time I had sunk into a deep depression. Sarah, my partner, who had been ambivalent about having a child, was angry at me for disappearing into this obsession. I had begun to consider more and more invasive procedures. I was both spinning out of control and standing in a dead stillness. I finally realized that I couldn't

continue. . . . I began the process of letting go. . . . For the last six months, we had been quietly considering international adoption. My partner had worried if she broached this topic, I might feel undermined in my efforts to bear a child biologically. . . . I saw that one way or another, a baby would enter our lives.

Some of us will always have a fierce desire to bear children. Part of the challenge in pursuing this desire is figuring out for ourselves where we draw the line with the available technologies. Another challenge for all of us is to determine the place for, and management of, assisted reproductive technologies.

Even under optimal social and economic circumstances worldwide, there will always be children whose biological parents cannot care for them. If we feel less pressure to give birth to our "own" children, some of us may be more apt to adopt or to become foster parents to those born to others, or to love, nurture, and be loved by the children of our neighbors, friends, or relatives. (For more on adoption and other options, see Chapter 17, "Considering Parenting.") Others will choose to pursue the new ARTs and will need to decide how far we are willing to go to have a child "of our own" and when to stop treatment.

Drawing the line with ARTs is both an individual and a social matter. As technologies continue to proliferate, ethical and social challenges multiply, with complex problems of justice and rights and conflicting principles continually raised. As a society, we are long overdue to discuss these issues and to guard against leaving them solely in the province of researchers and biotechnology entrepreneurs. We also need to devote resources and energies to identifying and removing the environmental causes of infertility. (For more on the social impact of emerging biotechnologies, see p. 730 in Chapter 31, "The Politics of Women's Health.")

NOTES

1. American Society for Reproductive Medicine "Fact Sheet: In Vitro Fertilization (IVF)," accessed at www.asrm.org/Patients/FactSheets/invitro.html on October 22, 2004.
2. Richard Scott Jr., M.D., and Pamela Madsen with the American Infertility Association, accessed at www.theafa.org/faqs/afa_whatmotherdidnotsay.html on October 22, 2004.
3. Ibid.
4. American Society for Reproductive Medicine, "Patient Information Booklets," accessed at www.asrm.org/Literature/patient.html on October 22, 2004.
5. *Cells to Selves: Biobehavioral Development* (Bethesda, MD: U.S. Department of Health and Human Services, Public Health Service, National Institutes of Health, National Institute of Child Health and Human Development, 2001).
6. Brady E. Hamilton, "Reproduction Rates for 1990–2002 and Intrinsic Rates for 2000–2001: United States," *National Vital Statistics Reports* 52, no. 17 (March 18, 2004): 1–12. Accessed at www.cdc.gov/nchs/data/nvsr52/nvsr52_17.pdf on October 22, 2004.
7. Richard W. Pressinger and Wayne Sinclair, "Environmental Causes of Infertility," Chem-tox.com, 1998, accessed at www.chem-tox.com/infertility/download/InfertilityFacts.pdf on October 22, 2004.
8. Genetics and IVF Institute, "Ovarian Reserve, FSH Levels, Clomiphene Challenge Tests, and Pregnancy Rates," accessed at www.givf.com/ovarian.cfm on October 22, 2004.
9. Ibid.
10. J. A. Collins, R. A. Milner, T. K. Rowe, "The Effect of Treatment on Pregnancy Among Couples with Unexplained Infertility," *International Journal of Fertility* 36, no. 3 (May–June 1991): 140–41, 145–52.
11. American Society of Reproductive Medicine, "Frequently Asked Questions About Infertility," accessed at www.asrm.org/Patients/faqs.html on October 22, 2004.
12. Centers for Disease Control and Prevention, "Assisted Reproductive Technology Surveillance," April 30, 2004. *Morbidity and Mortality Weekly Report* 2004: 53 (No. SS-1, 1).
13. Centers for Disease Control and Prevention, "Births: Final Data for 2002," *National Vital Statistics Reports* 10, no. 52 (December 2003).
14. Summarized from the website of the Johns Hopkins Genetics and Public Policy Center, accessed at www.dnapolicy.org on October 22, 2004.
15. Organization of Parents Through Surrogacy, accessed at www.opts.com/informat.htm on October 22, 2004.

Growing Older

■ **CHAPTER 26**

THE MIDDLE YEARS

As we grow older, we have the potential to live more fully and healthfully than any generation before us.* As a fifty-eight-year-old woman says:

My attitude towards aging has changed over the years. My youngest daughter was born when I was 42. She sees me as young, and I feel relatively young at 58. I can't believe that I thought my mother was old when she turned 38 and I was the

* A girl born in 2000 is expected to live 79.9 years. Women reaching 65 have an average life expectancy of an additional 19.5 years. The number of women 85 and older—2.3 million in 2000—is expected to reach 6.3 million by 2030. In 2030 one fifth of the total population will be 65 or older. (Compilations of census data and projections done by the Administration on Aging. Available at www.aoa.gov/prof/Statistics/statistics.asp.)

same age my daughter is now. My sense of the lifespan has increased, with an extended adulthood of active years and old age beginning around 80 or 85.

Midlife is a loosely defined period that covers the years from about forty-five until sixty-five. This time of life involves emotional, social, and physical changes; the biological transition of menopause is just one of its aspects. The middle years and beyond can be rich and fulfilling.

EXPLORATION AND GROWTH

With the advent of menopause, children leaving home, or the decline of a parent, we come to the end of familiar roles and ways of being and begin a different way of life.

All my life I was a secretary. Finally, at age 57, I took a year to attend school and become a licensed practical nurse. Seven years later, at age 65, I am happily employed as an LPN—my lifelong dream.

Midlife can bring a surge of energy or restlessness. Those of us whose children are grown may feel satisfaction with a job well done, or at least finished. This transition is harder for some than others. Even when you have other interests, your house may feel empty, with some essential vitality departed. Then again, you might feel wonderfully free. We can use this time to refocus, to acquire new skills, to refine old ones, to spend more time with our partner or friends, to work harder at a present job, or to find a job. As one woman put it, "It's getting ourselves back."

I just want more! More time free of kids to focus on my work; more time to myself; more passion in my marriage or from somewhere else.

Attitudes toward the middle years vary from one community to another and also by economic situation. If you work at a physically demanding job, you may experience an earlier onset of chronic conditions associated with aging that require you to slow down, while women who have had less stressful working conditions may be more interested in new outlets for activity.

Perspectives often change with a heightened awareness of time passing and the value of the time that remains.

I want to use my time well and live in a way that is true to my values. Some women face this question in college. For me, I just wanted to get married and have children. What do I want to do now? I want to feel I am leaving a legacy. It hit me full force at mid-life.

MYTH OR REALITY?

- *Once my periods stop being regular I can have intercourse without using birth control.*

Myth. For some of us, irregular bleeding patterns may continue for years, during which pregnancy is still possible. It is only after *a year without any bleeding* that you can be fairly certain you are postmenopausal and thus discontinue birth control.

- *Sex gets worse after menopause.*

Myth. During our postmenopausal years there is sometimes a gradual decline in sexual interest or frequency but generally not in orgasmic capacity or overall satisfaction. Some of us find that we enjoy making love more in the postmenopausal years. If vaginal dryness is an issue, using lubricant can help make sex more enjoyable.

It was a shock when a friend of ours, a middle-aged man, died suddenly. It got me thinking that I don't know how many years Dan and I have left together. . . . Work is still very important to me, but I no longer want it to absorb my whole life. I want to spend time together and have fun.

Coming to terms with life raises questions: What do I want to do? What am I not able to do? What can I control? Now that I know myself pretty well, how can I live as authentically as possible? What would I like to learn? How shall I balance my life? Midlife offers opportunities to reexamine your values, relationships, self-image, and health practices.

LOSSES, GAINS, AND CHALLENGES

Women face age discrimination at earlier ages than men do, sometimes even in our thirties. Western society overvalues youth and beauty, setting them as a sexist standard for measuring women's value, along with sexuality and reproductive ability. This devaluation and ageist attitude can make it more difficult for us to deal with losses that occur in the middle years.

Our biologic capacity to reproduce definitively ends at menopause, at the average age of fifty-one. Some of us who do not have biological children have to accept that we never will. Signs of aging can be upsetting and may challenge us to develop a new body image.

The most important signs of midlife for me were the physical changes that made me realize that I was not young; vision loss, lack of sexual appetite, hair texture thinning, skin changes, and some wrinkles. I couldn't count on my looks anymore. My body was changing; what was the rest of my life going to be like?

We become prime targets for often risky "anti-aging" treatments, from wrinkle creams and Botox to face-lifts and liposuction.

If we have children, they may be toddlers or adolescents, or they may be leaving home or raising children of their own. Sometimes they have trouble becoming adults. They may return home to save money, or after an illness, divorce, job loss, or other troubles. They may bring their children with them or move on and leave the grandchildren with us. They may die early in an accident or from disease, which may be devastating.

Other important relationships may change or end: Your partner or close friend may die, or you may divorce. Parents become ill or die. We become susceptible to chronic illnesses, such as arthritis, and to life-threatening conditions, such as heart disease.

These pressures can cause considerable emotional, physical, and financial stresses. They may bring us a heightened awareness of the passage of time and of human mortality.

When my father died this month, for the first time I really recognized that death is around the corner. It definitely makes me treasure life more than ever. . . . I try to slow down and force myself to feel and see and enjoy the world.

RELATIONSHIP CHANGE AND THE "DEPENDENCY SQUEEZE"

Midlife women belong to the "sandwich generation"—we may have both aging parents and dependent children in our lives. Conflicts can occur when parents or other close relatives need care at the same time that jobs are demanding, children are still at home or are returning home, or a partner is ill or needs care. With these multiple demands, there's barely enough time to care for everyone, or for ourselves. Responsibilities for aging and elderly parents also may last a long time, obliging us to give up or postpone long-awaited changes or adventures. (See "Caregiving and Needing Care," p. 568.)

Most of our important relationships are changing. We may become mothers-in-law and grandmothers, and enjoy seeing future generations being born. Some grandmothers are deeply involved with raising grandchildren. If your children leave their children for you to bring up, you may find yourself in an unexpected new role.

I was in my late 30s and my other children were all in high school, when one of my daughters developed a drug problem and I had to take her two little ones to raise. I was afraid I couldn't do it, but I felt it was my responsibility. I didn't want them to go to foster care. I arranged for day care so I could keep my job. The kids do see her sometimes. They think of her as an aunt. I am proud that both of my grandkids are doing well now, and that I was able to raise them.

When grandparents raise grandchildren, it is usually because of death, divorce, illness, joblessness, drug and alcohol abuse, incarceration, AIDS, or child abuse or neglect on the part of the parents. Today approximately 2.4 million U.S. grandparents are raising grandchildren. This situation is more than twice as common for African-American families than for white or Latino families.[1] Some of us may be involved in a legal battle for custody of our grandchildren or visiting rights. Grandparents are joining support groups and forming coalitions to bring about changes in law and to educate communities to help with these challenges (see "Resources").

If you have a partner, your relationship may change and need reevaluation. You might experience renewed pleasure in long-standing relationships.

Sex is better. David and I are able to give each other the benefit of the doubt and help each other through crises with compassion, without as much defensiveness or selfishness or confusion.

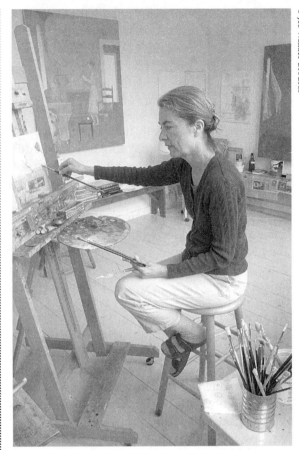

Artist Susan J. Walp paints at her home in Vermont.

You may have to redefine roles and relationships and develop new goals together. Sometimes, when the children leave, the "empty nest" discloses an unsatisfactory relationship. Divorce or separation may be exhilarating, a new beginning; you'll need courage to face living alone. If your partner leaves, separation can be devastating; it may take tremendous energy to rebuild your life.

Many women find new partners, going down unexpected roads. Some come out after years in the closet, often falling in love with another woman and turning to a community of women. Others, rich in relationships with old friends, are happy being single at this point.

Many of us have more energy to connect with our communities by working in nonprofit organizations (see "Resources").

MENOPAUSE: OUR "CHANGE OF LIFE"

Just as your body "changed gears" with puberty, so again you experience a transition as you pass from the reproductive years into your post-menopausal years. Many women scarcely notice menopause. The periods end, period. It can be a welcome end to bleeding, irregular periods, anemia, PMS (premenstrual syndrome), or concerns about pregnancy. If you have had uterine problems, such as heavy bleeding or fibroids, they may clear up without treatment when your hormone levels drop. Menopause is a normal part of these middle years, not a disease, and a self-help approach may alleviate most of its discomforts. You may need or prefer medical strategies for managing menopause. This chapter discusses various options.

Menopause is defined as the end of monthly bleeding (menstrual periods). It can begin as early as forty or as late as fifty-five or sixty and still be normal; the average age is around fifty-one. The entire transition period, which involves many physical and emotional changes for some women, is called the *perimenopause* ("peri" means "around") and can last anywhere from one to ten years. Women who smoke tend to go into menopause earlier than nonsmoking women.

Some physical changes occur because the ovaries are no longer producing enough estrogen to result in regular cycles (though other cells in the body do produce some estrogen). Lower estrogen levels may lead to other changes as well. There is nothing abnormal or diseased about these changes; they are simply signs of what's going on and do not necessarily require medi-

cal attention or treatment. A fifty-six-year-old woman says:

For me, menopause was wonderful! No more bloating, sore breasts, menstrual migraines, back pain, greasy hair, and zits. I now realize I felt like I had been pregnant for thirty-five years!

How women experience and think about menopause may vary with cultural background and lifestyle differences. One large U.S. multi-ethnic study found that African-American women were more likely to report hot flashes, white women to report more mood and memory changes, and women of Japanese and Chinese origin to report fewer menopausal signs in general.[2] Whether variations are due to genetic makeup, diet, expectations, or something else is still unknown, but it can be useful for you and your health care providers to be aware of them.

SURGICAL AND CHEMICAL MENOPAUSE

In women younger than the normal age range for menopause, surgical removal of the ovaries will lead to an abrupt drop in hormone levels, resulting in the same changes as those in natural menopause. Certain medical treatments such as chemotherapy, other cancer drugs, or drugs for heavy bleeding may also produce a menopausal state. Many younger women to whom this happens find it more difficult to adjust to menopausal changes, such as hot flashes or vaginal dryness, and may choose hormone replacement therapy (see "Hormone Therapy," p. 538).

WHAT HAPPENS DURING MENOPAUSE

Signs of aging are different from signs of menopause. For instance, graying hair occurs in both women and men and is a function of the aging process, not of decreased hormone levels. Neither aging nor menopause occurs at a predictable age or a regular rate, or lasts a predictable length of time. Perimenopause is a time of ups and downs. A fifty-one-year-old woman recalls:

I thought I was going crazy; one month I would have lots of hot flashes and no period at all, and then I'd start having periods again, and my signs of menopause would go away for several months.

Common perimenopausal signs include changes in bleeding patterns for periods, hot flashes, sleep disturbances, and vaginal dryness. Some women may experience changes in frequency of urination, memory or mood, or sexual feeling. Sometimes bone density decreases rapidly; this change is not strictly menopausal, as it also happens to men (see "Bone Loss and Osteoporosis," p. 546).

PREMENSTRUAL SYNDROME (PMS)

Some women report more severe premenstrual discomforts (PMS) during perimenopause, such as swollen or tender breasts, water retention (bloating), anxiety, or irritation. Whether you have had such discomforts for years or are beginning to have them now, you may look forward to relief as soon as your periods end and your hormone cycles level out.

CHANGES IN OUR PERIODS

Menstrual cycles may become longer or shorter; bleeding may be heavier or lighter and may last a shorter or longer number of days; and occasionally, a menstrual period will be skipped altogether for one or several months. With reduced amounts of estrogen and progesterone, the uterine lining gets thinner, which causes the flow to be lighter or last fewer days. Sometimes, with irregular ovulation, bleeding can actually be heavier, and periods may last longer. Hormone levels vary from day to day, so there is no single hormone test to indicate that you are in menopause. If the bleeding is extremely heavy, ask your health care provider to test you for von Willebrand disease, the most common inherited bleeding disorder (see p. 696).

Despite lighter or shorter periods, you can still become pregnant. If you don't want to, you will need birth control. For some women, irregular bleeding patterns may continue for years. You can be fairly sure you are no longer fertile when you've gone one year with no bleeding.

HOT FLASHES/NIGHT SWEATS

Hot flashes are legendary signs of menopause, though some women never have them at all. If you have them, you suddenly feel warm, then very hot and sweaty, and sometimes experience a cold chill afterward. Hot flashes are thought to be due to a change in the brain's control mechanism for body temperature as a result of declining estrogen. Some women experience a more rapid pulse rate, heart palpitations, and increased blood flow to surface blood vessels, which causes a visible reddening of the skin that moves from the chest up to the face.

Each woman usually has a consistent pattern of hot flashes, although every woman's pattern is different. Hot flashes can vary in frequency from almost never to several times an hour. Other conditions can mimic hot flashes, such as thyroid dysfunction or use of particular medications (for example, certain antidepression drugs).

An occasional hot flash may be easy to ignore, but some women find them acutely uncomfortable and embarrassing. We cannot know in advance what our own pattern will be. Hot flashes may begin twelve to eighteen months or more before menstrual signs of menopause and can continue for some years after periods end. They may occur even around your period or after childbirth. Forty-five percent of women still have them five to ten years after periods stop, and a few of us have them into our seventies.

One fifty-two-year-old woman describes her hot flashes:

It's not like I'm feeling "a little warm"—it's like I'm on fire, and I don't care if anybody else is around, I still want to strip off all my clothes to get cooler.

You may feel warmer at night before other changes begin. True hot flashes sometimes cause enough perspiration to soak nightclothes and sheets (night sweats), and they can disturb sleep.

Heavier women's hot flashes tend to be more frequent and severe than thinner women's, because the increased energy load creates more body heat, canceling out the effect of slightly higher estrogen levels in fatty tissue.

If hot flashes are bothering you, you can adopt various strategies to reduce discomfort.

- Dress in layers so you can shed or add clothes according to how you are feeling.
- Avoid spicy foods, hot drinks, alcohol, and caffeine, all of which can set off hot flashes. Identify your own triggers and avoid them.
- Carry cool water with you and drink it regularly. Keep your environment cool with fans or air-conditioning.
- Avoid stress as much as possible.
- Exercise regularly (it can help reduce hot flashes).
- Try paced deep breathing when a flash starts (which may make it less severe).
- Try to maintain a healthy body weight for your age and height. Heavy women tend to feel warmer faster.

- One woman put a cold pack under her pillow at night so when she woke up at night with a hot flash she could turn her pillow over and it was nice and cool.
- *Alternative remedies.* Sometimes health care providers suggest nutritional supplements (such as soy products), botanicals (such as red clover), antioxidant vitamins (such as vitamin E), and herbal preparations (such as black cohosh and St. John's wort), and many women use them. They've been found safe for short-term use (six months). Some of the remedies seem to help, but the studies have often been contradictory, and all show a placebo effect (as many as 30 percent or more of women feel better even on dummy pills), making firm conclusions impossible (for more on herbal remedies, see Chapter 5, "Complementary Health Practices").[3] Studies funded by the U.S. National Center for Complementary and Alternative Medicine are expected to report results in 2005.
- *Hormones.* Some of us have such severe and persistent hot flashes that we consider hormone therapy to make up for the loss of natural estrogen. Taking hormones has been shown to relieve hot flashes and some other menopausal symptoms, but it may also increase the risk for certain medical problems, especially over time (see "Hormone Therapy," p. 538).

SLEEP DISTURBANCES

Sleep disturbances in midlife may or may not be caused by menopause. The connection between hormonal changes and sleep mechanisms isn't clear, though researchers are investigating it. Aging itself may trigger sleep problems, although some women have sleep disturbances during the perimenopausal stage, but not before or afterward. Most commonly, a woman will fall asleep without a problem, then wake up in the early-morning hours and have difficulty getting back to sleep. Women who experience hot flashes or night sweats tend to have insomnia more often than those who don't. Sleeplessness can cause fatigue, irritability, and a feeling of being unable to cope.

Some women may find medication (sleeping pills, antidepressants, or hormone therapy) helpful. Whether you take anything or not, you may want to try these lifestyle changes:

- Cut out caffeinated beverages (coffee, tea, colas, and chocolate), especially after about three P.M., as caffeine stays in the bloodstream for up to six hours. Caffeine is a stimulant that interferes with sleep and increases the amount of urine in the bladder, which means you have to pee more often.
- Avoid smoking, especially in the evening. Tobacco is a stimulant.
- Avoid or limit alcohol. It becomes a stimulant as it is metabolized, resulting in fragmented sleep patterns and the need to urinate during the night.
- Go to sleep at about the same time every night.
- Exercise regularly. Exercising during the day or early evening can relieve tension and help promote sleep (see p. 545 for additional benefits).
- Take a hot bath, listen to music, or read.
- Filter out noise. Close doors and windows, use earplugs, or use a soothing sound machine.

If sleep disturbances persist, you may want to discuss medical relief with your health care provider. Low-dose antidepressants can relieve insomnia and hot flashes, as well as depression, for some women. Many people use melatonin to improve sleep, though it works best for jet lag, and not much data exist on its regular use. Valerian has long been used as an herbal sleep remedy. Sleeping pills can be habit-forming, so read their accompanying information sheet carefully and use them occasionally, not regularly.

VAGINAL CHANGES

As estrogen levels decline, vaginal walls frequently become thinner, drier and less flexible, and more prone to tears and cracks. Less vaginal lubrication is produced, and it also takes longer to become moist during lovemaking. Penetration may become less comfortable or even painful, and it sometimes leads to irritation and increased susceptibility to infection. If tissues become very delicate, vaginal wall bleeding may result from penetration. Women with what many doctors call *vaginal atrophy* may end up avoiding intercourse or other activities because of the discomfort. One fifty-six-year-old woman says:

Forget intercourse! After menopause, I couldn't even ride my bicycle anymore—my vagina always felt sore.

Some prescription and over-the-counter drugs may cause or contribute to dryness. Antihistamines, for example, dry vaginal tissues as well as nasal tissues. Douches, sprays, and colored or perfumed toilet paper and soaps can irritate vulvar tissues.

Ways to relieve vaginal dryness include:

- *Lubricants and vaginal moisturizers,* such as Silk-E, Albolene, or Astroglide, may be helpful at the time of lovemaking. Avoid scratching, which can irritate delicate tissues and lead to infections and further problems. Applying vitamin E oil or prescription ointments to the and pubic and vaginal area can relieve itching. Itching can be a sign of a yeast infection that needs treatment (see p. 653). If dryness persists, try an over-the-counter moisturizer, such as Replens, which may be used one or more times a week but *not* at the time of penetration. Remember that these products are not contraceptives, and they don't protect against sexually transmitted infections or HIV/AIDS.

- *Regular sexual activity* also helps maintain vaginal health, although it may take you much longer to become lubricated.
- *Drinking more liquids* each day (eight or more cups, according to most sources) may also help.
- *Low-dose local estrogens* such as Estring, Estrace, Vagifem, and Premarin cream prevent dryness. In these forms (silastic ring, vaginal tablets, vaginal creams), less estrogen gets into the bloodstream, which may limit the long-term risks. The ring delivers a minuscule amount of estrogen to the bloodstream, the tablets send a little more, and the cream can send a larger and somewhat unpredictable amount, depending how much and often it is used. Many women take hormones because of vaginal changes that disturb our sexuality or lifestyle (see "Hormone Therapy," p. 538).

Vaginal dryness at any age may simply mean that you are not ready for penetration. The slower arousal time of older people has compensations.

When Jay used to lose his erection, I would think that I had failed as a woman because I couldn't keep him aroused. But now I see that it can mean more time to play around and a chance to start over again so that lovemaking lasts longer.

URINARY CHANGES

Some midlife women leak urine involuntarily when straining, lifting, or laughing. Others complain of having to pee more often and needing to get up a few times during the night. Others feel an urgent need to empty a full bladder but can't make it to the toilet without leaking. When the inability to control leakage becomes problematic, it is called *urinary incontinence* (UI).

Urinary incontinence is more common at older ages, but it is not part of normal aging. Some sources say lower estrogen levels are a cause of UI, but studies are contradictory. Some medications and caffeinated beverages can make you pee more often. Mobility problems can be a factor, too, when you can't run to a toilet on your own.

Several types of UI can occur together. The most common type is *stress incontinence,* which occurs when you cough, sneeze, laugh, or exert yourself during strenuous activity. *Urge incontinence* is an involuntary flow after a sudden strong urge to urinate. These types of incontinence, as well as having to pee frequently, may be symptoms of a reversible urinary tract infection.

Declining estrogen levels can also result in thinning of urinary tract tissues and a weakening of the bladder and urethra (the tube from the bladder to the outside), increasing susceptibility to urinary infections. If you or someone you care for is having urinary problems, make sure to check for an underlying infection (see "Urinary Tract Infections," p. 692).

Incontinence can be successfully managed, treated, and sometimes even cured. Besides wearing panty liners, you can try these self-help and medical approaches:

- *Kegel exercises.* At all ages, strengthening the muscles of the pelvic floor will help control urine leaks. If you have never done Kegel (perineal) exercises, this is a good time to start and keep doing them (for details, see p. 235 in Chapter 13, "Sexual Anatomy, Reproduction, and the Menstrual Cycle").
- *Bladder training,* teaching yourself to go longer and longer without urinating, can also be very helpful. Sit on the toilet every two

hours, whether you have to go or not. Then, every two days, extend the interval by thirty minutes until you're doing it every four hours. Try to maintain the schedule whether or not you have an accident. If you have an urge to urinate, stay still and use the muscle-strengthening exercises until the urge passes, then move slowly to the bathroom. Sometimes it helps to relax the body rather than tense up all over in an attempt to hold the urine back. Avoid drinking a lot of fluid before you go out or while you're away from home, and catch up with liquids when you return home.

- *Medications* are available to help decrease bladder contractions (hyperactive bladder) that produce leaking. Some are relatively new, and they may not help your particular urinary problem, so it's a good idea to get more information before deciding to take them. Studies don't agree on whether estrogen reduces incontinence or makes it worse. Certain medications (Detrol and Ditropan) may impact memory and other central nervous system functions.

Other Treatments

If leaking is caused by an anatomic problem (see "Pelvic Relaxation and Uterine Prolapse," p. 649), a *pessary* (which resembles a diaphragm) can be inserted into the vagina to help keep the bladder and urethra in the correct positions and prevent leakage. One of several types of surgery might correct the defect, but if you are thinking about this, be sure you have a thorough discussion of the risks and benefits with an experienced gynecologic surgeon or specialist in female urology. Ask about the success rate, and whether you might need to repeat the procedure if it doesn't work.

Finding help can be challenging, because female reproduction and urology are separate medical specialties. Most urologists know little more than the basics about female reproductive organs, while not all doctors in either specialty know much about treating middle-aged and older women. Try to find a surgeon who specializes in female urinary problems (this new medical specialty is called *urogynecology*; see "Resources"). As with any recommendation for major surgery, understand what is proposed and get another opinion before agreeing to any procedures.

SEXUAL DESIRE

Menopause does not necessarily change sexuality, but as women age, both sexual desire and response may be affected by menopause-related problems such as heavy, unpredictable periods or urinary leaking; other health problems such as high blood pressure or diabetes; or life changes such as the death of a partner or a partner who is no longer interested in or able to engage in lovemaking. Address the specific health problem instead of blaming menopause. For example, if you or your partner take medication that seems to be reducing sexual desire, discuss your concerns with your health care provider. Often substituting a different drug will help. If sex is uncomfortable, have this evaluated.

Many women do experience a decline in sexual interest as a result of lower hormone levels. (This also happens when the ovaries are removed during a hysterectomy or damaged by chemotherapy or radiation.) Feeling less desire may be a welcome change for some of us, but it may be unwelcome for others or for our sexual partners. Lovemaking can sometimes be much more enjoyable in the postmenopausal years: no more periods or PMS symptoms, no fear of pregnancy, more privacy if our kids are grown and gone, and more spontaneity. Often how we feel about sex after menopause is no different from how we felt about sex before menopause (see "Sexuality and Aging," p. 541, and "Hysterectomy and Oophorectomy," p. 637).

MEMORY AND MOOD

Many women report memory gaps or lowered ability to concentrate around menopause, but no clear scientific evidence shows these changes to be related to lower estrogen levels. Occasional forgetfulness—those "senior moments" so many of us talk about—may reflect general stress, specific worries, depression, not having paid attention to the details, or being distracted by things like a phone ringing, a child yelling, or a dog barking. A fifty-two-year-old says:

With all the changes that are going on in my body, no wonder I can't remember other things! And no wonder I sometimes get a bit weepy—a whole part of my life is behind me now. Luckily, these feeling don't last long. I've heard that post-menopause is a breeze after perimenopause.

In fact, the brain's capacity to reorganize its cells and grow connections continues throughout life. Brain exercise such as reading, social activity, or stimulating conversation can improve memory.

If you consistently can't remember things you did five minutes earlier, forget the names of people or objects, or struggle with routine tasks or simple decisions, a careful medical evaluation might show whether it's just "brain overload" or an early symptom of a more serious condition. (To find out more, see "Memory Changes," p. 565.)

Depression

Some women report feeling depressed during perimenopause. Research shows that menopause does not cause depression, though it may

ARE YOU BEING ABUSED?

Abuse may be a factor in depression. According to the Women's Health Initiative (WHI), in a study of nearly 92,000 women ages 50 to 79, 11 percent suffered some form of physical or verbal abuse; 89 percent had been subjected to put-downs, severe criticism, and threats.[4] Women in their fifties were more likely to report abuse than older women. Black women were three times more likely to have been physically abused, but white women reported more verbal abuse. If you are being abused in any way, mention it to supportive friends, appropriate services, and your health care provider. (For more information, see Chapter 8, "Violence and Abuse.")

produce some mild and transient negative mood changes. Nonetheless, the transition can trigger severe emotional problems, especially if you struggle greatly with menopausal symptoms or have a prior history of depression (including postpartum depression) or severe PMS. Even if you've never needed counseling or medication, you may want to consider getting help if depression is disrupting your life. (For more information, see Chapter 6, "Emotional Well-Being.")

ABNORMAL BLEEDING

Some women bleed in a way that feels like one continuous period, so heavy that even "super" tampons or pads cannot contain it. Very heavy bleeding (sometimes called *hypermenorrhea, menorrhagia,* or *flooding*) is often just an annoying part of perimenopausal change. If you are bleeding heavily, you might be anemic or actually feel faint. Heavy bleeding may also be a sign of disease.

The hormonal ups and downs of peri-menopause may be the cause of almost any imaginable bleeding pattern. Relatively common causes of heavy bleeding are fibroids (noncancerous growths in the inner muscle wall of the uterus) or polyps (small noncancerous tissue growths that can occur in the lining of the uterus). However, unusual bleeding can be the only outward symptom of uterine cancer, which is uncommon but can be life-threatening if it is not found and treated early. Don't ignore heavy or prolonged bleeding—see your health care provider if it persists.

Health care providers may recommend a procedure such as an endometrial biopsy (done in the office with a thin plastic tube), a hysteroscopy (an exam with an optical device placed into the uterus from the vagina), a sono-hysterogram (a specialized ultrasound putting salt water into the uterus through the cervix to enhance the image), or even a D&C (dilation and curettage: surgical scraping of the uterine lining) to examine the uterine lining or contents and find out what's causing the bleeding. Physicians perform D&Cs less often now, since they are done "blind" and often require general anesthesia, which is expensive and risky. Some doctors push hysterectomy as a solution, but less invasive treatment options are often available. (For more about fibroids, abnormal bleeding, and hysterectomies, see Chapter 28, "Unique to Women.")

HORMONE THERAPY

Since the 1960s, hormone replacement therapy (HRT—now called hormone therapy, or HT) has been marketed and prescribed for two purposes: short-term relief from severe menopausal discomforts, and long-term prevention of conditions that can come with aging. Estrogen in pill, patch, ring, or cream form supplements the declining levels of estrogen made by the ovaries. Sometimes a progestin (natural or synthetic) is added to the mix to prevent growth of the uterine lining that may lead to endometrial cancer (unnecessary, of course, after hysterectomy). While numerous studies have shown that combined HT (the combination of estrogen and progestin) reduces hot flashes, vaginal dryness, and the gradual thinning of bones, many of its supposed long-term benefits have been either disproved or seriously questioned.

For decades, drug companies marketed hormones as a magic pill for maintaining youthfulness and preventing heart disease, despite conflicting reports about their long-term benefits and studies showing that prolonged exposure to estrogen increases the risk of breast cancer and blood clots. Recently, large-scale studies have shown that the long-term risks may outweigh the benefits. The Women's Health Initiative, with randomized trials of a popular combination of estrogen and progestin called Prempro, confirmed the risk for breast cancer and blood clots. The risk for cardiovascular disease and stroke was actually found to be higher for women taking combined hormones.[5] The risk of stroke was also higher for women taking estrogen alone.[6] When the first results of the WHI study came out in 2002, many women felt outraged at having been misled about both the benefits and the risks of these drugs—especially those of us who had been taking HT, sometimes for years.

The WHI was a very large and well-designed study, but it tested only one regimen of hormone therapy. (The dose and combination of hormones selected for the trial were the ones that the vast majority of U.S. women using hormone therapy had taken for years.) As a result, the trial findings did not answer all questions about the safety and effectiveness of hormone therapies. A third of the women in the WHI were in their fifties, making this the largest randomized controlled trial ever done of women in this age group. Although the majority of the participants were even older, it would be misleading to suggest that the trial's results apply only to older women. Future research may identify safer or more effective regimens than the one tested in the WHI, but for now, women should be cautious and even skeptical about unproved claims and theories on these drugs.

Another consideration is the type of estrogen used and ways in which it is delivered to the body. The human body makes three kinds of estrogen: *estrone, estradiol,* and *estriol.* Some hormone formulations (sometimes called *bio-identical,* because they resemble the body's own hormones more closely) or ways of taking hormones (patch, cream, ring) may be safer than the pill form, but that hasn't been proved. Pills in which some estrogen comes from mares' urine are commonly used in the United States. It is not yet known whether all the higher risks resulting from HRT are caused by estrogens, progestins, or both, or by how they are metabolized (they pass through the liver when taken in pill form). With each new study, our understanding of the balance between risks and benefits shifts, and there are still lots of unknowns. Conclusions from studies must be considered and applied individually for each woman.

Decades of drug company ads and promotions have influenced both women and health care providers. Though promotion of HT has decreased since the release of the WHI results, theories about unproved benefits persist, and many health care providers continue to downplay the risks. On a case-by-case basis, some women—particularly those with severe hot flashes—may still benefit from hormones.

The hormone controversy also raises an important bioethical issue. Many of us believe that the standards for using unproved treatments on healthy populations should be more stringent than those for treating people who are ill and choose to risk something new as a possible cure. Menopausal women are healthy. Medication may result in unanticipated dangers, as shown by the new findings about hormone treatment.

OTHER MEDICAL OPTIONS

Given the concerns about the health risks of hormone treatment, researchers are trying to develop new drugs that can provide the benefits of hormones without the negative effects. *Selective estrogen receptor modulators* (SERMs), such as raloxifene, can prevent bone loss and reduce the risk of bone fracture without stimulating either breast or uterine tissue to become cancerous. However, raloxifene does not reduce hot flashes, and it may even increase them; also, it has not yet been shown to prevent hip fracture.[7] *Bisphosphonates* (such as Fosamax) are another class of drug proved to reduce bone thinning and the risk of fracture. They do not affect hot flashes. Both bisphosphonates and SERMs seem to have fewer risks than hormones, but they are newer drugs, and their effectiveness and safety for healthy women have been studied only up to ten years.[8]

Since the risk of debilitating fractures becomes significant after age seventy, women who start taking these drugs at menopause will probably have to take them for decades for the benefit to become apparent. (For more about bones, see "Osteoporosis," p. 566.) A steroid called tibolone is widely used in European countries for hot flashes, night sweats, and improving bone density, but its effect on cardiovascular risk is uncertain; it is currently being tested in the United States, and the FDA may approve it by 2006. Some antidepressants appear to improve both mood and hot flashes in some women. The connection in the body between hormone levels and neurotransmitters—where antidepressants work—is not fully understood.

IS MENOPAUSE REALLY A MEDICAL ISSUE?

When health care providers see the normal changes of menopause as a deficiency state or a disease requiring medication, they may either overtreat or undertreat women. Some doctors attribute almost every symptom to menopause, rather than investigating symptoms that may point to other serious conditions. Some women hope a pill will keep us young, yet a healthy lifestyle and self-care are safer and probably more effective. We can learn from one another how to manage the typical discomforts that occur.

After ending hormone therapy, some women experience a return of hot flashes and other menopausal signs, and decide to go back to hormones. Others, out of safety concerns, try antidepressants such as Effexor instead. While antidepressants seem to reduce hot flashes, there is no evidence that using them for months or years is safer than hormone therapy.

Alternative therapies may help with the transition: vitamins, especially antioxidants such as vitamin E; herbs or botanicals, such as black cohosh; or food supplements, such as soy products. Often these products are touted as a "natural" way to cope with menopausal discomforts, yet studies are contradictory about their value. These remedies may not be produced in consistent strengths or doses, and they may not even be safe for everyone. The only thing researchers agree on is that soy in food has estrogenic effects. Some oncologists have concerns about soy for breast cancer survivors.

It's your decision whether to take hormones or not. Consider your own history, values, health status, and preferences, as well as what's known and not known about risks and benefits. Keep the risks in perspective. For most women, smoking, poor diet, and lack of exercise are bigger risk factors for breast cancer and heart disease than any form of hormone therapy.

If you choose hormones, discuss with your health care provider which brands and forms are most effective at the lowest possible dose and for the shortest period of time necessary. If you already have a history of heart disease or breast cancer, you will probably be advised against taking HT. If you decide to stop taking hormones, tapering off slowly may minimize the return of discomforts.

We must all must work together to find satisfactory and safe solutions for problematic menopausal signs. We also need to educate ourselves. You can keep up with new research findings through the National Women's Health Network and other women's health organizations (see "Resources").

HORMONES AND BONE DENSITY

Hormone treatments—both estrogen alone and estrogen/progestin combinations—have been shown to reduce the risk of osteoporosis and bone fracture in women. But because of the proven risks of taking hormones, the U.S. Food and Drug Administration now cautions women and health care providers that only women at significant risk of osteoporosis should consider taking hormones to prevent it.[9] Other medications are available (see "Osteoporosis," p. 564).

Even if you are in a high-risk category, you can do nonmedical things to reduce risk. Regular weight-bearing exercise, such as walking, running, or dancing, is crucial to the development and preservation of bone density.[10] Exercise also builds muscle mass and improves balance, thus helping to prevent falls and fractures. Quitting smoking; increasing your intake of calcium, vitamin D, and other nutrients; and eliminating excessive use of alcohol help maintain overall good health.

HORMONES AND MOOD

Though the ad campaigns of drug companies have touted—and individuals have reported—the positive effects of hormone treatment on mood, the Women's Health Initiative data showed that hormones had no clinically meaningful effect on vitality, mental health, or depressive symptoms. The only exception was among women ages 50 to 54 who were experiencing moderate to severe hot flashes. Women in that group got relief from hot flashes and insomnia, but reported no improvement in any of the other outcomes.[11]

HORMONES AND EYES

Dry eye syndrome, in which the eye doesn't produce enough tears for proper lubrication, may be experienced as a burning sensation or a feeling of grittiness or dryness in the eyes. It affects more than 3.2 million women in the United States aged fifty and older, but it is not a normal result of aging. It increases the risk for eye infections. Taking hormones after menopause is linked to dry eye, so avoiding them may prevent it. Consult an ophthalmologist if you think you have this problem. Common over-the-counter remedies include flaxseed oil (to be taken by mouth) and "artificial tears." Avoid fans and being in dry (air-conditioned or heated) air. There are sunglasses and regular glasses with protective sides and tops that limit air exposure to eyes. If you have dry eyes, get checked for Sjögren's syndrome (see p. 664).

FINDING THE RIGHT HEALTH CARE PROVIDER

One of the most important things you can do to improve your health care is to establish a relationship with a practitioner whose philosophy resembles yours, and who is knowledgeable, open-minded, and up-to-date. If possible, do so *before* menopause. A supportive provider can be a good source of information and encouragement. Women's physical needs in menopause are as varied and unique as our personalities. You need a provider who will listen to what you know and feel, and who will take the time to answer questions completely and without prejudice. If your current practitioner won't do that, ask friends, coworkers and other health care providers to recommend someone else. If you can't change, at least speak up, ask questions, and insist on participating fully in decisions concerning care. Sometimes the physician assistant or nurse has more time to answer questions. Also remember that the understanding of menopause—and human health in general—is a work in progress, and any decision on your health should be reevaluated regularly.

SEXUALITY AND AGING

Sexuality, unlike fertility, continues throughout our lives. It is a myth that sexual desire and activity have to fade as a natural, irreversible part of aging. While we do have to accommodate the changes in our bodies, sexual feelings often depend more on how we feel about our bodies and our relationships as we age.

I'm no longer worried about pregnancy; the children are gone; my energy is released. I have a new surge of interest in sex. But at the same time, the culture is saying, "You are not attractive as a woman; act your age; be dignified," which means, to me, be dead sexually. It's a terrible bind for a middle-aged woman. I say, acknowledge, applaud, and enjoy sexuality! Change the image of women to include middle-aged beauty and sexuality!

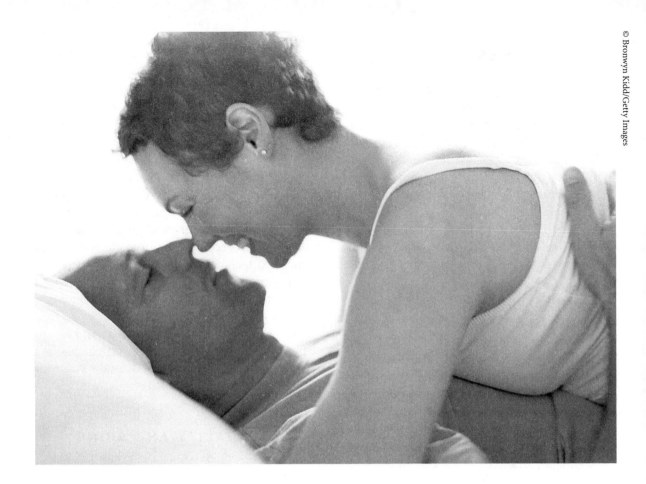

Some women enjoy lovemaking more, since it can deepen after many years of a committed intimate relationship. Others are less interested. Partners might lose interest, too, having slower arousal times or less frequent ejaculations. Adjustments, disruptions, or feeling less sexual can also result from chronic or acute illness or surgery. It can take a while to adjust to new circumstances and resume a pleasurable sex life.

If you are separated, divorced, or widowed and dating again for the first time, you might feel a bit awkward, unsure of what to expect. It may be hard to find a suitable partner. Straight women contend with a double whammy: With each decade of age, there are fewer men in our age range, and those men often prefer to date younger women. Some women have relationships with younger men.

We have to send out signals if a sexual relationship is what we want. . . . What really bothers me is my vanity—exposing a middle-aged body to a beautiful younger man.

The joy of making love with a young man who is so full of energy and straightforward is wonderful.

Some midlife or older women have sexual relationships with women for the first time. Others have been lesbian or bisexual for many years, some more or less openly, and others in secret (see Chapter 11, "Relationships with Women").

Now in my 50s, I am 18 years into what I hope will be a lifelong relationship with a woman. Sex for us is a steady friend. During our busy work-week, we cuddle, and that's good. On weekends and on vacations, we make time for lovemaking and cherish how it reconnects and refreshes us.

Many single women miss not just sex but touching and the excitement of romance, and express sexual feelings through masturbation and fantasy. Some women don't want sex at all. One seventy-three-year-old woman says,

I frankly don't need it, and I don't miss it at all. I had a very, very full sex life, and I was mad about my husband, which is a nice way to be. When he died, it was a real shock. I haven't discovered another person that I had that desire for in 25 years now. I'm used to my life the way it is now, and I don't think that my life is incomplete.

BIRTH CONTROL AND SAFER SEX AT MIDLIFE

If you are sexually involved with men, you can still get pregnant until your periods have stopped completely. If you do not want a child, keep using some form of birth control until your periods have ceased for two whole years, because you won't know until the second year whether you really have stopped.

If you are sexually active and are not in a mutually monogamous relationship with a partner who is free of sexually transmitted infections (STIs), you are at risk for getting an STI, including the HIV infection that causes AIDS. Many women don't think about this after menopause, but the problem is becoming more common as more of us explore our sexuality in later years. Thinning and/or dryness of the vaginal lining may result in small tears through which infection becomes possible. Practicing safer sex—that is, using condoms or latex dams for protection—

can reduce the risk of STIs. (For information on how to protect yourself, see Chapter 14, "Safer Sex.")

"SEXUAL DYSFUNCTION" IN WOMEN: MYTH OR FACT?

If you mention to your health care provider that you are experiencing sexual dissatisfaction, you may be offered medical treatment. Researchers are claiming that lowered sexual function is a medical condition in women as well as in men, and are testing possible treatments for women who complain of sexual problems. This approach seems to assume that women's sexual

HOW DRUGS AND DISEASE AFFECT SEX

Some drugs—such as Prozac and related antidepressants—depress sexual function or interest. Medication for high blood pressure can prevent erections, as can too much alcohol. (The depressive effect of alcohol becomes more pronounced as people get older.) Fear often interferes with sex after a heart attack or a diagnosis of heart disease, but most women find that after an initial recovery period, sex is as enjoyable as ever. Ask your health care practitioner and pharmacist about the effects on sexual interest, arousal, or functioning of any medications that are prescribed for you or your partner; look them up in the *Physicians' Desk Reference* or on MedlinePlus (http://medlineplus .gov). (For the "Sex and Disability" table showing effects of some conditions, see p. 218 in Chapter 12, "Sexuality.") If your clinician cannot answer your questions about sexuality, ask to be referred to someone who can.

physiology and attitudes resemble those of men. Pharmaceutical companies support some of these studies, in the hope of expanding the market for drugs already approved for erectile dysfunction (difficulty having and maintaining erections) or loss of libido (sexual desire) in men. Midlife and older women troubled by vaginal dryness or changes, lack of desire, or problems with arousal are among the targeted customers for these drugs.

Sildenafil (Viagra) and Similar Drugs

In 2004 the manufacturer of a much publicized program of clinical trials of Viagra for women stopped the program when researchers found what we have long known from experience: Desire and arousal are two different things. The drug, which improves blood flow to the genitals, increased the outward signs of arousal in some women, but those changes had little effect on women's desire to have sex. Viagra may help some women whose desire suddenly drops as a result of taking antidepressants, but it doesn't do much for the rest of us.

Estrogen

Hormone levels may affect women's sexual experiences. Many women find that taking hormones after menopause maintains lubrication and reduces pain associated with a dry vagina, making sex more pleasurable. Also, getting rid of hot flashes and insomnia may improve your sex life. Still, the effect of estrogen on desire independent of these factors is uncertain.

Testosterone

Testosterone may be prescribed for women on hormone therapy who have a decreased interest in sex. This hormone is called an *androgen* be-cause it occurs in higher levels in men. It contributes to muscle strength, appetite, a sense of well-being, and sex drive. It has been found to increase libido in women whose ovaries have been removed, but the effect on women going through natural menopause is still being studied. In studies with older men, exercise was more effective in improving sexual arousal.

Testosterone also has other effects: acne; increase in facial hair and clitoral size; permanently lowered voice; and decrease in bone density. Some women use low-dose testosterone cream or gel directly on the clitoris, to reduce the amount that gets into the body and thus limit side effects. However, even in low doses, these products have not been adequately tested for safety or effectiveness in women, even for short-term use.

(For more information, see "A New View of Women's Sexuality" [W58] on the companion website, www.ourbodiesourselves.org.)

CHANGING ATTITUDES AND COMMUNICATION

Our need for love and sex does not diminish with age. Yet we may have to overcome years of conditioning to initiate sex or consider alternatives to our customary patterns.

My libido was down, as was Tom's. We were having less frequent sex and I was waiting for him to take the initiative. Finally, I said to myself, "I can do something about this, I am a sexual being"— and I began to initiate sex and we had a great time.

It is possible to change old patterns, assumptions, misunderstandings, and miscommunications by talking and exploring together. We can have sex throughout our lifetime.

Do whatever pleases you both, even if it seems unusual or strange at first. If your partner is a man, forget about performance—getting erections, lasting longer, or being the "best lover"—and simply focus on enjoying each other. Genital sex is not all there is. Touching, kissing and caressing all over, mutual masturbation, and oral sex can give both women and men pleasure and satisfaction.

Talking frankly may be difficult at first. It requires practice, especially with a new partner. Consider getting some help together—or alone, if your partner is unwilling to go for counseling. A licensed sex therapist or counselor specializing in sexual issues probably knows more than a medical practitioner and can give useful advice.

We can also explore our sexuality without a partner, discovering what turns us on by stimulating ourselves.

(For more information, see "Sexual Issues in Menopause" [W59] on the companion website, www.ourbodiesourselves.org. For more about various aspects of sexual desire, pleasure, and satisfaction, also see Chapter 12, "Sexuality," and "Resources.")

TAKING CARE OF OURSELVES: PREVENTIVE HEALTH

Many of the changes of aging, once thought biologically inevitable, are preventable and sometimes even reversible. You can take active steps to maintain good health and lessen the impact of illnesses or chronic conditions. Acquiring healthy habits—quitting smoking; exercising more; eating healthfully; and reducing dependence on caffeine, sugar, alcohol, and tranquilizers—will help us all achieve the highest possible quality of life as long as we live.

ACTIVITY AND MOVEMENT

Physical activity becomes increasingly important in midlife. Without exercise, we lose muscle mass. The ratio of body fat to muscle mass increases as we grow older. Women typically begin to lose bone mass in our thirties, often because of physical inactivity and sedentary jobs. Happily, an increasing number of women of every age have rejected this norm and are on the move!

A woman in her fifties says:

I took up tae kwon do, Eastern self-defense, which appealed to me as a Japanese-American. To my amazement, after a few months of kicking and hitting an imaginary opponent, my chronic insomnia and stiff neck disappeared. Gone also were the painful attacks of gastritis. I began feeling more energetic. . . . That was more than five years ago. Today, all the ailments that I thought I would have to live with the rest of my life are gone.

Aerobic exercise—such as walking, jogging, and dancing—makes your heart work harder and strengthens muscles and ligaments supporting the skeleton. Weight-bearing exercise builds bone. Strength training—such as swimming, lifting small weights, and doing push-ups or other arm exercises—helps maintain muscle strength and improves balance. Yoga promotes flexibility and balance. There's exercise to fit almost any kind of physical limitation, including isometric muscle toning and "chair yoga" if you are not mobile. It's important to exercise the whole body, so as to keep strength up everywhere.

Exercise can lower blood pressure and reduce the risks of heart attack and stroke, arthritis, emphysema, and osteoporosis. It is central in maintaining a healthy weight. It can help improve sleep and bowel functioning, maintain strength and good posture, and relieve depression and hot flashes; and it generally makes most people feel better. In one study, women who engaged in moderate or heavy physical activity had more "good cholesterol" (high-density lipoprotein, or HDL) and less of a blood-clotting factor.[12] After exercise, blood rushes to the skin, bringing with it extra nutrients, raising skin temperature, and increasing the collagen content. Skin actually thickens, becoming more elastic and less wrinkled.

(For more information and some tips to help you keep moving even if you don't like exercise, see Chapter 4, "Our Bodies in Motion.")

BONE LOSS AND OSTEOPOROSIS

Bone, like all the other living tissues in our bodies, is constantly replacing itself throughout life. If we are physically active and eat a healthy diet with adequate calcium during our youth, we build bone when it matters most and give ourselves a lifelong advantage. Some bone loss is normal in women and men as the years go by. By the middle thirties, we start to lose bone more quickly than we replace it. Most women lose bone even faster during the first years after menopause. Another period of increased bone loss occurs in our seventies.

Not all bone loss is *osteoporosis,* a condition of extreme bone loss leading to fractures. Only 15 percent of women who are now fifty and who live to be very old will have osteoporosis, and many of us who develop osteoporosis will never know about it unless we break a bone. Publicity campaigns by drug companies give the impression that *all* women will get osteoporosis unless we take medication (although the ads mostly target middle-class women assumed to have money for these products). It is more important to prevent fractures than to prevent osteoporosis. In fact, most fractures are preventable with commonsense safety measures. (For more information, see "Bones, Falls, and Fractures," p. 564 and see "Prevention and Treatment of Osteoporosis in Women" [W60] on the companion website, www.ourbodiesourselves.org.)

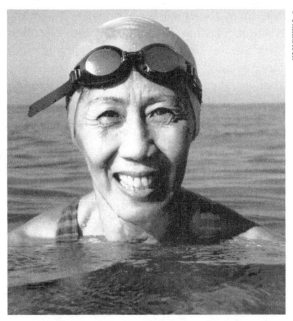

Do We Need Bone Density Tests?

Routine X rays (including of the teeth and jawbone) cannot clearly show signs of osteoporosis until 30 to 40 percent of bone is lost, but they may show reduced bone mass caused by other conditions. Bone testing is useful primarily for those at high risk, and even then it might not improve outcomes. Early detection is meaningless unless women learn how to reduce bone loss and make necessary changes in eating habits, exercise, and lifestyle patterns. Since these changes can benefit all women, we should be doing them anyway. Thus, the tests are unnecessary for many of us.

If you or your health care provider suspects early osteoporosis, you can have your bone mineral density measured by dual-energy X-ray absorptiometry (DXA). Following this test, some of us are told we have *osteopenia,* bone loss that is usual with aging and *could* lead to osteoporosis but presents no immediate danger. This diagnosis is controversial among medical practitioners, and the suggested treatments—hormone therapy or bisphosphonates (Fosamax, Actonel)—carry risks, some known and some unknown.

Prevention

It is never too late to begin strengthening your bones. Eat well, including adequate amounts of calcium; do weight-bearing exercise to build and maintain adequate bone, muscle mass, and balance; and avoid harmful habits such as smoking. You can also prevent early osteoporosis by avoiding, when possible, medical interventions that contribute to bone thinning, such as hysterectomy and/or oophorectomy (removal of the ovaries). Many women also try calcium, vitamin C, and vitamin D supplements; yoga, walking and weight training; special back exercise regimens; and physical therapy. Exercising in water offers beneficial resistance to movement while placing less stress on joints, but swimming itself is not weight-bearing, so it does not build bone strength.

EATING WELL

Although the same basic principles of healthy eating apply throughout life, nutritional requirements change somewhat with age. Good nutrition is essential to health, independence, and quality of life for women at midlife and older, and it is one of the major elements in successful aging. Eating well can also help prevent or manage chronic diseases and their complications, such as diabetes, heart disease, stroke, osteoporosis, and cancer.

Tastes can change as we get older. It may become more difficult to prepare healthy foods from scratch. Instead of buying processed, packaged food that may have too much fat, salt, and sugar in it, try cooking a larger quantity at once and freezing portions to heat up later. (For all but the following few items of special interest to midlife and older women, see Chapter 2, "Eating Well.")

CALCIUM, VITAMIN D, AND MAGNESIUM: A BALANCE OF NUTRIENTS

Calcium

This essential nutrient prevents bone loss, which can lead to osteoporosis. Since women over thirty-five absorb calcium less easily, it is important to exercise more (necessary to absorb calcium) and get enough calcium in your diet, along with other nutrients that help your body absorb calcium. If you can't tolerate milk products (lactose intolerance), don't worry; many other sources of calcium are available. Interestingly, long-term studies consistently show *no* reduction in fractures for people with high dairy product consumption. You can use calcium sup-

COMPARING CALCIUM SUPPLEMENTS			
COMPOUND	HOW MUCH CALCIUM	FORM	EFFECT ON DIGESTION
Calcium carbonate	40 percent calcium	Tablets	May upset stomach
Calcium citrate	21 percent calcium	Tablets	May be easier to digest
Calcium phosphate	39 percent calcium	Added to orange juice and soy milk	Easily absorbed without upsetting digestion

plements to fulfill the daily recommendation of 1,200 to 1,500 milligrams (use the lower figure if you are taking hormones). Calcium supplements come in various forms. Most experts do not recommend special magnesium supplementation.

Vitamin D

You need 400 to 800 IU a day for optimal calcium and phosphorus absorption. The main sources of vitamin D are sunshine, fish, fortified milk, and cereal. Yogurt and cheese, while good sources of calcium, contain no vitamin D. If you live in a northern climate, you may want to take a vitamin D supplement or a combination calcium/vitamin D pill during the winter months. When outdoors, be sure to take precautions for preventing skin cancer, such as walking in the early morning, staying out of the midday sun, and using sunscreen.

Magnesium

Calcium should be balanced with magnesium in a two-to-one ratio. If your magnesium level drops lower, calcium will be lost. Fruits and vegetables contain magnesium. Some calcium supplements also include magnesium.

VISION CHANGES

Eyes have less elasticity by midlife. It becomes easier to see better at a distance, and you may have to take off your glasses for close work, or you might need different glasses altogether.

I knew I needed bifocals when I was trying to sing a hymn one Sunday and couldn't read the music. Now I can guess age by how far away from your face you hold the page!

Glaucoma, a chronic eye disease, usually appears at midlife or later and affects women more than men. It occurs when fluid inside the eye exerts excess pressure that can damage the optic nerve, but it rarely causes early pain or symptoms. After age forty-five, some experts recommend getting an eye exam annually that includes a test for glaucoma (see p. 561).

PLANNING FOR EMERGENCIES

It is not too soon to think about making sure that someone you trust can take care of business and make health care decisions for you if you suddenly can't do it yourself.

• A *durable power of attorney* gives someone you trust the authority to act on your behalf in financial and other legal matters if you are unable to take action yourself.

• A *health care proxy document* gives someone you trust the authority to make medical testing and treatment decisions for you in case you are unable to make them for yourself.

• A *medical advance directive* can protect your right to refuse unwanted treatments and makes your wishes clear to your proxy person, other family members, friends, and medical care providers. This can be written as a letter to the person who has your health care proxy.

Give copies of these documents to the people authorized to act for you, your health care provider, your lawyer (if you have one), and your immediate family. State laws may vary as to the particulars. Check with your state attorney general's office for the specifics of your state laws and for copies of forms to use for advance directives and/or living wills.

SOCIAL AND POLITICAL ISSUES

AGEISM

U.S. society often separates people by age and fails to support and celebrate us as we get older. Getting older is equated with disease, and this medicalized view permeates all institutions. Once we are no longer "young," we may feel marginalized, ignored, and invisible. This may make it difficult for us to embrace this time in our lives and to maintain a sense of confidence, empowerment, and self-esteem.

Ageism is the systematic devaluation of and discrimination against a person because of her or his age. Ageism appears to be "just the way things are" until we name it and confront it. It doesn't have to be that way. Many cultures have a heritage of respecting life experience and celebrating the postmenopausal years as a time of wisdom.

We need to separate aging from disease. We can't deny the inevitable problems that arise with aging: chronic illness; new needs and increased dependence; possibly surviving our partner, relatives, and closest friends; and difficult decisions to make for the end of life. Still, the more we can take charge of our aging process, the better. Some biological changes that were once considered inevitable can be prevented, slowed, reversed, treated, or managed. We can plan ahead to try to avoid poverty, isolation, and ill health and to meet our long-term care, housing, and social needs.

PAY, PENSIONS, AND POVERTY

Older women are almost twice as likely to live in poverty as older men,[13] often receiving low wages from nonunionized jobs that offer few or no benefits, such as pensions. Poverty is a major cause of ill health and diminished well-being. Without enough money, it's hard to live well and healthfully. Women of color are more likely

DO WE NEED LONG-TERM CARE INSURANCE?

In midlife, people often start receiving promotions for insurance covering long-term care in case of chronic illness, frailty, or disability. It's cheaper to get it now than if you wait until your sixties or later, but it is not financially advantageous for everyone and does not cover everything you might need. (For more about this type of insurance, see p. 572 in Chapter 27, "Our Later Years.")

to suffer from these inequities. (For more information, see "Women's Work: Pay, Pensions, and Poverty" [W61] on the companion website, www.ourbodiesourselves.org.)

Everyone has a stake in supporting older women's demands and concerns: equal pay, paid family leave for caregiving, access to health care for all, flexibility in jobs, part-time work with benefits, and portability of pension benefits from one job to another. Whatever our differences, we must insist together on the changes that will recognize and reward our contributions to our families, our communities, and our society as we age.

INSURANCE AND ACCESS TO HEALTH CARE

Many midlife women in the United States face a gap in health insurance coverage, being too young for Medicare (under sixty-five) and not quite poor enough for Medicaid. The U.S. is the only industrialized country in the world that does not provide access to basic health care for all. Because most health insurance here is tied to benefits offered voluntarily by employers, unemployed people and even many workers are uninsured. Many women lose health insurance coverage after divorce. Asian-American, Pacific

Islander, and African-American women are twice as likely as white women to be uninsured, and Latinas are three times more likely to be without insurance.[14] It is increasingly difficult to keep jobs as we grow older. Then we are faulted for needing "entitlements" such as Social Security, Medicare, and disability benefits, though we may have been contributing to these funds for many years. Medicare is criticized as too expensive when it should be considered a model for a universal, single-payer health insurance system.

Advocates are organizing in many states and nationally to address these gaps in coverage. (For information about advocating for changes in the health care system, see below and Chapters 30 through 32.)

RESEARCH ON WOMEN'S HEALTH

Until very recently, medical research paid little attention to the health concerns of aging women. Even today it focuses on the medical aspects of menopause, as though reproductive organs were the center of a woman's life. It continues to overlook the basic biology of aging, occupational and environmental damage, racial and ethnic differences, and the influence of socioeconomic factors on our health. Studies, often designed and funded by corporate interests rather than objective researchers, focus on drugs. They rarely address the needs of women of color, which undermines the ability of health care practitioners to provide appropriate care. Two important studies are under way to remedy this long-standing neglect.

The Study of Women's Health Across the Nation (SWAN) includes 3,301 midlife women who were between the ages of forty-two and fifty-two when the study started in 1996. It compares the menopause experience in Latina, African-American, Caucasian, Japanese, and Chinese women. The study examines psychological, social, and economic factors, in addition to health and medical components, including ovarian aging, effects on bone and body composition, and risk factors for cardiovascular disease.[15]

The Black Women's Health Study, funded by the National Cancer Institute, enrolled fifty thousand African-American women. Although it focuses primarily on younger women, it is also looking at conditions more typical of midlife and older women, such as cardiovascular disease, diabetes, and breast cancer, which affect black women earlier and may reduce how long we live.

ADVOCACY

Women over fifty, individually and with advocacy organizations* such as the Gray Panthers, Raging Grannies, OWL: The Voice of Midlife and Older Women, Civic Ventures, and Generations United, are campaigning to improve the status and image of older people; to call on decades of wisdom and contributions; and to find ways to integrate all of us into the fabric of society. People born between 1946 and 1964 (the baby boom following World War II) will increase the over-sixty-five population to about one fifth of the total in 2030—enough to make an impact.

A fifty-five-year-old woman says:

Intellectually, I know some of my physical and mental capacities will diminish as I age, but I want to deal with this with a sense of self-acceptance [and] not lower expectations. I hope my generation of feminist boomers will not deny the limits of aging and not give in to internalized ageist attitudes towards others and ourselves as we age.

* AARP, which solicits members of both sexes age fifty and over, is a useful source of information about many aspects of adapting to aging, but it is also a powerful lobby for private insurance and pharmaceutical interests. Its recent positions on senior health issues are debatable.

Aging well is not just a matter of individual responsibility. Ageism often combines with sexism, racism, heterosexism, and discrimination against people with disabilities to make life a struggle for those of us who do not have the financial resources to age comfortably. We need to build support for ourselves and advocate for programs that will be responsive to midlife and older women's needs.

SUPPORT GROUPS

Support groups can be an especially important source of strength for midlife women, offering shared experience and information. They also may reduce feelings of isolation and give us some perspective.

I had never been in any kind of support group before. I thought it would be a discussion group and everyone would be an expert except me, and I'd be embarrassed because I wasn't an expert on anything. But that's not the way this group worked. There's a lot of mutual help; people really listen to each other and laugh a lot. Now I don't worry about menopause or growing older the way I used to.

Many of us find social engagement essential to our sense of well-being. Relationships of all kinds sustain us as we age.

I was brought up to believe that the people in my family were the most important people in my world. I'm still very attached to immediate family members, but I have consciously extended family to include "sisters" in the women's community.

We can live our lives more fully and expressively when we assert our pride in the experience and confidence of our years and stimulate communication within and across the generations.

Our growing numbers give us the potential to become a constituency with significant clout.

NOTES

1. Mary K. Bissell, ed., *The Kinship Care Source Book* (Washington, D.C.: D.C. Kinship Care Coalition, 1997). Available from the National Committee to Preserve Social Security and Medicare, Washington, D.C., 202-216-0420.
2. N. E. Avis, R. Stellato, S. Crawford, J. Bromberger, P. Ganz, V. Cain, and M. Kagawa-Singer, "Is There a Menopausal Syndrome? Menopausal Status and Symptoms Across Racial/Ethnic Groups," *Social Science & Medicine* 52, no. 30 (February 2001): 345–56.
3. F. Kronenberg and A. Fugh-Berman, "Complementary and Alternative Medicine for Menopausal Symptoms: A Review of Randomized, Controlled Trials," *Annals of Internal Medicine* 137, no. 10 (July 12, 2002): 805–13.
4. R. J. Rodabough, S. L. D. Rovi, et al., "Prevalence and 3-year Incidence of Abuse Among Postmenopausal Women," *American Journal of Public Health* 94, no. 4 (April 2004): 605–12.
5. Writing Group for the Women's Health Initiative Investigators, "Risks and Benefits of Estrogen Plus Progestin in Healthy Postmenopausal Women: Principal Results from the Women's Health Initiative Randomized Controlled Trial," *Journal of the American Medical Association* 288, no. 3 (July 17, 2002): 321–33.
6. WHI Steering Committee, "Effects of Conjugated Equine Estrogen in Postmenopausal Women with Hysterectomy: The Women's Health Initiative Randomized Controlled Trial," *Journal of the American Medical Association* 291, no. 14 (April 14, 2004): 1701–12.
7. P. D. Delmas, et al, "Effects of Raloxifene on Bone Mineral Density, Serum Cholesterol Concentrations, and Uterine Endometrium in Postmenopausal Women," *New England Journal of Medicine,* 337, no. 23 (December 4, 1997): 1641–47.
8. H. G. Bone, D. Hosking, J. P. Devogelaer, J. R. Tucci, M.D., R. D. Emkey, et al, for the Alendronate Phase III Osteoporosis Treatment Study Group, "Ten Years' Experience with Alendronate for Osteoporosis in Postmenopausal Women," *New England Journal of Medicine* 350, no. 12 (March 18, 2004): 1189–99.
9. U.S. Food and Drug Administration, Center for Drug Research and Evaluation. "Questions and Answers for Estrogen and Estrogen with Progestin Therapies for

Postmenopausal Women," updated April 19, 2004, accessed at www.fda.gov/cder/drug/infopage/estrogen_progestins/Q&A.htm on October 29, 2004.

10. "Osteoporosis Prevention, Diagnosis, and Therapy," NIH Consensus Statement, March 27–29, 2000, 17, no. 1: 1–45, accessed at http://consensus.nih/gov/cons/111/111_statement.pdf on October 29, 2004.

11. J. Hays, J. K. Ockena, R. L. Brunner, et al., "Effects of Estrogen Plus Progestin on Health-Related Quality of Life," *New England Journal of Medicine* 348, no. 19 (May 8, 2003): 1839–54.

12. G. A. Greendale et al., "Leisure, Home, and Occupational Physical Activity and Cardiovascular Risk Factors in Postmenopausal Women: The Postmenopausal Estrogens/Progestins Intervention (PEPI) Study," *Archives of Internal Medicine* 156, no. 4 (February 26, 1996): 418–24.

13. AARP and the International Longevity Center, *Unjust Deserts: Financial Realities of Older Women* (New York: International Longevity Center, 2003), 3.

14. Unpublished estimates by the Urban Institute and Kaiser Commission on Medicaid and the Uninsured, based on the March 2003 Current Population Survey, 2004.

15. M. F. Sowers, S. Crawford, B. Sternfeld, et al., "SWAN: A Multi-center, Multi-ethnic, Community-based Cohort Study of Women and the Menopausal Transition," in R. Lobo, J. Kelsey, R. J. Marcus, eds., *Menopause: Biology and Pathobiology* (San Diego: Academic Press, 2000), 175–88.

■ **CHAPTER 27**

As more of us live longer, we change the content and definition of these years and gain a new sense of the range of normal aging.* Our older years can be a good phase of life.

I'm 90 years old and in good health. My main problem is balance. I have always believed in lifelong learning, and I continue to take courses. A friend of mine who told me "Every decade I plan to have a project" inspires me.

A seventy-two-year-old woman says:

---

* Distinctions are now being made among the "young old" (ages 65–74), "old old" (ages 75–84) and "oldest old" (ages 85 plus). The oldest person on record was Jeanne Calment, a French woman who died at age 122 in 1997.

I am madly in love with a man whom I met since I became a widow. I can say that my feelings are just as intense, emotionally and physically, as ever they were at any of the other ages. . . . I love everything we do together sexually, and most of the time we both feel easy about where it leads, that it's different each time and doesn't always end the way experts describe.

The quality of our lives often depends more on our health than on our age.

When I was 65 I felt young. I started a new job and new activities. I am now 86, and I felt "young" up until a year ago. My memory is not so good now, and that really makes a difference.

Up through my 70s I did everything I always did. Now . . . I get tired more easily. Neither my husband nor I drive at night any more. We do keep up our interests and try to keep fit; [we] go to exercise two mornings, and once a week we swim.

There is much we can do to take care of ourselves and manage certain health conditions. Yet even when we eat well, exercise, and have strong social contacts, aging brings with it loss, decline, and illness. It's essential to incorporate this reality into our view of aging well, and to find ways to cope with new circumstances.

FEMINIZATION OF AGING

The population of people over sixty-five is overwhelmingly female. Women live, on the average, nearly seven years longer than men. And increasing numbers of women are living eighty or more years. Along with the benefits of longevity come certain problems: chronic illness, increased dependence on medical care, caregiving or needing care, insufficient economic resources, and possibly surviving one's partner, relatives, and closest

friends. Because women live longer, these are predominantly women's problems. Researchers and policy makers have mainly overlooked them.

One positive side of our growing numbers is our potentially greater clout as a political constituency. In 2000 women over forty-five constituted 18.6 percent of the adult U.S. population.[1] The government and the press are paying more attention to us. It's important to build upon this attention by demanding, creating, and fighting for programs that meet the needs of midlife and older women and the needs of an aging population.* Especially important are protecting and maintaining Medicare and Social Security programs and developing a long-term care policy to provide a continuum of services for our older years that acknowledge the diversity of our living situations and economic resources.

RETIREMENT

For those of us in the U.S. job market, the official retirement age (when we can collect full Social Security) is being phased upward. This legal change, implemented in 2003, increased the age of full retirement in gradual steps from age 65 to age 67. Depending on our economic circumstances, we may be working past 65; retiring at 62 and collecting reduced benefits; shortening our workweek; or shifting to part-time or more flexible schedules.

LOSS OF A PARTNER

Large numbers of us outlive our husbands or partners, often by a decade or two. Women sixty-five and older are more likely to live alone (41 percent as compared to 18 percent of men),

* OWL is an important national organization advocating for the concerns of midlife and older women (see "Resources").

• *Medicine will affect me differently as I get older.*

Reality. Aging may cause increased sensitivity to drugs, as they are metabolized more slowly. You may need lower doses adjusted to your size, age, and nutrition needs. Women at any age may require lower doses than men because of lower body mass and weight.

• *If my partner retires, I could lose my health insurance.*

Reality. Women who have health insurance under a spouse's employment-related health plan typically lose coverage when the spouse retires. Since the majority of women have partners who are older, many of us experience a gap in coverage after our spouse retires and before Medicare coverage begins. During this period, paying privately for a nongroup plan can be prohibitively expensive and pre-existing conditions may make it difficult to get any insurance at all.

while older men are more likely to be married in their older years (73 percent of men and 43 percent of women).[2] More than 11 million women constitute over 80 percent of the U.S. widowed population.[3] Millions more women have lost unofficial partners, male and female. The stress of widowhood can be enormous. Widows are particularly vulnerable to disease and often lose or cannot afford health insurance coverage just when it is most needed.

If you are recently widowed, you may have to negotiate insurance and other practical matters while still numb and shocked by loss. You will need people to phone you, visit, bring food, offer invitations, and perhaps help with tasks around the house—and to leave you alone when that's what you want. Some friends may pull back, embarrassed or frightened by your grieving or neediness, especially when the initial, formal mourning period has ended. Despite the stresses, it is sometimes more possible for women to adjust to widowhood than men, because we tend to have an easier time reaching out for help and making and keeping friends.

Grieving may be complicated when unconventional situations make it hard to be open about loss and to receive social support from friends and community.

Years ago, when Trudy discovered that she had cancer . . . she drove to the hills above our home early one Sunday morning and put a bullet through her heart. It pierced my heart, too, for it ended our eighteen years of life together. Because that life had been lived in such a deep dark closet, Trudy's death caused me to close the door in denial of my lesbian feelings. It took eleven years for me to begin to creep cautiously from the closet.

Losses may occur in quick succession, offering no breathing time to grieve and recover.

Diagnosis of heart arrhythmia led to insertion of a pacemaker. I needed time to assimilate the roller coaster of emotions—the high of being lucky to be alive and with no physical limitations, the loss of my youthful feelings of immortality. . . . But within weeks, my wonderful talented son experienced a breakdown. I had to put my issues aside, turn off my feelings, and shift into coping mode to make sure he got the help he needed.

The grieving process can bring you through to the other side—to a new sense of yourself.

My husband died after a seven-year period when his health had been deteriorating and I had been his primary caretaker. My mother died within six weeks of his death. I lost a part of myself, my role as a helping, caring person. . . . What I had left was the beginning of a new identity as a feminist and a woman [who] was growing older.

The medical impulse to prescribe medication for grief and loss can be enormous, as can be the temptation to accept it. Watch out for doctors who want to medicate away legitimate feelings of sadness and rage, or to label normal grieving as "pathological" if it takes "too long." It is a sign of strength to acknowledge feelings of despair, anger, guilt, emptiness, fear, relief, anxiety, and confusion.

I think now those tranquilizers suppressed or sent underground the pains of that period (divorce, death of mother, betrayal by a lover). These pains still surface with agonizing strength. Maybe if I had fully faced them and "digested" them at the time they happened, this would not be the case.

There is no time limit on how long grieving should last. Each woman has her own unique rhythm. Talking with women who have been there often helps, as do reminiscing, writing, and keeping a journal. It takes enormous energy to rebuild your life.

After my husband died, I got great support from women in my church. We have a women-over-70 group. We let down our hair and talk about our problems and help each other by providing a sustaining set of relationships.

Don't exhaust yourself trying to take care of the emotional needs of others. Take special care of yourself. You will probably need more rest

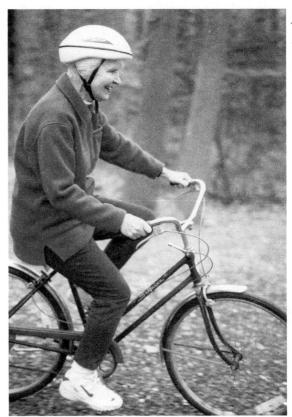

© Lynda J. Banzi

than usual. Go slowly—give yourself time to heal and to regain your trust in the world and in your own capacities.

GETTING MEDICAL CARE

Even though many of us are living longer, with later onset of diseases, we all need more health care as we age. Some of the normal conditions of aging can make daily living harder. Older women face physical, emotional, and social changes and challenges that require specialized training and care.

We may need a multidisciplinary team of people to help us manage our medical conditions so we can continue to be as vital, active, and independent as possible. These practitioners should have formal training in caring for older women and should understand how different medical conditions can interact. Unfortunately, there is a great shortage of doctors, nurses, psychologists, psychiatrists, social workers, occupational therapists, physical therapists, pharmacists, and dentists who are trained in caring for older adults.

Health care providers may judge older women's complaints and health problems to be neurotic, imaginary, or inevitable far more than men's, and at earlier ages. Sometimes providers do not fully treat chronic conditions, misdiagnose and fail to treat reversible conditions, overprescribe drugs, and have only limited time to spend with us. Managed care may limit access to certain tests, treatments, and health care practitioners. It is even more complicated for immigrant women, who may face barriers to proper treatment because of language, literacy and cultural issues, money, immigration status, cultural deference to physicians and other health care providers, and other concerns.

Take an active role with health care providers, and try to establish good communication with them. If your practitioner is not well informed about managing the diseases and chronic conditions of aging, or is not caring toward you, seek someone who can be more helpful. It's your body, and you have a right to know what is going on.

In certain circumstances, it makes sense to get a second opinion.

I had lower-back problems. My neurologist sent me to an orthopedic surgeon who told me to have an operation which, he informed me, had some risks. I didn't feel comfortable with his assessment and sought a second opinion. It was hard to find a doctor to do this. The opinion of the second doctor was that I didn't need an operation. I agreed, as did my husband and children. I started physical therapy and feel much better.

TIPS FOR MEDICAL APPOINTMENTS

- Make a list of all your questions ahead of time.
- Bring a friend or family member with you to act as advocate, if possible.
- Take notes, bring a tape recorder or someone to take notes, or ask the provider to take notes for you.
- Bring a list of all your medications (both prescription and over-the-counter) and supplements.
- Tell the pharmacist how many and which medications you are taking when you're filling a new prescription. Your health care provider and pharmacist can help you keep track of medications and check for drug interactions.

(For more information on getting appropriate medical care, see Chapter 30, "Navigating the Health Care System.")

HEALTH INSURANCE COVERAGE

Women who have health insurance under a spouse's employment-related health plan typically lose coverage when the spouse retires. Since the majority of women have partners who are older, many of us experience a gap in coverage in our mid-sixties, when paying privately for a nongroup plan can be prohibitively expensive and pre-existing conditions make it difficult to get any insurance at all. Coverage is available under COBRA,* but you must be able to pay for it yourself.

---

* COBRA is federal legislation requiring insurance companies to maintain the option of coverage at group rates for eighteen months after you lose your job (or your eligibility through a spouse). The eligible person must pay for the insurance out of pocket.

Medicare

If you are over sixty-five or permanently disabled, you are probably eligible for Medicare, the federal insurance program. Contrary to the assumption that Medicare will cover all health care costs, it covers only 80 percent of allowable costs (actual costs may be higher). Medicare's Part A (hospital insurance) is financed by a compulsory payroll tax as part of the Social Security finance tax; Part B (supplementary medical insurance), for which you pay a monthly premium, covers nonhospital care, including outpatient doctors' services and limited home care. Some providers do not accept Medicare patients because the reimbursement rate is too low. This means that at age sixty-five, you will have to pay for medical co-payments, your Part B premium, your deductibles, and all noncovered medical expenses—or you can purchase a private insurance policy to cover the difference (Medigap insurance). Medicare's major limitations are that it focuses on acute care and does not pay for long-term care, preventive health, and nursing homes. While prescription drug benefits are supposed to be included by 2006, the law (passed in 2003) does not limit prescription drug prices or provide significant savings for everyone. Many people believe it will encourage privatization of the Medicare program and threaten Medicare's universal benefits. (For more information, see Chapter 31, "The Politics of Women's Health.")

THE FOCUS OF MEDICINE: WHAT'S THE RIGHT APPROACH?

Medical institutions are organized primarily around acute care. Most chronic diseases do not respond to daring surgery or high-technology interventions, but they still have to be managed. Many women explore alternative approaches to healing, such as acupuncture, chiropractic, or herbs, but these are frequently not covered by health insurance or Medicare, and their efficacy is often unknown. Simpler things like diet, canes, physical and occupational therapy, and pain relief get less attention, even when we need them most, and emotional support is often neglected.

We need a continuous care system in which everyone receives care appropriate to her condition, provided promptly and efficiently and in the right amount, increasing or decreasing as her capability changes. Since conventional medical care does not come even close to these goals, we must keep pressuring policy makers in health institutions and government to fund the long-term health care and social services needed by an aging population. Better care for older people requires recognition and better pay for nonmedical providers who care for the chronically ill, such as social workers, case managers, and family members.

WRONG DIAGNOSIS, WRONG TREATMENT

Health care practitioners tend to blame physical and emotional problems on aging when women are over sixty, and especially when we are over seventy-five, and they may not look for treatable disorders. If you have ample financial resources and private physicians, this may happen less, but on the other hand you may be pushed to have unnecessary and risky treatments, such as expensive new drugs and cosmetic surgery.

Providers without adequate training may interpret emotional or mental confusion as senility when it may actually indicate poor nutrition, treatable physical problems, grief, or a reaction to inappropriate medication. Time after time, older women are given tranquilizers, sedatives, antidepressants, and hormones instead of being helped to discover what's really wrong.

TOO MUCH MEDICINE?

People over sixty-five take 30 percent of the medications prescribed annually in the United States, though they currently constitute only 13 percent of the U.S. population.[4] Many of us take several medications daily for various chronic conditions, often prescribed by different physicians. Health care providers sometimes neglect to find out what drugs we are taking, including over-the-counter products, before prescribing others. In the United States in any given year, as many as 35 percent of people have adverse reactions due to incorrect dosage or negative drug interaction, and 17 percent of older adults are hospitalized as a result.[5]

Aging may cause increased sensitivity to drugs, as they are metabolized more slowly. You may need lower doses adjusted to your size, age, and nutrition needs. Women at any age may require lower doses than men because of lower body mass and weight. The kidneys and liver excrete drugs more slowly, so they stay in the body longer. Also, drugs stored in fat tissue remain longer in the body, increasing the likelihood of harmful effects even from low or infrequent doses. Some drugs can cause depression (for which you may be offered more drugs) or mental confusion, though symptoms often stop when the medication is stopped. The toxic effects of drugs can be mistaken for mental illness. In nursing homes, many elderly people are tranquilized into quiet and compliance.

A 94-year-old friend who lives in a nursing home was recently diagnosed as having various ailments that require anywhere from three to ten pills a day. She was never told what the pills were or what they were for. When the nurse came to her room to give her the pills, my friend looked her squarely in the eye and said, "The doctor only knows my body and how it works for a short time. I know it for 94 years, and nothing is going in it until I know what it is!"

WHAT YOU CAN DO TO MONITOR MEDICATION

- Bring a list of all your medicines to your medical appointments, indicating doses and how often you take each. Regularly ask your health care provider and/or pharmacist to review all your medications.

- Ask about other approaches, such as heat, massage, acupuncture, or consulting a physical therapist.

- If you believe that you are (or a relative or friend is) being inappropriately or excessively medicated, talk to whoever is in a position to change the situation. Some states have a nursing home residents' advocate called an *ombudsman* to whom you can complain if health care providers or institutional staff are not responding.

PHYSICAL IMPAIRMENTS AND CHRONIC CONDITIONS

Each of us ages differently. Don't automatically assume that conditions affecting you are the inevitable result of aging. Be wary of any health care practitioner who dismisses complaints by saying, "What do you expect at your age?" Many problems are as treatable now as they are at any age. New medical techniques are successfully reducing problems that in the past would have limited our lives and independence. If you do have to modify a cherished activity because you can't see, hear, or move around as well as before, it will take time to get used to new limits and find alternative ways to manage.

GETTING AROUND

Devices

One woman in her seventies calls her cane her new "friend." Her approach counteracts the stigma attached to canes, hearing aids, walkers, and other assistive devices. To some people, they may make us look "old," but in fact, they can help us stay active and involved.

If you need to use a walker, get one that folds up (for travel) and has a seat (for resting) as well as a bag (for carrying small items). It's easier and more comfortable to use when you stand upright inside the space between the handlebars, not bent over, leaning forward with the whole thing in front of you like a shopping cart.

Transportation

U.S. society, organized around the nuclear family and the individual automobile, magnifies the isolation of older women, many of whom live alone. We need to work for more and improved public transportation and for communities in which it is safe to walk around.

Even if you have to limit driving (day or night), you may be able to find other ways to keep up cherished activities and social relationships. Invite others to share a cab, or ask for rides. Some councils on aging and community and religious institutions will help neighbors organize transportation for themselves, or they will recruit volunteers to provide rides. Many communities provide transportation services for older people and people with disabilities, and some offer taxi coupons at reduced rates.

Chronic Ailments

Many serious health problems affecting midlife and older women are discussed elsewhere in this book because they affect younger women, too (see Chapter 28, "Unique to Women," and Chap-

ter 29, "Special Concerns for Women," especially the sections on cancer, arthritis, hypertension, heart disease, and diabetes). Other problems and changes that sometimes come with aging are discussed on the following pages, including visual impairment, hearing loss, and osteoporosis.

If you are anywhere over fifty, a lifetime of exposure to occupational health hazards may have caused debilitating disease (see Chapter 7, "Environmental and Occupational Health"). This is even more likely for women of color, 40 percent of whom work in physically demanding or otherwise hazardous occupations, and who are at even higher risk for chronic diseases that become more common with age. One in three African-Americans has high blood pressure, compared with one in four among the population at large. One in five older African-Americans and one in three Latinos have Type 2 diabetes, compared with one in ten white people.

Social and Economic Factors

Just struggling for survival can be more disabling to health and well-being than medical conditions. Isolation from family and friends; caring for homebound relatives without outside help; and poor medical care due to high cost, lack of insurance coverage, inadequate medical understanding of aging, and, in some areas, not enough available doctors all can worsen health.

Money worries about limited income and cutbacks to Social Security, Medicare, and other government programs add greatly to the unhealthy stresses of daily living. Inadequate income also makes it harder to take care of ourselves in simple but crucial daily ways. It is harder to get exercise if sidewalks are not cleared of snow, if the streets are unsafe, or if indoor exercise facilities are too expensive or too far from where we live.

Poverty often causes health and medical problems. A tight national economy, drastic cuts in social programs, and so-called welfare reform have made this worse. Low income severely restricts access to medical care, especially in a time of reduced government aid. Support and services may be deliberately withheld from older immigrants.

SENSORY LOSS

Our senses may become less sharp as we grow older. These changes usually occur so gradually that we adapt without even noticing. Loss of taste and smell can lead to loss of appetite and even malnutrition. Decline in vision or hearing affects interactions with others more directly and may reinforce stereotypes of older people as "slow" or "stodgy."

Telling others what you need (though it may be difficult at first) helps them understand how they can help. Don't hesitate to ask someone to speak up or give you a hand—and let people know that your mind is still working.

EYESIGHT

In the United States, of more than a million blind people, seven hundred thousand are women. Many more women have some visual impairment, especially after age seventy-five. In industrialized countries, more women than men are blind because vision loss is more widespread as people get older, and women live longer. When women don't have decision-making authority or access to financial resources, getting eye checkups at a clinic or hospital may be difficult, and women's eye problems may be more advanced than men's when treatment does become available.

Distance

You may need glasses for the first time, or you may need stronger glasses, perhaps bi- or trifocals. It can be hard to adjust to them; some people are embarrassed about wearing them. "Dry" and "wet" *macular degeneration* are the leading cause of vision loss in people sixty and older. They occur when the macula—the center of the retina—deteriorates and a blind spot develops in the middle of the field of vision. Dry (deterioration of light-sensitive cells) is more common than wet (growth of leaky blood vessels, with bleeding inside the eye). Laser therapies that destroy leaking blood vessels can reduce vision loss. Taking zinc, vitamins A and C, and beta-carotene may slow down the advance of this condition.[6]

Cataracts

Cataracts, or cloudy lenses, may develop, usually after our fifties. Although there isn't much evidence that cataracts can be prevented, some eye care providers recommend taking vitamin E. When you plan to have cataracts removed, investigate options in advance. Recent improvements include laser surgery and having lens implants put in at the time of the operation, instead of contact lenses or new glasses afterward. An experienced ophthalmologist (a medical doctor who specializes in eye disease) must perform these procedures. It's a good idea to get a second opinion about eye surgery. Some doctors push operations when they aren't necessary, or sooner (or later) than is appropriate. Cataract surgery is usually done as an office procedure. If you are over sixty-five and financially disadvantaged, ophthalmologists will provide free care. (For information, call the National Eye Care Project hotline at 1-800-222-3937 between eight A.M. and four P.M. Pacific Time.)

Glaucoma

Glaucoma, a chronic eye disease, usually appears at midlife or later and affects more women than men. Excess pressure of fluid inside the eye can damage the optic nerve and cause blindness if not treated. Because glaucoma rarely causes early pain or symptoms, after age forty-five, *everyone should have an eye exam yearly that includes a test for glaucoma.* Tests done with a tonometer are quick and painless (though some people find them uncomfortable). Ophthalmologists have the most accurate diagnostic equipment and skills. Optometrists, who measure eye function, can do tonometry only in certain states. If detected early, mild glaucoma can be treated with eyedrops. More severe glaucoma requires surgical treatment with regular follow-up, since there's no permanent cure.

Detached Retina

If you experience sudden flashes of light, loss of side vision, and/or "floaters" (black spots) that don't go away, get medical attention at once. These could be symptoms of a detached retina—a medical emergency. Intermittent black spots should also be checked out, but they're not an emergency. If they become chronic, you can sometimes get rid of them by resting your eyes or doing eye-rolling exercises.

Diabetic Retinopathy

Diabetic retinopathy, or damage to the retina leading to blindness, is a common complication of both types of diabetes. The retinal blood vessels break down, leak, or become blocked, impairing vision. If you have diabetes, you need a thorough annual eye exam by an ophthalmologist. Controlling blood sugar levels, as well as laser treatments, can prevent or slow retinopathy.

HEARING

We may take hearing for granted until we suddenly notice that we miss what is being said or must ask people to repeat themselves more often than feels comfortable. Feelings of isola-tion can be as hard to deal with as the actual hearing loss.

Every once in a while, I miss out on parts of a conversation. . . . I discover, to my later discomfort, that occasionally I act as if I did hear—bright smile, nod of agreement.

Being hard of hearing is an invisible disability. Others don't know unless you tell them.

One of the most important things a hard-of-hearing person can do for herself, I have discovered, is to be very assertive. Tell each person you talk with to speak more slowly or more clearly, and force yourself to keep reminding that person if she forgets.

Hearing loss is not inevitable with aging, though it does seem to run in some families. It's the third most common chronic condition among older people. Sixty percent of people over sixty-five, and 90 percent of those over seventy-five, have some degree of hearing impairment.[7] The enormous increase in the volume and range of noise in an industrialized environment has contributed significantly to hearing loss in the present generation of people over sixty-five, especially among factory workers and city dwellers. People born after 1945 face additional risk from more years of exposure to loud music.

It is very important to get your hearing tested regularly and get an accurate diagnosis if it is impaired, because effective treatment depends on what kind of ear problem you have. Conduction deafness (related to transmission of sound inside the ear) can often be corrected with surgery, unlike nerve deafness (damage to the auditory nerve linking the ear to the brain).

Many of us deal with hearing loss by learning to watch others more closely for visual cues, and by reading lips when they speak.

A seventy-eight-year-old woman says:

I developed a new interest in foreign movies. I was missing a lot at the theater and in American movies, but when I go to a foreign movie, I can read the subtitles, so I don't miss a thing—and I'm expanding my horizons!

Don't let embarrassment cause you to hesitate to make your needs known. At public or social events, ask people to speak more loudly—and to look out at the audience instead of down into their chests. Remind them to avoid putting their hands in front of their mouths when they speak. If your hearing is worse in one ear, ask people to sit on the side of the "good ear." It also helps to eliminate background noise that interferes with hearing, such as music, TV or radio conversation, running water, and the clatter of pots or dishes.

Hearing aids can make a huge difference to social life and self-esteem. Although Medicare does not pay for hearing aids, some Medigap policies include partial coverage. Unfortunately, there are lots of misleading ads for gadgets that don't work, so do some research before you buy one. (For organizations that have helpful material, see "Resources" or ask your health care provider.)

Signing is a way to make cultural events accessible to people with hearing loss who use American Sign Language (ASL). If you are planning a cultural event, be sure to find someone who will sign.

JOINTS AND FEET

Arthritis caused by wear and tear on the joints *(osteoarthritis)* is the most common chronic condition; 25 percent of women past midlife have it. It causes pain but is not crippling, and it can often be relieved with early diagnosis, self-help, and medical treatment. Managing osteoarthritis involves a balance of exercise and rest, along with pain relief medication. Nonsteroidal anti-inflammatory drugs, including COX-2 inhibitors, have gastrointestinal and possibly cardiovascular side effects, so take the lowest effective dose.[8]

Exercise gently and slowly, and rest between repetitions when lifting weights. Gentle stretching two or three times a week can help reduce pain and maintain mobility. A warm bath or shower can ease morning stiffness and serve as preparation for stretching or limbering exercises. Swimming and exercising in water can also help. Build up slowly to half an hour of moderate activity every day, like walking, low-impact movement, or even household chores. Don't avoid exercise out of fear of pain, but don't do anything painful. If it hurts, stop and try another kind of exercise. Fortunately, it is never too late to start exercising. Weight-training programs in nursing homes have increased muscle strength in people in their nineties.[9]

People with arthritis are often sensitive to cold, dampness, and changes in barometric pressure, which alters pressure within joints. Keeping warm is best. If you are considering a move to a warmer, drier climate, try a visit first. Moving can be one of life's most stressful experiences. Changing your social life and leaving friends behind may feel worse than aching joints from bad weather. (For more information, see "Arthritis," p. 660.)

Foot Problems

If you notice aches and pains in your feet while walking or resting, you may have growths such as bunions or bone spurs. Shoe design and poor fit can cause foot problems. High heels distort women's gait and posture, and strain our legs, knees, backs, and necks. Pointy toes pinch, causing painful hammertoe and blisters. Any existing foot problems may worsen with age, especially if you are heavy or on your feet all day. Well-designed shoes with a firm supportive arch can make a big difference. Most managed care programs do not cover routine care by a podiatrist (foot doctor), but they will pay for problems caused by infection and neglect of routine care. Some podiatrists make house calls, and some eldercare programs offer these for homebound people with low incomes.

BONES, FALLS, AND FRACTURES

Osteoporosis (brittle bone disease) occurs when bones become less dense. Some bone density decline is normal in both men and women, but some women lose bone faster at menopause, and again in their seventies. Osteoporosis produces no symptoms, or only mild ones during early stages, such as backaches or back-muscle spasms. It becomes visible clearly on X rays only when 30 to 40 percent of bone density is lost. You may be unaware that you have osteoporosis until you fracture your spine, hip, or wrist in a simple fall.

Osteoporosis can be painful and difficult to manage in later stages, especially when it affects the spine. You may feel pain in the upper or lower spine that lasts for several days and then stops, caused perhaps by a damaged vertebra collapsing spontaneously or cracking (compression fracture). In a more advanced form, compression fractures in the upper spine cause curvature of the spine, commonly called "dowager's hump." In rare cases, the chest area is shortened, which may make digesting food and even breathing more difficult.

Fracture Prevention

Preventing falls is the simplest way to prevent fractures. Try to avoid overmedication, which is the main cause of falls for elderly people, and eliminate hazards in your home, such as scatter rugs and other obstacles. Keep stairs clear, and install grab bars in the shower or bathtub and anywhere else they are needed. In winter, have snow and ice cleared off steps and sidewalks promptly. One study of nursing home residents demonstrated that wearing hip padding to cushion falls significantly decreased the number of people who broke a hip.[10]

Medical Treatments

Several new drugs are now available to treat osteoporosis and fractures. *Bisphosphonates,* such as Fosamax, which inhibit bone breakdown, are a nonhormonal treatment for osteoporosis. These medications must be used very carefully, as directed, to avoid irritation in the esophagus (the passage from the throat to the stomach). The most effective way is to take a pill first thing in the morning and not to lie down again; it's important to remain upright. You may exercise or read for thirty to forty-five minutes before eating breakfast. Many people find the once-a-week dose more convenient than taking a pill every day.

Calcitonin, a hormone produced by the thyroid gland, regulates blood levels of calcium and thus contributes to building bone. Formerly available only by injection, calcitonin is now available in a nasal spray, which is less expensive and can be self-administered. Other potential treatments are being studied but have not yet been proved safe and effective long-term.

Starting drug treatment just to prevent fractures is somewhat controversial. Most hip fractures in women occur in our eighties, so it may make sense to take medication earlier only if we are at high risk for osteoporosis; if we are in our seventies; or after a fracture occurs (to prevent another one). Treatment could make a significant difference in quality of life for older women who have already suffered a fracture or have thin, brittle bones, are likely to fall for other reasons, or are starting to get dowager's hump. Possible bone loss should be taken more seriously in women who have rheumatoid arthritis, HIV, or eating disorders, or who take other drugs that increase the risk of osteoporosis. The best way to keep bones healthy is to eat a healthy diet with enough calcium and to engage in exercise tailored to individual abilities. Medications may be helpful, but beware of misleading drug ads that exaggerate benefits and minimize risks (see p. 729 in Chapter 31, "The Politics of Women's Health"). For more information, see "Bones, Falls, and Fractures," p. 564, and see "Prevention and Treatment of Osteoporosis in Women" [W61] on the companion website, www.ourbodiesourselves.org.

DEPRESSION

Being depressed is not typical of aging in general, though an ageist culture certainly doesn't help anyone's mental health. Because women live longer, we are vulnerable to life events that cause sadness and even depression: loss of a spouse or partner, poverty, chronic illness, loneliness, and isolation. If you lose your appetite, don't feel sexual, can't enjoy anything, sleep too much or not enough, have difficulty making decisions, or keep thinking about death or suicide—and if such symptoms continue for over a month and talking to friends doesn't help—you may be depressed.

Therapy

Many mental health professionals are not used to working with elderly people. We need more trained geriatric social workers, psychologists, and psychiatrists. You might have to persist to find a therapist who trusts your ability to grow and develop. You may do best with someone in your age range. Medicare coverage for mental health services is probably as good as under most private health insurance plans, but an HMO's rules will restrict your options, and most plans limit the number of visits covered. That makes fees for ongoing psychotherapy prohibitive for many of us.

Medication

Drug treatment can sometimes relieve depression, but be aware that older people experience more and greater effects from psychoactive drugs, and some drugs may even cause or deepen depression. Low thyroid function, common in older people, can feel or look like depression, but it should be treated as a thyroid problem. (For more information on depression, see Chapter 6, "Emotional Well-Being.")

MEMORY CHANGES

Though memory is sharpest and quickest in our first twenty-five years, the brain's capacity to reorganize and grow connections continues throughout life. We don't all remember the same way: Some people are more visual (some even have photographic memory), while others recall aural information better. Smells or tastes can bring up memories of long ago. Mental exercise sharpens that capacity, so we really do need to use it or lose it.

Memory problems are more pervasive as we age. It takes more conscious effort to gather, learn, and recall details. It may take a few moments to remember a name, and much later, it may take even longer for facts to surface. Occasional forgetfulness may reflect no more than distraction or not paying attention to details. Older people may lose some memory power as measured by tests, but generally do better than young people on tasks requiring experience and judgment. One ninety-four-year-old woman says:

There's nothing wrong with my memory—it's all in there. It's only the retrieval system that's a little slower.

PREVENTING MEMORY LOSS

Clear Input

Changes in hearing, smell, taste, vision, and touch may cause gaps or errors in information entering the brain. Eyeglasses, better lighting, eye-to-eye contact, taking mental snapshots, using a hearing aid, having conversations in a quiet room, checking with the speaker to verify what you just heard, writing things down and looking at your notes, and managing stress well may help you retain clearer information.

Brain Exercise

It helps to do word games, crosswords, and jigsaw puzzles; to learn something new each day; to write or draw with your nondominant hand; to eat a healthy diet; to exercise regularly; to participate in interesting and fun activities; to develop positive relationships; and to do something that makes you feel worthwhile. Mental stimulation (reading, social activities, or interesting conversations) can increase your ability to remember. With the right kind of stimulation and therapy, it's sometimes possible to recover lost brain function after injury, such as an accident or a stroke.

Brain Food

A healthy diet for the memory is similar to that for general good health (see Chapter 2, "Eating Well"). We need to pay particular attention to eating foods that contain the B vitamins, especially B_6 and B_{12} (yeast, wheat germ, green leafy vegetables, and lean animal protein), omega-3 fatty acids (olive oil and fish), antioxidants (brightly colored, ripe fruits and vegetables) and resveratrol (grapes and blueberries). Exercise as you can, and drink plenty of fluids each day (unless your doctor advises otherwise for specific reasons). Avoid tobacco and limit alcohol intake;

both alcohol and tobacco contribute to diseases that can impair memory.

Drug Watch

Medications or drug interaction may leave your mind fuzzy or confused. To avoid drugs that damage memory, deal with infections and other health problems as soon as possible. If you need to take a drug, ask your health care provider and pharmacist whether it has an anti-memory effect. Over time, cardiovascular (heart and circulation) conditions or diabetes will affect blood flow to brain cells. If you have these diseases, try to control your blood pressure and blood sugar (see "Cardiovascular Problems," p. 671, and "Diabetes," p. 680).

Studies are under way of anti-inflammatory medicines, vaccines, and beta-secretase-lowering substances for prevention of Alzheimer's disease. Hormone therapy has been shown to increase the risk of cognitive decline, including Alzheimer's, and it is no longer recommended for anything beyond hot flashes and other menopausal discomforts (see Chapter 26, "Midlife and Menopause").[11]

Early Checkup

If you have short-term memory loss, a careful medical evaluation with various tests can determine whether the change is treatable or reversible, can be slowed down, or is progressive.

TREATABLE OR REVERSIBLE MEMORY DISORDERS

Ten to 15 percent of memory disorders are treatable or reversible if caught early enough. Such conditions include changes in thyroid balance, vitamin deficiency (especially vitamins B_1, B_6, B_{12}, folic acid, and niacin), and confusion from taking medicines such as antihistamines (in allergy or sleep medicines) or anticholinergics (in some pain, sleep, or incontinence medicines)—including over-the-counter drugs. Memory problems from traumatic or accumulated stress, depression, anxiety disorders, alcohol or chemical dependency, or dehydration can also be treated. With proper diagnosis and treatment, symptoms may disappear. Neglect of such conditions may result in dysfunction resembling Alzheimer's disease.

DEMENTIA AND ITS IMPACT ON WOMEN

Dementia is the decline of thinking abilities while one is alert and awake. It may affect memory, knowledge, decision skills, or communication. It can change personality, too. People with dementia may struggle with routine tasks, such as driving or cooking, and they may forget something they have just done, such as mailing a letter or eating a meal. Almost half the U.S. population over the age of eighty-five has some kind of dementia.[12]

Because we live longer, more women than men have Alzheimer's disease. You may be left to struggle with it alone if you outlive your partner or your children. Alzheimer's and other dementias are also critical issues for women because caregivers are typically female (see "Caring for Someone with Memory Loss," p. 568).

VASCULAR DEMENTIA: TIA AND STROKE

A stroke is really a "brain attack" resulting in loss of oxygen. Any sudden changes such as abrupt memory loss, slurred speech, clumsy movements, numbness, tingling or weakness in any part of the body (especially on one side), or sudden personality changes are signs of stroke. Some people lose consciousness. People who suffer a stroke may have permanent difficulty remembering facts. *Stroke is an emergency situation, and immediate treatment is critical to minimize brain damage.* Moments of dizziness, caused by lack of blood getting to the brain, may indicate a transient ischemic attack (TIA, or mini-stroke), but sometimes there's no warning. A person who has shown signs of a stroke should be monitored for a few days; a second stroke may occur within forty-eight hours.

PROGRESSIVE DEMENTIA: ALZHEIMER'S

Alzheimer's disease, Pick's disease, and Lewy body disease are all progressive dementias. Alzheimer's, the most common one, affects more than 4 million Americans. Because the number of cases increases with age and more people are living longer, the number of people living with the disease at any time is also increasing. About 10 percent of people over sixty-five have it.[13] The cause of Alzheimer's is unknown, but research is looking at connections among inflammation, metabolism, genetics, and brain damage. Alzheimer's disease is not contagious, nor is it caused by seepage from aluminum pots and pans.

Forgetfulness, the first stage, can be dealt with by using reminders, calendars, timers that buzz, and routines that become habits. Forgetting where you put your keys is not Alzheimer's; forgetting that keys open doors might be. Confusion, the second stage, can cause clumsy movements, problems remembering time, and difficulty understanding statements or questions. Home help may be needed for daily routines such as meals or bathing. In the third stage, severe dementia, constant assistance and supervision are needed.

TREATING MEMORY LOSS

Memory loss is often very distressing, both for anyone who has it and for loved ones. There is no cure for Alzheimer's, although vitamin E and antioxidants may help by reducing cell and circulatory damage, and several types of medicines

CARING FOR SOMEONE WITH MEMORY LOSS

Dealing with [Mom] used to be like dealing with a six-year-old, and now it reminds me of taking care of a two-year-old. The odd thing is, peeping out from under the Alzheimer's are bits of her personality—she's still a trouper when it comes to facing medical procedures, she still loves going out to dinner, she is still happy to see me—although she is beginning to struggle with my name.

It may be harder to deal with the person's emotional reactions than with forgetfulness. Avoid confronting or repeated questioning—it's not likely to improve the situation. What does help is being emotionally present and loving in the moment. Communicate with touch, pictures, and humor. People with serious memory loss may try to make sense of what is confusing or try to fill in the gaps, so they may seem to be lying or making things up, but they aren't.

In later stages, safety measures are essential, since a person with Alzheimer's may wander from home or get lost (see "Safe Return Program" and other suggestions in "Resources"). If a person with Alzheimer's becomes violent, get professional help immediately. Most families try to cope at home as long as possible, then find they need to reconsider.

Early education of the primary family caregiver and planning with the whole family unit (and perhaps a clergyperson and neighbors) can help with long-term care management and unexpected issues. Working with health experts, community, and support organizations can provide emotional support and pragmatic, simple suggestions about care.

The wife of a man with Alzheimer's says:

No one person can handle dementia care alone. Let me repeat: You cannot do Alzheimer's alone. Don't even try.

The daughter of a man with Alzheimer's says:

We're putting my father in a nursing home in a week or so. He's declining so rapidly, mentally, my mother can't cope any more. The rapidity of his decline is what shocks me. At Christmas [four months ago] he was still reading The Wall Street Journal.

may improve functioning. More research needs to be done on treatments and cure.

CAREGIVING AND NEEDING CARE

GIVING CARE: FOR WOMEN WHO ARE CAREGIVERS

Women have been the primary caregivers throughout the generations. With increased longevity, a growing number of us are lucky to see our parent(s) live to old age as we ourselves age. The resulting responsibilities have to be balanced with workplace and other family commitments. Many of us care for parents, in-laws, spouses, and relatives for more years than we spend rearing children.

There are 44.4 million caregivers in the United States, each of whom provides care for an adult eighteen years or older; 79 percent of these are taking care of someone fifty or older. Sixty-one percent of all caregivers are women;

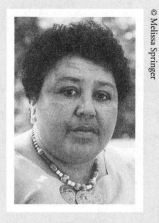

© Melissa Springer

"I AM A CONFLICTED CAREGIVER"

JUDY SIMMONS

After evading marriage and children (the two were linked in my formative years), I am at age 51 in my fifth year of tending to my mother. She needs help to live with Alzheimer's disease and I am it. . . .

In a Reader's Digest*-like version of our heartwarming story, I would be the family-values heroine who gives up a high-powered New York media career and discovers the true meaning of life wiping bowel movement off her feisty 70-something mother, the spunky most unforgettable character of the month. My less genteel version of this travail casts Momma as indeed a game person playing a poor hand with determination, but I am a conflicted caregiver. . . .*

I have at every point underestimated what I've let myself in for in choosing to care for a loved one with Alzheimer's disease. Remaining rational from moment to moment, day to day, takes unusual effort. The unpredictability of Momma's condition undermines my ability to order my life. I can't have expectations about her comprehension and ca-pabilities, and it's surprising how much expectation figures in life: the sun will rise; the ground won't open up and swallow us at our next step; she pulled down her underwear when she went to the toilet this morning so she'll do the same this afternoon . . . I wish. I'm called on to live in the moment, as metaphysicians often advise, but that can be anxiety-producing. And, for someone like me who is used to a lot of autonomy, such interdependence and lack of control generate a fair amount of frustration and resentment. . . .

At least Mom has a livable income, and she has me; still we are pressed. She needs physical therapy, for instance, but doesn't qualify under strict Medicare criteria and our budget doesn't stretch. . . .

My biggest challenge is emotional control. The sustaining rage of my life is my undoing now. It's my response, my defense, my coping mechanism, my motive power, has been for much of my life. Rage against segregation, injustice, amoral capitalism, against petty greed, lyin', cheatin' hearts, and fundamentalists of all kinds. Noble, artistic rage that fueled my ambition to write world-changing poems. Idealistic, pioneering rage that drove me to hurt myself proving that a woman and a Black person could cut it in Fortune 500land.

But the rage that propelled me to socially constructive acts of art and freedom struggle is incompatible with and destructive to the domestic, nurturing enterprise I have undertaken. Yet I still have it. So many frightening realities are bearing down on me that I maintain the little sanity I lay claim to by taking it one day, one hour, one minute at a time—when I can think clearly enough to remember that, when I can hold myself that still.*

* To read the complete essay from which this excerpt was taken, see "I Am My Mother's Keeper" (W62) on the companion website, www.ourbodiesourselves.org. The original essay was published in *Ms.*, July/August 1996, and is reprinted with permission of the author.

41 percent of these women are working full-time, and 14 percent are working part-time. Sixty-five percent of working women who are caregivers have had to make workplace adjustments, such as going in late or leaving early, taking a leave of absence, moving from full-time to part-time, giving up work entirely, giving up job benefits, turning down a promotion, or choosing to retire early.[14] Nonetheless, our caregiving is often taken for granted, and we receive little validation, support, or appreciation.

Research shows that caregivers have higher rates of depression, chronic disease, infection, and exhaustion than peers the same age who don't look after others. One of a caregiver's greatest challenges is to balance her own needs with her multiple responsibilities. Caregiving may raise the question of who will be there to care for us.

We rushed my husband to the hospital with a stroke, and it was a medical miracle. Now I am not so sure it was a blessing. He is not always rational and cannot be left alone. . . . I had to give up my job. Financially, we are in terrible shape, but disaster will strike when he dies. I am 57 and won't be eligible for anything. I can't see my way out.

Many resources exist to help caregivers, but we need to advocate for more comprehensive public policies that would ease the burdens of care-giving.

Caring for Parents

Caring for parents offers a final opportunity to work on relationships, communicate what you want to, and be at peace. It can involve hands-on care, assistance with tasks of daily living, and knowledge about the medical, legal, and financial aspects of long-term care. It can create stress, physical strain, and exhaustion. Often family caregiving still means that you will be providing care in isolation, without pay or supportive services, with no one to take over when you need a break, and possibly without job retraining, a pension, Social Security, tax credits, or even health insurance. You may have some help, but that help can be expensive. It's often difficult to find time for yourself.

There is also a tremendous range in living situations: Parents might live independently, in assisted living, in continuing care communities, or in nursing homes locally or long-distance. They may live with you, or you may move in with them.

Caring for parents in their old age can be extremely satisfying. A fifty-three-year-old daughter says:

I admire my mother's adaptability at age 82. It's wonderful having her close by. I feel blessed to have this time with her.

Getting Help with Caregiving

With increased numbers of women in the workforce, fewer siblings to share caregiving, geographic distance between family members, and more years of caregiving, it is often difficult for primary caretakers to get help. Yet we cannot do it alone.

Respite care, even for a weekend, can help you if you work full-time. *Adult day care* can help with an elderly relative living at home by providing support and company during the day. The

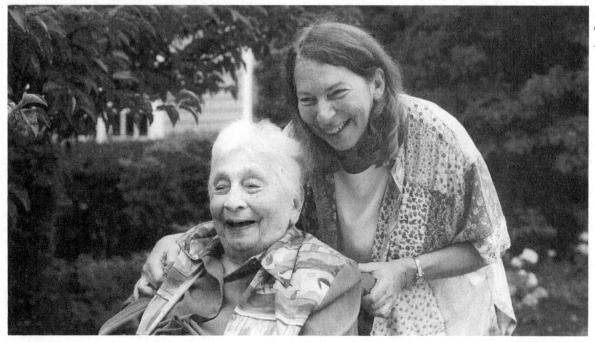

© Jörg Meyer

National Family Caregiver Support Program* is the first universal federal program providing some support for caregivers. (For information in your area, call the Eldercare Locator, 1-800-677-1116.)

Long-term care services are currently fragmented and expensive. Out-of-pocket expenses for long-term care represent the greatest financial risk for older adults, especially those who have cognitive, physical, or mental problems. *Medicare* covers only short-term home care or nursing home care for acute illness after a hospital stay. All other expenses must be paid out of pocket, including long-term care at home, in the community or in a nursing home. *Medicaid* is a primary source of funding for home care and nursing home care, but only those of us with very low incomes or who spend down all our assets until we become low-income are eligible. *Private long-term care insurance* usually has strict limits on the kind of care covered and where it must occur for it to be reimbursed. Most people sixty-five or older lack adequate coverage for long-term care. Also, most long-term care insurance covers only skilled nursing and some help with bathing, dressing, and using the toilet, not the housekeeping help many older people need (such as shopping, cooking, and laundry).

Those of us who care for aging parents need flextime, part-time work, job sharing, leave without penalties, and a tax break. We also need affordable help. The Family and Medical Leave Act† is a good start but needs to be expanded. Recognition of family caregivers and funding for

---

* The National Family Caregiver Support Program, created in 2001, provides information, support, counseling, respite, and other services to all family caregivers.

† The Family and Medical Leave Act (1993) requires employers to grant twelve weeks of unpaid leave each year to care for a newborn or adopted child or a seriously ill family member or to recover from one's own serious health condition. It does not cover temporary or part-time workers and applies only to companies with more than fifty employees.

TIPS FOR FAMILY CAREGIVERS

1. Recognize signs that you need help. Household chores or personal care may require two people. Fatigue means that you need more rest, help at home, a better diet, exercise, improved sleeping conditions, less stress, and time off (respite care).
2. Get a medical evaluation for the person needing care to identify any problems and how to treat them. Learn about the condition you are dealing with, and how to manage it. Locate local resources for assistance.
3. Discuss spiritual values and preferences, especially choices about final health care and death. Take care of legal matters early, especially durable power of attorney and health care proxy (see "Advance Directives," p. 579, and "Planning for Death," p. 580). Share the information with at least one trustworthy person who does not live in the same home as you.

long-term care policies and programs that support and supplement families as caregivers for elderly relatives should become a priority for public policy.

Needs of Paid Caregivers

Workers in long-term care occupations—such as nurses, nurses' aides, personal care attendants, and home care workers—are mostly women and are grossly underpaid. Women of color and recent immigrants often occupy the lowest-paid jobs. These jobs require a lot of standing and lifting, and workers are more likely to develop chronic conditions such as leg and back pain. Those of us who do these jobs may require care sooner than middle-class white women, but are less likely to have the money or insurance coverage to pay for it. We may also have to leave our own parents or kids at home to take care of other people's loved ones.

All women concerned with caregiving, whether as family caregivers or as paid workers, must join together to affirm the value of this work and demand a decent wage with good benefits.

ACCEPTING CARE: FOR THOSE OF US WHO NEED CARE

Women accept and even expect that others will depend on us, yet many of us fear becoming dependent ourselves. Chronic illness or a new disability may be a blow to our pride and habits of self-sufficiency.

If we haven't had to do so before, we face learning to accept assistance without resentment or loss of pride. It helps when those providing care do so without taking over or taking away all choices. And it helps when those needing care can accept offered help graciously.

An eighty-two-year-old woman says:

As a widow at age 80 I had been living alone, and it was becoming harder for me to get around. A lot of my friends had died. . . . The solution for me was to relocate to a long-term care community close to my daughter. This gave me independence with family support nearby. My move has enabled my daughter and me to renew our relationship. We have built up a friendship based on a deep understanding of each other. I truly treasure this in my old age.

It's a good idea to plan ahead with family members or friends about the kind of care and living situation you want if you can no longer manage at home. Then, if a crisis occurs, they will have all the information they will need.

IMPORTANT PAPERS

Certain documents and information may be needed by whoever is taking care of you and your possessions in the event of illness or death. Make sure those closest to you know where the following papers are:

- Social Security number and benefits information
- Health insurance information for Medicare, Medicaid, Medigap, and long-term care
- Will, durable power of attorney, health care proxy, advance directive/living will
- Insurance: auto, homeowners, liability, disability, and life
- Financial: checkbook, savings account passbook, stock and bond certificates, trust and/or estate planning information, pension plan documents, 401(k)/IRA information
- Mortgage papers, property deed, home equity loan papers
- Automobile title document
- Income tax returns
- Burial plot deed and any prepaid funeral agreement

LIVING ARRANGEMENTS

LIVING INDEPENDENTLY

Despite differences in well-being, living conditions, and income levels, most women want to be self-sufficient and to live at home as long as possible.

I have a great abhorrence for nursing homes. I would rather struggle with overcoming physical difficulties in my own home than be put in the hands of people that I'm paying and then have to please them so they'll be nice to me.

A variety of community services can help individuals and couples to stay at home. Visiting nurses, social workers, physical therapists, occupational therapists, and home health aides may be available to perform needed services. Other services include local or municipal transportation programs; Meals on Wheels, which delivers hot lunches to older people at home, usually five days a week; community meals and other activities at senior centers, community centers, or houses of worship; telephone reassurance; counseling services; adult day care; and hospice. Emergency response systems offer rescue services to older people with potentially life-threatening conditions who live alone, and some phone companies have special services.

Long-term-care services are not available everywhere. When you are seeking home care, it can be challenging to judge quality. If you hire someone through an agency, you may not be able to interview the worker in advance. In recent years, policy makers have touted home care services as a way to save money on expensive nursing homes. But home care services are subject to budget cuts. Too many of us are without any services, and our caregivers without respite. Many are on waiting lists nationwide.

For information about resources in your area, call Eldercare Locator at 1-800-677-1116 (www.eldercare.gov). Nearly all regional and local agencies and councils on aging will send a trained social worker to evaluate your situation and identify the resources and services that are available to you. Many communities have senior housing subsidized by federal, state, or local agencies, as well as day programs.

ALTERNATIVE LIVING ARRANGEMENTS

As we grow older, living with others is not only cost-effective but also care-effective, because housemates can look out for one another, rather than paying others to do so. Options include cooperative, intergenerational living with relatives or friends; congregate housing (a managed home with some supportive services where residents have private rooms and share meals and activities in common space); turning part of a house into an "in-law" apartment; building a separate unit on the same land for a friend or relative; and small group homes. Many older women have the strength, will, and independence of spirit to make the changes required for new living arrangements. While many of us enjoy the company of our own generation, some prefer mixed-age housing.

If you want or will need alternative housing for yourself or a family member, start planning early. Attractive places are hard to find and have long waiting lists. Also, applicants often need to be in good health. Waiting until you are sick limits your options.

ASSISTED LIVING

These facilities provide rooms or apartments as well as a range of services in a communal setting, a middle ground for elderly people who need daily assistance but not full-time skilled nursing care. Assisted living facilities may also be called boarding care, congregate living, or residential care facilities. They are usually not subject to the same regulations as nursing homes, and they may refuse those who need nursing care or who do not meet their requirements. For some people, the flexibility and nonmedical approach of assisted living is a plus.

Privately run boarding facilities are an informal mode of assisted living, especially in states with few regulations. They may be suitable when you do not need nursing or case management but prefer not to be alone.

Assisted living facilities are more available in some areas than others, and for many of us, the cost may be out of reach. Community activists for affordable housing can help by including assisted living apartments in the developments they propose. This type of affordable housing will be needed increasingly as the over-sixty-five population increases.

LIFE CARE OR CONTINUING CARE COMMUNITIES

These communities offer apartment living for people in relatively good health, with medical and social services nearby and assisted living units and a nursing home on the premises—in other words, a continuum of care from minimal to round-the-clock. For an entrance fee and monthly charges, residents are guaranteed a permanent place to live and a specified package of medical and nursing benefits to suit changing needs. Some have units specializing in memory loss for people with dementia. Such communities enable people to keep up activities and relationships and to obtain health care without having to move.

Whether nonprofit or for-profit, life care communities should be regulated by law. Before signing up, always get a written agreement specifying the care and living alternatives available; your rights to terminate the contract and receive a refund; and the conditions under which you might be discharged. Find out whether the money you invest goes to the corporation or is returned after your death to your heirs (that's what should happen in communities that emphasize private ownership of units). Get everything in writing, and have the community's financial statement reviewed by your accountant, estate planner, or lawyer.

Only you can decide whether a facility is right for you, and whether the amount of energy you will need to assert your rights there is worth it at a time of limited energy and need for support. Unfortunately, many of these places are so expensive that they serve only the upper and upper-middle classes. Some communities are run as co-ops by the residents, which allows them to avoid federal guidelines prohibiting discrimination against disabled people and minority groups. Some staff and residents may hint that people from the working class or a different religion or culture will not feel "comfortable" at a particular facility. Some do not welcome gays and lesbians, who may go back into the closet upon moving in. Still, when continuing care communities are truly welcoming, inclusive, attractive, and well-run, they provide a terrific model that we as an aging society could adopt to make the older years a time of activity, growth, and safety for all of us.

A seventy-two-year-old writes:

I have always said that when I became frail, I would rather be in a nursing home singing around the piano with other residents than alone in my house. I have picked out a continuing care community that helps people stay in their own units and whose nursing home, when needed, is run on the Eden philosophy [see p. 576] with pets, more resident control, and a less medicalized atmosphere. That's where I'll go when I sell my house in a few years.

NURSING HOMES

If we need fairly constant nursing care, we may have to go into nursing homes. On any given day, only 5 percent of elders live in nursing homes, but 75 percent of those who do are women. One quarter of all women eighty-five years and older live in nursing homes.

The biggest problem with nursing homes is

that routines, schedules, and medicalization limit daily life. Many facilities refuse to let couples share a room or have any privacy, and staff attitudes about sex among older people may be demeaning to residents. There are exceptions, though. A fifty-eight-year-old woman says:

When my wheelchair-bound mother-in-law was 88 and living in a nursing home, she met the only ambulatory man there, age 85. They fell in love. The nursing staff came to her and said that they could move him into her room, and she said, "Oh no, I want to maintain my independence."

Often, in the interest of "efficiency," routines that are designed for only the sickest residents limit healthier people's options. Lacking any meaningful decisions to make, residents of conventional nursing homes may become depressed, withdrawn, confused, and disoriented. Physical and mental abilities deteriorate without mental stimulation or chances to exercise and carry out simple tasks independently.

We need to evaluate nursing homes carefully, since quality of care varies tremendously. Look for group activities, posted calendars of events, and individualized rooms where residents keep some of their own furniture and possessions. Inquire about staff training, staff turnover, the ratio of nurses to residents, and the range of activities. Ask visitors how their relatives are treated. A good source of information is the ombudsman at your state or area eldercare agency or council on aging. Some are cautious about challenging the nursing home administration and will give only positive recommendations, saying little about the bad ones. Some may give hints, such as "You may prefer to try another one." Some more progressive places have tried to provide for the needs of women from diverse cultures by offering more varied meal menus and cultural exchange programs:

My mother was much better able to cope with Western food when she could look forward to occasional Eastern meals at the nursing home's new "international nights." Her health and attitude improved, and she began talking to other residents and staff about her native Korean recipes.

Some aspects of conventional nursing home care, such as the skyrocketing costs, impersonal care, medicalization of everyday life, and lack of privacy and choices for residents, are negative. Care is sometimes inadequate, with owners putting profits ahead of quality, underpaying workers, and skimping on patients' needs. Patients are often discharged as quickly as possible from hospitals, while home care services have been reduced. The result is waiting lists for admission, or premature admission for people who would stay at home if services were available. Some residents could return home if home care services existed. But because nursing home care is essential for some, the quality of life and care needs to be improved so that residents have more control. A new advocacy organization working with long-term-care professionals and family members to enliven nursing home life is called the Eden Alternative.[15]

State and federal laws provide protection for nursing home residents. The 1987 Nursing Home Reform Act sets standards for quality of life and quality of care, and provides for unannounced inspections. Residents also have specific rights, including rights to self-determination and information. To find out more about advocating for the rights of nursing home residents, contact the National Citizens' Coalition for Nursing Home Reform (see "Resources").

Planning Ahead

It's best to begin talking about health care and new living arrangements when you are in good health, and to involve the whole family. Family meetings can help clarify what you expect of one another. If communication is difficult, ask an outside person such as a social worker or a member of the clergy to join you. Many families avoid such meetings, dreading the unpleasant subjects of illness and dependency. You can't predict the future, but the more prepared you are, the more likely your wishes will be respected (see also "Advance Directives," p. 579). A health care institution that will not honor your wishes must, according to federal law, tell you so upon admission so that you can go elsewhere.

ELDER ABUSE

In a violent society where women's safety is often threatened, you may be even more vulnerable because of frailty, immobility, or unwillingness to believe that anyone could wish you harm. Those of us who are older are mugged on the street or attacked in our homes by burglars who think we won't or can't fight back. Many of us in hospitals, rehab facilities, or nursing homes are afraid to complain about problems, fearing that staff members will take it out on us. And, if you are accustomed to trusting people and the printed word, you may become a victim of scams, ordering merchandise you don't need or donating to bogus charities. Here are ways you can protect yourself:

- Verify the identity of anyone you don't know before opening your door or giving out any information. Don't let strangers in, even if they claim to be "lost" or "not feeling well."
- Don't give your Social Security or bank account number to anyone over the phone.
- Don't give credit card numbers over the phone unless you have called the merchant yourself.
- Ask people you know and trust to check on you regularly.

- If you are badly treated by staff anywhere, report it and have a family member or friend file a complaint.
- If you are abused by a member of your family, call the police (911).

END-OF-LIFE DECISIONS

Increasingly, we confront the reality of death. Parents, children, and people we love die. Acceptance of the reality of our own death comes for many of us as we grow older.

A seventy-eight-year-old woman says:

We don't talk about dying. So, our denial of death and dealing with death gets us into a lot of traps. Sometimes we clutch life and are not really being able to create choice about where we will be for our last days and minutes. If we stop aging, we die. Yay for aging!

For some of us, this stimulates a deepening of religious faith or, if we haven't been religious, an increased interest in spirituality. Another woman, also seventy-eight, says:

I am more aware of a mystery and beauty in life since I have accepted death as a personal eventuality for me. . . . That has released me for more vivid living. I reach out more. . . . I do not look to the future with dread. It has to be shorter than my past, but it does not have to be less rich.

It's also common to feel ambivalent and scared about acknowledging death or to have difficulty coming to grips with its reality. One seventy-four-year-old woman explains:

Intellectually, I'm very glib about it, but in my gut, I can't accept that one day I won't be here.

An eighty-five-year-old woman says:

*I doubt that when I die, my life will be over—my
life with all its loving and caring and striving.
Can it be that all my loved ones—mother, sister,
other relatives—can all this love be gone? Nothing
in nature disappears. Out of our bones, our skele-
tons, new life comes in some other way.*

Medical science, rather than concern for quality
of life, often shapes dying and death these days.
Women are more likely to face end-of-life circumstances with chronic disease and disability
in hospitals or nursing homes. Doctors frequently use every medical means possible to
defy death and prolong life for its own sake without considering whether there is any hope of recovery. Some even ignore the ill person's wishes
for palliative (comfort) care.

MAKING DECISIONS ABOUT OUR DEATH

We cannot control whether or when we die, yet
we can sometimes exercise elements of choice
and control with end-of-life decisions. New life-
sustaining medical technologies, such as respirators and feeding tubes, benefit some but burden
others. It's up to you to say what you want or
don't want. It may be possible to choose where
you die—at home or in a hospital or hospice facility. You may choose medical care that relieves
extreme pain and allows you to keep your dignity, instead of accepting aggressive treatment
inappropriate for terminal illness. Compassionate end-of-life care is essential.

Though legal, medical, and theological con-
troversies abound, the right to make decisions
about what constitutes a tolerable quality of life

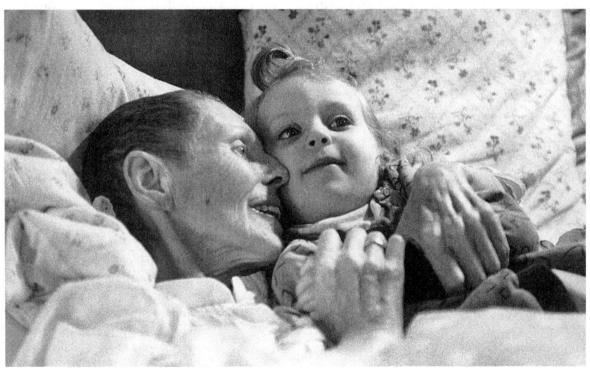

© Paula Lerner

A dying woman holds her granddaughter close.

and worthwhile existence is part of our basic right to control our bodies and our lives.

A woman in her seventies says:

I have been searching for a doctor who would let me participate not just in my health care but in my own death, too.

Another woman says:

I've had a lot of things done to my body, and I'm 73. I've made up my mind that enough has been done to me. If something bad happens, something major, I'm not sure I want to be repaired again. No more tampering with my body! I don't want to live to be 100 if I'm all botched up.

ADVANCE DIRECTIVES

You may actively decide to avoid a long, drawn-out period of illness and dependence, or a medicalized death in which life is prolonged by artificial means. All fifty states and the District of Columbia authorize some type of advance directive, living will, or health care proxy (appointment of a health care agent). The Patient Self-Determination Act requires hospitals, nursing homes, and other health care facilities to ask people whether they know they can make advance directives and to provide necessary information and documents. Yet in practice, few people complete advance directives, and many doctors don't encourage discussion. Some doctors ignore requests to avoid "heroic measures" such as mechanical ventilation or feeding tubes, or they delay writing up "do not resuscitate" (DNR) orders.

Living wills, much less specific than advance directives, are valid only in cases of terminal illness, not for slow degenerative disease or for a very old person whose vital organs just give out ("multiple systems failure"). They are also not useful for the person who wants to have every possible treatment tried. For all of these situations, a durable power of attorney for medical affairs ("Planning for Death," see p. 580) is more useful.

RIGHT TO DIE

Some of us want to choose the occasion and means of our death. U.S. constitutional and common law in all states supports the right of any competent adult to refuse medical treatment in any situation, but this is not the same as the right to commit suicide or to aid someone in ending his or her life. At the same time, our flawed and inadequate medical care system promotes abuse of the "right to die." Advocates for low-income communities are concerned that if this right is adopted without recognition of a "right to care," those without money or insurance will be pressured to choose the cheaper alternative. One study found that people whose funds were running out were more likely to reject life-prolonging care.[16]

Permitting suicide should not be a way for the medical system to shirk its responsibility to provide support and comfort to the dying. Also, some people who say they want to die are really saying they can't bear living with severe pain or depression—which may be treatable, making life much more bearable.

Some people prefer to die surrounded by family and friends. Some may be thinking about taking a fatal substance. You may even not tell loved ones about your plans, to avoid legal hassles for them. An important way to gain the power to choose our own death is working through advocacy organizations to change the laws and social attitudes related to death and dying and challenging legal, medical, and religious control.

Claiming the right to make decisions about the end of life in no way minimizes the seriousness or the finality of the decision, nor the pain

PLANNING FOR DEATH

1. Designate a health care proxy. Pick someone (eighteen or older) to act for you in the event that you are unable to make health care decisions. Make sure this person knows your end-of-life wishes and is willing to carry them out. Fill out and sign the forms with two witnesses, keep the original, and give copies to your health care proxy, family, doctor, lawyer, and clergyperson.

2. Write an advance directive stating your end-of-life wishes. Specify the situations in which you do or don't want life-sustaining efforts (feeding tubes, ventilators, etc.). Such documents are not binding in all states but can provide guidelines for your health care proxy and doctors.

3. Ask your doctor to fill out a comfort care/do not resuscitate (DNR) form if you do not want to be "brought back" should your heart or breathing stop. Give your loved ones copies, and make sure the form is in your file if you are in a hospital, rehab, or nursing home.

4. Meet with a spiritual or religious adviser and discuss spiritual values and choices about final health care and death.

5. Make a will, set up trust funds if appropriate, and choose how you want your property distributed. Decide if you want to donate organs such as kidneys and corneas for transplant, and put those instructions in a separate statement.

6. Decide on funeral arrangements, and discuss with family what kind of memorial service you want, if and where you want to be buried, or if you want to be cremated.

and grief of those we leave behind. The issues are complex. It is certainly more appropriate for you, rather than any outside authority, to weigh all the factors involved and then decide whether your life is worth living.

HOSPICE CARE

Hospices—and hospice services at home—are intended as a humane alternative to hospital or nursing home end-of-life care. Hospice aims to comfort people who are dying, rather than to prolong life. Hospice workers help manage pain. They can also assist with dying comfortably at home, if primary caregivers are available, or in hospice facilities, which may be self-contained or attached to a hospital. They provide services for the rest of the family as well as the dying person, offering support, understanding, respite, and attention to spiritual and emotional needs as well as physical ones. Bereavement counseling may continue for a substantial length of time beyond a family member's death. Medicare pays for hospice services only when someone is expected to live for six months or less. But even doctors can't always be sure whether an illness is terminal. These services may be needed earlier and over a longer period of time, though most people use them for a shorter time.

Hospice services cannot be provided to a person living alone in her own home unless there are family members or others available to be with her, or money to hire extra help around the clock. Hospice services are now available in many nursing homes. The nursing home continues to provide round-the-clock staff and regular care while the hospice agency provides additional pain control, special workers, supervision, and services to the family, just as if the nursing home resident were in her own home or in a special hospice facility.

GROUP SUPPORT FOR A DYING PERSON

Some of us want to be connected with friends and community when we are very sick and dying.

When Esther, longtime friend and member of our women's group, was dying of breast cancer, she drew upon the love of her three communities, her family, her synagogue, and ourselves. . . . We took turns doing whatever was wanted or needed. We attended her, sat with her, her husband and sons. We brought cooked food, planted the spring garden she loved, helped her finish the book she was writing. Accepting our offerings, she presided over all activities in a clear firm way, seated in her living room chair. It was a sad, peaceful rich time; she made it easier for us. She had a gift for giving to each of us in the measure that we gave to her, down to the smallest details, up to the very last moment when she died peacefully with her family around her. It gave us ease to surround her with love.

BEREAVEMENT

The death-denying culture of the United States has a long way to go to provide emotional, spiritual, and physical comfort for dying individuals and grieving families. Religious and ethnic customs and rituals may help people deal with terminal illness, and enable those of us left behind to express grief and celebrate the life that has ended. Many hospices, hospitals, community centers, and houses of worship offer bereavement groups. It's important to remain available for our friends as they adjust to life without their loved ones.

SURVIVAL SKILLS

We are adaptable. We may never "get over" setbacks, but it's possible to continue living well.

A seventy-seven-year-old woman says:

The seventies have been the best decade of my life. From what I have seen with my friends, it is either the best or the worst. My creative work as an artist is what keeps me alive; my friends keep me happy and contented. If I had to give up people, I would never have another happy day, but I would stay alive if I could work.

We can't deny human mortality and the physical changes we experience. But we can slow down, reverse, treat, and manage some of them, and age well. We can redefine "old" and empower ourselves through our attitudes and lifestyles.

There's a discrepancy between my image of an older person in her 70s and the way I feel. In fact, there's no connection. My concept of a grandmother was of someone who didn't do much. But I became a grandmother at 47. I started a vigorous exercise program at 43 and am still running every day at 76 and love it.

In our later years many of us feel more entitled than ever before to do what pleases and satisfies us, to slow down, to let go of the strain of former obligations, and to express thoughts and feelings more strongly than ever before.

A sixty-five-year-old woman says:

Getting old can be wonderful if you're not imposed on by other people's rules about how you should be when you're old. I consciously break as many as I can, because then I'm breaking through oppression.

A seventy-eight-year-old woman says:

I savor life more often. Elemental things of life have assumed greater importance. . . . I am more aware of the importance of touching (both physical and emotional), of communication, of tenderness. Space and time for quiet reflection are more available for me now. In a strange way, impossible to put into words, I am experiencing a unity beyond space and time.

CONTINUING EDUCATION AND LIFELONG LEARNING

Many educational opportunities are available in our later years, often at modest cost. Community colleges and public universities, institutes for learning in retirement, and organizations such as Elderhostel have programs in which to learn new subjects and skills, and to keep our minds alert. This is also a good way to share an interest with new friends. (To find more information on education programs, see "Resources.")

SPIRITUALITY AND EMOTIONAL WELL-BEING

Staying in touch with yourself helps you reach out to others, cope with difficulties, and continue to grow. There are many ways to connect with your deepest feelings—writing in a journal, meditating, spending time outdoors, taking a long hot shower or bath. Some women are strongly connected with a spiritual community:

Last week, at age 73, I sat in a group of older women discussing religion and spirituality and was reminded of our midweek prayer meetings 60 years ago. . . . I nourish my spirit through music,

nature study, and meditation, but mostly through relatedness to people I love.

Four years ago, at age 81, I got diabetes. It has impaired my living condition, but it doesn't get me down. In fact, I have always had the feeling that the more we have to fight and overcome, the stronger we are. . . . That's part of life, and it gives us a good feeling that we are not just little ants, we are fighters. Sometimes a frail body can draw its strength from a courageous mind.

FRIENDS, SUPPORT GROUPS, AND COMMUNITY ACTIVITY

Friendship is valuable not only for happiness and mental well-being but for physical health and survival. Many of us know well how to form and sustain friendships. It's possible to overcome loneliness and isolation by reweaving and changing family relationships, nurturing old connections, and reaching out to new friends.

It is never too late to form a support group. Joining advocacy organizations builds our communities and has the wonderful benefit of forging supportive networks of friends and colleagues.

Going to the March for Women's Lives was one of the most thrilling and exciting things I have ever done in my 85 years. The local League of Women Voters had organized buses that would drive from our retirement community to Washington, D.C., and then drive along slowly at the rear so that those of us who couldn't walk that far could participate. Being part of such an important event with all those young women was electrifying.

We must build a society that empowers and supports us as we age, fosters interdependence among the generations, and strengthens the connections in our families, communities, and institutions that sustain people from life to death. What we do as we age will influence people, policy, and attitudes for future generations.

NOTES

1. U.S. Bureau of Census 2000, compiled by the Administration on Aging.
2. Administration on Aging, U.S. Department of Health and Human Services, "Profile of Older Americans: 2003," accessed at www.aoa.gov/prof/statistics/profile/2003/2003profile.pdf on October 29, 2004.
3. Alliance for Aging Research, *Will You Still Treat Me When I'm 65?* (Washington, D.C.: 1996), 9.
4. Alliance for Aging Research, *Medical Never-Never Land: Ten Reasons Why America Is Not Ready for the Coming Age Boom* (Washington, D.C., 2002), 13.
5. International Longevity Center U.S.A., *A National Crisis: The Need for Geriatrics Faculty Training and Development: Toward Functional Independence in Old Age* (New York: 2002), 4.
6. D. S. Friedman, N. G. Congdon, J. Kempen, J. M. Tielsch, B. O'Culmain, *Vision Problems in the U.S.: Prevention of Adult Vision Impairment and Age-Related Eye Diseases in America*, 4th ed. (Schaumburg, IL: Prevent Blindness America, 2002), 18.
7. American Association of Retired Persons, "Facts About Hearing Loss," *AARP Disability Initiative: Fact Sheet*, 1992.
8. J. M. Wright, "The Double-edged Sword of COX-2 Selective NSAIDs," *Canadian Medical Association Journal* 167, no. 10 (November 2002): 1131–37.
9. Maria A. Fiatarone et al., "High-Intensity Strength Training in Nonagenarians: Effects on Skeletal Muscle," *Journal of the American Medical Association* 263, no. 22 (1990): 3029–34.
10. J. B. Lauritzen et al., "Effect of External Hip Protectors on Hip Fractures," *Lancet* 341 (January 2, 1993): 11–13.
11. S. A. Shumaker, C. Legault, S. R. Rapp, et al., "Estrogen Plus Progestin and the Incidence of Dementia and Mild Cognitive Impairment in Postmenopausal Women: The Women's Health Initiative Memory Study: a Randomized Controlled Trial," *Journal of the American Medical Association* 289, no. 20 (May 26, 2003): 2651–62.
12. D. A. Evans, H. H. Funkenstein, M. S. Albert, et al., "Prevalence of Alzheimer's Disease in a Community Population of Older Persons," *Journal of the American Medical Association* 262 (November 10, 1989): 2551–56.
13. Alzheimer's Association, "Statistics About Alzheimer's Disease," accessed at www.alz.org/AboutAD/statistics, on October 29, 2004.
14. National Alliance for Caregiving and AARP, "Caregiving in the U.S.," accessed at www.caregiving.org/04final report.pdf in April 2004.
15. William H. Thomas, *Life Worth Living: How Someone You Love Can Still Enjoy Life in a Nursing Home* (Acton, MA: VanderWyk & Burnham, 1996).
16. Kenneth E. Covinsky et al., "Is Economic Hardship on the Families of the Seriously Ill Associated with Patient and Surrogate Care Preferences?," *Archives of Internal Medicine* 156, no. 15 (1996): 1737.

Medical Problems and Procedures

CHAPTER 28

This chapter includes information on certain procedures and problems specific to women's bodies and organs. Chapter 29 covers medical conditions that affect large numbers of women or for which it is difficult to get reliable, women-centered information elsewhere. Both chapters include some alternatives to conventional medical treatments. Please be aware that information is constantly changing as a result of new research. (For related information, see Chapter 5, "Complementary Health Practices," and Chapter 30, "Navigating the Health Care System.")

The sections of this chapter are:

ROUTINE PHYSICAL EXAM AND BASIC TESTS

A routine physical exam, also called *well-woman care* or a *health maintenance exam,* provides an opportunity to uncover health problems that may not be obvious, and to review important preventive health measures. The annual checkup can also help you establish a more comfortable, ongoing relationship with your health care practitioner.

During any physical exam, your health care provider should take the time to explain exactly what she or he is doing and why. You are entitled to learn more about your body and to ask questions if you are unsure about anything. If your practitioner seems rushed or impatient, ask her

or him to take more time, either at this visit or some other time. If she or he is not responsive, consider switching to another provider. You might also bring along a friend or family member to act as your advocate. If you have a practitioner who is respectful, gentle, and informative, you will find it easier to relax during the exam. Although health care providers cannot guarantee the outcome of any exams, tests, or procedures, they have a responsibility to give you all the available information. If you have doubts or feel you need more information, seek another opinion.

A thorough general examination should include some or all of these features:

- Questions about individual and family history regarding medications, medical problems, work, family, and living circumstances
- Checks of blood pressure, pulse, height, and weight
- Examination of the eyes, nose, throat, skin, and nails
- Listening to the heart and lungs with the stethoscope
- Examination of the abdomen, nerves, muscles, and bones
- Manual breast examination
- Pelvic exam, including a rectal exam (especially if you are over forty)
- Pap test (taking a smear from the cervix with a swab)
- Tests for chlamydia and gonorrhea (swabs in the cervix) and possible screening for syphilis and/or HIV (blood tests) (see also Chapter 15, "Sexually Transmitted Infections")
- Blood test (hematocrit) to check for anemia, and a blood lipids analysis to measure fats such as cholesterol
- Blood sugar check if you have a family history of diabetes
- Urine test, which can detect infection, diabetes, and other problems

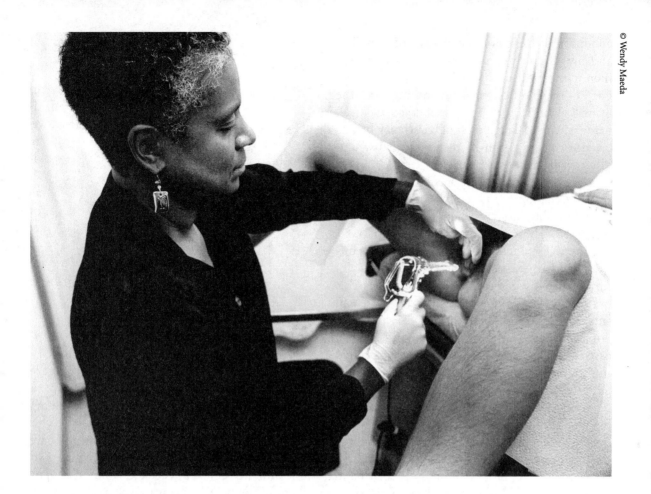

If you use traditional herbal medicine and/ or spiritual healing, inform your health care provider. It will enable him or her to help you make better use of Western medicine and to avoid negative interactions between prescription drugs and the remedies you are using.

PELVIC EXAM

A routine gynecological checkup should include an examination of your external genitals (vulva), a vaginal exam aided by a speculum, a bimanual internal exam, and a rectal examination. If you have been doing regular vaginal self-exams (see p. 591) or charting your menstrual cycle (see "Fertility Awareness," p. 245), you will be able to tell your health care provider about any changes you have noticed, or simply help her or him understand what is normal for you. If it's your first pelvic exam, say so. Ask the practitioner to go slowly and explain what she or he is doing. Be sure to empty your bladder before the exam. Also, your practitioner should put two gloves on the hand that touches your vulva while putting in the speculum, then take off the top glove before doing the internal exam (see next page) to make sure germs don't get inside you.

When examining the vulva, your provider will first check visually for irritations, discoloration, swelling, bumps, skin lesions, size and condition of the clitoris, hair distribution, lice, and any unusual vaginal discharge. She or he will then check internally with a finger for any Bartholin's gland cysts or pus coming from the Skene's glands. She or he will ask if you ever leak urine when you laugh or cough (urinary incontinence can be a sign of uterine prolapse and other problems; see p. 649).

Next, a metal or plastic speculum will be inserted in the vagina to hold the walls apart. (The speculum should be warmed, if metal, and put in gently.) The practitioner will examine your vaginal walls for lesions, inflammation, or unusual discharge; check your cervix (now visible) for unusual discharge, signs of infection, discoloration, damage, or growths; and take a Pap smear to examine for abnormal cervical cells. Sometimes a smear of vaginal discharge is taken as well, to test for certain sexually transmitted infections (see Chapter 15, "Sexually Transmitted Infections").

Some women experience pressure in the bladder or rectum with a speculum in place. Relaxing your muscles may help. If it doesn't, ask the practitioner to readjust the speculum or try a different size. Some practitioners keep a hand mirror available. If you wish to watch the exam to learn more, ask for help in positioning the mirror and light source. After removing the speculum, the practitioner will insert two fingers of one hand into your vagina; place the other hand on your lower abdomen; and press down on the abdomen, manipulating with the fingers in your vagina in order to locate and determine the size, shape, and consistency of the uterus, ovaries, and tubes. She or he can also locate any unusual growths, tenderness, or pain. Pressure on the uterus is usually painless, but pressure on the ovaries sometimes causes discomfort. The ovaries are difficult to find, and often the twinge of pain you feel is the only way the practitioner is aware that he or she is touching them. The bimanual examination will be more comfortable

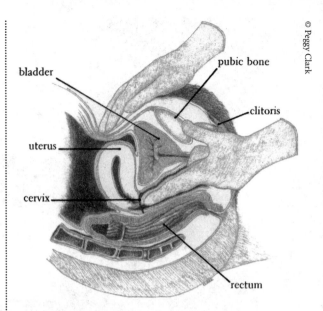

A bimanual pelvic exam

for you and easier for the practitioner if you are able to relax your neck, abdomen, and back muscles and breathe slowly and deeply, exhaling completely.

To do the rectovaginal exam, the health care provider inserts one finger into the rectum and one into the vagina, to check the tone and alignment of the pelvic organs as well as the ovaries, tubes, and ligaments of the uterus. This exam also helps detect rectal lesions, and tests the tone of the rectal sphincter muscles. If you are over thirty-five, the practitioner should also check for masses or blood in the rectum (sometimes an early sign of colon cancer). Some women find the rectovaginal exam unpleasant; others don't mind it. You may feel like you are having a bowel movement as the practitioner withdraws his or her finger from your rectum. Don't worry—you won't.

Some practitioners are much more sensitive and skilled in internal exams than others; some women find it easier to relax than others. You can do Kegel exercises (see p. 235 in Chapter 13, "Sexual Anatomy, Reproduction, and the Menstrual Cycle") and practice inserting a tampon or speculum before an internal exam to help with relaxation.

SELF-EXAMINATION

Over the years, an increasing number of women have discovered the benefits of doing vaginal and cervical self-exams. By examining yourself regularly, you can learn more about what is "normal" for you: what your discharges look like; the color, size, and shape of your cervix; and the changes in your mucus during the different stages of your menstrual cycles. Using a speculum ourselves, we can demystify a small piece of medical technology and learn more about our bodies. Some of us have taken self-examination a step further by talking about our experiences and sharing our knowledge with other women in self-help groups. For cervical self-examination, you will need only a few basic items:

- A light source that can be directed, such as a strong flashlight
- A speculum (plastic speculums are inexpensive and easy to get; if your pharmacy doesn't have them, you can order one online [see "Resources"])
- Lubricant, such as K-Y jelly or Lubifax, or warm water
- A mirror with a long handle
- Antiseptic soap or alcohol

Find a comfortable setting and familiarize yourself with the speculum, then get into a relaxed position on the floor or couch. Some women use a pillow behind the back for support. Lie back with your knees bent and your feet wide apart. You may want to lubricate the speculum. Hold the speculum in a closed position with the handle pointing upward. Or you can put the speculum into the vagina sideways and then turn it.

Experiment to see what feels most comfortable for you.

Once you have fully inserted the speculum, grasp the handle and firmly pull its shorter section toward you. This opens the blades of the speculum inside your vagina. Now hold the speculum steady and push down on the outside section until you hear a click; that tells you it's locked into place. For some women, placing the speculum and finding the cervix may take some effort. Breathe deeply and manipulate the speculum gently while looking into the mirror. Focus the light source on the mirror to help you see better. (A friend or partner can help by holding the flashlight and/or the mirror.)

With the speculum in the correct position, you will be able to see both the folds in the vaginal walls and your cervix, which looks pink, bulbous, and wet. (If you are pregnant, your cervix will have a bluish tint; if you are menopausal or nursing, it may be quite pale.) Depending on where you are in your menstrual cycle, your secretions may be white and creamy or clear and stretchy. By learning what is "normal" for you, you can easily identify any changes that may indicate ovulation, an infection, or pregnancy (to find out more, see Chapter 13, "Sexual Anatomy, Reproduction, and the Menstrual Cycle").

Some women prefer to remove the speculum while it's still open; others close the blades first. Clean it afterward with antiseptic soap or alcohol, and store it for later use.

PAP SMEAR

The *Pap smear* is a way to distinguish normal from abnormal cells of the vagina, uterus, and cervix. It is most accurate for cervical cells. To take a Pap smear, during the pelvic exam, the practitioner uses a *cytobrush,* or spatula, to get one or more samples of cervical tissue from the outside of the cervix and just inside the cervical canal. You may feel a slight scraping sensation.

The sample goes to a cytology laboratory for analysis. Medical practitioners don't always agree about treatments for various kinds of abnormal cells detected by Pap smears, so it can help to understand more about Pap test technology and treatment options.

DIAGNOSTIC TESTS AND TREATMENTS

Before giving your consent for any of the procedures and/or tests described here, ask your health care practitioner the following questions (see also "Informed Consent and Informed Decision Making," p. 702):

1. Why does she or he think you need the procedure?
2. What are the benefits of the procedure over others? What are the alternatives?
3. How is it done?
4. What are you likely to feel during and after the procedure?
5. What are the risks involved?
6. What are the negative effects? Will it affect your ability to have children?
7. What may happen if you don't have it done?
8. How experienced and skilled is the practitioner in doing this procedure? How many does she or he perform in a year?

DILATION AND CURETTAGE

Dilation and curettage (D&C) may be used to find the cause of uterine bleeding or to treat it, especially in emergencies. It is also used to diagnose uterine fibroids, endometrial polyps, and uterine cancer. It may help to diagnose cervical cancer, or it may be done to prevent infection following an incomplete abortion or after delivery, if part of the placenta is left in the uterus. The diagnostic

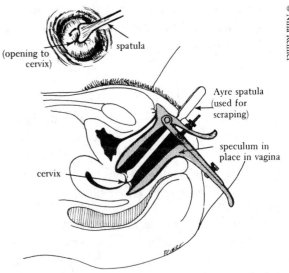

© Nina Reimer

Placement of speculum for a pelvic exam. Spatula scrapes cervix for Pap smear (this is usually painless).

D&C is rapidly being replaced by vacuum aspiration or endometrial biopsy (see next page).

Many physicians still prefer to do a D&C in a hospital, using general anesthesia, but this is not necessary. It can be done in a doctor's office using local anesthesia, thereby minimizing the risks and expense, which are both greater with general anesthesia.

D&C involves enlarging (dilating) the opening of the cervix by inserting a series of tapered rods that become progressively wider in diameter. The practitioner then inserts a long, thin metal instrument with a spoon-shaped end (curette) through the cervix into the uterus to scrape out some of the uterine lining (and sometimes a tissue sample from the cervical canal). The procedure should take five to fifteen minutes. Most women have some bleeding following a D&C and may also pass small clots and/or have cramps for a couple of days. The risks, which are generally slight, include infection, hemorrhage, perforation of the uterus or surrounding internal organs, and complications related to the anesthesia used.

VACUUM ASPIRATION

For diagnostic purposes, vacuum or *endometrial aspiration* is more common now than the D&C. It involves inserting a small cannula (a flexible tube) into the cervix and removing the uterine lining by means of low-pressure suction. This procedure can be done in an office with local anesthesia, thus eliminating the risks of general anesthesia. It usually causes the same mild to moderate cramping as the D&C.

CERVICAL AND ENDOMETRIAL BIOPSY

In a biopsy, a sample of tissue is clipped from the cervix or scraped from the endometrial lining to be examined under a microscope as an aid to diagnosis. A *cervical biopsy* is done on abnormal areas of the cervix that appear through visual examination with a colposcope (see "Colposcopy," below). An instrument that looks like a paper punch removes the tissue sample from one or more sites on the cervix. The biopsy may be done on an outpatient basis, generally without anesthesia. Most women experience some cramping during the biopsy and spotting afterward.

In an *endometrial biopsy* (which can also be done on an outpatient basis, with local anesthe-

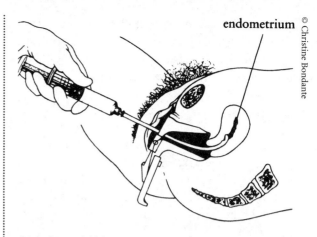

endometrium

© Christine Bondante

An endometrial biopsy

sia, if necessary), usually a pipelle (a plastic device) is used to obtain a sample of the uterine lining. The procedure may be part of an infertility work-up. It is fairly accurate when used to diagnose cancer of the uterine lining (endometrium).

COLPOSCOPY

This procedure uses a *colposcope* (a lighted magnifying instrument resembling a small mounted pair of binoculars) to examine the vaginal walls and cervix for abnormalities. It is used with acetic acid wash. A biopsy specimen is usually taken from any abnormal areas for more accurate diagnosis. Colposcopy is useful in the diagnosis of abnormal bleeding. (For colposcopy guidelines for DES [diethylstilbestrol] daughters, see p. 627.)

Colposcopy is an office procedure that usually involves little or no discomfort. However, it is often combined with a cervical biopsy, which may be painful. Also, it is a prolonged speculum exam, which for some women is physically or psychologically uncomfortable. It is wise to remain lying down for five to ten minutes after a colposcopic exam.

When colposcopic equipment is not avail-

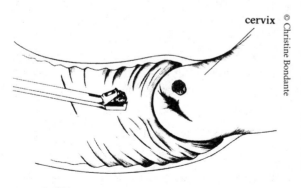

cervix   © Christine Bondante

A cervical biopsy

able, a less specific test (Schiller's test) is sometimes used. In this procedure, an iodine solution is used to determine areas of the vagina or cervix from which a biopsy specimen should be taken.

CONIZATION OR CONE BIOPSY

Conization removes a cone-shaped section of the cervix. It is often recommended when a woman has severe dysplasia or cancerous cells confined to the cervix. A diagnostic conization may turn out to be therapeutic if it removes all the abnormal tissue.

A major surgical procedure, cone biopsy is done in a hospital under general anesthesia. Though the edges of the coned area are sutured or cauterized, bleeding and infection are fairly common short-term complications. The removal of too many mucus-secreting glands may affect fertility by causing a decrease in cervical mucus. Sometimes pregnant women suffer a miscarriage after conization because muscle tissue has been removed, though cerclage treatment (which keeps the cervix from opening prematurely) may be possible.

Another option is treating the abnormal area of the cervix with a laser. Laser techniques cause few complications and promote faster healing. Laser destroys tissue, however, making it unavailable for laboratory analysis. After a laser treatment, a Pap smear may show atypical cells for four to six weeks. You should have two follow-up smears at three-month intervals and two more at six-month intervals before returning to your regular Pap smear schedule.

CAUTERIZATION AND CRYOTHERAPY

Cauterization involves destroying abnormal tissue with a chemical such as silver nitrate, or with an electrically heated instrument. It is used to treat abnormal cell development (dysplasia), lo-calized cervical cancer, or cervical erosion (a reddened area that develops around the cervical opening). Sometimes cauterization is used to treat chronic cervicitis, vaginal or vulvar warts, or endometriosis involving the cervix or vagina. Cauterization can be done in a doctor's office, preferably right after the menstrual period. The practitioner inserts a speculum and applies the instrument to the affected area. After treatment, a scab forms, allowing healthy new tissue to grow. The scab falls off in a week or so, and complete healing takes seven or eight weeks. Side effects include swelling of the cervix and profuse discharge for two or three weeks. Rarely, infection or infertility can result if the cervical glands are damaged.

Cryotherapy (cryosurgery, cold cautery) uses liquid nitrogen to destroy abnormal tissue by freezing. It can be done in an office and takes only a few minutes, but it may cause a profuse watery discharge and temporary changes in the cervical mucus. Many practitioners would rather do a loop electrosurgical excision procedure (LEEP, see below) so they can obtain tissue for diagnosis at the same time (cryotherapy, laser treatment, and cautery all destroy tissue).

After either cauterization or cryotherapy, you should not douche, use tampons, or have sexual intercourse for ten to fourteen days while your cervix heals. Until healing is complete, Pap smears will be inaccurate and difficult to interpret. Cauterization and cryotherapy both may cause narrowing of the cervical opening, which makes future Pap smears difficult to do. As with all procedures for treating cervical dysplasia, there is a very small risk of damaging the cervix and causing infertility problems.

LOOP ELECTROSURGICAL EXCISION PROCEDURE

For treatment of cervical abnormalities, the *loop electrosurgical excision procedure* (LEEP) has largely replaced conization, cauterization, cryotherapy, and carbon dioxide laser. During a LEEP procedure, a low-voltage, high-frequency radio wave is run through a thin wire loop, which is used to remove abnormal tissue from the cervix. The loop scoops out the targeted tissue in a matter of seconds. The excised tissue is then examined in the lab to determine whether the abnormal cells are cancerous. A major advantage of LEEP and similar techniques is that they combine diagnosis and treatment in the same visit to the medical practitioner. Local anesthesia is used. The procedure may involve minor discomfort. Cervical healing takes about a month for routine cases.

LAPAROSCOPY

The *laparoscope* is a lighted tubelike instrument that is inserted through a small incision made below the navel, allowing the physician to see the uterus, tubes, and ovaries. Laparoscopy is useful to diagnose and treat ovarian cysts, ectopic (tubal) pregnancy, infertility caused by blocked tubes, unexplained pelvic pain or masses, and endometriosis, and in recovering an IUD that has perforated the uterus. It is also used in some female sterilization techniques. Much gynecological surgery is now being done laparoscopically, because this approach can make recovery easier and quicker. Laparoscopy is usually done in a hospital, under either general or local anesthesia. Before inserting the laparoscope, the practitioner inflates the abdomen with carbon dioxide to move the intestines out of the way and see the pelvic organs better. With local anesthesia, you may experience an uncomfortable pressure or fullness. You may feel some pain under your ribs for the first few days after a laparoscopy as your body gradually absorbs the excess gas.

HYSTEROSCOPY*

Hysteroscopy involves inserting a telescope-like instrument through the vagina into the uterus so it can be examined from the inside, either directly or on a video screen. Hysteroscopes are available for both office use (often without anesthesia) and surgery (with general or regional anesthesia). Reasons for using them include abnormal uterine bleeding, infertility or repeated miscarriage, abnormal growths (fibroids and polyps), and lost IUDs. Complications are rare; they include pelvic infection, perforation, allergic reaction to the gas or liquid used to distend the uterus, excessive uterine or cervical bleeding, and negative reactions to the anesthesia. A few deaths from excess fluid absorption have been reported, but death is even rarer than complications.

BENIGN BREAST CONDITIONS

Women's self-images are often affected by our own and others' reactions to our breasts. Our feelings, both positive and negative, are reinforced by our society's obsessive fixation on breasts and the way they are used to sell everything from cars to whiskey. This may make it difficult to think about our breasts as functioning parts of our bodies.

Breasts come in all sizes and shapes: large, small, firm, saggy, lumpy. Your breasts may be slightly different in size or shape. Nipples may lie flat, stick out, or retract (be inverted). The areola (the area surrounding the nipple) may be large or small, darker or lighter, and it usually has little bumps just under the skin. Sometimes there are

* For an excellent fact sheet on hysteroscopy (stock no. CO-016), send a stamped, self-addressed envelope to: Harvard Vanguard Medical Associates, Central Ob-Gyn, One Fenway Plaza, Boston, MA 02215-2523.

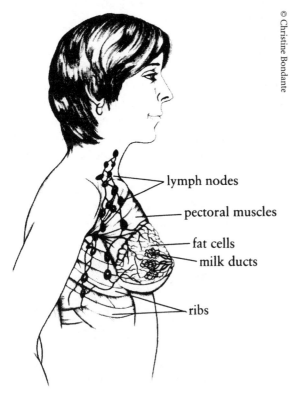

© Christine Bondante

A breast, showing the structure of milk ducts, lymph nodes, and fat cells.

hairs near the edge of the areola. These individual differences, along with the changes caused by age and menstrual cycles, can produce needless anxiety. We may worry that every change or pain is a symptom of cancer, when in fact most conditions causing change, lumps, or pain are benign (not cancerous). (For more information, see "Our Breasts," p. 238.)

BREAST CHANGES THROUGHOUT LIFE

Our breasts are dynamic organs—they change considerably during our lifetime in response to changes in our body's hormone production. Understanding these changes can help reassure us when we think something is going wrong.

In girls, around the time the ovaries begin producing estrogen (a year or two before menstrual periods start), the breasts respond by growing. At first there's a firm mass directly behind the nipple—the *bud.* As puberty progresses, the ductal tissue in the bud grows out into the fatty tissue, forming branches and lobules to make up the glandular portion of the breast. The fatty and fibrous tissues that support it *(stroma)* also increase during puberty. Most of this growth happens early, but slower growth

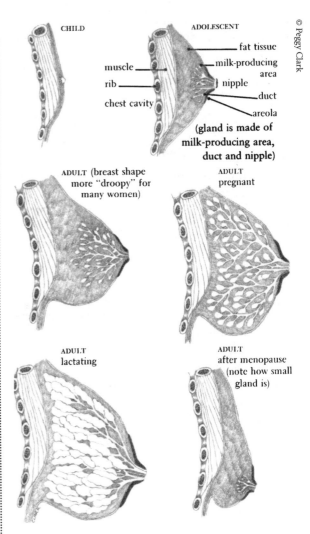

© Peggy Clark

Breast changes over a lifetime.

continues during the teen years. One breast may develop more quickly than the other, and it's not uncommon for a woman to have breasts of different sizes.

The breasts continue to respond to estrogen and progesterone during the menstrual cycle, with growth and fluid retention that may be barely noticeable for some women but painful for others. Most lumpiness at this stage is just stroma. Small cysts (dilation of a lobule or duct with fluid inside) may form, but they are usually smaller than a pea. Benign (noncancerous) tumors, such as fibroadenomas, may form in the teens and twenties and grow large enough to feel—like smooth, mostly round, rubbery marbles that can be moved back and forth in place.

By our fifties, glandular tissue and dense stroma decrease *(involution),* and fatty tissue increases. Small cysts may fill up further with fluid, sometimes causing tenderness and growing to sizes that can be felt with the fingers. As menopause approaches, hormone levels begin to fluctuate, and our usual cycles may become irregular. The effect of hormone changes on the breasts may be increased pain and lumpiness. That can be distressing if we are looking for signs of breast cancer. Cancer rarely forms within cysts, but we may feel anxious while awaiting proof that a cyst is not cancer.

Some women's breasts remain lumpy after menopause. Most benign lumps are caused by hormone stimulation, so if you are taking hormones after menopause, the breasts will continue to feel as they used to. Cysts rarely form after menopause, but if a new lump does form, it's a good idea to have it checked. Breast pain in the postmenopausal years may be coming from the chest wall, arthritis of the spine, or, possibly, cancer. (For more information about benign breast conditions and normal breast development, see "Our Breasts," p. 238.)

SCREENING FOR BREAST CANCER

Three screening methods are used to detect breast cancer: breast self-exam; examination by a health care practitioner; and mammograms.

BREAST SELF-EXAM

Almost all breast lumps (90 percent) are discovered by women or our partners, usually while washing, dressing, making love, or engaging in other daily activities, and sometimes through breast self-exam. This technique to check your own breasts for suspicious lumps is recommended by many health care practitioners, with the idea that finding cancer early may improve the outcome. However, recent studies found no difference in breast cancer survival rates between women who did regular breast self-exam and those who didn't. Women who do self-exam regularly find more lumps and have more biopsies, but most of those turn out to be benign.* The problem is that by the time you can feel a lump, most cancers—if there is one—have been present for six to eight years, so whether you find it this month or next month is not crucial. Most American women (60 percent or more) do not do breast self-exams regularly, although many have tried it.

If you want to become more familiar with any changes in your breasts, you can check them once a month, right after your period ends, when your breasts are not tender or swollen. If you don't have regular periods or no longer menstruate, examine your breasts about the same time every month. The technique is the

---

* The U.S. Preventive Services Task Force found insufficient evidence to recommend for or against teaching everyone to do breast self-exam; its Canadian counterpart concluded self-exam should not be taught.

same whether you do it standing up or lying down. First, look in the mirror to check for any visible changes. Then, with your arm behind your head on the side you're examining, hold the fingers of your other hand flat and feel for lumps or thickening, moving your hand in a circle, up and down, or from the center out. (For a step-by-step guide, see "Breast Self-Exam" [W63] on the companion website, www.ourbodiesour selves.org.)

WHAT IF I HAVE A LUMP?

Words are hardly adequate to describe the anxiety we feel if we find a lump that wasn't there before. Often cancer is the first thought that flashes into our mind. That thought can be terrifying. Some of us go to the doctor immediately. Others of us are so afraid it's cancer that we say nothing about it for a while. Indeed, finding a lump requires taking some decisive actions for yourself and your health. It's a good idea to tell someone you love about your concerns, so you can get some support and not have to go through the next steps alone. Then contact your health care provider and make an appointment for a clinical exam or mammogram. Tell the appointment person or nurse that you have found a new breast lump, and ask to be seen promptly.

While all lumps need to be checked out, remember that more than 80 percent of all lumps are *not* cancer, especially in women under forty. Lumps in our breasts big enough to feel may be cysts; benign tumors such as fibroadenomas; pseudolumps; or cancers, and it's impossible to tell the difference with physical examination alone. A lump that gets smaller over time is unlikely to be cancer. A lump that remains the same size or gets bigger could be cancer, so it should be medically evaluated (see p. 599).

Your doctor will do a clinical examination of your breasts and determine whether further evaluation is necessary. She or he may suggest following the lump for a few months, schedule you for diagnostic breast imaging (mammogram or ultrasound), or refer you to a breast specialist (usually a surgeon). If still further evaluation is indicated, a biopsy may be recommended, since only a tissue sample determines for sure whether a lump is cancerous or benign.

This can be a very stressful time. Even though chances are that a breast lump is benign, statistics don't always calm our fears when it's our body and our lump. It helps to speak frankly with your health care provider about your concerns and to have the support of loved ones. It is also important to have confidence in your doctor. If you are not comfortable with his or her recommendations, particularly a "wait and see" approach, be sure to say so. Getting a second opinion may be a good idea in this situation.

BREAST LUMPS

Cysts are fluid-filled sacs that develop from dilated lobules or ducts, most commonly in those of us in our forties or fifties. They can be identified by ultrasound or by removing the fluid and making sure no lump remains. You don't have to get simple cysts treated unless they are causing pain or are so big that you can't feel the surrounding breast tissue.

Treatment involves numbing the skin (local anesthetic), inserting a thin needle into the cyst, and drawing the fluid into a syringe *(aspiration)*. The fluid may look gray and cloudy, dark and oily, or clear yellow or green. If a lump remains after aspiration, or if the fluid looks dark and bloody, you'll need to have the area biopsied (see p. 602). Cysts may refill with fluid after aspiration.

Fibroadenomas are benign fibrous growths that form mostly during our teens and twenties; some that form early may last throughout life. They may develop in one or both breasts. A fibroadenoma that's getting larger is usually removed surgically. These growths sometimes shrink at menopause, as hormone levels decrease. Fibroadenomas are rarely associated with cancer, although some breast cancers can feel like fibroadenomas. The younger you are, the more likely it is that your doctor will assume any lump you have is a fibroadenoma and not a cancer, but there is no way to be certain except by doing a biopsy and looking at it under a microscope.

Pseudolumps are areas of dense normal breast tissue. They develop in many women during the premenopausal years. To make sure there is no cancer, these areas should be evaluated with good breast imaging and follow-up exams.

Cancer in the breast usually feels firm and hard. It often does not have clear edges but blends into the surrounding breast tissue. Breast cancers are usually about one centimeter (half an inch) in size before you can feel them; in women with firmer, lumpier breasts, they must be even larger to be felt.

CLINICAL BREAST EXAMS

Having your breasts examined by a health care provider is widely recommended, along with mammograms, though a clinical exam by itself is not enough to diagnose cancer. The practitioner should inspect your breasts carefully for skin changes while you are sitting up, as you raise your arms over your head and then lower them to your sides. Your breasts should also be examined while you are lying down. This is very important, as a lump can sometimes be detected in only one of these positions.

In a study of women ages 50 to 59, clinical exams were better at ruling out cancer than at finding all the cancers that later showed up on mammograms. In younger women—whose breasts are denser—it's even harder to tell from a clinical exam what kind of lump is there. That doesn't mean you shouldn't get a clinical breast exam; it means only that to be sure whether a breast lump is or is not cancer, other tests are also needed. Even if you have already had a mastectomy, getting checked can be useful, because chest surgery does not remove all breast tissue, and there's still a small risk of cancer. Transgendered people, both male to female and female to male, may benefit from breast exams, too.[1] Telling your health care provider your natal sex may help to make sure your risks are not neglected.

MAMMOGRAMS

Mammograms are X rays of the breast, done with a special machine, to *detect* breast cancer;

they do not *prevent* breast cancer. *Screening* mammograms check women without any symptoms or breast problems for evidence of cancer at a stage when it may be more treatable. *Diagnostic* mammograms are done when a woman has a symptom, such as a lump, to find out what it is. Before getting a biopsy of a lump, your doctor may want you to have a mammogram to evaluate it further and help determine whether other areas need to be biopsied. Sometimes other imaging techniques, such as MRI or ultrasound, may be used to investigate an area of concern that has shown up on a mammogram.

Technicians may tell you not to wear perfume, powder, or underarm deodorant when you come in for a mammogram, because particles in some of these products may appear on the film and be misread as breast calcifications. If you have moles on or just under your breasts, ask the technician to put adhesive spots on them, to make sure they are not mistaken for suspicious growths when the film is read.

SCREENING MAMMOGRAMS

Mammograms detect some cancers that are not yet palpable (easily felt); serve as a map or guide

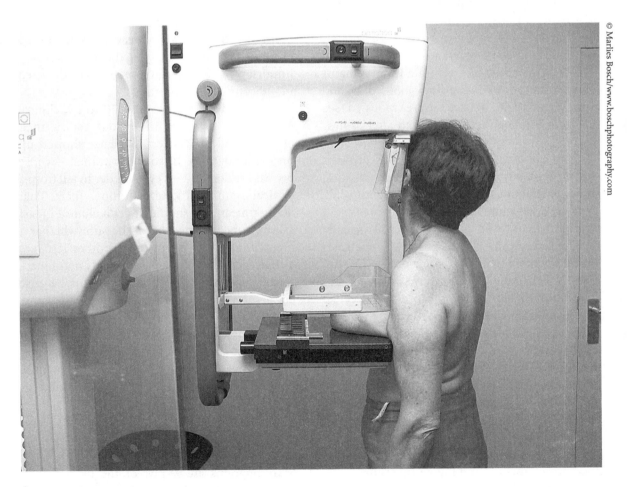

A woman gets a mammogram.

to surgeons; and provide a baseline against which later mammograms can be compared to see whether any unusual changes have taken place over time. Some of the cancers that are detected on mammograms can be successfully treated before they become invasive—but not all. There has been controversy over the years regarding the effectiveness of screening mammograms for finding breast cancer early enough to improve the survival rate.

Mammograms are not a perfect tool—there's a small chance they can miss cancers that are there, or mistakenly identify benign areas as cancerous—partly because breast tissue density varies individually and with age, and partly because of variations in the skill of technicians reading the film. Premenopausal women have denser breasts, which makes reading the film more difficult and errors more likely.

When to begin and how often to have routine screening mammograms is controversial. There is a risk—though a very small one—that exposure to radiation from a mammogram may induce breast cancer. Younger women's breasts may be more susceptible to radiation damage than those of older women, and starting annual or frequent mammograms early increases the lifetime amount of radiation exposure, thus increasing the risk.

The decision whether or not to have screening mammograms is more complex if you are between forty and fifty and have no suspicious lumps but are at high risk for breast cancer. Many doctors argue that high-risk women are more likely to have cancers for mammography to detect, and so have the most to gain. Others say women with breast cancer risk factors may also be more vulnerable to the effects of radiation. These are questions for which we have no answers.

Public health experts' recommendations vary as to the best age for starting regular mammograms and whether the interval between mammograms should be one year or two.* One of the issues is the test's effectiveness for screening women in a particular age group or risk category. Another issue is the cost of doing it, and whether health insurance covers it. A federally funded breast (and cervical) cancer screening program is available in all fifty U.S. states for women over forty who have no health insurance and meet certain income guidelines. If you need it, ask your health care provider about it.

For premenopausal women, clinical breast exams are the most appropriate screening method. Magnetic resonance imaging (MRI) may be useful in younger women, but it's very expensive. Newer breast imaging technologies are being more widely used, but they have not yet replaced mammograms for screening. In the absence of strong evidence that routine screening mammograms can catch breast cancer in time to treat it successfully and prolong survival, some women are deciding not to have them. To help you decide what is best for you, consult "Resources" and discuss the issue with your health care provider.

Remember that mammograms just indicate possibly cancerous areas. Only a biopsy (a procedure to remove part or all of a lump and examine some cells under a microscope for evidence of cancer) can tell for sure (see "Which Biopsy Method?," p. 602).

(For more information, see "Mammography Screening Controversy" [W64] on the companion website, www.ourbodiesourselves.org.)

---

* The U.S. Preventive Services Task Force recommends a screening mammogram every one to two years for women age forty and over. Trans people over forty with breast tissue may benefit from mammograms, too, because taking hormones may increase cancer risk. The Canadian Task Force on Preventive Health Care recommends screening every one to two years over age fifty and states there is insufficient evidence to recommend for or against screening in women ages 40 to 49.

MEDICAL EVALUATION OF A BREAST PROBLEM

If your mammogram shows a suspicious area, the next step is further evaluation with more imaging and a biopsy. Try to schedule your appointment after your period. Your breasts may be lumpy at other times in your cycle, and the health care practitioner may miss a lump hidden by general swelling. The examination may be uncomfortable but is generally not painful. Cancers usually feel more irregular, harder, and less freely moving than benign growths. The practitioner's judgment on whether the lump feels like cancer is bound to be subjective. Even if a mammogram and/or ultrasound is also done, only a biopsy can determine with certainty whether a growth is cancer.

Although your lump (or whatever is on the mammogram) will probably turn out to be benign, you may want to ask your health care provider to refer you to a breast specialist (usually a surgeon) who has had considerable experience with both cancer and benign conditions, just to make sure the diagnosis is accurate.

DIAGNOSTIC BREAST IMAGING

Diagnostic breast imaging can help identify a lump that can be felt or an abnormality seen on a screening mammogram. The methods currently used are mammography and ultrasound.

Diagnostic mammograms include special angle, spot compression, and magnification views to see hidden areas better and determine what any masses might be. For denser breast tissue, ultrasound may be more useful than a mammogram. Although mammography can show a mass, it can't tell the difference between a solid lump and a cyst.

Diagnostic breast ultrasound is now widely used. In addition to distinguishing between a solid mass and a cyst, the latest ultrasound technology can look through dense glandular tissue and show what's underneath. This may confirm a separate mass or show that it is only a pseudo-lump (see p. 599). Other techniques such as MRI (magnetic resonance imaging) and MIBI scans (which use injected radioactive material to light up a cancer) are also used for breast imaging. Imaging is an important tool for deciding whether an area should be biopsied, but it never provides a definitive answer. If a biopsy is not done right away, ask your doctor why, and be sure you are comfortable with the answer. If the area is to be watched over time, be sure you stick to the recommended schedule for follow-up. If you don't want to wait and see, it's your right to get a second opinion. For your peace of mind, you may even wish to insist on having a biopsy, even if your insurance will not cover the procedure.

WHICH BIOPSY METHOD?

The purpose of a biopsy is to obtain tissue from the abnormal area for evaluation under the microscope. Today four methods are being used.

Fine-needle aspiration can be done in the doctor's office. Local anesthetic is used to numb the area. A thin needle is placed into the target area, and cells are drawn into the syringe for examination under the microscope. A normal result is reassuring but should not be considered definitive; your practitioner should keep checking the breast. If there are abnormal cells, you'll need a biopsy that samples more tissue to find out exactly what they are. You can get a false positive result (cells thought to be cancer but which turn out to be benign), so it is important to confirm the diagnosis.

Core-needle biopsy (also called true-cut biopsy) can also be done in the doctor's office or in the mammography suite, with special equipment or ultrasound guidance. You'll get local anesthesia for it. The needle is thicker than the one used for fine-needle aspiration. This procedure is very accurate for finding cancer.

Incisional biopsies are less commonly performed today. In the doctor's office or ambulatory surgical suite, with local anesthesia, the practitioner makes a surgical incision in the skin and removes a piece of the abnormal area. It's done when removing the whole target area would deform the breast tissue. Core-needle biopsy has largely replaced this technique.

Excisional biopsy is the most common surgical biopsy. It can be an office procedure but is most often done in the ambulatory surgical suite. You'll get local anesthetic, with or without some sedation (although some surgeons still use general anesthesia). A surgical incision is made in the skin, and the entire lump or abnormal area is removed and sent for microscopic examination.

Before the biopsy, you may want to ask the surgeon to cut so as to leave the smallest possible scar, as sometimes doctors are not careful about this. Depending on the size and location of the lump, the incision can sometimes be made along natural wrinkle lines, along the edge of the areola, or under the arm. How your breast will look afterward depends on the length and location of the scar as well as how much tissue was removed. Any scar, discoloration, or distortion usually become less noticeable over time, though this varies significantly from one woman to another. The breast usually aches in that area for a few days to a week, with some bruising.

This is the most definitive technique for diagnosis, but also the most invasive and painful. If the area to be removed is something that can't be felt during a physical exam, it must be located for the surgeon using a mammography or ultrasound technique called *wire localization* (or needle localization). You'll be given local anesthetic before a radiologist puts fine, flexible wire into your breast through a needle, to mark the area where the biopsy should be done. Some women find the wire insertion more painful than the incision.

Accurate placement of the wire decreases the amount of tissue the surgeon must take out, minimizing change in the shape of your breast. The tissue removed with the wire is examined with X rays and under the microscope. If the abnormality is missed (which happens in 5 to 10 percent of cases), the procedure should be repeated after the breast has healed well enough for you to have another mammogram.

The information you get from the surgeon can help you decide which form of biopsy to have. The least invasive procedure may not always be the best choice, since you may need additional procedures to get a definitive diagnosis.

RESULTS OF THE BIOPSY

Waiting for the results of a biopsy can be very stressful. Ask when the results will be ready and whether the doctor's office will call you or you should call first. If you haven't heard by the appointed day, call. If there are further delays or you feel you are getting the runaround, be your own advocate and assert your right to get the information you need. You may wish to ask a partner or friend to help you. If the results are negative, it means no cancer was found, though a follow-up exam may still be recommended. Positive results mean that cancer was found (see "Breast Cancer: Treatment," p. 607).

If you are premenopausal, the doctor may say that the lump is just *fibrocystic,* a word that has unfortunately become a catchall term for noncancerous lumps of fibroglandular tissue in younger women. You may be so relieved not to have cancer that you don't ask any more questions. However, it's helpful to ask what "fibrocystic" means for your lump. You'll want to know what condition was detected, whether this type of growth tends to recur, and whether it's associated with an increased risk of breast cancer. *Atypical ductal* or *lobular hyperplasia* is linked to a moderately increased risk of breast cancer. If you have one of these, plus a first-degree family member (mother, sister, daughter, father, brother, or son) with breast cancer, your risk is even higher.

You have the right to obtain a copy of your medical records, and it's a good idea to keep a copy of the biopsy results (pathology report). Having your own copy helps if you get a second opinion or change doctors. The information may also be helpful in years to come as new data become available about which, if any, types of lumps might lead to cancer.

BREAST CANCER RISK

"Breast cancer is every woman's fear, and one in eight women's grim reality," said the late congresswoman Bella Abzug, who died of the disease. With lifetime risk now standing at one in seven, most women still *won't* get breast cancer. Women over sixty are 80 percent of those who die of it. Younger women can get the disease, however; it's the leading cause of cancer death in women 35 to 54 years old, because women in that age bracket do not have a high death rate in general. Breast cancer can interrupt our lives and those of our families at a time when we often have multiple responsibilities at home and in our jobs and communities. Also, it affects a part of our body that's important to many of us, for reasons related to our sexuality and self-image, as well as to nursing our babies.

WHO GETS BREAST CANCER?

Any woman can get breast cancer.* Most women who get breast cancer have no family history or known genetic risk, and 70 percent have none of the known risk factors besides age. Only 5 to 10

---

* Although men also get breast cancer, they make up only about 1 percent of the total numbers of cases.

WHAT FACTORS INCREASE THE RISK OF GETTING BREAST CANCER?

The evidence is strong or very strong that breast cancer risk goes up with the following (not necessarily in this order): age (77 percent of cases occur in women over fifty); family history of breast cancer in a mother, sister, or daughter diagnosed before menopause; lack of physical activity in adolescence and adulthood; taking hormones, including the estrogen and progesterone in hormone treatment for menopause and DES; younger age at menarche (first menstrual period) or older age at menopause; being overweight; never having given birth, or being older at the time of a first full-term pregnancy; breast density after menopause; alcohol use greater than one drink a day; race (white women's risk is higher); radiation to the chest (including X rays); and certain genetic mutations (see next page). Some evidence suggests that recent oral contraceptive use slightly increases risk of breast cancer among women under thirty-five years old.[2]

It seems likely that some aspects of diet affect breast cancer risk, but so far research hasn't proved it. Hormone levels in the womb may influence breast cancer risk, too. For example, when a woman is pregnant with twins, she has higher levels of estrogen circulating in her uterus, and if she has twin daughters, then they have an increased breast cancer risk.[3]

None of the breast cancer risk factors is a "smoking gun," as cigarettes are for lung cancer. The increased risk associated with each factor is modest.

percent of cases are in women with high-risk mutations of the BRCA1 and BRCA2 genes.

About 267,000 women per year will get a diagnosis of various kinds of breast cancer. The rate at which new cancers are diagnosed has increased over 40 percent since the early 1970s, and the number of cases continues to rise in the United States and internationally. Some of the numbers are due to more women having mammograms, which leads to more cases being found, but most researchers agree that the real incidence is increasing. Rates are increasing most rapidly in the developing world and among immigrants to the United States from low-risk nations, and the daughters of such immigrants. Breast cancer risk is four to five times greater in the United States and Europe than in Asia and Africa. These historical and geographic patterns suggest that factors in modern industrial societies increase breast cancer risk. Many people believe that the industrial processes and environmental damage that began during or after World War II played a role in rising rates of breast cancer in Western countries. There is cer-

tainly more to learn about why some women get breast cancer and others don't.

GENETIC TESTING AND INHERITED RISK

Breast cancer, like other cancers, develops when changes occur in genes in breast cells. In that sense, all breast cancer has a genetic element. But "genetic" does not mean "inherited." Only an estimated 5 to 10 percent of breast cancer cases result from an inherited genetic predisposition to the disease. In other words, over 90 percent of all breast cancer cases result from factors that are not inherited and, in many cases, are unknown.

Blood tests have been developed—and are now aggressively marketed commercially—that can identify mutations in the BRCA1 and BRCA2 genes. But a positive test result (having one of these mutations) does not mean that an individual will develop breast cancer. (Those of us who have an inherited BRCA1 or BRCA2 mutation have a 35 to 85 percent chance of developing breast cancer during our lives.)[4] Nor does a

CAN BREAST CANCER RISK BE REDUCED?

Even though the cause of most breast cancer is unknown and nothing is guaranteed to prevent cancer, some studies have shown that certain health strategies are associated with lower risk.

- Be physically active—get over three hours of exercise every week.
- Eat more fruits and vegetables and less fat. Limit alcohol to no more than one drink a day.
- Carefully weigh risks and benefits before using hormones such as birth control pills,

fertility drugs, and hormone treatment for menopause discomforts.
- Breast-feed babies—longer is better—not only because it develops their immunities to disease but also because lactation reduces cancer risk in the mother.
- Microwave in glass or ceramics, not plastic. Don't let plastic food wraps touch high-fat foods such as cheese or meats during heating.

Research suggesting that aspirin may reduce risk by inhibiting estrogen production needs to be confirmed by long-term studies.[5]

negative test mean that a woman won't develop breast cancer; it means only that her lifetime risk is the same as that of most other women in the industrialized world. And so far, there's no way to tell how strong the connection is between the various mutations that exist and the risk of getting breast cancer, or how aggressive (or nonaggressive) the disease will be if it develops in a woman with one of these genetic mutations.

Genetic testing should be considered only in limited circumstances. Women most likely to benefit from genetic testing are those of us who believe—because of a family history of two or more first-degree relatives (mother, sister) with breast or ovarian cancer—that we may be mutation carriers and, if so, want to take some action

to try to reduce our cancer risk. All genetic testing should be accompanied by complete information about benefits and risks, professional counseling, and comprehensive written informed consent. We need to approach genetic testing with extreme caution until science can tell us more about the results and public policy can protect us from discrimination in employment, insurance coverage, or other areas on the basis of genetic information. (For more information, see "Genetic Testing and Inherited Risk" [W65] on the companion website, www.ourbodiesourselves.org.)

ENVIRONMENTAL POLLUTION AND BREAST CANCER

The consistent link between estrogen and breast cancer is one reason that scientists and activists have recently called for more study of the many environmental pollutants that can mimic or disrupt estrogen and other reproductive hormones. One theory is that exposure to light at night—for example, from shift work or simply from living in the industrialized world—may increase breast cancer risk by reducing the body's levels of melatonin, a substance that suppresses tumor growth.[6] Studies have failed to show a link with electromagnetic fields from electric power distribution systems, appliances, and other electric equipment, but some activists are still looking for evidence. (For more information, see "Environmental Pollution and Breast Cancer" [W66] on the companion website, www.ourbodiesourselves.org.)

Even with strong evidence that chemical pollutants may affect breast cancer risk, it's difficult to apply what we've learned in the lab to studies of girls and women. For one thing, it would be unethical to design a study where half of the participants were exposed to a chemical and the others were not, just to find out whether it caused cancer. Also, researchers need to be able to estimate a woman's exposures to multiple

PROPHYLACTIC (PREVENTIVE) MASTECTOMY

Because there is no known way to prevent breast cancer (only to reduce cancer risk), some women at high risk have both breasts removed to avoid breast cancer. A mastectomy performed for preventive purposes should be a total, not a subcutaneous, mastectomy (subcutaneous leaves the nipple as well as more tissue under the skin). Although it seems to make sense that mastectomy would be effective, even the best surgeons leave some breast tissue behind under the skin and around the edges, so some risk remains. Breast reconstruction may be performed at the same time or later. Women who choose preventive mastectomy should continue to be checked regularly. Your feelings about having a mastectomy and your options for breast reconstruction afterward are likely to resemble those of women who do it for cancer treatment or other reasons (for further discussion, see p. 612).

chemicals dating back to the years when a tumor started. We can't really know what's in our processed food and drinking water, what's off-gassing from the new carpet, or what's being tracked into homes from the outdoors. Finally, corporations hesitate to fund research unless patentable chemotherapies or medical procedures are likely to emerge from it. Public and philanthropic support is needed to fund environmental studies investigating underlying problems and their relation to cancer. To find out how you can get involved with a breast cancer or environmental advocacy organization and make a difference for future generations, see Chapter 32, "Organizing for Change."

BREAST CANCER: TREATMENT

When you find out you have cancer, it's normal to feel shock, disbelief, fear, and anger. This trauma comes exactly when you need to focus all your energy on learning about your treatment options. The most important thing is to remember that a diagnosis of breast cancer is not an emergency.

Doing whatever your doctor suggests may be appealing at a time when you need to be taken care of, but it has not always resulted in the best care. Although most doctors have good intentions, they tend to offer only the treatment they know best. It's wise to get a second opinion before committing yourself to a course of treatment, even if you feel confident with your first doctor. Some physicians may be slow to accept new therapies until there's more experience with them; some may be unwilling or unable to discuss all available treatments. Some states, including Massachusetts, California, and Minnesota, have laws that require patients to be informed of all the medical options.

Even though you may have a good relationship with your health care provider, if you live in a small town, you may want to consider going to the nearest large city with a research-oriented or university hospital that keeps up with ongoing studies; uses a "team" approach; and may be more flexible about treatment. A team involving medical oncologists (cancer specialists), surgical oncologists, and radiation oncologists may offer a combination of treatments for your individual situation. A local women's health center, the National Cancer Institute, or the American College of Surgeons can help you find appropriate cancer centers and specialists. Certain centers offer more treatment choices, including experimental therapies (see "Our Rights as Patients," p. 702). If you meet income guidelines and were diagnosed under a federally funded screening program for uninsured or underinsured women, Medicaid will cover treatment for breast cancer. Some communities have local support groups for women with cancer, where you may be able to get help with transportation to medical appointments and with child care, as well as encouragement from other women who have had or are having similar experiences.

It's okay to take several weeks to adjust and find out about your options. Surgery within six to eight weeks of the biopsy is usually recommended. In some cases, chemotherapy is used over several weeks or months to reduce the size of the tumor prior to surgery (see p. 615). You may or may not need to have radiation.

When you are trying to decide about treatment, the most pressing question is likely to be "How can I maximize my chances of disease-free survival?" But after years of disease-free survival, you may be more concerned about minimizing the long-term effects of treatment. To decide on the best treatment, you also need to know the size of the tumor, whether or not there's cancer in the lymph nodes, the hormone status of your tumor, and other tumor characteristics (see the following pages). Most of this information is available after the biopsy and is used to recommend systemic therapies (endocrine/hormone therapy or chemotherapy) and/or radiation.

Evaluating these factors with a team of specialists helps you to explore your treatment options most effectively. Ask as many questions as you need to. You're the one who has to live with the results.

It is important to learn about all the available options. The entire field of breast cancer medicine is changing rapidly as old, established theories and treatments are being questioned, while newer techniques have not been used long enough to be completely evaluated. This book points out some directions to pursue and some pitfalls to avoid. Also see "Resources"; *Dr. Susan Love's Breast Book* is especially helpful.

STAGES OF BREAST CANCER

Cancers are "staged" (classified) to get an idea of prognosis for an individual, as well as for comparison of treatments and outcomes in different populations. Staging for breast cancer is based on three elements: tumor size or extent (T); which lymph nodes, if any, contain cancerous cells (N); and metastases, cancer detected by X rays or scans in other parts of the body (M). When cancer is first diagnosed, it is staged by physical exam and some testing for metastatic spread (clinical stage). After surgery, lab analysis of the breast tissue and lymph nodes removed will determine the pathologic stage. The stage is important because doctors usually base their recommendations for treatment on how well other women with cancer at the same stage and similar history have responded to the treatments. The TNM stage is then grouped into five categories or overall stages.

CARCINOMA IN SITU: NOT QUITE CANCER

Seen under a microscope, *in situ tumors* (sometimes called calcifications) are made up of cells that look like but are not behaving like cancer. They remain within their normal environment—inside the duct or the lobule. There are no blood vessels or lymphatic vessels there, so these cells have no access to other parts of the body. In contrast, *invasive* (also known as infiltrating) breast cancer goes through the walls of the ducts and lobules, invading the surrounding fatty/fibrous portion of the breast tissue where blood vessels and lymphatic vessels lie.

BREAST CANCER STAGES

STAGE	SIZE	TUMOR EXTENT AND LOCATION	NODES AFFECTED	METASTASIS
O	Varies	Localized (in situ) DCIS (ductal carcinoma in situ)/ LCIS (lobular carcinoma in situ)	None	None
I	≤2 cm.	Small	None	None
II	2-5 cm.	>5 cm. if no nodes	1-3	None
III	>5 cm.	Smaller if in skin or chest wall or involving 4-plus nodes	Yes	None on scan or X ray
IV	Any	Spread; treat to control symptoms	Variable	Yes

Lobular Carcinoma In Situ

LCIS is not really cancer now—it's considered a risk factor for the development of breast cancer some day. Because LCIS is not pre-invasive, there's no need to remove it. However, in studies of women with LCIS, 20 to 40 percent developed cancer (mostly invasive ductal carcinomas) over twenty years or more. That's a substantial risk. Such cancers may occur anywhere within either breast, not only in the area where the biopsy was done.

Treatment of LCIS

If you have LCIS, you currently have three options. One is to be monitored closely with breast exams and yearly mammograms. The second option is to have the same close follow-up and take the drug tamoxifen for five years to try to reduce your risk of developing cancer. Tamoxifen, like all medications, has its own risks, as well as side effects (see "Endocrine [Hormone] Therapy," p. 617). Each woman must weigh the risks and benefits for herself. There are also ongoing studies of other medications for risk reduction that you might want to participate in (for information, contact the NCI Cancer Information Service: 1-800-4-CANCER or www.cancer.gov). Another, far more drastic option is to have a preventive (or prophylactic) mastectomy. But even if you have the breast removed, some breast tissue is always left behind, and it may still be at risk for cancer.

Ductal Carcinoma In Situ

DCIS may never become cancer, but it is sometimes considered a risk factor for breast cancer. More women get this diagnosis now because improvements in technology have made it possible to find more DCIS with screening mammograms. Of women diagnosed with DCIS, 70 per-cent will be treated for a cancer that never would have become life-threatening; only 30 percent are likely to need treatment, but there's no way yet to tell which women really need it. If you receive this diagnosis, get a second pathology opinion before agreeing to any treatment.

Treatment of DCIS

Over 90 percent of us who have DCIS will still be living ten years after diagnosis, regardless of what treatment we have. Treatment aims to eliminate DCIS and reduce the chance it will recur. With a procedure similar to lumpectomy, called *wide excision,* even if the operation removes all the DCIS (which is called having *clear margins*), there's a 5 to 10 percent risk of developing either DCIS again or an invasive cancer in the next five to ten years. Having radiation therapy after wide excision may decrease local recurrences by about half. This leaves a 2.5 to 5 percent risk of invasive ductal cancer. Many women find this level of risk acceptable. However, the latest big study comparing treatments found only a very small difference in recurrence rate between women given radiation therapy and women treated with surgical excision alone.[7] The same study found that taking tamoxifen didn't significantly lower the chance of recurrence, though in other studies, it reduced risk by as much as 65 percent in women whose DCIS had estrogen receptors *(estrogen-receptor positive).*

Some women decide to have a mastectomy (see p. 606) in the hope of preventing invasive cancer. Doing this does not guarantee you will live any longer than if you don't remove the breast, so breast-conserving surgery is a very reasonable alternative. Of women who have a mastectomy for DCIS, 1 to 2 percent die of cancer. You'll want to think about how much uncertainty you are willing to live with.

INFLAMMATORY BREAST CANCER

This is a rare and aggressive form of invasive ductal breast cancer. The first symptom is redness of the skin, which is why it is called inflammatory. It is treated with antibiotics. When it doesn't get better, a biopsy of the breast and the skin will diagnose the cancer. The usual treatment is chemotherapy first, followed by mastectomy and radiation (see below).

OVERVIEW OF BREAST CANCER TREATMENTS

As researchers discover more about the biology of breast cancer, treatment theories change. Breast cancer, in general, grows slowly. Most breast cancers have been growing for six to ten years before they are large enough to be seen on a mammogram or felt during an exam. During this time, cancer cells could be spreading (metastasizing), through blood vessels and the lymphatic system, to other places within the body. This doesn't always happen—not all breast cancer cells survive outside the breast. Also, the size of the cancer doesn't always correspond to how aggressive it is; the type of cells in it will af-fect what happens, too. However, there is no sure cure. The classic saying among breast cancer survivors is that you don't know you're cured until you die from something else. Women who have been successfully treated "so far" refer to being "NED," or having no evidence of disease.

Current treatments for breast cancer are either *local* (therapy to the breast) or *systemic* (therapy to the whole body). Surgery and radiation are local therapies; chemotherapy, endocrine/hormone therapy, and biologic/targeted therapy are systemic therapies. Almost all women with breast cancer get some kind of local therapy. The two usual surgical treatment options are lumpectomy (breast-conserving therapy), followed by localized radiation to the affected area or mastectomy. Survival depends on whether cancer cells have already spread beyond the breast, and on the effectiveness of systemic therapy. Local therapy may make a difference in recurrence, or how likely the cancer is to come back within the breast/chest area.

Whether or not it's a good idea for you to have systemic therapy depends on whether the cancer might spread and on how you feel about the risks and side effects.

Unfortunately, there are currently no tests

BREAST CANCER TREATMENTS

TREATMENT	IMMEDIATE EFFECTS	SHORT-TERM SIDE EFFECTS	LONG-TERM SIDE EFFECTS
Radiation	Fatigue, swelling, skin burns	Swelling, blood clots in vein, tightening of shoulder muscle	Small risk of other cancer
Chemotherapy	Fatigue, nausea, vomiting, anxiety, hair loss	Memory and reasoning problems, hot flashes, sudden menopause	Hot flashes, nerve damage
Aromatase inhibitors	Diarrhea	Muscle aches, hot flashes	Muscle aches, hot flashes

that show which cancers will spread. Doctors try to predict the likelihood of metastasis from other factors, rather than waiting for more cancer to show up later on X rays or scans. Currently, the strongest predictor is the axillary (underarm) lymph nodes on the side of the tumor. When breast cancer cells are found in those lymph nodes, it is more likely there are breast cancer cells elsewhere in the body. Even when the nodes are negative (no breast cancer cells are seen), some women may still have metastatic cancer, so several other predictors are also used. (For more information on these, see the section on systemic therapy, p. 614.)

LUMPECTOMY OR MASTECTOMY?

Studies evaluating treatment of early (Stages I and II) breast cancer have shown no difference in survival rate between the group of women who had mastectomies and those who had lumpectomies with radiation. Which you choose may be affected by how you feel about losing a breast or facing the likelihood of having to deal with cancer again in the future, but it won't change how long you can expect to live.

The larger the amount of breast tissue removed, the more the shape or size of the breast will be affected. If the breast tissue removed has clear margins (no cancer cells at the edge), you won't need more surgery. If the margins are not clear, that means the entire tumor was not taken out the first time, and you may have to go back for another procedure. Approximately 70 to 75 percent of women diagnosed with breast cancer need only a breast-conserving lumpectomy, yet many women in the United States still undergo mastectomy. If over a quarter of the breast needs to be removed, a mastectomy is usually recommended.

After I and the guy I live with had spent almost two hours with the surgeon, we came away con-vinced that simple mastectomy was the only sensible treatment. . . . Then I went to Boston for a second opinion. . . . It turned out that the "other side" [lumpectomy plus radiation] was equally convincing. . . . I felt like a statistic that was being wooed by both sides. . . .

Even after mastectomy, radiation may be recommended if the cancer was larger than 5 centimeters or if the lymph nodes contained cancer. Radiation decreases the risk of local recurrence and possibly improves survival. Studies are under way to find markers that would identify cancers that could be eliminated without radiation; so far, no such markers have been found.

Deciding what treatment to have is never easy. Some women are devastated by the idea of having a breast removed, particularly because of the role of breasts in body image, sexuality, and breast-feeding. Others prefer removing a breast to living with a higher degree of uncertainty about recurrence. Sometimes one physician seems more reasonable; sometimes your intuition will point strongly to a certain option. A particular choice may be more convenient, or a friend's experience may convince you. We each have to make the best decision we can, in our own way, hopefully with well-informed and friendly support.

Ten years ago, when I had the first lumpectomy, they didn't get clear margins, so I said, "Look, let's just take it off and be done with it." Also, I wanted to avoid radiation and just have chemo afterward. When they did the mastectomy, they found six cancer sites—it wasn't just the lump I found myself—so I'm glad I did it.

REMOVAL OF LYMPH NODES

Axillary lymph nodes (under the arm) are sampled at the time of breast surgery, to aid in decision making about systemic therapy. Years ago, when surgeons removed all the nodal tissue from the armpit, drainage was blocked, and many women developed permanent arm swelling (lymphedema). Now, in most cases, only some lymph nodes are removed, and surgeons avoid stripping (removing) the lymphatic vessels, to lower the risk of swelling. Many surgeons also try not to injure the underarm nerve near the nodes being removed, and all surgeons try to avoid injuring nerves that go to muscles.

A newer procedure, *sentinel node biopsy,* removes only the first nodes that get lymphatic drainage from the tumor area, on the theory that those are the ones most likely to have cancer in them. This reduces how much surgery you need to check for cancer spread, and the risk of swelling is much smaller (though it can develop years later). This procedure is over 95 percent accurate. However, if the sentinel nodes are positive, the surgeon may remove more nodes until negative nodes are found.

To find the sentinel nodes, a dye is injected into the breast tissue surrounding the tumor, then traced to the lymph nodes. One of the dyes used in the United States is radioactive, so the sentinel nodes are identified with a sterile "Geiger counter" probe. The other available dye, which is blue, may cause an allergic reaction that can be quite severe in one person out of a hundred. Recovery time from the sentinel node procedure is much quicker than axillary dissection; you may be back to full activity in three to five days.

DEALING WITH MASTECTOMY

Once the anesthesia wears off after mastectomy, you may experience intense pain.

The muscles in my back and right shoulder began to screech as if they'd been pulled apart and now were coming back to life slowly and against their will. My chest wall was beginning to ache and burn and stab by turns. My breast which was

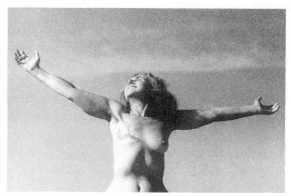

© Hella Hammid

Writer Deena Metzger with a tattoo over her mastectomy scar.

no longer there would hurt as if it were being squeezed in a vise. . . . The pain grew steadily worse and I grew more and more furious because nobody had ever talked about the physical pain.[8]

Medication will help, especially if you insist on getting enough to control the pain.

How we feel about losing a breast will be different for each of us. Some women accept it more matter-of-factly than others. Our age, feelings about body image and breast-feeding, even the size of our breasts may affect our reactions. Nearly everyone who has a mastectomy finds that the chest area becomes numb. Some skin sensation returns, but the area will still feel different than it did before surgery.

PROSTHESIS, RECONSTRUCTION, OR SCAR?

Some women who have had a mastectomy feel comfortable doing nothing to "fill in" the place where a breast is missing, choosing not to get an external prosthesis or have breast reconstruction surgery.

I refuse to have my scars hidden or trivialized behind lambswool or silicone gel. . . . I refuse to hide my body simply because it might make a woman-phobic world more comfortable. . . . I am personally affronted by the message that I am only acceptable if I look "right" or "normal." [9]

Others of us don't want a visible scar, and some worry that other people may be repelled by it. Some decide to use a prosthesis inside a bra, to fill in the area and "match" the other side under clothing. Some prefer to have breast reconstruction done by a plastic surgeon; this is done by using your own tissue and/or an implant.

With an *external prosthesis,* you may look as if nothing has changed, as long as you wear your bra, which holds the prosthesis in place. It may shift under your clothes or feel heavy; it may be hot in the summer and cold in the winter. However, the feel, fit, and comfort of prostheses are continually improving. Stores and online companies that specialize in prosthesis fitting can custom-make one to fit your anatomy. You can get a temporary prosthesis after surgery; once your scar has healed, you can be fitted for a permanent one. Many health plans cover all or part of the cost of a prosthesis. Medicare will pay for one every year or two if you get a prescription from your doctor. If you have health insurance, ask your insurance company what costs it will cover.

Breast reconstruction is a surgical option either at the time of the mastectomy or later. If you feel you have too many decisions to make all at once—sorting out your cancer therapy as well as whether to have reconstruction and what kind—then don't rush into it. You will also want to learn about important safety considerations, especially regarding silicone breast implants (see below).

Surgical reconstruction involves using either an *implant* under the chest muscle or your own tissues, with blood vessels, moved from your back, abdomen, or buttocks to your chest area (called a *flap reconstruction*). Sometimes an implant is used to supplement the tissue transfer

operation. Reconstruction is not without risks, both during surgery (blood loss, infection) and later on, but it also may have physical and emotional benefits.

An *implant* is a flexible synthetic envelope filled with salt water (saline) or silicone gel. The implant is placed behind the pectoral muscle or flap of your own tissue, then the skin is sewn together. If there's not enough space for the implant, a flexible expander is put in first to stretch the overlying tissues with saline injections during a time frame of three to six months. Once it's the right size, the expander is removed and replaced with a permanent implant.

Many women have developed debilitating conditions after breast implant surgery. One breast implant manufacturer reported the following findings for women with breast cancer who were followed for two to three years after breast implant surgery: 46 percent needed additional surgery within two or three years; 25 percent had their implants removed; 6 percent had substantial breast pain; 6 percent had necrosis (death of tissue); 6 percent had ruptured implants, often with "silent" and prolonged leakage of silicone into their bodies. The manufacturer also noted an alarming increase in many symptoms associated with autoimmune diseases for *all* implant patients, including joint pain, fatigue, hair loss, and muscle pain. [10]

We need more research on women who have had breast implants for at least eight to ten years, since most leakage or rupture occurs after that period of time. Some research already indicates an increase in fibromyalgia among women with leaking silicone gel breast implants. [11]

There's considerable controversy about the safety of silicone implants. (For more information, see "Breast Implants" [W67] on the companion website, www.ourbodiesourselves.org.)

Make sure you consult a board-certified plastic surgeon to find out what type of reconstruction offers the best match to your other breast. If the reconstruction uses muscle from somewhere else on your body, you will lose strength at the spot it came from. Ask how often the transferred tissue dies (its *necrosis rate*) in the kind of operation being recommended. If you smoke or have diabetes, complications may be more likely, as your blood vessels may be narrower or damaged, and healing can be more difficult. If you are active, especially in a particular sport, ask your surgeon to try to make it possible for you to return to this activity eventually. Once you get a recommendation, ask to speak with other women who have had the same procedure, both with this surgeon and with others. You can find other women to talk to through breast cancer support groups, oncology social workers, and other organizations (see "Resources").

Make sure the surgeon understands what you want; she or he may have something different in mind. It's important to mention what size you would like to be and how you feel about having a second scar where your own tissue was taken for the operation. Your body size and how much flesh you can spare may be a factor, too. Ask about newer procedures that may be less damaging. Take the time to become as well informed about reconstruction as you are about treatment.

Whatever type of reconstruction you choose, the surgeon can create a nipple and areola using darker, grafted skin or a tattoo. This is usually done several months after the reconstruction surgery. Sometimes, with one breast removed, plastic surgeons recommend reducing the remaining breast or changing its shape to match the reconstructed one more closely. Consider the possible problems that can result from additional surgery and its risks, plus further recovery time and side effects, such as loss of nipple sensation, before you agree to do this.

RADIATION

Most doctors recommend radiation immediately after lumpectomy and sometimes after mastectomy to try to prevent spread or recurrence and possibly improve survival. Treatment involves trips to the hospital or medical center. Your skin will be marked to show the radiologist where to apply the beam. Radiation doesn't hurt, but possible side effects include skin burns (reddening), extreme sensitivity to the sun, and sores that don't heal.

SYSTEMIC THERAPY

Drug treatment is given to women whose breast cancer has or may spread (*metastasize*). Studies have showed that survival rates improved when women whose lymph nodes tested positive for cancer at diagnosis got systemic treatment, even though cancer cells could not yet be found elsewhere. Approximately 25 percent of node-negative women eventually show signs of metastatic disease, too, so as many as 90 to 95 percent of women in this group are also treated, in the hope of catching the 25 percent who do have metastases. Many women are in fact being overtreated, and oncologists do not always make the risks, benefits, and side effects clear.

Neither chemotherapy nor hormone therapy guarantees a cure—it's more like insurance. The key concept is that how much you benefit is directly related to the risk of damage. The higher your risk, the bigger the benefit. Chemotherapy may reduce the risk of metastatic recurrence by about 35 to 40 percent, and endocrine (hormone) therapy may reduce the risk by almost the same amount. A combination of both may reduce the risk by almost 50 percent. For example, if you have many positive lymph nodes and about a 60 percent risk of metastasis, combined chemo and hormonal therapy would reduce that risk to about 30 percent. Some women would be willing to take the drugs to lower such a high risk. If your tumor is small and node-negative, and your risk of metastatic disease is estimated at 12 percent, combined systemic therapy would reduce the risk to about 6 percent. In other words, if your risk is already low, systemic therapy after surgery doesn't offer much additional benefit.

Systemic therapy is often given before surgery *(neoadjuvant therapy)* to women who have Stage III breast cancer. It may also be given to shrink larger tumors and make breast-conserving treatment possible.

CHEMOTHERAPY

The best timing for chemotherapy is not known. Usually, it is given after healing from surgery; chemotherapy may be interrupted by a course of radiation, or the radiation may be given after the chemo (doing both together increases the side effects). The optimal choice of drugs, dose, and length of therapy is still being studied as medical oncologists try to find ways to tailor treatments to particular tumor characteristics. That means the second and third opinions you get from medical oncologists may result in completely different recommendations. Therapy using a combination of drugs—especially the combinations called CA (cyclophosphamide and adriamycin) and a taxane (taxol or taxotere)—gave better results in studies than one drug used alone. Different women may react differently to particular drugs.

Most chemotherapy drugs are given intravenously (an IV drip to your veins) in a hospital or clinic, several days a week over several weeks or months. Treatment can usually be arranged to fit into your life.

I waited a while to set up my schedule and tidy things up at work. Take charge of your treatment and tell them what you need.

You'll need to consider how you're going to get to the hospital for treatment. It's a good idea to line up somebody to go with you, since afterward you may feel nauseated or unable to drive yourself home.

As the drugs build up in your body, you may recover more slowly from each successive treatment. Ask your oncologist about adding medications to the infusion to offset nausea and build up your white blood cells (see "Anemia," p. 659). Drinking lots of water during the chemo session may help to reduce some side effects.

Newer chemotherapy drugs that can be taken orally are being tested and have been shown to be useful in women with Stage IV breast cancer. More studies of women who are in earlier stages are needed. Chemotherapy can cause early menopause, an important consideration if you still want to get pregnant.

LIVING THROUGH CHEMO

Anyone who's been through chemotherapy will tell you it's no picnic. Most of the drugs used to treat breast cancer have side effects—nausea and vomiting, fatigue, and hair loss are the most common, along with a metallic taste in the mouth. Increased risk of infection and anemia are also possible. But the chemo experience is different for everyone. Some women breeze through it while working full-time. Others find it difficult and exhausting. Still others are someplace between these extremes. You won't know what your experience will be like until you're there. It depends on what drugs are prescribed for you and how your own system reacts to them.

Inform yourself about the specific drugs, their known side effects, and how to offset them. Ask whether you will receive chemotherapy orally or by intravenous infusion or injection, and how long each treatment will take. If your veins are hard to find, will you need to have a catheter or a shunt? It's a good idea to have someone with you for the first twenty-four hours after your first treatment, just in case you have a severe reaction.

Some women have found naturopathic remedies and massage helpful during chemo. If you are not already in a cancer support group, this is a good time to find one. Sharing the experience can give you both encouragement and ideas for dealing with the treatment.

Fatigue

Both chemotherapy and radiation can cause fatigue. That's a signal saying your body needs more rest. Pay attention to it and give yourself a break. You're going through a tough time, and you need nurturing and naps. The fatigue may last for several weeks after treatment is finished, so listen to your body and rest when you need to. Explain to friends and family that you need their help. When people ask, "What can I do?," tell them. Whether it's by babysitting, cooking a meal, running an errand, or driving your child to an activity, willing friends can make your life a little easier. Helping you also helps them deal with their own anxiety about your illness.

Nausea and Vomiting

Fortunately, these unpleasant reactions to chemo can now be minimized and sometimes even eliminated with newer medications such as Zofran (ondansetron), Kytril (granisetron), and Ativan (lorazepam). If your oncologist doesn't prescribe one of these drugs, ask for it before your first treatment so you can prevent nausea and vomiting. Anti-nausea medications can cause constipation, so you may need to make changes in your diet or use a mild laxative or stool softener. Marijuana reduces nausea for some patients, but obtaining it for medical purposes is still problematic.

Acupuncture can also help prevent or relieve nausea and vomiting. It's important to find a licensed acupuncturist who has experience in treating patients with breast cancer.*

* For a list of acupuncturists in your area, go to www.medical acupuncture.org or call 213-937-5514.

Low Libido, Infertility, Early Menopause

Chemotherapy can also affect sexuality, intimacy, and fertility. It's not just being bald, tired, and nauseated—chemo can cause vaginal dryness and discomfort during sexual activity and send your sex drive packing. If you haven't yet reached menopause, chemo may hit the fast-forward button. The closer you are to natural menopause, the more likely you are to have hot flashes, vaginal dryness, mood swings, sleep disturbances, and, down the line, increased risk of osteoporosis. The younger you are, the more likely you'll have periods again once treatment is finished.

"Chemo Brain"

Almost every woman who's experienced chemotherapy talks about the forgetfulness, loss of concentration, and fuzzy thinking that often accompany treatment. Women taking tamoxifen also show symptoms of chemo brain. Research shows that these symptoms are real, not imaginary,[12] and can last ten years or more. Before beginning treatment, you may want to ask chemo veterans about ways to cope with this problem. Some women find chemo brain a minor nuisance. Others of us have such serious memory and attention problems that we stop driving until treatment is finished. It helps to take a friend with you when you see your oncologist. One of you should take notes or record the conversation on tape.

Infection

Chemotherapy lowers your resistance to infection because the drugs attack the white blood cells that are part of your immune system as they attack the cancer cells. To reduce your risk of infection, take extra precautions: Avoid crowds and people (especially children) with colds or other illnesses; protect your hands when cooking or gardening; attend promptly to cuts or burns. You will also need frequent blood tests to monitor your white blood cell count, and possibly a drug to boost it.

Hair Loss

Not all chemotherapy drugs cause complete loss of hair. Ask your oncologist if yours will. The important thing is to do what makes you feel most comfortable, but you probably won't know in advance. Many women recommend getting a wig, just in case, and then supplementing with scarves and hats.

If you want a wig, ask your hairdresser, friends, oncologist, social workers at the hospital, or women in your support group to recommend a stylist. Having the wig fitted before you start chemo makes it easier to find one that resembles your natural hairstyle and color, if that's what you want. Some women never buy a wig at all and are comfortable being bald and/or covering up with scarves and hats (beware of silk—it's very slippery on a bald head).

Shortly after your first treatment, usually in a couple of weeks, your scalp will become tender and uncomfortable. The hair will fall out in large clumps. It won't hurt, but many women find this process distressing. Instead of waiting for it to happen, you may prefer to have someone shave your head. Shaving may give you a feeling of control over the process.

Once your treatments are finished, your hair will start to grow back; how quickly that happens varies with the individual. Sometimes the new hair is different—curlier, straighter, or a slightly different color—but many women's hair grows back exactly the same as before. If you colored your hair prior to treatment, doctors usually recommend waiting until there's at least an inch of new hair before coloring it again.

ENDOCRINE (HORMONE) THERAPY

Normal breast cells have estrogen receptors. When estrogen attaches to these receptors, growth is stimulated. Breast cancer cells may also have estrogen receptors. Treatments that change the hormonal environment of the tumor can stop its growth and even reverse it.

Tamoxifen is the most common hormone therapy for women of all ages. It is a synthetic estrogen that usually has anti-estrogen effects. The current recommended dosage is 20 milligrams daily for five years. Side effects include hot flashes in 20 percent of the women who take it, as well as fatigue. A small percentage of women may have depression, or blood clots resulting in stroke, heart attack, or death. One in a thousand may develop uterine cancer.

Aromatase inhibitors block the enzyme that converts androgens (produced by the adrenal gland) into estrogen. This slows the growth of estrogen-positive breast cancer. These drugs appear to be as effective as tamoxifen, maybe better, but they increase fracture risk and cause muscular pain and hot flashes within three years. Their long-term side effects are not known. They work only in postmenopausal women or women whose ovaries have been taken out surgically.

Oophorectomy (surgical removal of the ovaries) may slow cancer growth in premenopausal women, especially those with a breast/ovarian cancer gene mutation. If your ovarian cancer risk is not high, you might consider a drug that puts you into a temporary menopausal state for three years; this gives you the potential to regain your fertility later.

BIOLOGIC/TARGETED THERAPIES

A new type of drug targets certain characteristics of cancer cells. These seem to be useful for breast cancer, with fewer side effects than traditional chemotherapy, though they can affect normal cells, too. For example, Herceptin blocks the HER-2/neu receptor, a protein on the surface of cells that promotes growth when a particular substance attaches to it. It was effective in studies of women with Stage IV breast cancer and is now being studied in women with earlier stages of breast cancer.

TREATMENT OPTIONS FOR METASTATIC BREAST CANCER (STAGE IV)

Breast cancer is called stage IV, or metastatic, when breast cancer cells have migrated to other parts of the body. Most commonly, metastases show up in the lungs, liver, bones, or brain. Unless the tumor is causing bleeding problems or infection inside the breast, there is no reason to have a mastectomy once the cancer has metastasized. Treatments at this stage start with the least toxic therapy that can control symptoms and prolong life. Although the average survival is eighteen months, women may live much longer if the cancer responds to treatment. In other cases, more treatment may not extend life or even make you feel better. As you think about what treatment to have, you'll want to consider your goals—not just living longer but also relieving your symptoms and maximizing the quality of your life.

FUTURE PROMISE: THE PROGNOSIS FOR BREAST CANCER

As things stand now, about three quarters of women who get breast cancer are still alive ten years later, and almost two thirds are still alive fifteen years later. More than 200,000 new cases are diagnosed every year in the United States; more than 44,000 women in the United States die of breast cancer each year. However, some women live long, healthy lives after a breast cancer diagnosis. Even with all the indicators available, it is difficult to make predictions for any specific woman. An individual's immune system and general health are part of the picture, but there are still many unknown factors. Current research is focusing on biomarkers (proteins in the blood that indicate the presence of cancers and how they will behave); ways to keep cancer cells from reproducing, such as cutting off the blood supply to tumors and changing the genetic instructions that make them grow out of control; and developing drugs that can target cancer cells without killing healthy ones. In the foreseeable future, further work in these areas may result in more appropriate and effective treatments—and perhaps even a cure. Right now it may seem hard to be hopeful, but we can still go forward with the positive aspects of our lives in whatever time we have.

BENIGN UTERINE CONDITIONS

ABNORMAL UTERINE BLEEDING

This term for a common problem includes several different patterns: excessive monthly flow; bleeding between periods; and periods with very little blood or none at all. Excessive and/or irregular bleeding is a nuisance for many of us; it may also result in iron deficiency anemia, and fatigue. Possible causes are hormone imbalance, pregnancy, using birth control pills (which contain hormones), fibroids in the uterus, infection, and, more rarely, precancerous or cancerous growths. It is also the most common symptom of von Willebrand disease, an inherited bleeding disorder (see p. 696). Bleeding from the vagina may also be originating in the urinary or gastrointestinal tracts. Which might be the cause of your abnormal bleeding depends in part on your age. Irregular bleeding is normal in women approaching menopause, or during the first year of taking hormones for menopausal hot flashes (see Chapter 26, "Midlife and Menopause").

It's a good idea to consult a health care provider if you have several periods lasting three days longer than usual or fewer than twenty-one days apart; if you bleed after intercourse or after putting anything inside your vagina; if you soak through a pad or tampon every hour, especially with clots; if you spot or bleed between periods, or after six to nine months of taking hormones for hot flashes; or if you go three months without a period.

DIAGNOSTIC TESTS

To find out what's wrong, your health care provider can do a pelvic exam and a Pap smear; look at your other symptoms, such as pelvic pain or hair growth; and test your blood for anemia, hormone levels, and pregnancy. If the bleeding is severe, ask to be screened for von Willebrand disease. Depending on what those exams show, you may have further tests. A *transvaginal ultrasound* produces an image of the inside of your uterus so your provider can detect polyps (growths on the lining) or fibroids (growths in the muscle), or rule out endometrial cancer (cancer of the uterine lining). A *sonohysterogram* is ultrasound with an infusion of salt water through a tube into the uterus, which makes any growths easier to see. If necessary, your provider may suggest having a *hysteroscopic exam,* using a flexible telescope inserted through the vagina into the uterus, to see what's inside and possibly to remove any abnormal growths such as fibroids or polyps (see "Hysteroscopy," p. 595). Endometrial hyperplasia (pre-cancer) is a serious concern for female-to-male (FTM) trans men whose uterus is intact; if a pelvic exam is too demanding for you psychologically, ask to have a transabdominal ultrasound first.

If your provider suspects a pre-cancerous condition, you may need an *endometrial biopsy* to check. This is an office procedure in which a thin tube with a suction device is inserted through your vagina and cervix into the uterus to withdraw samples of uterine cells for analysis. It's quick, but it can also be uncomfortable or painful, so you may want to ask for pain medication. If the biopsy finds abnormal cells, you will probably want to read "Uterine Cancer," p. 637, before deciding on a treatment.

TREATMENTS FOR ABNORMAL UTERINE BLEEDING

What to do about abnormal bleeding will depend on what's causing it; how uncomfortable it is; how much it's disrupting your life; your age; and how you feel about having children in the future. Many health care providers still suggest having a hysterectomy for heavy bleeding, but this is rarely necessary. Be sure to get a clear diagnosis of the problem, as well as a second opinion. There are usually other things you can try instead of rushing into an operation.

Self-Help

If you are premenopausal, you may be able to stabilize your menstrual flow by reducing stress and changing your diet. Cutting down on animal fat and adding fiber helps to restore normal hormonal balance by lowering cholesterol, which is converted to estrogen in your body. Soy protein, which contains phytoestrogens (from plants), can help to regulate periods. Supplements of vitamins A, E, and C with bioflavonoids may also help if your diet does not include enough of these vitamins.[13] (Take no more than 10,000 IU of a vitamin A supplement twice a day, since larger doses can be toxic. One carrot contains 8,000 IU, and dark green leafy vegetables contain a lot, too, so you can get enough vitamin A from food.) If you are bleeding heavily, increase your iron intake to prevent anemia (see p. 659).

Acupuncture might help to restore hormonal balance. A holistic nutritionist may be able to advise you about herbs that might help. If you are approaching menopause, the bleeding may stop by itself as your hormone levels get lower.

Medical Treatments

Various medications can reduce or regulate abnormal bleeding and relieve pain. *Nonsteroidal anti-inflammatory drugs* (such as ibuprofen) for pain may also reduce bleeding. *Birth control pills* make the cycle more regular and reduce bleeding. An *IUD* (intra-uterine device) treated with a progestin (a hormone used for birth control) can be even more effective for bleeding than pills. Some other drugs, such as danazol and Lupron, reduce bleeding even more but also have serious negative side effects; they are usually used only for a short time, to postpone or prepare you for surgery.

Surgical Treatments

A procedure called *endometrial ablation* removes the lining of the uterus, reducing or stopping the heavy bleeding. Some newer techniques for ablation can be done in a doctor's office under local anesthesia. Most women recover quickly, and some are even able to have children after having endometrial ablation, though there's no guarantee you will be able to get pregnant. Whether you will ever need to repeat the operation will depend on what technique is used and how skilled your practitioner is. If your bleeding is caused by fibroids, there are other surgical treatments available to remove them, without removing the uterus (see "Fibroids," p. 630). *Hysterectomy,* surgery that removes the uterus, permanently stops bleeding and relieves related symptoms, but it also eliminates your ability to bear children (see p. 637).

CERVICITIS

Cervicitis is a general term for inflammation or infection of the cervix. A Pap test report may mention it, but it's not always a real disease or disorder. It can also result from a break in the tissue (lesion) of the cervix caused by an IUD insertion, abortion, or childbirth. Cervicitis is occasionally a sign of a common vaginal infection, sexually transmitted infection (see Chapter 15), or pelvic inflammatory disease (PID, see p. 646). Sometimes scar tissue and normal discharge are mistaken for cervicitis.

Symptoms

You may notice increased vaginal discharge, pain with intercourse, an aching sensation in the lower abdomen, fever, and/or the need to urinate more frequently. When you touch your cervix, it may feel warmer and larger than usual. Moving it with your finger may also be uncomfortable. If you examine yourself using a speculum, your cervix will look red and swollen, and you may observe a discharge. If only the cervical canal is affected, your cervix will look normal, but you may see a yellowish discharge coming from the cervical opening (the os).

When you have a medical exam, be sure to tell your health care provider your medical history and whether or not your discharge seems normal for you. A Pap smear will be taken, and a test for human papillomavirus (HPV) may also be done. Examination of the cervical cells in the lab can tell you whether you have a bacterial infection or a sexually transmitted infection (see Chapter 15, "Sexually Transmitted Infections"). Finding out exactly what is causing the inflammation should lead to more appropriate treatment.

Medical Treatments

If tests show that the inflammation results from STIs such as gonorrhea, syphilis, or chlamydia, you will get oral or injected antibiotics. For mild cervicitis not involving a disease, medical treatment may be pointless. For more severe cases, some physicians recommend cryosurgery or electrocautery (see "Cauterization and Cryotherapy," p. 594). Have these only as a last resort, as they can be painful, can lead to fertility problems, and may take about six weeks for healing. Your provider will probably recommend not using tampons, not inserting anything else in the vagina, and avoiding intercourse during healing from surgical treatment.

Self-Help Treatments

When symptoms are mild and not related to PID or STIs, the following remedies may help: goldenseal douche (¼ teaspoon to 1 quart of water two times a day for two to three weeks), vitamin C douche (500 milligrams in 1 quart of water daily for three to four weeks), or vinegar douche (for more information on herbal remedies, see Chapter 5, "Complementary Health Practices," and "Resources").

To speed healing and strengthen the immune system, and for future prevention, you may want to try oral doses of vitamin C (500 to 1,000 milligrams a day), zinc (25 milligrams a day), and vitamin E (400 milligrams a day). You can also apply vitamin E directly to your cervix with your finger. You can use slippery elm as a douche or paste, applied directly to the cervix in a diaphragm or on the end of a tampon.

Whatever treatment you use, try to combine it with extra rest and good nutrition. Avoid using tampons or putting other objects into your vagina. If you do have intercourse, use a condom.

CERVICAL EVERSION

Cervical eversion (also called ectropion) means that the kind of tissue lining the cervical canal also grows on the outer vaginal part of the cervix, making it red, with a bumpy-looking texture that is smooth to the touch. This is a common physical variation among women. Most women do not have any symptoms. Eversion requires no treatment unless it is accompanied by infection. Those of us whose mothers took DES during pregnancy are more likely to have this condition (see "DES," p. 626).

CERVICAL EROSION

True cervical erosion looks like a large or small pinkish-red sore on the cervix, beside the cervical opening. This condition causes little discomfort, and it is rare. Most cases referred to as erosion in the past were really eversion.

A Pap smear can distinguish cervical erosion, which is benign, from cervical cancer or precancerous changes in cervical cells. If erosion is the diagnosis, your health care provider may recommend having Pap smears more frequently than the usual one a year. Ordinarily, no treatment is needed. Some practitioners may suggest cauterization or cryotherapy (see p. 594), but there's no reason to do that if your Pap smear is normal.

CERVICAL POLYPS

Cervical polyps consist of excess cervical cells that "pile up" within the cervical canal. They appear as bright red tubelike protrusions from the cervical opening, either alone or in clusters. Polyps are very common. Most polyps contain many blood vessels with a fragile outer wall, so bleeding may occur after intercourse or other vaginal penetration, douching, or self-exam. Polyps may also bleed during pregnancy, when hormonal changes stimulate growth of excess cervical tissue.

Cells from the polyps should be collected as part of a Pap smear (see below). Cervical polyps are almost never cancerous. Occasionally, however, they look like cervical cancer or precancer. You can have a colposcopy (p. 593) and biopsy to tell for sure. If the polyps extend inward into the uterus, an evaluation of the uterine cavity (hysteroscopy, p. 595) may also be recommended.

Treatments

Polyps do not necessarily require treatment. When they are small and there is little or no contact bleeding, you can usually just keep track of them with regular self-exams. You may want to have them removed if your symptoms change or if the polyps begin to grow. A polyp can usually be removed in a doctor's office. The practitioner twists the polyp off and cauterizes the base. If your polyp is very large, or if you have several of them, you may have to go to the hospital for removal. Sometimes polyps grow back after removal.

CERVICAL DYSPLASIA AND CERVICAL CANCER

If your test result is not normal, you may see "dysplasia" on the lab report. That means abnormal (dys) cell growth (plasia). Cervical dysplasia, cervical intraepithelial neoplasia (CIN), and squamous intraepithelial lesion (SIL) are all terms used to describe abnormal cells on or near the cervix. In most cases, there are no symptoms.

Most cervical cancers can actually be prevented by finding pre-cancerous conditions of the cervix with Pap smears or similar tests and treating them. Having a regular Pap smear or other screening test as often as recommended for your age and situation is the best prevention strategy.

WHO NEEDS A PAP SMEAR AND OTHER TESTS, AND WHEN?

Almost all women should have regular Pap smears or other cervical screening tests throughout our lives. Because most of the cellular abnormalities we call dysplasia are thought to be caused by HPV (human papillomavirus), there have been some recent changes in how often Pap smears are recommended.

Young women should start having Pap smears at age eighteen *or* about three years after starting any sexual activity near or in the vagina—whichever happens first. That includes oral sex, intercourse, and fingering, because all of these (not only intercourse) can expose you to HPV infection.

Women under thirty should have a pelvic exam and Pap smear annually. If the Pap results are normal, it's the only test needed. Because most young women *do* have mild and nondangerous forms of HPV, the special new test for HPV is not recommended for screening until you are over thirty.

Women on oral contraceptives should have traditional Pap smears, not the newer Liquid-Based (LB) Pap, because the Pill affects the LB Pap outcomes. The LB Pap produces more false positives in women on the Pill.

Women over thirty should have the new combination LB Pap smear and HPV DNA test *once*, unless you have had only negative Pap smears. By this time, your immune system will usually have fought off HPV infections, and the test will tell you so. (If results are normal, combined tests need not be taken more often than every three years.)

- *If the results of both the Pap and HPV tests are normal,* you do not need to be tested again for two years unless you think you have been exposed to HPV since the test. If so, keep having annual Pap smears.

- *If the Pap test is negative (normal) but the HPV test is positive,* this can alert you and your provider that you are at risk, even *before* abnormal cells show up on your Pap smear. Have another Pap smear and an HPV test in six to twelve months.
- *If both tests are positive,* talk with your provider about what to do next. Further tests and colposcopy may be suggested (see "Medical Treatments for Cervical Dysplasia," p. 625).

Women who are not sexually active, or who are monogamous *and* whose partner is monogamous, can follow a different path. If you have three annual Pap smears that are normal, *and* you have none of the risk factors noted above, you can have a Pap smear every three years for as long as your situation remains the same.

Women over sixty-five account for nearly 25 percent of all cervical cancer cases. About 40 percent of women over sixty-five have not had a Pap smear in the last three years. Because HPV can live in the body for many years before becoming active, regular Pap smears are now recommended for women over sixty-five, even if you are not having sex or have had a hysterectomy (see below). If you have had normal Pap smears for three years, every three years is enough. Once you have had normal smears for a ten-year period, you can stop screening if you want to (unless you have new partners during this time), because it seems to take about ten years for an HPV infection to produce serious cervical abnormalities. If you have had recent abnormal test results, get annual Pap tests or what your provider recommends. Medicare now covers the cost of cervical screening every year for women over sixty-five at high risk, and every two years for those not at high risk.

Women who have had hysterectomies should usually continue to have Pap smears, especially if the cervix was left in place. If it wasn't, the smear is taken from the vaginal wall. Follow the guidelines for women over sixty-five. Many women don't know exactly why and what kind of hysterectomy was done or how much of the cervix was removed. When you go for a checkup, bring whatever records you might still have from your surgery. With records and an examination, your provider will be able to tell what kind of hysterectomy you had and whether or not you need to continue to have Pap tests. If your uterus and cervix were removed because of a benign condition, you probably don't.

GETTING AND UNDERSTANDING A PAP SMEAR

During a pelvic examination, with a speculum in place, the provider collects cells from the cervix, at the end of the vagina. Your cells are sent to a lab for analysis, and you can get the results by phone or mail. To make sure the lab has the right kinds of cells, have the Pap about two weeks after the start of your last menstrual period (*never* during your period); don't douche or use tampons, birth control foams, jellies, or other vaginal creams during the three days before the test; and don't have intercourse or put anything else in your vagina during the twenty-four hours before the test.

The results of the Pap smear are classified according to what kinds and degrees of cell changes you have, if any. Four different classification systems are currently in use, but most labs now use the Bethesda System SIL. Dysplasia occurs along a scale, with "all normal" at one end and "invasive cancer" at the other end. It can be difficult to distinguish one stage or grade of dysplasia from the next, and different laboratories or practitioners may label a given cell sample differently. Different systems also use different names for what they find. So, diagnosis is often uncertain, and treatment decisions can be controversial and hard to make.

As many as 40 percent of all tested women will have an abnormal Pap smear at some time during our lives. We often feel anxious when we hear this, because we fear cancer, but there is no need to panic. Most cervical cell changes are very slow. Dysplasia is not cancer, and in about 80 percent of cases, dysplasia does not develop into cancer. The cells of most women diagnosed with mild dysplasia will return to normal. But *all* cases of diagnosed dysplasia should be watched closely—with repeated Pap smears and other recommended procedures—and treated if they progress.

Some health care providers may want to rush you into treatment if you test positive for HPV along with dysplasia. Because the diagnostic tests are not always accurate, and because medical practitioners vary in their diagnoses and preferred treatments, it can be important to get a second opinion about your condition. Also, sometimes the immune system fights off HPV on its own.

WHAT INCREASES MY RISK OF DYSPLASIA AND CERVICAL CANCER?

Most dysplasia (cellular abnormalities) and cervical cancer are now understood to be caused by certain kinds of human papillomaviruses (HPV; see "Cervical Cancer and HPV," p. 634). Other conditions may also increase your risk:

1. *Never having a Pap smear* or not having had one for five or more years. Over half of new cervical cancer diagnoses every year are in women who don't get this screening test and therefore do not get early intervention to prevent cancer from developing.

2. *History* of sexually transmitted infections, especially chlamydia (see Chapter 15, "Sexually Transmitted Infections").

3. *Family history* of cervical dysplasia or cervical cancer.

4. *Older age,* possibly because time increases the chances of being exposed to diseases.

5. *Smoking* is linked to cervical cancer in large population studies.

6. *Synthetic hormones* (such as DES, hormone therapy, or the Pill).

7. *Having unprotected sex at an early age.* If we start having intercourse before softer and more vulnerable cells in the vagina are gradually replaced by tougher cells in our late teens, our cells are more vulnerable to whatever may cause cervical abnormalities.

8. *Exposure to infection.* It takes only one sex partner to get an infection, but more sex partners mean more chances to catch HPVs, STIs, and other germs. If you or your partner or both of you have (or have had) multiple sex partners, your risks of developing abnormal cervical cells are greater. Barrier contraceptives (especially condoms) may reduce such risks. The female condom provides better coverage (see p. 336).

9. *Contact with cancer-causing substances* (in mining, textiles, metalwork, or chemical industries), or sexual contact with a partner(s) who has worked with these substances.

10. *A protein substance in sperm,* or having a sex partner with cancer of the penis. Using a condom or cervical cap for intercourse may reduce such exposure.

11. *A compromised immune system,* especially if you are HIV-positive or have AIDS. Get a Pap test twice during the first year after diagnosis.

If the results are normal, annual smears are enough.

12. *A weakened immune system* from being pregnant, taking drugs like tamoxifen, or having chemotherapy.

13. *Unhealthy living and working conditions and environmental hazards,* often the result of low income. Women without access to a safe, clean environment are more likely to have dysplasia and cancers, and at an earlier age, than middle-class women.

HOW CAN CERVICAL PROBLEMS BE PREVENTED OR REVERSED?

Using an IUD or a barrier method of contraception (such as the condom or diaphragm) along with or instead of oral contraceptives (the Pill) may help to prevent dysplasia or, if you already have it, to allow cells to return to normal by preventing further infection. This is important, because HPV and other STIs put women at greater risk for cervical dysplasia and cancer (see Chapter 14, "Safer Sex," for prevention methods). Access to screening (Pap test) may prevent cervical cancer by finding abnormalities early and treating them.

Eating fruits and vegetables high in vitamin C (see Chapter 2, "Eating Well") and/or taking supplements may help prevent dysplasia or cervical cancer. After a diagnosis of cervical abnormality, taking folic acid (1 milligram per day) and vitamin C (1,000 milligrams per day) may help reverse the condition. Quitting smoking may also help maintain cervical health.

You may want to get tested again after six months to see whether any dysplasia has cleared up.

Medical Treatments for Cervical Dysplasia

Treatments for dysplasia vary widely. You'll want to get appropriate treatment for your condition and to avoid unnecessary or pointless diagnostic tests, treatments, and surgery. Different practitioners may have varying "preferred" treatments for each diagnosis. That's why second and even third opinions may be important. Procedures such as colposcopy (see p. 593), punch biopsy, and cone biopsy (see p. 594) should be done only by medical practitioners who have special training, skills, and a lot of experience.

Watchful waiting is the least drastic approach, with repeat Pap smears and HPV tests, other tests, and/or colposcopy and punch biopsy to monitor your condition. Trying a self-help approach for six months to a year—such as regular condom use for intercourse—may reverse dysplasia and will prevent new infections. The next step is *destruction of abnormal cells* by cryotherapy, laser, loop electrosurgical excision procedure (LEEP, see p. 594), or a similar technique called large loop excision in the transformation zone (LLETZ or ELECTZ).

Cone biopsy (conization or conical) is often recommended when repeated Pap smears or colposcopies confirm severe dysplasia or localized cancer (cancer in situ or CIS), and if the abnormal area extends into the cervical canal (where it cannot be reached for colposcopy or cryotherapy). The cone-shaped piece of tissue removed by this procedure is examined to ensure that all borders of the abnormal area were completely removed. If the abnormal area extends beyond the edge of the cone, a second conization may be recommended, to remove a larger area.

These treatments can be uncomfortable and occasionally painful. After cone or punch biopsy, cryotherapy, laser treatment, or LEEP, do not use tampons, douche, have intercourse, or put anything else into your vagina for at least three weeks. This minimizes both pain and the risk of infection. Some women experience cramping, tenderness, bleeding, and/or discharges.

Hysterectomy is usually recommended as the appropriate treatment for invasive cancer (see "Uterine Cancer," p. 637). This is major surgery, with serious risks and other health consequences (see "Hysterectomy and Oophorectomy," p. 637, and "Surgery," p. 689).

Cone biopsy may weaken the cervix, so it can be harder to carry a pregnancy to term. A hysterectomy permanently ends a woman's ability to bear children. While both may be appropriate for severe dysplasia and can save women's lives, you should seek a second or even third opinion and ask what other treatment options may be available if you are concerned about future childbearing.

(For more information, see "Cervical Health" [W68] on the companion website, www.our bodiesourselves.org.)

DES

DES (diethylstilbestrol) is a powerful synthetic estrogen that crosses the placenta of pregnant women and may damage the reproductive system of the developing fetus. DES may also affect other body systems: endocrine, immune, skeletal, and neurological. This drug was prescribed to an estimated 4.8 million American women between 1938 and 1971, in the mistaken belief that it would prevent miscarriage. In fact, DES was untested for pregnancy use or safety, and studies showing that it did not prevent miscarriage were ignored for almost two decades. It was aggressively marketed and used worldwide, under more than two hundred brand names, in pills, injections, and suppositories, until it was found to be linked to a rare form of vaginal cancer in daughters of women who had taken it.*

* DES was used until 1975 in England and the Netherlands, 1977 in France, 1981 in Spain and Italy, and 1983 in Hungary.

Large studies on DES mothers, daughters, and sons are now under way as a result of efforts by DES advocacy groups.

WHO IS EXPOSED AND HOW TO FIND OUT

Several million people have been exposed to DES, most without knowing it. If you were born between 1938 and 1971, try to find out whether your mother had problems with any of her pregnancies or remembers taking anything when she was pregnant with you. (DES was most widely used between 1947 and 1965, when "wonder drugs" were so popular.) If a woman doesn't know or can't remember whether she took DES, she may be able to ask the doctor she saw, or it may be on the medical record at the hospital where the birth took place (though some health care providers or facilities no longer have old records or refuse to give out the information). Any woman unsure about her mother's exposure can get a special exam (see p. 627) from a medical practitioner knowledgeable about DES exposure (see DES Action, www.desaction.org, for referrals).

MEDICAL PROBLEMS AND CARE FOR DES DAUGHTERS

One out of every thousand DES daughters is likely to develop *clear-cell adenocarcinoma*, a rare type of vaginal or cervical cancer. It has occurred in girls as young as seven and women up to age forty, with the peak at ages 15 to 22. Although the number of cases of clear-cell cancer has declined in the last two decades (mirroring decreased use of DES in the 1970s), it continues to be found in DES daughters, some in their 50s. If you are a DES daughter, you need to continue to get special DES exams (see p. 627) for the rest of your life.

Regular DES exams can find clear-cell cancer early, so that it can be treated. This cancer grows quickly and sometimes has no symptoms in the early stages. Typical treatment for clear-cell cancer may include a radical hysterectomy, surgical removal of all or part of the vagina, and reconstruction of the vagina. Radiation treatment may be added. Eighty percent of women survive this extreme treatment, but most find it very hard to adjust to.

Recent studies show that DES daughters have a greater risk for a more common vaginal cancer, *squamous cell carcinoma.*[14] You may also have *adenosis*—columnar cells where the usual squamous cells should be—around the cervix. If you do, you may be more vulnerable to precancerous or cancerous changes. Annual colposcopy monitoring may be recommended until any adenosis is healed, which usually happens by a woman's late thirties; discuss this with your gynecologist. *Dysplasia* (abnormal cell change) is more common among DES daughters, but normal cell changes may be mistakenly seen as abnormal when your cervix is checked, leading to unnecessary treatment with possibly harmful effects. That's why it's important to find a health care provider with experience in DES screening.

Structural changes in the uterus and cervix are common in DES daughters. Cervical "collars" or "hoods" *(adenosis)* do not have to be treated and may disappear after age thirty. A *smaller* or *T-shaped uterus* may contribute to pregnancy problems (see below).

If you are a DES daughter over age forty, your risk for *breast cancer* may be two and a half times greater than that of unexposed women.[15] DES mothers, too, have developed more breast cancers than unexposed women—sometimes as long as twenty years after exposure—so both mothers and daughters should get a professional breast exam every year, in addition to doing self-exam.

Contraception for DES daughters poses some special considerations. Birth control pills may be risky, since they increase estrogen exposure in someone already at higher risk of hormone-related cancer. IUDs may not be safe because of cervical and uterine abnormalities. Barrier methods (condom, diaphragm) are probably the safest choice overall.

Pregnancy problems may result from structural abnormalities in the uterus and cervix of DES daughters. You might have trouble conceiving, or be more likely to miscarry, deliver prematurely, or have an ectopic (tubal) pregnancy (in the fallopian tube instead of the uterus). A pregnant DES daughter needs high-risk obstetrical care. Checking early in pregnancy for signs of problems may help prevent serious complications.

The doctor who was doing my DES exams didn't know anything about pregnancy problems for DES daughters. So I brought him seven articles that DES Action gave me. We both read them, and as a result, he checked my cervix at every prenatal visit. It took 15 seconds and took away tons of anxiety.

Other problems, including endometriosis, menstrual irregularities, and PID have been reported by many DES daughters. DES sons and grandchildren may have problems, too.

THE DES EXAM

DES daughters should see a medical practitioner experienced in DES screening, because changes caused by DES do not usually show up in regular pelvic exams or Pap smears. Ask whether your health care provider is monitoring other DES daughters and is familiar with the techniques described here. The exam should include careful visual inspection of the vagina and cervix, gentle palpation of the vaginal walls, separate Pap smears from the cervix and from the surfaces of the upper vagina, and a bimanual pelvic exam (see p. 590). Iodine staining (Schiller's test) of the vagina and cervix can distinguish normal tissue (which stains brown) from adenosis (which does not stain). These tests will indicate anything that might need further testing by colposcopy or biopsy.

ENDOMETRIOSIS

Endometriosis is a puzzling hormonal and immune system disease in which tissue like that of the uterine lining (*endometrium*) grows outside the uterus (the tissue is sometimes called nodules, tumors, lesions, or implants). It affects girls and women from as young as eight to past menopause and can cause pain, infertility, and other problems.

The most common locations of endometrial growths are in the abdomen—on the ovaries, fallopian tubes, ligaments supporting the uterus, area between the vagina and the rectum, outer surface of the uterus, and lining of the pelvic cavity. Sometimes growths arise in abdominal surgery scars, on the intestines, in the rectum, or on the bladder, vagina, cervix, and vulva (external genitals). Rarely, they develop in the lung, arm, thigh, and elsewhere. Endometrial tissue outside the uterus responds to hormone cycles but has no way of leaving the body. The result is internal bleeding, degeneration of the blood and tissue shed from the growths, inflammation of surrounding areas, and the formation of scar tissue (*adhesions*). Other possible complications include rupture of cysts (which can spread endometriosis to new areas), intestinal bleeding or obstruction, or interference with bladder function. Symptoms seem to worsen with time, though cycles of remission and recurrence are sometimes the pattern.

Women and girls with endometriosis are at greater risk for cancer, particularly melanoma and ovarian and breast cancer, and for autoimmune diseases such as hypothyroidism, rheumatoid arthritis, and lupus (see p. 661). However, endometriosis lesions rarely become cancerous. Because of these risks, and because endometriosis can be life-disrupting, we should not ignore symptoms.

"Don't be a baby, honey; all girls get cramps. Take two aspirin and go back to class," the nurse at my high school told me when I was bent over double in tears. . . . I'm not a baby. I'm not a hypochondriac. . . . It took six years to find out. Looking back, I wish I had been a more aggressive patient. I should never have allowed myself to believe these occurrences were all in my head. . . . Don't listen to the people who tell you to go away. Be persistent. Listen to your body.

The most common symptoms of endometriosis are pain before and during menstrual periods and sexual activity, infertility, and heavy bleeding. Other symptoms may include fatigue, painful bowel movements or lower-back pain with periods, diarrhea and/or constipation, and intestinal upset with periods. Many women with endometriosis also have allergies, asthma, and eczema. The degree of pain is not necessarily related to the extent or size of the growths. Even tiny growths can produce substances called *prostaglandins* that are involved in pain (as well as menstrual cramps). About 30 to 40 percent of women with endometriosis experience infertility.

Endometriosis is annoying for many women because it is chronic and its seriousness is often not understood. In one survey of four thousand women who had it, 79 percent said that they were unable to carry on normal work and activities at times, yet 69 percent had been told by a gynecologist that nothing was wrong.

I was diagnosed too late, though I complained bitterly about very painful, heavy periods since my mid-teens. I think it's disgraceful that doctors aren't more interested in treating this disease before things get so out of hand. . . . I am thirty-six and too destroyed (physically and emotionally) to carry on the fight to preserve my fertility.

Both medical literature and the popular media have labeled it a "[white] career woman's disease" and have blamed the victim, a myth that probably developed because these were the types of women who had the resources needed to get a correct diagnosis. However, women of color do have endometriosis, and many women experience symptoms before age twenty; more teenagers and girls are being diagnosed. And, contrary to medical myth, early pregnancy—even teenage pregnancy—does not prevent endometriosis. Another problem is that many doctors still don't take menstrual pain seriously and are slow to diagnose endometriosis.

Diagnosis requires a laparoscopy, though growths can sometimes be detected during a manual pelvic exam. Endometriosis is sometimes confused with other disorders that have similar symptoms (PID, ectopic pregnancy, cysts, appendicitis, diverticulitis, or even cancer). To get the right treatment, you need a correct diagnosis. The Endometriosis Association (www.endometriosisassn.org) has a diagnostic kit that helps.

Choosing a treatment is rarely simple. In the process, you may want to consider your age, your symptoms, where and how severe the growths are, whether or not you want to get pregnant, your past experiences with hormones, and your family history.

Hormonal treatments aim to stop the ovary from producing estrogen and also to stop menstruation. They include gonadotropin-releasing hormone (GnRH) analogs, danazol, progesterone-like drugs (Provera), oral contraceptives, and new drugs currently in development. Most are very expensive. All cause side effects that are problematic for some women. Also, all tend to work while you are taking them, but when you stop, the condition usually comes back within a short time.

Surgery ranges from conservative (scraping, cutting, cauterizing, or lasering the growths) to radical (hysterectomy and removal of the ovaries). Radical surgery has been called the definitive cure for endometriosis, but the disease can continue or recur even with removal of the ovaries. Less invasive surgery through the laparoscope has largely replaced major abdominal surgery.

Complementary medicine, especially nutritional approaches, traditional Chinese medicine, and other treatments, have proved helpful

THE ENVIRONMENTAL CONNECTION

A new theory about the cause of endometriosis is that dioxin, often called the most toxic chemical ever made by humans, is involved. Dioxin and similar chemicals disrupt hormones and stimulate immune system reactions. Dioxin accumulates in our food from environmental sources, including pesticides and herbicides, industrial waste, and incineration. This suggests that endometriosis may be triggered or worsened by the environment in which we live. It's also possible that endometriosis is just one of a group of diseases resulting from exposure to these chemicals. If so, we may be able to prevent endometriosis and related diseases in our children.

The Endometriosis Association, an international self-help organization founded in 1980, has developed the world's largest research registry on the disease, using data gathered from thousands of women. It conducts research collaboratively with the National Institutes of Health and Vanderbilt University School of Medicine, and its Open Research Fund supports twenty scientific projects in seven countries. (For more information, see "Resources.")

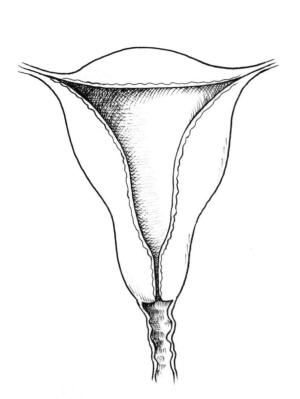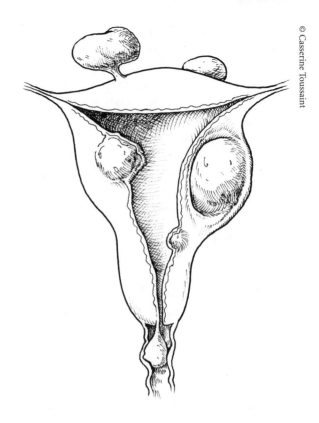

A uterus without fibroids, left, and a uterus with fibroids (benign growths), right.

for some women. Contact the Endometriosis Association for more information plus a comprehensive book (see "Resources").

Pregnancy is not a cure, though it may offer temporary relief. If you know you want a child, be aware that delay may make pregnancy less likely if the disease advances.

Getting Support

Joining a support group can decrease feelings of isolation and provide opportunities to counteract misinformation or a lack of information, as well as to share experiences with others who understand what you're going through. The Endometriosis Association can help you find a group (see "Resources").

FIBROIDS (LEIOMYOMAS, MYOMAS)

Fibroids are solid benign tumors* that appear, sometimes in groups, on the outside, inside, or within the wall of the uterus, often changing the size and shape of it. About 30 percent of all women get fibroids by age thirty-five; black women are more likely to have them, and to get them at a younger age. The cause of fibroids is unknown, but these growths seem to be related to estrogen production. They may grow more

* The word "tumor" is very scary to most of us. It used to be a euphemism for cancer, but in fact, tumors are just growths of cells that serve no purpose. Over 90 percent of all tumors are benign (not cancerous) and harmless.

quickly if you are pregnant, using oral contraceptives, or taking estrogen for hot flashes (all of which raise estrogen levels in the body).

Fibroids may be discovered during a routine pelvic exam. Because fibroids can grow, they should be monitored. If they haven't grown any more by the time you have your next monitoring exam several months later, a yearly checkup will be enough. Ultrasound can give more definite information about the number and size of fibroids, but this is not always necessary.

Often fibroids don't cause symptoms. However, some fibroids may cause pain, bleeding between periods, or excessive menstrual flow.[16] If you have fibroids and abnormal bleeding, be sure to get carefully checked for other possible causes of the bleeding (see p. 618). Depending on their size and location, fibroids can also cause abdominal or back pain, urinary problems, and constipation, and your belly may look bigger. Large fibroids sometimes make it difficult to conceive or to sustain a full-term pregnancy.

SELF-HELP TREATMENTS

If you are taking estrogen in any form, you may be able to reduce large fibroids by not taking it anymore. Some women try to prevent or reduce fibroids by avoiding processed foods and the hormones usually found in commercial meat, dairy, and egg products. If your fibroids cause heavy bleeding, see the self-help treatments in "Abnormal Uterine Bleeding" (p. 618). Yoga exercises may ease the feelings of heaviness and pressure; some women find visualization techniques helpful, too.

MEDICAL TREATMENTS

In many cases, no treatment is necessary for fibroids; this is called *watchful waiting*. If you have excessive bleeding, pain, urinary difficulties, or problems with pregnancy, you may want to have an operation to remove the fibroids (*myomectomy*). This usually requires an abdominal incision, but sometimes it can be done with less invasive techniques (laparoscopy or hysteroscopy), which also means less anesthesia and therefore less risk. Even large, multiple fibroids can be removed with a myomectomy. Depending on where the fibroids were growing, myomectomy may make it harder or easier for you to get pregnant. In at least 10 to 25 percent of cases, new fibroids grow. Given enough time and continued hormone stimulation, most women with fibroids are likely to develop new ones.

Embolization of the uterine arteries is a newer, less invasive technique that cuts off blood supply to the fibroids and makes them shrink. It reduces bleeding, other symptoms, and tumor or uterus size in most women who have it done, and the complication rate is low.[17] This procedure is done by radiologists. The recovery time is shorter, and for women close to menopause, it is probably safer. For women still intending to have children, the effects on pregnancy and childbirth are not yet known.

Many physicians recommend *hysterectomy* (removal of the uterus) as a treatment for fibroids in women who are past childbearing age or who do not want more children. This surgery may be unnecessary, particularly if you are nearing menopause, when the natural decline in estrogen levels usually shrinks fibroids. Moreover, hysterectomy, like any major surgery, carries some risks. (For more information, see p. 637.) Embolization or myomectomy—done by a skilled practitioner—avoids some of the problems associated with hysterectomy and poses no greater risks. New laser techniques for dissolving fibroids are also being investigated.

Sometimes the drug Lupron is recommended to women approaching menopause or planning to have surgery, to help shrink fibroids. Many practitioners now consider Lupron inappropriate to use for longer than six months, because its negative side effects include menopausal symptoms and bone thinning.

The newest treatment, having a *medicated IUD* (intra-uterine device) put into the uterus, can reduce bleeding and may shrink fibroids, possibly enabling you to avoid surgery.[18]

OVARIAN CYSTS

Ovarian cysts are relatively common and may result from normal ovulation. They develop when a follicle has grown large but has failed to rupture and release an egg. Most of these cysts are filled with fluid. Often, cysts don't cause any symptoms or discomfort, but you may experience a disturbance in the normal menstrual cycle, an unfamiliar pain or discomfort in the lower abdomen at any point during the cycle, or pain during intercourse. They're often found by a routine bimanual pelvic exam, then diagnosed with ultrasound. Cysts usually disappear by themselves, though some types may have to be removed.

To determine whether a cyst requires treatment, wait a cycle or two for it to disappear. If it persists, a medical practitioner may use ultrasound to monitor it. Practitioners disagree about whether removing benign cysts is necessary, but small ones do not usually cause problems and may be left alone. A large cyst is more of a health risk because it can rupture, causing severe abdominal pain and sometimes bleeding. A large cyst may also twist and damage the blood supply to the ovary. These two uncommon situations require prompt surgery. Pathological cysts, such as a dermoid cyst, a cyst of endometriosis, or cancer, should usually be removed.

If your physician advises removal of the ovary along with a benign cyst, get a second opinion. Removing the ovary, though a conventional practice, is unnecessary in many cases. Ovaries perform many functions, even after menopause.

Recurrent cysts may indicate a hormonal imbalance and/or life stresses. Changing your diet, learning how to reduce stress, and using acupuncture may also help to get your system back in balance.

POLYCYSTIC OVARY SYNDROME

Polycystic ovary syndrome (PCOS, or Stein-Leventhal syndrome) is a complex condition of hormonal imbalance that occurs in 4 to 6 percent of women. It may start around puberty or become noticeable in the twenties or thirties. Women are affected by it in different ways.

Some common concerns are a history of no periods (amenorrhea); irregular periods; hair thinning at the forehead; acne; excess weight, especially around the waist; and trouble getting pregnant. Other signs that help medical practitioners diagnose PCOS are hormone imbalances; slightly enlarged ovaries with many small benign cysts (visible on ultrasound); insulin resistance, with higher risk of developing diabetes (see p. 680 in Chapter 29, "Special Concerns for Women"); and a family history of PCOS.

The cause of PCOS is unknown, and there may be several different forms. If you have it, your levels of two hormones that drive ovulation—follicle-stimulating hormone (FSH) and luteinizing hormone (LH)—may be out of balance. Your body may make more androgens (hormones such as testosterone, which women have in small amounts) than usual. That can block egg growth and ovulation and cause acne, receding hairline, and excess face and body hair.

PCOS was named after the many tiny ovarian cysts once considered its main characteristic. Researchers disagree as to whether or not these cysts are immature eggs that didn't get released during ovulation. Not every woman with PCOS has them, and not every woman who has them has PCOS.

OTHER PROBLEMS LINKED TO PCOS

You may be most concerned about irregular periods, face and body hair, or infertility—what brought you to your health care provider in the first place. Unfortunately, the hormonal imbalance underlying this syndrome may cause other medical problems, too. PCOS is related to higher risks of diabetes, heart disease, and endometrial cancer (cancer of the uterine lining). Which of these risks may apply to you depends on how PCOS affects your body (for more about cardiovascular disease, see p. 671; for more about diabetes, see p. 680; for more about endometrial cancer, see p. 637).

Diabetes Risk

Insulin, a hormone made by the pancreas, turns food sugars into energy. If you have insulin resistance, a normal amount of insulin isn't enough to do this, and the body starts making more, resulting in a condition called *hyperinsulinemia* (too much insulin). Women who are insulin-resistant are more likely to develop Type 2 and gestational diabetes (diabetes during pregnancy).

Cardiovascular Risk

Triglycerides—a type of fatty acid in the bloodstream—may be higher than normal in some women with PCOS. The total cholesterol count may be higher, too. HDL, the "good" cholesterol, may be lower than normal. This raises the risk of heart attacks, because it can result in plaque that narrows or clogs arteries and other blood vessels over time.

Cancer Risk

Women with PCOS who have infrequent periods are slightly more likely to develop endometrial cancer, because abnormal cells may build up in the lining of the uterus when it is not shed regularly. Eventually, some of these cells may turn cancerous. Women with PCOS who ovulate and have regular periods do not have a higher risk of endometrial cancer.

TREATMENTS FOR PCOS

Generally, treatment depends on how PCOS affects you. Eating a healthy diet and exercising regularly will lower your risk of developing heart disease and diabetes. If you are overweight, getting closer to normal body weight for your age and height may help you start ovulating again and decrease insulin resistance. Medical treatments to restore ovulation or target insulin resistance may help reverse many of the problems linked to PCOS. However, it is currently not known whether any of these therapies can stop or reverse the long-term effects of PCOS.

Birth control pills make periods more regular and help prevent endometrial cancer. By lowering the androgen levels in the bloodstream, they may also prevent balding and decrease facial hair and acne. While some women with PCOS have trouble getting pregnant, this is not true for everyone. If you do not want to get pregnant, be sure to use birth control every time you have intercourse. *Androgen blockers* such as spironolactone (Aldactone) may also be prescribed. *Diabetes drugs* that decrease insulin resistance can help balance reproductive hormones, too. Preliminary studies of insulin-resistant women with PCOS show that these drugs may restore ovulation and reduce face and body hair, acne, balding, and weight.

Fertility drugs such as Clomid (clomiphene citrate) may be prescribed to trigger egg growth and ovulation if you want to get pregnant. If that doesn't work, stronger drugs such as Follistim, Gonal-F, or Fertinex may help. You might also consider having in vitro fertilization (IVF). (For more information, see p. 520 in Chapter 25, "Infertility and Assisted Reproduction.")

Surgical techniques that make small holes in one or both ovaries may restore ovulation, though not always permanently. Adhesions—scar tissue that can twist the ovaries or make them cling to other organs—may result. This is more likely to happen when surgery is done on both ovaries.

CERVICAL CANCER

Each year in the United States, about 17,500 women are diagnosed with cervical cancer. Of the 5,000 women who die annually of cervical cancer, 50 percent have never had a Pap test and therefore are more likely to have cancers that were caught later in their development. Some studies show an elevated risk of cervical cancer in women who are smokers, farm workers, cooks, cleaners, maids, and the wives of coal miners. (For more discussion of the causes and prevention of cervical cancer, see "Cervical Dysplasia and Cervical Cancer," p. 622.)

If severely abnormal cells have spread beyond the upper tissue layer (surface epithelium) of your cervix into the underlying connective tissues, you have invasive cervical cancer. A Pap smear followed by a biopsy can determine whether that has happened. At first the spread is very shallow and may not involve the lymph or blood systems. In its early stages, cervical cancer is almost always curable (depending on the severity of the lesions and the treatment used).

Treatment

Most physicians recommend a *hysterectomy* (removal of the uterus; see p. 637) with close follow-up for invasive cervical cancer. If the cancer has spread into the lymph or blood systems, doctors usually suggest radiation or hysterectomy plus removal of the ovaries (*oophorectomy*). Sometimes a combination of the two is

CERVICAL CANCER AND HPV

Today certain types of human papillomaviruses (HPVs) are understood to be the cause of cervical dysplasia (abnormal cell growth) and cervical cancers. HPVs are very common, and most men and women will be infected with one of these viruses at some point. Of approximately one hundred types of HPV, only about thirty infect the genital area. HPV16 is believed to cause half of all cervical cancer cases, and HPV18 is responsible for another 20 percent. Another type causes condyloma warts in the genital area, in both women and men.

In most cases, an individual's immune system can control HPV or eliminate it from the body. However, HPV can be present for weeks, months, or decades after initial infection. If HPV persists or is not controlled, it can lead to cervical abnormalities in some women. Scientists do not know why some women are able to fight off HPV while others cannot, but they think there are additional factors that can increase women's risks.

The link to HPV has changed recommendations for screening, especially who is considered to be at risk. An annual Pap smear is now recommended for any girl or woman who is having sex (see "Who Needs a Pap Smear and Other Tests, and When?" p. 622). Sexual behavior is more of a real factor in risk than a woman's age. (For more information on HPV, see p. 288 in Chapter 15, "Sexually Transmitted Infections.")

used (chemotherapy is not as effective as local radiation).

Radiation treatment is given in two ways. If the tumor is large, you will get external radiation daily over a period of several weeks. This will mean daily trips to the medical center or hospital, which can be exhausting and cause you considerable inconvenience, depending on how far away you live. You may need to ask family and friends to go with you, help with your other commitments, and provide support. Negative effects of the radiation treatment—which are usually temporary—include diarrhea, skin changes, rectal bleeding, and fatigue. Because each person reacts to radiation differently, the amount may have to be increased or decreased depending on your response.

When the radiation treatment has reduced the size of the growth, radioactive materials are placed inside your uterus or in the upper portion of your vagina. You will be admitted to the hospital and given general anesthesia for this procedure. The implants are left inside your body for one to three days, while you are in the hospital. This treatment directs a greater amount of radiation to a smaller area. Depending on the size of the tumor and how much it has spread, 60 to 90 percent of women who have radiation treatment for cervical cancer survive for five years.[19]

You should be involved in your treatment and have the final say in all decisions. If you have any doubts about treatments recommended by your health care provider, try to get second and third opinions.

OVARIAN CANCER

Cancer of the ovaries results in more deaths (14,000 in the United States) each year than any other cancer of the female reproductive system, even though the lifetime risk of getting it is only about 1.7 percent. Although the incidence of ovarian cancer increases with age (a high percentage of cases is found in postmenopausal women), women of any age may develop it. More than 26,700 new cases are diagnosed an-

nually in the United States alone. One reason the death rate is so high is that most ovarian cancer is found in the later stages, when it is harder to treat effectively. When it is found early, over 90 percent of the women who have it survive.

The exact causes of ovarian cancer are still unknown. Possible risk factors include a family history of ovarian cancer; few or no pregnancies; the use of fertility-stimulating drugs; a history of breast, colorectal, or endometrial cancer; exposure to industrial products, including asbestos, or to high levels of radiation; a diet high in fat; and the use of estrogens other than the birth control pill. Using talcum powder in the genital area has long been suspected as a risk factor, but studies haven't proved it. Oral contraceptive use and multiple pregnancies may lower a woman's risk for ovarian cancer.* Having a tubal ligation (tying the fallopian tubes) also appears to reduce risk.[20]

Diagnosis

Ovarian cancer does not always have clear symptoms. Its warning signs—which may be vague and are frequently dismissed as "stress" or "nerves"—include indigestion, gas, bowel disturbances, loss of appetite or weight, a feeling of fullness, enlargement or bloating of the abdomen, lower abdominal discomfort or pain, unexplained weight gain, frequent urination, fatigue, backache, nausea, vomiting, nonmenstrual vaginal bleeding, or pain during intercourse.

If you have persistent symptoms or a family history of ovarian cancer, make sure your gyne-

---

* Removal of the ovaries has been proposed as an option to prevent ovarian cancer. Although the benefit of prophylactic oophorectomy is not certain and a small risk remains, some specialists suggest this surgery for women whose risk is very high—those who have certain gene mutations (see "Genetic Testing for Ovarian Cancer Risk," p. 636).

colologist does a thorough evaluation for it.* In some cases, you may need to be referred to a gynecological oncologist, who specializes in cancer diagnosis and treatment. The tests now available are not accurate enough for ovarian cancer screening (routine testing in women with no symptoms and no risk factors). A blood test for a protein called CA-125 is not enough to diagnose ovarian cancer, because many other conditions can also raise the level of CA-125 in the blood—it needs to be used in combination with other tests.

Diagnostic tests for cancer of the ovaries include pelvic ultrasound, computerized tomography (called *CT* or *CAT scan*), magnetic resonance imaging *(MRI),* and surgery, the only conclusive diagnostic tool. Exploratory surgery *(laparotomy)* is used for diagnosis, staging, and, frequently, tumor reduction. (For more information on stages and different types of ovarian cancer, including borderline tumors not likely to become malignant, consult "Resources.")

MEDICAL TREATMENTS

Early detection, prompt diagnosis, and accurate staging are necessary for the successful treatment of ovarian cancer. What treatment may work depends on the stage of the disease at the time of diagnosis, the type of cells that make up the tumor, and how fast the cancer is growing. The current standard medical options for treating ovarian cancer include surgery, chemotherapy, and/or radiation. Immunotherapies, including interferon, interleukin, bone marrow or stem cell transplants, and monoclonal antibodies, are also available in clinical and/or research settings. Although not necessary for every patient, second-look surgery may be indicated for

---

* A Pap smear should be part of the pelvic exam, as it may reveal malignant ovarian cells, but it is not a reliable test for ovarian cancer.

GENETIC TESTING FOR OVARIAN CANCER RISK

Two known genes, BRCA1 and BRCA2, have been related to an increased risk for ovarian and breast cancers. Evidence of mutation does not mean that a woman will get ovarian or breast cancer. The role of any specific mutation in the development of cancer is still being researched.

About 5 to 7 percent of ovarian cancer cases are possibly associated with an inherited risk factor. Although genetic testing may be helpful to some women with two or more first-degree relatives (mother, sister, daughter) who have ovarian cancer, it has become the subject of great controversy. First, these tests are becoming a lucrative business and may be promoted to women who don't need them. Second, they may lead to discrimination in insurance and health care. Third, because there is no clear preventive therapy for a woman whose risk for ovarian cancer is high, many people question the whole point of testing. Women who want to be tested need to consider the potential medical, legal, and psychosocial implications of genetic testing. Comprehensive genetic counseling can be useful, since genetic counselors are trained to offer honest and balanced information (see "Resources").

women at high risk for persistent tumor. (For more about surgical removal of the ovaries, see "Hysterectomy and Oophorectomy," p. 637.)

New cancer therapies become available to patients through clinical trials. Information about some of these investigational treatments is registered with the National Cancer Institute (see "Cancer" in "Resources"). Many women explore supplemental or alternative treatments, alone or in conjunction with mainstream treatments.

Grassroots women's health activists are beginning to lobby for increased funding for ovarian cancer research and awareness. More efforts are needed to help reduce mortality from this disease and ultimately to prevent it.

UTERINE CANCER

Cancer of the lining of the uterus (endometrial cancer) is the most common pelvic cancer, affecting fourteen out of every ten thousand women yearly. Most women with this cancer are over fifty and past menopause; 10 percent are still menstruating. If you are very heavy; take synthetic estrogen; or have diabetes, high blood pressure, or a hormone imbalance that combines high estrogen levels with infrequent ovulation, your risk of uterine cancer is increased. During the early 1970s, there was a sharp rise in the incidence of uterine cancer, brought about by increased use of estrogen to relieve menopausal symptoms.

Symptoms

Bleeding after menopause is the most common symptom of uterine cancer. For women who are still menstruating, increased menstrual flow and bleeding between periods may be the only symptoms. Unfortunately, the Pap smear, while effective at detecting cervical cancer, is not reliable for detecting uterine cancer. If you have the above symptoms, your medical practitioner will probably recommend an aspiration or endometrial biopsy to sample the uterine lining. In some cases, a D&C is suggested, but most experts now prefer aspiration over D&C. Make sure that you have discussed the risks and benefits of all these alternatives before making a decision.

PREVENTION AND SELF-HELP

Because endometrial cancer appears to be influenced by factors such as obesity, hypertension, and diabetes, controlling these conditions with self-help methods may prevent this type of cancer from developing or spreading. Exercise and a healthy diet, with plenty of fruits and vegetables, is the best strategy.

MEDICAL TREATMENTS

Medical treatment for uterine cancer includes surgery, radiation, and chemotherapy. There is wide disagreement about which is best. Outside the United States, radiation is used frequently with good results. In this country, hysterectomy is the most common treatment, sometimes with follow-up radiation after surgery if the tumor was large, if spread to the lymph nodes was suspected, or if the cellular changes were greater than usual. If the cancer comes back after one of these treatments, progestin treatment may help slow it down. When uterine cancer is found early, the success rate of conventional treatments is very high.

HYSTERECTOMY AND OOPHORECTOMY

The United States has the highest hysterectomy rate in the industrialized world. About one third of all American women have had a hysterectomy by the age of sixty. Today about 90 percent of hysterectomies are done by choice and not as an emergency or lifesaving procedure. Various studies have concluded that anywhere from 10 percent to 90 percent of those operations were not really needed, but many physicians continue to recommend them. Certainly, they have saved lives and restored health for many women, but unnecessary operations have exposed women to risks needlessly. Health care providers should recognize the value of a woman's uterus and ovaries, even when the woman is in midlife or beyond.

Both procedures are considered major surgery and may have long-term effects on our health, sexuality, and life expectancy. Because of the controversy over hysterectomy and oophorectomy rates, many insurance plans now require a second opinion from another physician before agreeing to pay for the procedures. Be-cause some surgeons recommend hysterectomy routinely, we need to know when it is truly necessary (see box).

Fortunately, diagnostic techniques such as sonography, Pap smears, hysteroscopy, and laparoscopy make it possible to avoid or delay many hysterectomies that might have been done in the past. Unfortunately, most surgeons do not use them enough, believing there is no advantage to saving a uterus, especially if a woman is past her childbearing years.

WHEN IS HYSTERECTOMY NEEDED?

Hysterectomy may be recommended for several life-threatening conditions:

1. Invasive cancer of the uterus, cervix, vagina, fallopian tubes, and/or ovaries. Only 8 to 12 percent of hysterectomies are performed to treat cancer.
2. Severe, uncontrollable infection (PID).
3. Severe, uncontrollable bleeding (rare, usually associated with childbirth).
4. Rare but serious complications during childbirth, including rupture of the uterus.

If you have any of these conditions, hysterectomy may save your life. It may also free you from significant pain and discomfort.

Hysterectomy may be justified as treatment for some conditions that are not life-threatening:

1. Pre-cancerous changes of the endometrium, called *hyperplasia*. (Remember, however, that most hyperplasia can be reversed with medication.)
2. Severe pelvic infections unresponsive to antibiotics.

3. Extensive endometriosis causing debilitating pain and/or involving other organs. (More conservative surgery and/or medication is usually an effective treatment.)
4. Fibroid tumors that are extensive, large, involve other organs, or cause debilitating bleeding. (However, fibroids can be removed by myomectomy, thereby preserving the uterus.)
5. Pelvic relaxation (uterine prolapse) that is causing severe symptoms. (Another treatment option in this case is uterine suspension surgery.)

Depending on their severity, many of these conditions can be treated without resorting to major surgery. In some cases, observation and explanation are enough.

Hysterectomies should not be performed for mild abnormal uterine bleeding, fibroids without symptoms, and pelvic congestion (menstrual irregularities and low back pain). These problems can usually be treated with cheaper and safer alternatives. If your doctor insists on hysterectomy for one of these conditions, consider changing to another health care provider.

The most recent data suggest that African-American women have a somewhat higher hysterectomy rate than white women, possibly because African-American women are more likely to have fibroids (see p. 630). For many years, hysterectomy was performed solely for the purpose of sterilization among many poorer women and women of color in the United States. This abuse led to federal sterilization guidelines in 1979.

Whenever you have any doubts about the need for a hysterectomy and/or oophorectomy, seek one or more other opinions about possible alternative approaches (such as a myomectomy, which removes fibroids without removing the uterus).

RISKS AND COMPLICATIONS OF HYSTERECTOMY AND OOPHORECTOMY

Although the death rate from hysterectomy is low (under 1 percent), surgical complications include the following:

1. *Infection.* Most infections can be treated successfully with antibiotics, but some can be severe or even uncontrollable.
2. *Hemorrhage* at the time of surgery or afterward (a transfusion or second operation may be necessary).
3. *Damage* to your internal organs, most frequently the urinary tract and sometimes the bowel. Sometimes there is damage to the ureter (tube connecting the kidney to the bladder) or the bladder.

Less common surgical complications include blood clots, complications from the anesthesia, and intestinal obstruction from post-surgical scarring.

LONG-TERM RISKS

For those of us who are in our early forties or younger, removal of the uterus and ovaries may increase the risk of heart attack. Even if our ovaries are not removed, there is an increased chance of an earlier menopause. This is usually due to the decreased supply of blood to the ovaries, so that they lose their ability to produce hormones, either immediately or over time. Many physicians assure us that we can avoid these risks by taking estrogen, but estrogen therapy does not substitute for functioning ovaries (see "Hormone Therapy," p. 538).

Hormonal effects of hysterectomy vary from one woman to the next. Some women suffer severe hot flashes and lack of lubrication; others don't. Some women use hormone therapy for a while, then gradually taper off. Other long-term risks include constipation, urinary incontinence, bone and joint pain, and pelvic pain. Depression can occur after hysterectomy, though the most likely cause is not the operation itself but how you feel about losing your uterus and ovaries.

HYSTERECTOMY, OOPHORECTOMY, AND SEXUALITY

Many women are concerned about the effect that hysterectomy, with or without oophorectomy, will have on sexual response. Physicians and popular literature tend to insist that any sexual difficulties we may experience are "all in our head." In fact, there is some physiological basis for these problems, and in some studies, about 25 percent of women report some sexual problems after this surgery.[21] Many women experience orgasm primarily when the penis or a lover's fingers push against the cervix and uterus, causing uterine contractions and increased stimulation of the abdominal lining (peritoneum). Without the uterus or cervix, that kind of sensation may be lost. Also, if the ovaries are removed before menopause, hormone levels drop sharply, and that can affect sexual feeling.

I had a hysterectomy two years ago at the age of 45. I went from being fully aroused and fully orgasmic to having a complete loss of libido, sexual enjoyment, and orgasms immediately after the surgery. I went to doctors, all of whom denied ever having seen a woman with this problem before and told me it was psychological. Before surgery, my husband and I were having intercourse approximately three to five times a week, simply because we have an open and loving relationship. Now I find that I have to work at becoming at all interested in intercourse. And I no longer have the orgasm that comes from pressure on the cervix, although I still have a feeble orgasm from clitoral stimulation.

Testosterone, a hormone that contributes to muscle strength, appetite, a sense of well-being, and sex drive, can increase sexual desire in women whose ovaries have been removed, but it may have masculinizing side effects, such as lowered voice, acne, and facial hair. Using low-dose testosterone cream or gel can reduce the amount that gets into the body and thus limit the side effects. However, even in low doses, these products have not been adequately tested for long-term safety or effectiveness in women.

Vaginal lubrication tends to lessen after hysterectomy and oophorectomy, and the local effects of surgery may occasionally cause problems. If your vagina has been shortened by the operation, intercourse may be uncomfortable. Scar tissue in the pelvis or at the top of the vagina may make intercourse painful.

However, for a majority of women, sex is unchanged or even more enjoyable after hysterectomy, since painful symptoms are gone. In the words of a woman who had a hysterectomy because of huge fibroids:

I had terrible cramps all my life and genuine feelings of utter depression during my periods. My ovaries were not removed, and my libido was not affected. My sexual response, if anything, improved. I also had for the first time no fear of unwanted pregnancy and more general good health.

You may weigh the benefits of surgery against the possibility of changes in sexual desire or response that can't be predicted in advance. Treatments less drastic than a hysterectomy can usually reduce pain and bleeding from benign uterine conditions and improve overall well-being.

OOPHORECTOMY: REASONS AND RISKS

Oophorectomy is removal of either one (unilateral) or both (bilateral) ovaries. The fallopian tube(s) may be removed as well. When both ovaries are removed, a hysterectomy is usually done at the same time. Common reasons for oophorectomy include ectopic pregnancy (outside the uterus), endometriosis, malignant tumors on the ovary, and pelvic imflammatory disease (PID). If you are past menopause and have an enlarged ovary, have it checked right away, since it could be cancerous.

If only one ovary is removed and not your uterus, you will continue to be fertile and have menstrual periods. However, you may experience an earlier menopause. If both ovaries are removed, you will experience surgical menopause. Even if one or both ovaries are retained, you may have menopause-like symptoms due to loss of blood supply to the ovaries. The ovaries usually continue to produce some hormones after menopause, and other cells in your body produce some estrogen.

Routinely removing the ovaries of women over forty-five during hysterectomy, whether or

HYSTERECTOMY PROCEDURES

- *Total hysterectomy,* sometimes called complete hysterectomy. The surgeon removes the uterus and cervix, leaving the fallopian tubes and ovaries. You may continue to ovulate but will no longer have menstrual periods; instead, the egg is absorbed by the body into the pelvic cavity.

- *Total hysterectomy with (bilateral) salpingo-oophorectomy.* The surgeon removes the uterus, cervix, fallopian tubes, and ovaries. One ovary may be left in, if it is not diseased. In rare cases (usually to treat widespread cancer), the surgeon will remove the upper part of the vagina and perhaps the lymph nodes in the pelvic area. This is called *radical* hysterectomy.

- *Supra-cervical (or subtotal) hysterectomy.* This procedure leaves in the cervix, to limit the effect of surgery on the function and anatomy of the vagina. It's also less likely to interfere with nerves and arteries. If the cervix is left in, you still need Pap tests.

- *Abdominal or vaginal?* The uterus can be removed either through an abdominal in- cision or through the vagina. Surgeons sometimes prefer an abdominal approach because it enables them to see the pelvic cavity more completely. The incision is made either horizontally, across the top pubic hairline, where the scar hardly shows afterward; or vertically, between the navel and the pubic hair- line. Vertical incisions tend to heal more slowly.

Vaginal hysterectomy has the advantage of a shorter recovery period and faster healing. Because the incision is inside the vagina, you won't have a visible scar. Laparascopically assisted vaginal hysterec- tomy (LAVH) enables the surgeon to see an image of the pelvic cavity. Vaginal hysterec- tomies are performed less frequently and require greater skill, so it's important to find a surgeon who does it regularly. Mistakes during surgery can result in permanent urinary tract difficulties. Other disadvan- tages include a possible shortening of the vagina, which can result in painful inter- course afterward, and possible temporary but severe back pain. Many surgeons now order antibiotics routinely before either abdominal or vaginal hysterectomy, to avoid infection.

not they are diseased, is one of the most contro- versial practices in gynecology. Those in favor of it argue that oophorectomy prevents the possi- bility of future ovarian cancer, which strikes one in a hundred women over forty and can be fatal if not found and treated early. But studies show that the actual risk of ovarian cancer following hysterectomy is fairly small (about one in a thousand). Other physicians think the cancer risk is insignificant compared with the risks in- volved in losing your ovaries: circulatory disease, premature osteoporosis, sudden menopause, and the risks of taking hormone therapy (see p. 538 in Chapter 26, "Midlife and Menopause").

SELF-HELP: RECOVERING FROM HYSTERECTOMY/OOPHORECTOMY

After a hysterectomy, you may be in the hospital a few days, depending on the kind of procedure and the amount of anesthesia you had. For the first day, you will probably have an IV and a catheter inserted in your bladder. You will usually be given medication for pain and nausea. Within a day, you can expect to be on your feet and encouraged to do exercises to get your circulation and breathing back to normal. You may also be told to cough frequently to clear your lungs. (Holding a pillow over an abdominal incision, or crossing your legs if you had a vaginal incision, will help reduce pain from coughing.) You may also have gas pains to contend with. A self-help technique to dispel abdominal gas uses heat applied to an acupressure point beneath the navel. Walking, holding on to a pillow and rolling from side to side in bed, and slow deep-breathing exercises may help, too. You can begin to have light solid foods, as well as fluids, when you feel able to keep them down. Hospital stays are shorter and shorter. This can be scary, but once your IV is out and you can keep down oral pain medications, being at home with good help may provide many comforts and avoids the risk of catching an infection in the hospital. Plan ahead to make sure you have the support you need (family, friends, or community support services).

Recovery at Home

After you go home, you will have light vaginal bleeding or oozing that gradually tapers off. You may also have hot flashes caused by estrogen loss, even if your ovaries were not removed. You will probably continue to have some pain that painkillers may not relieve entirely. Consult your medical practitioner if you have fever or discharge, as this may signal an infection.

Try to arrange for someone to take care of you for the first few days. You can expect to feel tired, so ask family and friends for help with household chores and children for at least the first few weeks. Your health care provider may tell you to avoid tub baths, douches, driving, climbing, or lifting heavy things for several weeks. If you have to drive or need to carry small children, ask for suggestions about how to do these tasks safely.

Full recovery generally takes four to six weeks, but some women feel tired for as long as six months or even a year after surgery. Most medical practitioners also recommend waiting six to eight weeks before resuming sex and/or active sports, but some women return to them earlier. Start with light exercise, such as walking, and gradually build up to your old routines.

Emotional Reactions

Some women feel only relief following hysterectomy, especially when the operation eliminates a serious health problem or chronic, disabling pain. But even if you were prepared for it and did not expect to feel depressed, you might cry frequently and unexpectedly during the first few days or weeks after surgery. This may be due to sudden hormonal changes. Many of us are also upset by losing any part of ourselves, especially a part that is so uniquely female. You may feel robbed. If you are premenopausal, you might resent the fact that you can't have children. Acknowledging feelings of anger and grief after losing a part of yourself or some of your sexual responsiveness is an important part of the recovery process.

Some gynecologists recommend psychiatric help and prescribe tranquilizers (or other habit-forming drugs) while ignoring treatment of underlying physical or sexual conditions caused by the surgery. We or our caregivers also may not recognize post-hysterectomy depression promptly. If you are depressed, try to find a women's group where you can talk about your feelings in a supportive atmosphere. If you can't find a group through a local women's health center, consider starting a post-surgery group of your own. (For information on support groups, see "Resources.")

OTHER PELVIC CONDITIONS

OBSTETRIC FISTULA

Obstetric fistula is a childbirth injury that typically affects girls and women living in acute poverty throughout Africa and South Asia. Fistula is caused by prolonged and obstructed labor when the constant pressure of the baby's head against the soft tissues of the vagina creates a hole between the bladder and the vagina, and sometimes between the rectum and the vagina. This leaves girls and women leaking urine and/or feces continuously from the vagina. It may also cause serious nerve damage to the legs, making it difficult or impossible to walk. Girls and women with fistula are often isolated and highly stigmatized. In most cases, the cost of an operation and the distance to a medical facility providing fistula services make surgical repair impossible. Fistula is entirely preventable, and it rarely or never occurs in the developed world. Women with this condition who immigrate to the United States or Canada may encounter health care providers who have never seen it before. (For more information, see "Obstetric Fistula" [W69] on the companion website, www .ourbodiesourselves.org.)

FEMALE GENITAL CUTTING

Female genital cutting (FGC)—also called female genital mutilation or female circumcision—is a traditional cultural practice in more than twenty-five African countries and some Asian communities. It involves cutting parts of the external genitals of girls or young women as a rite of passage into womanhood and to curb sexuality. FGC may consist of removing the hood of the clitoris, part or all of the clitoris and/or labia minora (inner lips), and, in some cultures, part or all of the external genitalia. The vaginal opening may also be narrowed or stitched (infibulation). Pricking, piercing, burning, scraping, slashing, or corroding the female genitals are also considered to be FGC by the World Health Organization. As a result of an influx of refugees and immigrants, thousands of women in the United States are living with the results of these practices.

Short-term health complications of FGC include excessive bleeding, infection, and shock, mostly due to unsanitary conditions, failed procedures by inexperienced circumcisers, or inadequate medical services once a problem occurs. Long-term health complications are abscess formation, scar neuromas, dermoid cysts, keloids, recurrent urinary tract infections, painful sexual intercourse, and vulval adhesions that block the vagina. In women who are infibulated, obstruction of the urethra and vagina by scar tissue may result in urine retention and urethral and bladder stones, irregular or prolonged menstrual flow, chronic urinary tract infections, and chronic pelvic inflammatory infection, which often leads to scarring of the fallopian tubes and infertility. Sexual and psychological issues are likely to emerge over time. Many women who have been circumcised may seek treatment for problems or issues related to the circumcision but may not acknowledge the connection. Some of us who are circumcised have felt that the way we have been treated by doctors in the United States has caused us more pain than the cutting itself. Providing access to sensitive health care is crucial.

It is important to understand the social and

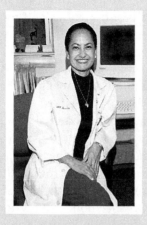

© Mainframe Photographics, Inc.

"FEMALE GENITAL CUTTING IS BOTH A HEALTH AND HUMAN RIGHTS ISSUE"

NAWAL M. NOUR, MD, MPH

As a physician and an advocate for the elimination of female circumcision, I walk a fine line between doing what is best for my patients and hearing their needs. As an Arab-speaking Sudanese, I understand my patients' culture from within without judging them. But I don't cover my hair or follow Islam the way many others do. And as a feminist and a Harvard-educated physician, I believe in providing the best health care for women worldwide.

I opened my practice in 1999, when I saw a need for circumcised women to obtain holistic care. Although 90 to 95 percent of my patients are circumcised, for many, that is not an issue. They are living healthy lives. When health providers focus only on women's circumcision, they neglect the need for a Pap smear, mammogram, or information on how to get health insurance. In fact, when I conduct community-needs assessments, many of the major concerns I hear are family planning, dental care, and interpreter services.

I started seeing circumcised women when I was an obstetric-gynecology resident. I wanted to work in the community, but the women said they wanted to be treated at a major hospital, because "that's where rich women go." So now I do both: go out and conduct workshops in the community, and direct the African Women's Health Center at Brigham and Women's Hospital in Boston.

Initially, 8 to 10 women came in an afternoon; now it's up to 20 to 25. They range from an eighteen-year-old who wants surgical reconstruction to women in their sixties who have no issue with circumcision but need general gynecologic, postmenopausal care. Women want a doctor who will not judge them but rather, understand and listen to them.

In the past, Western feminists sounded judgmental. It is harsh for women to listen to their tradition described as horrific or barbaric, or hear that they have been mutilated. "I feel beautiful, clean," some tell me. Now Western advocates are becoming more sensitive.

Since many of my patients are pregnant, I can spend nine months with them to try to convince them not to circumcise their daughters. Some want to perpetuate the practice because they think Islam ordains it. At times I suggest reading the Koran and hadith together to show them that it says nothing on the topic. I tell them that few women are circumcised in Saudi Arabia—home of Islam's holy cities of Mecca and Medina.

Some women defend female genital cutting as a tradition: They want their daughters to look like them or believe it will make them more marriageable. There is also a lot of miseducation about the clitoris: that it is a toxic organ that must be removed to protect the baby during delivery, or that it continues to grow until it touches the ground. And so I challenge them, "What do you think American women do? Why aren't all their daughters dead? Do you think their clitorises are so long they have to roll them up?" Humor is a nonconfrontational method of education.

I have found it incredibly helpful when I can involve husbands. Some have been in America longer, have been exposed to Western women, and see the pain or discomfort that their circumcised wives suffer. Some are helpful in stopping the practice because they want to make sure their daughters are pain-free, healthy, and happy.

My goal is to provide excellent holistic and preventive care to my patients and to ensure that their daughters are never circumcised. Female genital cutting is both a health and human rights issue; it must be stopped.

To read more about Dr. Nour, see "Nawal Nour and the African Women's Health Center" (W70) on the companion website, www.ourbodiesourselves.org.

cultural aspects of FGC and not to frame it exclusively as a medical or health problem. Efforts to outlaw the practice may not be effective if they are perceived as the government or a cultural majority imposing its will upon those who perpetuate the practice for complex reasons. Empowering African women to have more input in family and community decision making can help reduce FGC. The African-led RAINBOW (Research, Action and Information Network for the Bodily Integrity of Women) and the African Women's Health Center at Brigham and Women's Hospital focus on such empowerment initiatives. (For more information, see "Resources.")

PELVIC INFLAMMATORY DISEASE

I had been complaining of the same problem— pain in my lower right abdomen—for a couple of years. I had severe menstrual irregularities, fevers, bleeding between periods, bleeding after intercourse, pains, and general malaise. Several times I was treated with antibiotics, which brought only some temporary relief. Never was the issue resolved as to what was causing this. Never were my sexual partners or practices mentioned.

Pelvic inflammatory disease (PID) is a general term for an infection that affects the lining of the uterus (endometrium), the fallopian tubes (salpingitis), and/or ovaries (oophoritis). It is caused primarily by sexually transmitted diseases that spread up from the opening of the uterus to these organs (see Chapter 15, "Sexually Transmitted Infections"). Nearly a million women in the United States develop PID every year, and three hundred thousand women are hospitalized for it. This may be a low estimate, because so much PID is not diagnosed.

Symptoms

The primary symptom is pain in the lower abdomen. It may be so mild that you hardly notice it, or so strong that you may not even be able to stand. You may feel tightness or pressure in the reproductive organs, or an occasional dull ache. You may also have some, most, or none of these other symptoms: abnormal or foul discharge from the vagina or urethra, pain or bleeding during or after intercourse, irregular bleeding or spotting, increased menstrual cramps, increased pain during ovulation; frequent or burning urination, inability to empty the bladder; swollen abdomen, sudden high fever or low-grade fever that comes and goes, chills, swollen lymph nodes, lack of appetite, nausea or vomiting, pain around the kidneys or liver, lower back or leg pain; feelings of weakness, tiredness, depression, or diminished desire to have sex.

The intensity and extent of the symptoms depend on which microorganisms are causing the problem, where they are (uterus, tubes, lining of the abdomen, etc.), how long you have had it, what if any antibiotics you have taken for it, and your general health. Doctors characterize PID as acute, chronic, or silent (when symptoms are not noticeable).

Causes

Most cases of PID are caused by microorganisms responsible for sexually transmitted infections. They can get into the body during sexual contact with an infected man or woman* and also during miscarriage, childbirth, abortion, or other procedures involving the uterus, such as endometrial biopsy, hysterosalpingogram (X ray of the reproductive tract), IUD insertion, or donor insemination. If you have chronic PID and antibiotic treatment doesn't help, your sexual part-

* The incidence of PID is very low among lesbians.

ner(s) may be reinfecting you. Men can be carrying the organisms that can cause PID without having symptoms, so they must be tested and treated, too, and they should use a condom for intercourse.

The risk for developing PID is higher if you are exposed to infected secretions—especially infected semen—during menstruation and ovulation, when your cervix is more open and your mucus is more penetrable. Women using IUDs are also at higher risk during the first four months after insertion. In some parts of the United States, gonorrhea still causes most PID. In other areas, microorganisms such as chlamydia and mycoplasma, which can live in the genital tract for years, are being found in women with PID. Current guidelines recommend annual chlamydia screening for women age twenty-five and under who are having sex, to find and treat it before it causes PID.

The complications of PID can be very serious. If untreated, PID can turn into peritonitis, a life-threatening condition, or a tubo-ovarian abscess. It can affect the bowels and the liver *(perihepatitis syndrome)*. Months or years after an acute infection, infertility or ectopic pregnancy can result if your fallopian tubes were damaged or clogged by scar tissue. PID can also cause chronic pain from adhesions or lingering infection. In the most extreme cases, untreated PID can result in death.

PREVENTING PID

Preventing PID is like preventing STIs, because so much PID is caused by sexually transmitted organisms. Birth control foams, creams, and jellies kill some bacteria that enter the vagina during intercourse. If possible, don't have intercourse without using a protective barrier (condom, diaphragm). If you have already had an STI or PID, or if you and/or your male partner(s) have had more than one sexual partner, try to use condoms and avoid using an IUD. (For more on STIs, see Chapter 15, and for more on safer sex, see Chapter 14.)

DIAGNOSTIC TESTING AND TREATMENT

If you could know right away exactly which organisms were causing your PID, you could get the right antibiotics. But pinpointing the organisms often takes some tests that may be expensive and not readily available. Sometimes organisms infecting the uterus and fallopian tubes don't show up in a cervical culture. You may be told that your chronic cystitis is caused by trauma to the urethra during intercourse, when it's really a sign of PID; or that you got infected by wiping yourself from back to front, when you really have a sexually transmitted infection. You may be told that you have a spastic colon or an emotional, not a physical, problem, when that is not really true. Try to have your situation thoroughly assessed.

Blood tests can indicate whether or not you have an infection but not always which one. Sometimes an endometrial biopsy can find hard-to-culture organisms, but if it is not done carefully, this procedure can spread germs from the cervix and vagina to the uterus. In some cases, ultrasound, including vaginal ultrasound, may be useful. A definitive diagnosis often requires laparoscopy (see p. 595).

Treatments

Most experts seem to agree that since your health and fertility are at stake, you should not delay, but get treatment while waiting for test results. Some STD/STI clinics and fertility specialists are giving accurate and up-to-date tests and treatments for PID. Call the National STD Hotline, 1-800-227-8922, to find out about tests and clinics.

As with STIs, both you and your partner must be treated. If your partner continues to carry the microorganism(s), you will be reinfected. Taking the wrong drugs can make organisms more difficult to get rid of. However, the practical strategy is to begin treatment, then adjust it according to what cause is found. Once you start taking antibiotics, you cannot get an accurate culture again until at least a couple of weeks after you stop taking them.

Therapy lasts at least ten to fourteen days, because PID is a serious infection. You should receive two different kinds of antibiotics, since more than one organism may be involved. Remember to take all your antibiotics, even if your symptoms are gone, so that antibiotic-resistant strains of microbes will be less likely to develop. The Centers for Disease Control offers the most current information about effective antibiotics.

Antibiotics can cause yeast overgrowth in the vagina, so you may need something to keep the yeast in check while trying to cure the much more serious PID. Try unsweetened live-culture yogurt or acidophilus capsules (ingesting and/or inserting into the vagina) to restore beneficial bacteria that can offset the yeast.

Many experts recommend that all women with PID be hospitalized for treatment, but not all physicians follow these recommendations. Most women are hospitalized in the event of an acute attack, to get intravenous (IV) antibiotics. If you're still not cured, it may be because you got the wrong antibiotic, have a pelvic abscess, or were reinfected by a partner.

You may be urged to have a hysterectomy if the doctor thinks that PID has damaged your pelvic organs beyond repair. Also, emergency hysterectomies are done in some cases of acute PID (for example, when an abscess ruptures). If the infection is in your urinary tract, which it often is, then hysterectomy does not eliminate it. Hysterectomy is rarely necessary for PID, except in cases of persistent, debilitating PID.

SELF-HELP FOR HEALING

There are many things you can do to help heal yourself while you wait for test results to come back and for antibiotics to start working. Very hot baths and a heating pad applied directly to the lower abdomen help relieve pain and bring disease-fighting blood and drugs to your pelvis. You can soak a cotton cloth in castor oil, place it on the abdomen, cover it with plastic to prevent greasiness, and then put a heating pad or hot water bottle on top to bring a maximum amount of heat to the pelvic area. Ginger root compresses and taro root poultices may relieve pain, eliminate accumulated toxins, keep the area loose and freer from adhesions, and dissolve already formed adhesions. (These are strong medicines and are best used with the guidance of a holistic health practitioner.) Do not douche or use tampons; to do so may force microorganisms up into your uterus. Do not reuse a douche bag that may be harboring infectious organisms.

Certain herbs and teas may be useful against infection of the reproductive and urinary tracts. Raspberry leaf tea can strengthen the reproductive system; cranberry juice may help with UTIs. Try to eat wholesome, fresh foods, and manage and reduce stress as best as you can. Eliminating or restricting sugar, dairy products (to lessen mucus production), coffee, alcohol, tobacco, and other drugs that lower your resistance to disease, as well as taking vitamins C, A, D, B-complex, and zinc, may be helpful. You may be unusually tired and run-down, so get plenty of sleep. Complete bed rest is recommended but is difficult to achieve. Sometimes it takes months to feel better after PID.

Avoid intercourse until you have felt completely well through an entire monthly cycle and your partners have had negative test results for all STIs. You can have short bouts of PID months after the initial infection is cleared up, particularly if you don't keep up daily health routines or are under too much stress.

The most critical element in your healing will be the antibiotic treatment. Remember that PID is an extremely serious problem that needs prompt and skilled attention.

PELVIC RELAXATION AND UTERINE PROLAPSE

Pelvic relaxation is a condition in which the muscles of the pelvic floor become slack and no longer support the pelvic organs properly. In severe cases, the ligaments and tissues that hold the uterus in place may also weaken enough to allow the uterus to fall (prolapse) into the vagina. Women sometimes experience pelvic relaxation and/or uterine prolapse after one or more very difficult births, but the tendency can also be inherited. Uterine prolapse is often accompanied by a falling of the bladder (cystocele) and rectum (rectocele).

The first sign of pelvic relaxation is often a tendency to leak urine when you cough, sneeze, or laugh suddenly. If your uterus has fallen into the vagina, you may have a dull, heavy sensation in your vagina or feel as if something is falling out. You may have constipation, difficulty accomplishing a bowel movement, or the inability to control your bowels. These symptoms are usually worse after you have been standing for a long time.

PREVENTION AND SELF-HELP TREATMENTS

The best way to prevent pelvic relaxation and uterine prolapse is to do regular Kegel exercises and leg lifts, which strengthen the muscles of the pelvic floor and lower abdomen (see "Kegel Exercises," p. 235). Some women use Femina weights to do these exercises. Check whether your pelvic muscles are in good shape by trying to start and stop the flow of urine while sitting on the toilet. If you can't stop the flow, you need to do more Kegels. Some health care providers recommend doing them up to a hundred times a day, especially during pregnancy, when the pelvic muscles are under particular stress. You may also strengthen a slightly prolapsed uterus by relaxing in the knee-chest position (kneeling with your chest on the floor and your bottom in the air) several times a day. Some women find that certain yoga positions, such as the shoulder stand and headstand, relieve the discomfort of a prolapsed uterus.

MEDICAL TREATMENTS

Medical intervention is usually not necessary for pelvic relaxation or even mild uterine prolapse. If the prolapse is severe enough to cause discomfort, you can ask your doctor to insert a pessary (a rubber device that fits around the cervix and helps to prop up the uterus). Disadvantages include difficulty in obtaining a proper fit, possible irritation or infection, and the need to remove and clean the pessary frequently. A surgical procedure called a suspension operation can lift and reattach a descended uterus, and often a fallen bladder or rectum as well. Many medical practitioners recommend hysterectomy for prolapsed uterus, but it is usually unnecessary and should be done only as a last resort in appropriate cases. It's best to consult a physician who has expertise in this area and keeps up with new research.

VAGINA AND VULVA

VAGINAL INFECTIONS (VAGINITIS), GENERAL

All women secrete moisture and mucus from the membranes that line the vagina and cervix.

This discharge is clear or slightly milky and may be somewhat slippery or clumpy. When dry, it may be yellowish. When a woman is sexually aroused, under stress, or at midcycle, this secretion increases. It normally causes no irritation or inflammation of the vagina or vulva. If you want to examine your own discharge, collect a sample from inside your vagina—with a washed finger—and smear it on clear glass (such as a glass slide).

Many bacteria normally grow in the vagina of a healthy woman. Some of them, especially lactobacilli, help to keep the vagina healthy, maintaining an acid pH and controlling overgrowth of potentially bad bacteria. When infections occur, you may have an abnormal discharge, mild or severe itching and burning of the vulva, chafing of the thighs, and (in some cases) frequent urination. (Chronic vaginal symptoms sometimes result from skin conditions of the vulva and vagina, such as eczema or psoriasis.)

Vaginal infections may be due to lowered resistance (from stress, lack of sleep, poor diet, other infections in our bodies); douching or use of "feminine hygiene" sprays; pregnancy; taking birth control pills, other hormones, or antibiotics; diabetes or a pre-diabetic condition; cuts, abrasions, and other irritations in the vagina (from childbirth, intercourse without enough lubrication, tampons, or using an instrument in the vagina medically or for masturbation). We can also get infections during sex with a partner who has them (see Chapter 15, "Sexually Transmitted Infections"). Chronic vaginal infections may be a sign of serious medical problems such as HIV infection and diabetes.

PREVENTING VAGINAL INFECTIONS

1. Gently wash your vulva and anus regularly. Pure, unscented mineral oil cleans well and does not dry out the tissues as soap can. Pat your vulva dry after bathing, and try to keep it dry. Also, don't use other people's towels or washcloths. Avoid irritating sprays* and soaps (use special cleansers for sensitive skin). Avoid talcum powder, since some studies have linked it to ovarian cancer.[22]

2. Avoid nylon underwear and panty hose—they retain moisture and heat, which help harmful bacteria to grow faster. Wear clean underpants, preferably all cotton. Launder all underwear in hot, soapy water. Be sure to rinse thoroughly.

3. Avoid pants that are tight in the crotch and thighs.

4. Always wipe your genital and anal area from front to back, so that bacteria from the anus won't get into the vagina or urethra.

5. Make sure your sex partners are clean. A man should wash his penis daily and especially before making love. Using a condom can provide added protection. If you or your male partner is being treated for a genital infection, make sure he wears a condom during intercourse. Better yet, avoid intercourse until the infection has cleared up.

6. Use a sterile, water-soluble jelly if you need lubrication (K-Y jelly or Astroglide, *not* Vaseline). Spermicidal gels and creams, which usually contain nonoxynol-9, may cause irritation and are no longer recommended for preventing infections (see p. 269 in Chapter 14, "Safer Sex").

7. Avoid any kind of vaginal penetration that is painful or abrasive.

---

* Feminine hygiene sprays may irritate or cause an allergic reaction in the skin of the vulva. They are at best unnecessary and are often harmful. The FDA has suggested, and may soon require, that all feminine hygiene sprays carry a warning on the label.

8. Cut down on coffee, alcohol, sugar, and refined carbohydrates. Diets high in sugars can increase sugar in the vagina, which feeds bacteria.

9. Avoid douching of any kind unless specifically recommended by your health care provider. Although you may feel cleaner, douching can destroy the "good" bacteria in your vagina.

10. Avoid inserting yogurt to relieve mild symptoms of vaginal infections, other than yeast infections, because this can prevent proper diagnosis and may even contribute to chronic vaginal problems.

11. Eat well and get enough rest! Not taking care of yourself makes you more susceptible to infection.

12. Avoid using tampons, especially if you have a history of frequent vaginal infections.

MEDICAL OR ALTERNATIVE TREATMENTS?

The usual treatment for vaginitis is some form of antibiotic. As you use those drugs, however, they disturb the delicate balance of bacteria in the vagina and may actually encourage some infections (such as yeast) by altering the vagina's normal acid/alkaline balance (pH). Some antibiotics also have unpleasant or even dangerous side effects.

As an alternative to antibiotics for vaginitis, many women are turning to natural and herbal remedies that help to restore the normal vaginal flora and promote healing, though for most, there are no studies showing how effective they are. You can use herbs to make soothing poultices or sitz baths (sitting in the tub with just enough water to immerse your thighs, buttocks, and hips). You should not rely on these remedies if you have a serious STI (see Chapter 15, "Sexually Transmitted Infections"), or an infection that involves your uterus, fallopian tubes, or ovaries.

VULVITIS

Vulvitis, an inflammation of the vulva, may be caused by external irritants, an injury, oral sex, a bacterial or fungal infection, using a hot tub, or an allergy to common commercial products such as soaps, powders, deodorants, sanitary napkins, synthetic underwear, panty hose, and medicated creams. Vulvitis often accompanies other infections such as vaginitis or herpes. Stress, inadequate diet, and poor hygiene can make you more susceptible to vulvitis. Women with diabetes may develop vulvitis because the sugar content of the cells is higher, increasing susceptibility to infection. Postmenopausal women often develop vulvitis because as hormone levels drop, the vulvar tissues become thinner, drier, and less elastic and therefore susceptible to irritation and infection.

Symptoms of vulvitis include itching, redness, and swelling. Sometimes fluid-filled blisters form that break open, ooze, and crust over (they may resemble herpes). Scratching can cause further irritation, pus formation, and scaling, as well as secondary infection. Sometimes, as a result of scratching, the skin whitens and thickens. In diabetic vulvitis, the skin may look beefy red; in postmenopausal vulvitis, sores and red, irritated areas often appear.

Women with this problem tend to overclean the vulva, contributing to further irritation. Wash once a day with warm water only. To prevent vulvitis, see "Preventing Vaginal Infections," p. 650.

SELF-HELP TREATMENTS

Discontinue using any substances that might be a cause of vulvitis. All commercial preparations may be irritating, including antifungal agents and lubricants containing propylene glycol. Keep your vulva clean, cool, and dry—and remember to wipe from front to back. Hot boric acid compresses and hot sitz baths with comfrey tea are soothing. Use unscented toilet paper and soft cotton or linen towels and cotton underclothes, to prevent chafing. Cold compresses made of plain, unsweetened, live-culture yogurt or cottage cheese also help relieve itching and soothe irritation. Calamine lotion also helps relieve itching. Aveeno colloidal oatmeal bath can be very soothing. Use a sterile, nonirritating lubricant such as K-Y jelly or Astroglide during intercourse and other genital sex. Finally, try to eat well, get more rest, and find ways of coping with stress.

MEDICAL TREATMENTS FOR VULVITIS

Depending on the cause of vulvitis, your health care provider may prescribe antifungal creams or antibacterial treatment. Cortisone cream or other soothing lotions can relieve severe itching. (Low-dose cortisone creams are good for a short time. Fluorinated ones cause thinning and atrophy of the skin if used for a long time.) Postmenopausal women may be given topical estrogen cream, but it should not be used for prolonged periods without adding progesterone to reduce the risk of uterine cancer. If you have a vaginal infection or herpes, treating these problems will usually clear up the vulvitis as well.

If the vulvitis persists or worsens, you may need a vulvar biopsy to rule out the possibility of cancer or chronic vulvar conditions such as lichens sclerosa. This can be done in the practitioner's office with local anesthetic.

VULVODYNIA

Vulvodynia is a chronic pain condition. Women with vulvodynia experience severe burning, pain, itching, stinging, and/or irritation in the vulva (external genitals). There are two subtypes. In *dysesthetic* vulvodynia (also called generalized vulvar dysesthesia), symptoms occur in different areas of the vulva, at various times and sometimes even when the vulva is not being touched. In vulvar *vestibulitis* syndrome (also called localized vulvar dysesthesia), women feel pain mainly in an area between the labia (the vestibule), and only when that area is touched or pressed. (For more information about the anatomy of the vulva, see Chapter 13, "Sexual Anatomy, Reproduction, and the Menstrual Cycle.")

As many as 9 percent of women may experience significant vulvar pain.[23] Even so, it can be hard to get a proper diagnosis for it, let alone successful treatment. If your vulva hurts, it is important to find a health care provider who is familiar with vulvodynia. During a pelvic exam, the practitioner will lightly touch areas on your vulva with a cotton swab (Q-tip) to see where it's sensitive. As this may be painful, make sure your provider does it gently. Feel free to bring a close friend or partner with you into the exam room.

It started within the first few times I ever had sexual intercourse. Here I was with this wonderful partner, but the sex hurt so much it made us both cry—me from the physical pain, him because I hurt so much. Once it started, the pain would come back whenever something touched my vulva: a tampon, a finger, a speculum (that was the worst). I saw several nurses and doctors; the first doc told me I was just "tight" and needed to relax. Did she have any idea how insulting, demoralizing, and belittling that was? Finally, I found a physician who respected me, recognized that my pain was real, and was able to give it the label of vulvodynia. Even having a name for it helped. I've since tried many treatments, some more successful than others. Three years later, I'm thrilled to report that my wonderful partner and I are able to have pain-free sexual intercourse (as well as continue to share other kinds of physical intimacy)—my vestibulitis isn't totally gone, but it's on its way out!

Because the causes of vulvodynia remain uncertain, there is no standard treatment. Options include biofeedback techniques; diets low in oxalates (found in spinach, rhubarb, strawberries, chocolate, wheat bran, nuts, and beets); calcium citrate; tricyclic antidepressants; various topical treatments; interferon; and surgery (called *vestibulectomy*). Find a supportive practitioner who has the time and knowledge to explore treatment options with you. If you have a partner, it is important to educate him or her about vulvodynia and, together, explore options for physical intimacy (see Chapter 12, "Sexuality"). Also consider connecting with a support group of women to share stories and successes. The National Vulvodynia Association can help you find referrals to clinicians as well as connect you to support groups of women with vulvodynia in your area (see "Resources").

VULVAR CANCER

Women who have had HPV infections (see p. 288 in Chapter 15, "Sexually Transmitted Infections") seem to be at greater risk for vulvar cancer, although it is relatively rare. Some experts believe that vulvar cancer rates will rise sharply in the future, largely because of increased rates of HPV infections. There is no screening test for vulvar cancer, and many women are treated for other conditions before realizing a biopsy should be done.

Be aware of changes in your vulvar area (especially lesions), and request a biopsy if you find a suspicious lump or lesion. Because vulvar cancer typically grows slowly, early detection can mean the difference between minor surgery and the more emotionally and physically devastating experience of losing one's genitals. The surgery can also cause problems with sexual functioning, and if lymph glands have been removed, fluid buildup in the thighs can cause swelling, making mobility difficult.

Daughters of women who took DES are at higher risk for certain vaginal cancers and should have regular checkups by a knowledgeable medical practitioner (see p. 627).

OTHER VAGINAL INFECTIONS

YEAST

Candida albicans, a yeast fungus, grows in the rectum and vagina. It grows best in a mildly acidic environment. The pH in the vagina is normally more than mildly acidic. When we menstruate, take birth control pills or some antibiotics, are pregnant, or have diabetes, the pH becomes more alkaline. In a healthy vagina, the presence of some yeast may not be a problem. When our system is out of balance, yeastlike organisms might grow profusely and cause a thick white discharge that may look like cottage cheese and smell like baking bread. Drinking unsweetened cranberry juice every day is the simplest way to keep the vaginal pH balanced. If juice is too acidic for you, you can try cranberry capsules.

Diagnosis

The only way to be sure that an infection is caused by candida and not something else is to have vaginal secretions analyzed under a microscope. In some cases, it helps to get a lab culture done. Several other conditions (vulvitis, herpes) may respond temporarily to treatment for candida and then recur a short time later, so accurate diagnosis is important. Self-diagnosis is inaccurate over half the time, so it is usually wise to go ahead with self-treatment only after diagnosis by a health care provider.

Treatment

Treatment usually consists of some form of vaginal suppository or cream. Antifungal external creams such as clotrimazole may reduce or even eliminate the symptoms, sometimes without actually curing the infection. (A vaginal wet mount and yeast culture can determine whether the infection is really gone.) For severe, chronic cases, some of the newer oral antifungal medications may be necessary. Prolonged treatment should be based on a yeast culture. Suppositories and creams have fewer side effects than oral medications, and they can be used during pregnancy. If a woman has a yeast infection when she gives birth, the baby will likely get yeast in its throat or digestive tract. This is called *thrush* and is treated orally with nystatin drops.

Other treatments for candida infection involve boric acid capsules or painting the vagina, cervix, and vulva with gentian violet. This is bright purple and it stains, so a sanitary pad must be worn. This procedure can really help, but in occasional cases, women have a severe reaction to gentian violet.

Self-Help Treatments for Yeast

Some of us have had success with the following remedies: acidifying the system by drinking eight ounces of unsweetened cranberry juice every day, or taking cranberry concentrate supplements; inserting plain, unsweetened, live-culture yogurt in the vagina; inserting garlic suppositories (to prevent irritation, peel but don't nick a clove of garlic, then wrap in gauze before inserting). An effective and inexpensive treatment for candida infection is potassium sorbate, commonly used as a preservative in home brewing of beer. Dip a cotton tampon in a 3 percent solution (15 grams of dry potassium sorbate in one pint of water), then insert into the vagina at night and remove in the morning.

Also try to reduce sugar in your diet, get more rest, don't douche, don't use tampons for your period, and get extra rest. If you have a male sex partner, have him apply antifungal cream to his penis twice a day for two weeks, especially if he's not circumcised.

For a long time I felt as though I were on a merry-go-round. I would get a yeast infection, take Mycostatin for three weeks, clear up the infection, and then find two weeks later that the itching and the thick, white discharge were back. Finally, I discovered that reducing my sugar intake and drinking unsweetened cranberry juice would help prevent repeat infections.

TRICHOMONIASIS

Trichomonas vaginalis, or "trich," is a one-celled parasite that can be found in both men and women and that causes the disease trichomoniasis. Women with trich may have symptoms of vulvar itch and increased discharge, or no symptoms at all. Often there is a thin, foamy vaginal discharge that is yellowish green or gray and has a foul odor. If you also have another infection, the discharge can be thicker and whiter. Trich is usually diagnosed by examining the vaginal discharge under a microscope. It can also cause a urinary infection. Most people get it through intercourse (thus, trichomoniasis can be considered an STI), but it can also be passed on by moist objects such as towels, bathing suits, underwear, washcloths, and toilet seats.

The usual treatment for trich is metronidazole (Flagyl), several pills in one dose. Women with blood diseases, central nervous system disorders, or peptic ulcers should not take this drug. Pregnant and nursing mothers should also avoid metronidazole, as it can pass through the placenta and breast milk to the baby. Many women who take it experience unpleasant effects, such as nausea, headache, diarrhea, metallic taste, joint pain, and numbness of the arms or legs. Avoid alcohol while taking metronidazole, as the combination can make the effects of both worse.

In some cases, trich can be treated with clotrimazole, which has a 60 percent cure rate. If you have a stubborn case that has not responded to single-dose treatments and decide to use metronidazole, ask for a single oral dose instead of a three-to-seven-day course of pills. This usually works better, with far fewer negative effects. Because men can also carry and transmit the infection, male sex partners should also be treated. Female partners should be examined, and treated if trich is diagnosed.

Self-Help Treatments for Trich

Although some women have used douches made from vinegar, goldenseal and myrrh, chickweed, and other substances, douching can push organisms farther up into your reproductive system, causing even more serious problems. Douche only with the recommendation and guidance of your medical practitioner.

Garlic suppositories inserted every twelve hours may also help (see "Self-help Treatments for Yeast," p. 654). Taking tub baths, wearing loose clothing (since exposure to air destroys parasites causing infection), and avoiding tampons, douches, and vaginal sprays may help prevent recurrences. Also, use condoms with new male sex partners.

BACTERIAL VAGINOSIS

Bacterial vaginosis (BV) is a disturbance of the ecology of the vagina, with an overgrowth of certain microorganisms (possibly including mycoplasmas, gardnerella, and anaerobic bacteria). Many women with BV are unaware that they have it. Some practitioners believe it can be caused by routine douching; it may also be trig-

gered by infections, including STIs. The symptoms are similar to those of trich, though the discharge tends to be creamy white or grayish and is especially foul-smelling ("fishy") after intercourse.

Treatment is usually either metronidazole or clindamycin, taken orally or vaginally for five to seven days. Single-dose oral metronidazole may also be effective but less so (40 to 60 percent cure). Metronidazole is sometimes used first, because it spares the lactobacilli in your vagina and is less likely to trigger a yeast infection. Vaginal treatment avoids systemic side effects but is more expensive than the five-to-seven-day pill regimens. Some women will have another BV outbreak within nine months of initial treatment. Long-term condom use may help to prevent recurrent infection. Women with BV have more frequent infections following gynecologic surgery, and some studies suggest it increases the risk of giving birth prematurely if you have it during pregnancy. BV may also increase a woman's risk of getting PID or HIV (see Chapter 15, "Sexually Transmitted Infections").

Self-help Treatments

Self-help treatments include general vaginitis prevention measures (see p. 650) and taking extra vitamins B and C. You can help prevent recurrences by minimizing the use of tampons, avoiding douching, and using condoms (this offsets the alkaline effect of semen). Alternative treatments may provide temporary relief but not an actual cure. Vaginal and oral use of yogurt doesn't help for BV.

NOTES

1. National Coalition for LGBT Health, "Cancer and the LBGT Community," "Access to Quality Healthcare," "Love Your Body! A Transwoman's Guide to Health and Wellness," and "Respect Your Body! A Transman's

Guide to Health and Wellness," accessed at www
.lgbthealth.net/awarenessweek04/materials/all_facts.bw
.pdf on November 8, 2004.

2. M. D. Althuis, D. D. Brogan, R. J. Coates, et al., "Breast Cancers Among Very Young Premenopausal Women (United States)," *Cancer Causes and Control* 14, no. 2 (2003): 151–60.

3. James R. Cerhan, et al., "Twinship and Risk of Postmenopausal Breast Cancer," *Journal of the National Cancer Institute* 92, no. 3 (February 2, 2000): 261–65.

4. American Cancer Society, "Detailed Guide: What Are the Risk Factors for Breast Cancer?" accessed at www .cancer.org/docroot/CRI/content/CRI_2_4_2X_What_ are_the_risk_factors_for_breast_cancer_5.asp?sitearea on November 1, 2004.

5. M. B. Terry, M. D. Gammon, F. F. Zhang, et al., "Association of Frequency and Duration of Aspirin Use and Hormone Receptor Status with Breast Cancer Risk," *Journal of the American Medical Association* 291, no. 20 (May 26, 2004): 2433–40.

6. Scott Davis, Dana K. Mirick, and Richard G. Stevens, "Night Shift Work, Light at Night, and Risk of Breast Cancer," *Journal of the National Cancer Institute* 93, no. 20 (October 17, 2001): 1557–62. See also Eva S. Schernhammer, Francine Laden, Frank E. Speizer, Walter C. Willett, David J. Hunter, Ichiro Kawachi, and Graham A. Colditz, "Rotating Night Shifts and Risk of Breast Cancer in Women Participating in the Nurses' Health Study," *Journal of the National Cancer Institute* 93 (October 17, 2001): 1563–68.

7. J. Houghton and U.K. Coordinating Committee on Cancer Research (UKCCCR), Ductal Carcinoma in Situ (DCIS) Working Party, DCIS Trialists in the UK, Australia, and New Zealand, "Radiotherapy and Tamoxifen in Women with Completely Excised Ductal Carcinoma in Situ of the Breast in the UK, Australia, and New Zealand: Randomised Controlled Trial," *Lancet* 362, no. 9378 (July 12, 2003): 95–102.

8. Audre Lorde, *The Cancer Journals* (Argyle, NY: Spinsters Ink, 1980), 38.

9. Ibid., 60, 64.

10. Diana Zuckerman, Elizabeth Santoro, and Nicole Hudak, "Symptoms and Complications from Silicone Gel Breast Implants: FDA's October 2003 Summary of Research on Inamed Implants," accessed at www.breast implantinfo.org/what_know/oct03_summary.html on November 2, 2004.

11. S. L. Brown, G. Pennello, W. A. Berg, M. S. Soo, M. S. Middleton, "Silicone Gel Breast Implant Rupture, Extracapsular Silicone, and Health Status in a Population of Women," *Journal of Rheumatology* 28 (May 2001): 996–1003.

12. K. A. Phillips, J. Bernhard, "Adjuvant Breast Cancer Treatment and Cognitive Function: Current Knowledge and Research Directions," *Journal of the National Cancer Institute* 95, no. 3 (February 5, 2003): 190–97.

13. Adriane Fugh-Berman, *The 5-Minute Herb and Dietary Supplement Consult* (Philadelphia: Lippincott Williams & Wilkins, 2003), 322, 328, 352.

14. J. Verloop et al., "Prevalence of Gynecologic Cancer in Women Exposed to Diethylstilbestrol in Utero," *New England Journal of Medicine* 342, no. 24 (June 15, 2000): 1838–39. See also E. E. Hatch et al., "Incidence of Squamous Neoplasia of the Cervix and Vagina in Women Exposed Prenatally to Diethylstilbestrol (United States)," *Cancer Causes and Control* 13, no. 9 (November 2001): 837–45.

15. J. R. Palmer et al., "Risk of Breast Cancer in Women Exposed to Diethylstilbestrol in Utero: Preliminary Results (United States)," *Cancer Causes and Control* 13 (October 2002): 753–38.

16. S. A. Lippman et al., "Uterine Fibroids and Gynecologic Pain Symptoms in a Population-Based Study," *Fertility and Sterility* 80, no. 6 (December 2003): 1488.

17. J. Golzarian, S. Murgo, M. Laureys, et al., "Uterine Fibroids Embolization: A Review," *Journal Belge de Radiologie* 85, no. 1 (2002): 7–13. See also S. Murgo, P. Simon, J. Golzarian, "Embolization of Uterine Fibroids," *Revue Medicale Bruxelles* 23, no. 5 (October 2002): 435–42; and J. B. Spies, A. Spector, A. R. Roth, et al., "Complications After Uterine Artery Embolization for Leiomyomas," *Obstetrics and Gynecology* 100, no. 5 (part 1) (November 2002): 873–80.

18. V. Grigorieva et al., "Use of a Levonorgestrel-Releasing Intrauterine System to Treat Bleeding Related to Uterine Leiomyomas," *Fertility and Sterility* 79, no. 5 (May 2003): 1194–98. See also A. E. Lethaby, I. Cooke, M. Rees, "Progesterone/Progestogen Releasing Intrauterine Systems for Heavy Menstrual Bleeding," *Cochrane Review* no. 4 (2004); and R. Nagrani et al., "Can the Levonorgestrel Intrauterine System Replace Surgical Treatment for the Management of Menorrhagia?" *British Journal of Obstetrics and Gynecology* 109, no. 3 (March 2002): 345–47.

19. American Cancer Society, "Statistics for 2004," accessed at www.cancer.org/docroot/STT/stt_0.asp on November 8, 2004.

20. F. Modugno, R. B. Ness, J. E. Wheeler, "Reproductive Risk Factors for Epithelial Ovarian Cancer According to Histologic Type and Invasiveness," *Annals of Epidemiology* 11, no. 8 (November 2001): 568–74. See also S. A. Narod, P. Sun, P. Ghadirian, H. Lunch, C. Isaacs, et al., "Tubal Ligation and Risk of Ovarian Cancer in Carriers of BRCA1 or BRCA2 Mutations: A Case-

Control Study," *Lancet* 357, no. 9267 (May 2001): 1467–70; and S. E. Hankinson, D. J. Hunter, G. A. Colditz, W. C. Willett, M. J. Stampfer, et al., "Tubal Ligation, Hysterectomy, and Risk of Ovarian Cancer: A Prospective Study," *Journal of the American Medical Association* 270, no. 23 (December 1993): 2813–18.

21. A. Katz, "Sexuality After Hysterectomy," *Journal of Obstetric, Gynecologic, and Neonatal Nursing* 31, no. 3 (May–June 2002): 256–67. See also K. Kieser, "Sexuality After Hysterectomy," *Obstetrics and Gynecology* 95, part 2, no. 6 (June 2000): 1045–51; and K. J. Carlson, B. A.

Miller, and F. J. Fowler, "The Maine Women's Health Study I: Outcomes of Hysterectomy," *Obstetrics and Gynecology* 83, no. 4 (April 1994): 556–65.

22. B. L. Harlow et al., "Perineal Exposure to Talc and Ovarian Cancer Risk," *Obstetrics and Gynecology* 80, no. 1 (July 1992): 19–26.

23. B. L. Harlow and E. G. Stewart, "A Population-Based Assessment of Chronic Unexplained Vulvar Pain: Have We Underestimated the Prevalence of Vulvodynia?" *Journal of the American Medical Women's Association* 58, no. 2 (Spring 2003): 82–88.

CHAPTER 29 ■ ■ ■ ■ ■ ■ ■ ■ ■ ■ ■ ■ ■ ■ ■ ■

This chapter discusses medical conditions, diseases, and procedures that affect both men and women but have a particular impact on women, either because primarily women get them or because men's and women's bodies develop or respond to them differently.

The sections of the chapter are:

ANEMIA

The hemoglobin molecule in red blood cells carries oxygen to every part of the body. Anemia results from a shortage of red blood cells and/or their low hemoglobin content, so that our tissues get less oxygen. It occurs four times as often among women as among men. The symptoms, often vague, may include chronic fatigue, irritability, dizziness, memory problems, shortness of breath, headaches, and bone pain. Dark-skinned women may look grayish, and light-skinned women may look very pale. Mild anemia may have no noticeable symptoms.

IRON-DEFICIENCY ANEMIA

This anemia is by far the most common form in women. It can be caused by losing blood from our stomach or intestines, and also by heavy menstrual periods, miscarriage, abortion, childbirth, or surgery for fibroids. Pregnant women are especially prone to anemia because the fetus absorbs much of the iron the mother takes in.

The best prevention is an iron-rich diet. Cooking foods in iron pots increases their iron content. If you are still anemic, you may want to take supplements. (Some medical practitioners recommend them routinely for pregnant women.) Ferrous gluconate and chelated iron are the most easily absorbed forms (though some of us find out, through blood test results, that we cannot absorb them). They work best on an empty stomach, but if they cause nausea or cramps, take them with food. Taking vitamin C at the same time will increase absorption of the iron. Iron pills can cause very dark, sticky-textured stools or constipation, which can be remedied by eating more whole grains, bran, and fruit and drinking lots of water. Eating blackstrap molasses has helped some women. Iron interferes with the absorption of vitamin E, so if you take vitamin E, wait at least six hours before taking iron. Iron can be given by injection for severe deficiency.

VITAMIN-DEFICIENCY ANEMIA

This anemia results from a lack of folic acid, an essential B vitamin. Pregnant women, women who have had many children, women taking oral contraceptives, and malnourished women can become anemic this way. Symptoms may include burning or weakness in the legs. You can prevent or treat this deficiency by eating whole grains and dark green vegetables and/or taking folic acid supplements. Vegetarians who eat no animal or dairy products sometimes suffer from anemia caused by lack of vitamin B_{12} (present in all animal products). Adding brewer's yeast (which often contains vitamin B_{12}), a fortified bran cereal, spirulina (a microalga), or fermented foods like miso, tempeh, or fermented sprouts to your diet will help. Women who lack a protein called the *intrinsic factor,* necessary for oral absorption of vitamin B_{12}, get a particular type of vitamin deficiency anemia called *pernicious anemia.* Those women will need monthly injections of this vitamin.

HEREDITARY AND OTHER TYPES OF ANEMIA

Some forms of anemia can be inherited. *Sickle-cell anemia* is found in some people of African ancestry, and *thalassemia* affects people of Mediterranean descent. Also, some African and Mediterranean (especially Italian) women inherit a deficiency in an enzyme called glucose-6-phosphate-dehydrogenase, which results in the development of *hemolytic* (red-blood-cell-destroying) *anemia* if sulfa, aspirin, or antimalarial drugs are taken. This condition can be fatal. Finally, anemia can result from chronic illness such as kidney disease, thyroid disease, arthritis, or cancer. Exposure to certain drugs, chemicals, or metals, or to radiation, can occasionally cause anemia.

TESTING FOR ANEMIA

The *hematocrit* is a basic, inexpensive screening test for anemia. It measures the percentage of red cells in your blood. The normal hematocrit for a woman who is not pregnant is 37 to 47 percent. If your hematocrit is low, ask for a complete blood count, a lab test done on blood drawn from a vein in your arm. In some cases, other specialized, expensive tests may be needed. Any new onset of anemia should be thoroughly evaluated, as iron deficiency may not be the problem.

ARTHRITIS

"Arthritis" is a term used for many different joint diseases. Women, who get arthritis three times more often than men, most often develop either osteoarthritis or rheumatoid arthritis.

OSTEOARTHRITIS

Osteoarthritis is a degenerative disease in which the cartilage—usually in the knees, hips, ankles, or spine—gradually wears away. It affects about 16 million women in the U.S., usually after the age of forty-five or fifty, and usually is not crippling. Common symptoms are swelling, redness, and stiffness around the joints.

In *rheumatoid arthritis,* which affects about 3 percent of adult women, the body's own immune system attacks the membranes covering the joints. The symptoms include pain; swelling; redness in the fingers, knees, hips, and back; fatigue; anemia; fever; and weight loss. A blood test can distinguish rheumatoid arthritis from other forms of the disease. For more information about rheumatoid arthritis, see p. 662.

PREVENTION AND SELF-HELP TREATMENTS

Exercise, relaxation, and nutrition can both prevent and treat osteoarthritis, sometimes reducing or eliminating the need for medical treatment. Regular exercise—such as yoga, walking, or swimming—stretches, strengthens, and may help preserve the joints. Daily rest is especially important when arthritis is severe. Some studies suggest that a diet low in fats can dramatically reduce pain, swelling, and stiffness. Testing can determine what foods trigger an attack; it varies with the individual. Since many foods and substances (such as beef, pork, milk, sugar, chocolate, monosodium glutamate, pepper, alcohol, and artificial preservatives) actually trigger attacks, eliminating from your diet whatever triggers your arthritis can help prevent attacks. Some women find that regular consumption of alfalfa (sprouts, tea, or pills) prevents flare-ups of osteoarthritis, but alfalfa may cause rheumatoid arthritis to worsen. Acupuncture and supplements of B vitamins, vitamin C, and glucosamine (a component of connective tissue) may also be helpful.

Arthritis pain can also be accompanied by stress and depression, making us less motivated to take care of ourselves and thus causing more pain, setting up a cycle that is difficult to break. Meditation, yoga, relaxation exercises, and biofeedback may help us break the stress-depression-pain cycle. The symptoms sometimes abate temporarily during pregnancy. Some menopausal women find that osteoarthritis improves with hormone therapy.

MEDICAL TREATMENTS

The most common treatment for mild arthritis is aspirin, which relieves both inflammation and pain. Too much aspirin can cause stomach irritation and bleeding, but taking it with food or in specially coated (enteric) form reduces these risks. Nonsteroidal anti-inflammatory over-the-counter drugs (NSAIDs) such as ibuprofen and naproxen are also helpful but can cause the same stomach problems, as well as kidney and heart problems. COX-2 inhibitors are widely advertised for arthritis pain and claim to be safer, but they do have gastrointestinal, kidney, and cardiovascular side effects over time, so take the lowest effective dose.[1] Some studies found them no more effective than much cheaper drugs.

AUTOIMMUNE DISORDERS

Normally, your body forms antibodies against foreign substances that get into it (known as *antigens*) and renders them harmless so they cause no problem. Autoimmune disorders occur when your immune system mistakes something in your own body for an antigen and attacks it, causing injury and greatly interfering with daily life. The autoimmune diseases most common in women are discussed below. The root cause of these disorders is not known, but some researchers think that following a viral infection, the immune system mistakes human proteins for similar proteins that were in the virus.

HASHIMOTO'S THYROIDITIS

The pituitary and hypothalamus glands in your brain stimulate the thyroid gland to make certain hormones (T3, triiodothyronine, and T4, thyroxine) that are needed for metabolism. Chronic autoimmune thyroiditis, commonly called *Hashimoto's thyroiditis*, occurs when the immune system attacks the thyroid gland, resulting in low levels of these hormones (hypothyroidism). Symptoms include fatigue, slow movement and speech, intolerance to cold, constipation, irregular or absent menstrual periods, and weight gain. Other signs of underactive thyroid include puffy face, coarse hair and skin, eyebrow thinning, swollen neck or tongue, and brittle nails.

Hashimoto's thyroiditis is seven times more common in women than men, and the most common cause of underactive thyroid in developed countries. A combination of environmental factors (stress, pregnancy) and genetics may predispose women to this condition. It's permanent in most cases, though some women have it temporarily after pregnancy and childbearing. If not treated, it can cause high cholesterol, anemia (low red blood cell count), heart failure, and fertility problems.

Blood tests for diagnosis show high levels of thyroid-stimulating hormone (TSH) trying to make up for low levels of T3 and T4. Most patients will also have certain antibodies (anti-thyroglobulin or anti-thyroid peroxidase) in the blood because the immune system is attacking the thyroid gland. Treatment with medication replaces the missing hormones: Thyroxine (T4, Synthroid) is given in a once-daily pill, and combinations of T3 and T4 are being studied. Usually, you will feel better in a few weeks, but it may take several months for your symptoms to clear up. Eating a lot of soy can interfere with thyroxine, so you may need to rethink your diet if your soy intake is high. Taking too much thyroxine can result in thinning bones, or osteoporosis (see p. 564 in Chapter 27, "Our Later Years") and abnormal heart rhythms.

GRAVES' DISEASE (OVERACTIVE THYROID)

The most common underlying cause of overactive thyroid (hyperthyroidism) is Graves' disease, an autoimmune condition in which the patient's own immune system turns against the thyroid gland. This condition affects women much more often than men (about eight to one). Often called *diffuse toxic goiter* because the entire gland is enlarged, it's more common in the thirties and forties and tends to run in families, but the reason it develops is not known.

Symptoms

The most common symptom of hyperthyroid is visible enlargement of the gland (goiter). You may also have swelling around the eyes caused by inflammation, thickened skin over the lower legs, tremor, weight loss, anxiety, and palpitations. Most people's eyes feel irritated or look as if they are staring. About one out of twenty suffer more severe eye problems, which can include bulging, severe inflammation, double vision, or blurred vision.

Treatment

Tremor and palpitations, which are caused by excess thyroid hormone acting on the cardiac and nervous system, can be improved within a few hours by medication. *Beta-blockers* do not decrease the amount of thyroid hormone produced, but they may prevent some of these symptoms. *Anti-thyroid medications* prevent the thyroid from producing hormones. When taken regularly, these drugs are usually very effective within a few weeks. Anti-thyroid drugs can have side effects such as rash, itching, or fever, but these are uncommon. Rarely, these medications can cause a drop in blood cell counts.

Radioactive iodine is the most widely recommended permanent treatment. Because iodine does not concentrate in any other cells, there's very little radiation exposure (or side effects) for the rest of the body. Radioactive iodine can be taken by mouth, so you don't need to go to the hospital. Most patients are cured with a single dose. The only common side effect of radioactive iodine treatment is underactivity of the thyroid gland.

Some of us with Graves' have *surgery* to remove the thyroid gland because we cannot tolerate medication or do not want to take radioactive iodine. The surgery usually requires general anesthesia and an overnight hospital stay. Sometimes partial thyroidectomy can be done as an outpatient procedure, under local anesthesia with the aid of IV sedation. There is a very small (1 percent) risk of injury to structures in the neck near the thyroid gland, including the nerve to the voice box *(recurrent laryngeal nerve)*.

If hypothyroidism occurs after treatment of an overactive thyroid gland, it can be effectively treated with *levothyroxine*. This medication, one pill a day, usually does not cause side effects or complications.

RHEUMATOID ARTHRITIS

Three times as many women as men have some kind of arthritis. In rheumatoid arthritis, antibodies attack the membrane (synovium) that lines and lubricates a joint. The result is breakdown of cartilage and bone, leading to deformity and disability. It's not the same disease as osteoarthritis, which results from wear and tear on the joints as we age (see "Arthritis," p. 660). Rheumatoid arthritis affects about 3 percent of adult women, usually young to middle-aged. It typically starts in the hands and feet, and it can also affect the wrists, elbows, shoulders, neck, ankles, knees, and hips. In severe cases, the heart, lungs, blood vessels, and kidneys can be affected. Much of the joint damage that results in disability begins early, so early diagnosis and treatment are essential to reduce inflammation and prevent injury.

Symptoms include morning stiffness, symmetric joint swelling (equal on both sides) and redness, and nodules on the elbows or fingers. Diagnosis involves X rays and a blood test for markers of inflammation. Treatment aims to relieve pain, to reduce inflammation, to stop or slow down joint damage, and to improve function and well-being, but there is no cure. A balanced mix of rest, exercise, and occupational/physical therapy can help. Medications such as aspirin, acetaminophen, ibuprofen, COX-2 inhibitors, steroids, and narcotics can control pain and inflammation. Anti-rheumatic drugs may be able to reduce or prevent joint damage and preserve function. Newer drugs such as etanercept (Enbrel) and infliximab (Remicade) treat immune system chemicals that cause inflammation; in a recent study, a combination of drugs produced even better results than methotrexate or etanercept alone.[2] In the severest cases, surgery may be needed. (For more information and support groups, see the Arthritis Foundation's website, www.arthritis.org.)

LUPUS

Lupus erythematosus is an autoimmune disorder with symptoms that usually include a combination of skin, joint, blood, kidney, and neurologic problems. Close to a million U.S. women have it, ten times more than men. Two out of three women with lupus are African-American, Native American, or Asian-American. Lupus is characterized by unusual fatigue, a sign of general inflammation, with flare-ups and remissions. It usually develops in the twenties or thirties, though it may be diagnosed between ages fifteen and forty-five.

Lupus shows up in so many different ways that it may take months or years to piece them all together and come up with an accurate diagnosis. There are two types, *discoid* and *systemic*. Talk to your health care provider if you have any of these symptoms:

- Facial "butterfly" rash across cheeks and bridge of the nose
- Disclike skin lesions or rash marks
- Mouth or nose ulcers
- Arthritis without deformity
- Shortness of breath or chest pains indicating inflammation of the lungs (pleuritis) or the heart (pericarditis)
- Rash triggered by exposure to the sun
- Whitening of fingers after exposure to cold (Raynaud's phenomenon)
- Convulsions or psychosis

Symptoms that can be detected only with lab tests include low red or white blood cell or platelet counts, repeated false-positive results on syphilis tests, excessive protein or cellular casts in the urine, and certain antibodies in the blood. Other signs include low-grade fever, muscle weakness, joint pain and/or redness, hair loss, and persistent fatigue. Skin symptoms may be less noticeable in African-American women, which can delay diagnosis. Kidney damage is the most serious complication; it is treated with medication and hemodialysis. Although it can be extremely disabling, lupus is not usually life-threatening.

There is no cure for lupus, but treatment may control severe flare-ups and reduce their frequency and severity. It helps to avoid potential triggers such as smoking, sun exposure, and certain antibiotics, and to get exercise and supportive emotional care. Minor joint symptoms are treated with rest and nonsteroidal anti-inflammatory drugs. Anti-malarial drugs such as hydroxychloroquine may help for joint symptoms and rashes that don't respond to anti-inflammatories. In more severe cases, you may be given corticosteroids such as prednisone for anemia, low platelet counts, neurologic problems, and heart or lung inflammation. These drugs often improve symptoms, though there are some long-term risks (osteoporosis, weight gain, peptic ulcers, and high blood pressure). Immunosuppressants can reduce the need for steroids and lower the risk of kidney damage.

Women with lupus who get pregnant may have flare-ups after the birth or be more likely to miscarry. Because symptoms come and go, other people may not realize how this disease is affecting your life, so support groups are a key resource for coping (see "Resources").

SCLERODERMA

Scleroderma means "hard skin" and is a group of diseases, thought to be autoimmune in origin, involving the abnormal growth of connective tissue. In localized scleroderma, the skin hardens in abnormally colored, thickened patches. Three out of four people who have it are women. Most also have Raynaud's phenomenon, in which cold-induced spasm of blood vessels makes the hands and feet ache and turn pale. Changes in physical appearance and loss of hand function are common. Scleroderma can also spread to the blood vessels and internal organs, causing arthritis, muscle inflammation, gastrointestinal slowdown, dry eyes, and dry mouth. Severe scarring on the lungs, as well as heart and kidney problems, can cause death.

Treatment that targets the affected organs can be effective, though there is no cure. Certain blood pressure, migraine, and antidepressant medications reduce blood vessel spasm, and it helps to avoid smoking and keep your fingers warm. Drugs that suppress the immune system,

followed by anti-fibrotics to reduce scarring, can help but may have serious side effects. (For information and support groups, see "Resources.")

SJÖGREN'S SYNDROME

This autoimmune disorder of unknown cause occurs when the immune system destroys mucus-secreting glands, especially the salivary and tear-producing glands, leading to dry eyes and dry mouth. Common complaints also include burning throat, trouble chewing and swallowing, and a gritty, sandy, or filmed-over feeling in the eyes. Other symptoms may include tooth decay, joint pain, digestive or kidney problems, dry nose and skin, lung problems, vaginal irritation, burning tongue, and extreme fatigue. Over 90 percent of those who have Sjögren's are women. A recent study found that women with Sjögren's have low levels of hormones called androgens, which may be a factor in dry eye.[3]

Diagnosis may be difficult, as some symptoms can occur with other diseases, too, and not all of them occur at the same time. Some people have an additional tissue disease such as rheumatoid arthritis, lupus, scleroderma, or inflammation of the muscles or arteries. There is no single test for Sjögren's, but a primary care provider or rheumatologist can arrange to measure tear and saliva production, X-ray major salivary glands, biopsy minor ones in the lip, and do blood tests to determine whether it is what you have.

Artificial tears and salivas, ointments, and anti-inflammatory drugs can reduce discomfort. Using a humidifier at home and goggles outdoors may also help. High-quality dental and eye care are extremely important. If you don't know anyone else who has this condition, emotional support and information can make a real difference (see "Resources").

CHRONIC FATIGUE IMMUNODEFICIENCY SYNDROME/MYALGIC ENCEPHALOMYELITIS

Chronic fatigue immunodeficiency syndrome (CFIDS), also referred to as myalgic encephalomyelitis (ME), affects people of all ethnicities and income groups. Like many autoimmune and chronic pain conditions, it is more common in women (as many as 70 percent of patients) than in men. The causes of CFIDS are unknown. One theory is that it starts with an infection or is a neurological reaction to infection; the condition may result from a defect in an enzyme (Rnase-L) that the body uses to inactivate viruses. Symptoms can include incapacitating exhaustion, generalized weakness, cognitive problems, increased viral symptoms, nonrestorative sleep, exercise intolerance (when exercise makes symptoms worse), chemical sensitivities, and chronic physical pain. Some of us who have CFIDS are able to function at a reduced level, while others of us are completely disabled.

After four years of struggling up these three flights of stairs to my classroom, I can't do this anymore. Everything hurts. I am out of breath. It's only 8:00 in the morning. I will try to cover up my mind-numbing exhaustion, but when? My brain shuts down, my speech slurs and I feel like I am trapped in a bad charade. As I give all of myself to someone else's children, I am incompetent. Then, I go home with nothing left for my own kids.

Researchers and clinicians are not sure whether CFIDS is the same illness as ME or, possibly, fibromyalgia. The World Health Organization (WHO) defines ME as a neurological illness and uses two alternate names for it, chronic fatigue syndrome (CFS) and post-viral fatigue syndrome (PVFS). Subsets of patients display differences in the onset, symptoms, and severity of illness. Many patients may not get an accurate diagnosis, because CFIDS/ME is one of several conditions with similar body pain and weakness (post-polio syndrome, which occurs in survivors of both paralytic and nonparalytic poliomyelitis; chronic Lyme disease; fibromyalgia; multiple sclerosis; and lupus). It may also overlap with migraine, temporomandibular joint disorder (TMJ), irritable bowel syndrome, and multiple chemical sensitivities. Also, many practitioners are skeptical about CFIDS/ME and dismiss women with a referral to a psychologist.

My doctor said, "All working women with kids are tired. I can't find anything wrong. Things okay at home?" I look pale as candle wax with about as much energy as a doorknob. . . . That [appointment] started doctor shopping that yielded no results. To be a cooperative patient, I tried several long trials of antidepressants only to end up feeling progressively worse each time.

Symptoms

You may feel overall weakness and exhaustion and experience arm and leg muscle tremors. This lack of stamina and energy interferes with the ability to participate in normal daily activities. Rest does not relieve symptoms. Simple activity can lead to pain or the whole body aching, starting twenty-four to thirty-six hours after exertion. Aerobic activity can cause total relapse.

I was a successful rising scholar when I collapsed ten years ago. I was active, loved to ski, [and was] involved in the lives of my two children. It has been as if I had to watch my own death. If I had not had children, I would have committed suicide long ago, particularly during the periods of intense pain when all I could do was lie in bed. For years I did not have a single day I felt well. Imag-

EPIDEMIC, HISTORY, AND DEBATE

CFIDS/ME is not a rare disorder. It affects 422 out of 100,000 people ages 18 to 69, or about 800,000 people in the United States. It is three times more common than HIV infection in women (125 out of 100,000) and twenty-five times as common as AIDS among women (12 out of 100,000). The risk of getting it is considerably higher than a woman's lifetime risk of getting lung cancer (63 out of 100,000).[4]

Reaction to this epidemic has revealed many inadequacies and prejudices of the U.S. health care system, particularly fears of "hysterical" women. In 1988 the U.S. Centers for Disease Control and Prevention (CDC) labeled the illness "chronic fatigue syndrome" instead of the more global name, myalgic encephalomyelitis. Although this established it as a real, physical disease instead of a mental disorder, patients felt that the word "fatigue" minimized their symptoms. CFIDS/ME was dismissed as "yuppie flu" or an illness of middle- and upper-class white women (those most likely to be able to afford care), even though Latinas and African-Americans appear to be disproportionately affected.[5] Symptoms were brushed off as manifestations of midlife crisis or boredom. Even the women's movement was slow to acknowledge this as a disease affecting people of all races and classes. International scientists began to adopt the term "CFS," cementing that attitude into the global psyche. Patients and advocacy groups, mostly women, protested. These "difficult, unreasonable, and hysterical" women were held up as further evidence that people with CFIDS/ME needed cognitive behavioral therapy, as well as graded exercise programs and antidepressants. Those are still accepted treatments, but their effectiveness is the subject of debate.

ine the worst flu you ever had, and it never goes away—you think it can't get worse, but it does.

Exertion or standing for periods of time may bring on dizziness, light-headedness, and nausea with an irregular heartbeat (orthostatic intolerance). You may become sensitive to light, sudden noise, and odors. Some people feel jittery or anxious. Conversation might be difficult because of slurred speech and problems with recall, word retrieval, and understanding. It may become difficult to sort, sequence, and organize ideas and objects. Confusion and time disorientation can make it hard to finish tasks.

There is a test where patients are asked to put one foot in front of the other, hold their arms out, and close their eyes. A patient with CFS cannot hold that position for any length of time (I would im-

mediately fall over). A very few get dizzy; most of us just do not know where we are in space.

Changes in appetite, weight, and reaction to food can occur, including intestinal and bladder disturbances, irritable bowel syndrome, and new food sensitivities. You may have low blood sugar (hypoglycemia). Headaches, overall body pain, irritability, and mood swings are common. CFIDS/ME patients are often unable to get good-quality sleep, which makes symptoms feel worse. Some people have bouts of viral symptoms such as sore throat, tender lymph nodes, and sinus congestion. Some report hypersensitivity to medications and chemicals, and antibiotics are usually not effective. (To learn more, see "CDC Criteria for Diagnosing CFIDS" [W71] on the companion website, www.ourbodiesourselves.org.)

Nonroutine brain scans and blood tests of people with these symptoms sometimes show abnormalities, but these tests are not always available. Most advocacy organizations can provide information about tests and research, as well as hope and support for those of us struggling to cope with a complex and poorly understood condition.

Treatment

There is no cure for CFIDS/ME, but there is a range of therapies that may be helpful for symptoms such as headaches, pain, and sleep and balance disorders.

Since those with CFIDS respond differently to different strategies, you may have to try many treatments. Do your own research, network with others, listen to your body, and use trial and error. Feeling desperate after years of illness can make us vulnerable to "magic bullet" cures. When considering a new treatment, use caution, double-check information, and consider safety, benefit, and expense.

Rest, Exercise, and Nutrition

Moderating your activity level is crucial. Regular periods of uninterrupted rest are essential, but not complete bed rest, which can cause muscle atrophy and increasing muscle weakness. When you do feel better, don't rush back to normal activity, because pushing the body too hard or too quickly can result in a serious relapse. Mild stretching exercises and walking to keep your body in motion will help you maintain your physical conditioning. Don't push when your body tells you not to!

Diet

Dietary changes may help with stomach and intestinal symptoms. Certain foods may make you feel worse, particularly alcohol, caffeine, sugar, wheat, and food additives. A high-protein diet and magnesium supplements may be beneficial. You might want to investigate vitamins B_6 and B_{12}, folates, SAM-e, glucosamine, and essential fatty acid supplements, especially the omega-3 fish oils. Other supplements that support mitochondrial (energy) function are beneficial for some people.

Drugs

Antidepressants are commonly prescribed to treat the underlying chemistry of many types of pain and fatigue. Low-dose antidepressant medications such as Elavil and Sinequan often improve sleep quality. Other drugs can be tried to manage pain and cognitive symptoms. Because many of us with CFIDS are very sensitive to drugs, it is best to start out with the lowest possible dose and increase if necessary. Experimental drugs—such as Ampligen—show promise, but they are available only in clinical trials and have not yet been approved by the FDA.

The pain and confusion are gone, and I can walk a mile (with the aid of a brace on one leg). After six months on the medication, which I must take via IV twice a week . . . I was driving a car and beginning an exercise program. Within two years I was hiking a bit again! I could walk on the beach! It was wonderful. But expensive.

About one third of people with CFIDS recover almost fully, but no one knows why. Some get a little better; others recover minimally if at all; still others have progressively worse symptoms over time. For many of us, the illness waxes and wanes, with periods of relative health interspersed with relapses. If you are very ill, a good support person in your life who can help you keep track of what seems to work and what doesn't is extremely important. Support groups and websites can help you sort through symptoms, treatments, and coping methods, including information on how to apply for disability benefits (see "Resources").

CHRONIC PAIN CONDITIONS

Pain interferes with the lives of so many people that it's the most common reason for consulting a health care provider.[6] Sometimes it's the result of a disease or injury, but often (as with back pain or chronic headache) the cause is unknown. That doesn't make the pain any less real. Pain is considered chronic when it persists for over a month beyond the usual recovery period for an illness or injury; continues as a result of a chronic condition; or keeps coming back even when there's no evidence of illness or injury. It is a subjective experience, but it is certainly not just "all in your head." Chronic pain is a major source of disability in this country, especially for women. While chronic pain is often devastating, both self-help and medical strategies may help you manage pain, reduce suffering, and improve the quality of your life.

SELF-HELP FOR PAIN MANAGEMENT

Acknowledging that you're in pain and that you may not be able to relieve it completely can actually help you deal with it. Studies have found that acceptance of pain results in less disability and depression, while always seeing the negative in everything ("catastrophizing") may make pain worse.[7] Accepting that you are in pain doesn't mean giving up on your efforts to manage and treat it; in fact, it is the first step in creating a self-management approach.

Exercise prompts your body to release natural painkillers called *endorphins* that block pain signals from reaching the brain (that's the mechanism that produces "runner's high"). You may not be able to do strenuous exercise if you're hurting, but you can try gentle stretching, strength training, and endurance and stabilization exercises, especially if it's supervised. Your physical functioning is likely to improve, and you may even feel less pain.

Mind-body techniques such as relaxation training, meditation, biofeedback, and hypnosis may improve your response to stress, reduce anxiety and suffering, and enable you to do more physically. Starting these practices early may, in some cases, prevent long-term disability by keeping acute pain from becoming chronic.[8] The effectiveness of such techniques varies with the individual, so it's important not to blame yourself if they don't work for you.

Yoga combines body postures and breathing exercises in a way that may improve mood, flexibility, and strength. While there's not much evidence for the effect of yoga on pain, you may find it helpful. The National Center for Complementary and Alternative Medicine (NCCAM) is doing a study comparing yoga and exercise for pain. *T'ai chi* and *qi gong,* two Chinese mind-body disciplines, improved pain symptoms and quality of life for people with fibromyalgia in small studies;[9] now the National Institute of Arthritis and Musculoskeletal and Skin Diseases (NIAMS) is doing a larger study of t'ai chi.

"ALTERNATIVE" TREATMENTS

In addition to or instead of taking drugs, many people try nonmedical interventions to relieve pain and improve the ability to function. These techniques may not be covered by all insurance plans, but unlike drugs, alternative treatments usually have few side effects. Often they work best in combination. Every person responds differently, and it's up to you to decide what works best for you. You should know after the first few visits whether the treatment is helping. (For information on acupuncture, chiropractic, and massage, all of which may relieve pain, see Chapter 5, "Complementary Health Practices.")

MEDICAL TREATMENT FOR PAIN

A wide variety of medications can be used to relieve chronic pain. Their effects are not the same for everyone, so you may have to try different types to find something that helps. Also, doctors typically prescribe medications "off label" for pain, without specific FDA approval for that particular condition. Often the effectiveness of such medications is a matter of trial and error.

Bear in mind, too, that what works for one type of pain may not work for another. There may also be a "placebo effect"—that is, some people (about 30 percent) feel better even when taking dummy pills, as a result of increases in the body's own endorphins.

Most pain medications fall into four categories: analgesics, antidepressants, anticonvulsants, and anesthetics.

Analgesics include nonsteroidal anti-inflammatory drugs (NSAIDs), such as aspirin, ibuprofen, and naproxen; acetaminophen; COX-2 inhibitors; and opioids. NSAIDs and acetaminophen, which are available without a prescription, are widely used for back pain and headaches, and COX-2 inhibitors are heavily marketed for arthritis pain. Nausea, sleepiness, and constipation are the side effects most often reported. NSAIDs and COX-2 inhibitors may also cause stomach pain and bleeding, as well as heart and kidney problems.

Many people dislike the idea of taking prescription opioids because they fear becoming addicted. However, there is an important difference between addiction, which happens to a minority of pain patients, and tolerance (the drug has less effect over time, resulting in the need for a larger dose) or dependence (development of withdrawal symptoms if you stop taking the drug). Addiction involves relying on drugs to escape from (not cope with) life's realities, not just to relieve pain. Most medical practitioners recommend opioids only when other medications don't help and when they can improve how well you function without causing serious damage. Some opioids reduce sexual desire and response, and their long-term effects have not been adequately studied. They should never be taken with other narcotics, tranquilizers, alcohol, or anything that induces sleepiness. (For more information, see "Advantages and Possible Side Effects of Analgesics" [W72] on the companion website, www.ourbodiesourselves.org.)

Tricyclic antidepressants may relieve some types of chronic pain, but selective serotonin reuptake inhibitors (SSRIs), such as fluoxetine (Prozac), won't. A newer type, venlafaxine, seems to be more effective. If you're depressed, you may not have the energy to deal with pain. Treating depression, which often coexists with chronic pain, can improve both mood and ability to function.

Anticonvulsant (antiseizure) drugs such as valproate (Depakote) have long been used for pain management. However, they can make you dizzy or sleepy and cause swelling of the hands and feet, and you may not be able to drive a car while taking them. Weight gain is also very common. Newer anticonvulsants are gabapentin (Neurontin) and topirimate (Topamax).

Anesthetics such as lidocaine may relieve chronic pain if other types of medication don't work. Most have to be injected, and how well they work in the long term varies. A benefit is that they have minimal side effects and are non-addictive. Some can now be taken in ointment, patch, or nasal spray form.

ATTITUDES, VALUES, AND SUPPORT SYSTEMS

While you might never be able to get rid of the pain completely, you may develop strategies to manage it. Creating such strategies requires patience and observing how your body responds. Try different treatment approaches. Set realistic goals for daily activity, and focus on what you *can* do instead of what you can't. Build up strength and flexibility as you are able. Adapt your work space and home furnishings for greater comfort, pace your activity, rest frequently, and do things at a time of day when your energy level is higher. Try to be clear and assertive with your friends and coworkers about your limits.

Having understanding relatives, friends, and health care providers, as well as a support group of people with similar experiences, can help you stick to your strategy. (For more information on pain programs and support groups, see "Resources.")

FIBROMYALGIA

Fibromyalgia is a syndrome of diffuse pain, aching, and muscle stiffness, often accompanied by fatigue and sleep disturbance. It can be distinguished from other chronic pain syndromes by its well-defined, characteristic pattern of tender points: unusually painful spots in muscles and in areas where muscles join tendons. To diagnose it, the practitioner applies pressure to each of these sites and observes the person's pain response. If you have at least eleven out of eighteen painful tender points, with a history of widespread pain for at least three months, you meet the classification criteria for fibromyalgia. However, people with fewer tender points may be diagnosed with the syndrome. Lab tests and neurological and joint exams generally come up normal in the absence of any other disease.

While the location of tender points is generally consistent in everyone who has fibromyalgia, the everyday pain experienced by each individual varies considerably in location and intensity and may not always correspond to ten-

der point sites. The quality of pain can also vary, from intense aching to widespread burning. Pain often results from intolerance to exercise, so muscles remain tired and stiff after exertion, sometimes for several days. However, short periods of inactivity, such as standing or sitting in one position, can also cause pain and stiffness. Some of us find we can relieve it somewhat or prevent it by changing positions frequently. Most people also report stiffness when getting up in the morning; it may wear off in several hours or last throughout much of the day. Other symptoms of fibromyalgia can include headaches, sensations of numbness and tingling, a subjective sense of swollen hands and feet without any visible signs of swelling, irritable bladder, difficulty concentrating, and generalized hypersensitivity to environmental phenomena, such as changes in temperature, humidity, and barometric pressure as well as noise and odors.

Although the cause is unclear, some evidence suggests that decreased responsiveness of the hypothalamic, pituitary, and adrenal glands and of the sympathetic nervous system may play a role. Studies have repeatedly shown that the central features of fibromyalgia occur independently of psychological status, although pain may get worse with stress, as in other illnesses. Increasingly, health care providers are recognizing the physical basis of fibromyalgia, so we are less likely to be told that our problems are in our head.

Managing Fibromyalgia

Some of us with fibromyalgia find the following strategies helpful:

1. *Gentle, daily aerobic exercise,* starting from as little as three to five minutes and increasing to twenty minutes. It may be difficult to exercise while experiencing fatigue and aching, and it can take over two weeks before the benefits outweigh

the side effects. When they do, you can also try low-impact graded aerobic exercise (swimming, walking), gentle massage, and hot baths. If you also have CFIDS, go very slowly and monitor the effects before continuing.

2. *A consistent bedtime with enough sleep,* and one of several drugs that enhance deep sleep. You may have to try different medications in succession and combination before finding what works best for you. Doctors may also prescribe pain relievers or mild antidepressants that produce serotonins and enhance sleep. The doses you get for fibromyalgia are often one tenth of those used to treat depression, which suggests that the underlying problem isn't just depression. If you have brief relapses, a temporary increase in medication may be necessary.

3. *A healthy diet.* Some women feel better after eliminating caffeine and refined sugar.

4. *Massage and mind-body techniques* (see "Chronic Pain Conditions," p. 668).

Fibromyalgia is sometimes chronic and relapsing but not always disabling. With the right combination of medications, exercise, and regular sleep, many women can be helped. Learning as much as you can and becoming actively involved in your own treatment decisions can help you achieve as much recovery as possible. Support groups can provide up-to-date information, doctor referrals, and encouragement in coping (see "Resources").

Another syndrome often confused with fibromyalgia is *myofascial pain syndrome.* It is distinguished by localized rather than diffuse pain and tenderness. Instead of tender points, it has trigger points that, when palpated, result in referred pain at other locations. The referred pain can usually be eliminated by injecting a local anesthetic at the trigger point.

CARDIOVASCULAR PROBLEMS

"Cardiovascular" refers to the heart and blood vessels that together make up the circulatory system. Cardiovascular disease (CVD), heart attack, and stroke are the leading causes of death in women over age fifty in the United States and Canada. More women than men die within one year after a heart attack,[10] and more women than men die of stroke, possibly because fewer women than men are diagnosed and treated correctly.[11,12] Most research on CVD has focused on white men. Only in recent years have large numbers of women been included in clinical studies, and white women have been studied more than women of other races. Cardiovascular conditions include the following:

- **Atherosclerosis** is a type of thickening and hardening of the arteries *(arteriosclerosis)* in which deposits called *plaque* build up in the arterial walls. Plaques contain cholesterol, cellular waste products, calcium, and *fibrin* (a clotting agent in the blood). There are no specific symptoms.
- **Hypertension** means high blood pressure, above 140 over 90. It's a major risk factor for CVD, stroke, and congestive heart failure in women.[13] Although blood pressure tends to increase somewhat with age, hypertension is not normal. A blood pressure reading of 120–139 over 80–89 is a sign of developing hypertension. Many people's blood pressure rises from sheer nervousness in the doctor's office, a phenomenon called "white-coat hypertension." You may have to have your blood pressure measured several times to get an accurate reading.

Hypertension has been called "the silent killer" because people often have no symptoms, or only unexplained headaches or dizziness. In most cases, the cause can't be determined, but contributing circumstances include age, race, and weight (see chart on risk factors, p. 674). A healthy lifestyle can greatly reduce your chances of developing hypertension. If you already have hypertension, it can often be controlled with diet and exercise and, if necessary, with medication.

- **Coronary artery disease (CAD),** also called coronary heart disease, ischemic heart disease, or cardiovascular disease (CVD), results from atherosclerosis of the arteries that feed the heart, so the heart muscle doesn't get normal levels of oxygen and nutrients. One of the more common symptoms is *angina,* pain that develops during physical exertion or emotional stress, when the heart muscle is working harder and needs more oxygen. Angina usually disappears with rest. Women with angina may feel pain in the neck, jaw, back, or abdomen, as well as nausea and breathlessness. This may lead to misdiagnosis by health care providers who are familiar with only the typical symptoms men have (uncomfortable pressure, fullness, squeezing, or pain in the center of the chest).

- **Congestive heart failure (CHF)** occurs when the heart loses strength and is unable to pump enough blood to meet the body's needs. As outward blood flow slows, blood returning to the heart backs up, causing a buildup of fluid (congestion) in the tissues. CHF's more common symptoms are swollen legs or ankles or difficulty breathing (especially when lying down), or weight gain when fluid builds up. People with CHF become short of breath and tired, and can't exert themselves. Mild or moderate CHF can usually be treated with a combination of rest, proper diet, modified daily activities, and medication.

- **Heart attack,** which medical practitioners call *myocardial infarction* (MI), coronary thrombosis, or coronary occlusion, can happen if a blood clot completely blocks blood flow through a coronary artery. The clot usually

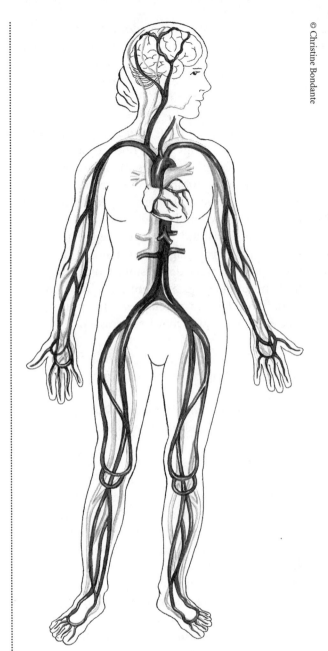

© Christine Bondante

The cardiovascular system

develops at the location of a plaque (fatty deposit inside an arterial wall). If the blockage lasts longer than twenty minutes, the heart muscle supplied by that artery is damaged and may die. Blood clots take only a few minutes to form, which is why heart attacks often occur with little warning. Pain is the most common symptom of a heart attack. It may last longer than a few minutes and does not go away with rest.

Women's symptoms may be different from men's,[14,15] so you, your health care provider, or the emergency room staff may not always realize that you are having a heart attack. Although many women have symptoms similar to men's (sudden strong crushing pain and shortness of breath), others feel tightening and ill-defined pain in the chest, extending into the neck, jaws, and shoulders; a heartburn-like feeling, nausea, and/or vomiting; shortness of breath, weakness, dizziness, pallor, anxiety, and sweating. Unexplained fatigue may be an advance warning sign of a heart attack. Symptoms may appear and then disappear spontaneously, and you may not have all of them.[16] If you experience any of them, call 911 or alert a friend and get to a hospital. Do not attempt to drive yourself.

- **Stroke** is a "brain attack," a cutoff of oxygen to the brain because of atherosclerosis leading to a blood clot in a blood vessel supplying the brain. Bleeding inside the brain *(cerebral hemorrhage)* may also cause stroke. Stroke can cause serious disability, so it is good to know the warning signs. Symptoms are sudden and include numbness or weakness of the face, arm, or leg (especially on one side of the body); confusion; slurred speech or trouble understanding; blurred vision in one or both eyes; dizziness and/or loss of balance or coordination; and severe headache with no known cause. If you or someone with you has one or more of these signs, call 911 immediately. Check the time when the first symptoms appeared—you need to act quickly, because a clot-busting drug can reduce long-term disability for the most common type of stroke if it is given within three hours of the start of symptoms.[17] A *transient ischemic attack* (TIA),

also called a mini-stroke, is a less severe version, lasting only a few moments and causing less damage, but having one may lead to memory loss and other problems. If you suddenly feel dizzy or lose balance, get immediate medical attention.

RISK FACTORS FOR CARDIOVASCULAR DISEASE, HEART ATTACK, AND STROKE

Some risk factors for cardiovascular problems can't be changed, such as our sex, age, and family background. However, others can be modified to prevent or reduce the risk of developing high blood pressure, heart disease, and stroke.

Weight, diet, and exercise can affect people's risk for both cardiovascular disease and diabetes by contributing to a metabolic process that's just starting to be understood. CVD can sometimes be prevented. Reducing the risk factors you can control (diet, smoking, alcohol and drug use, physical activity, dealing with stress) is a good place to start. Useful guidelines from the American Heart Association are available online at www.americanheart.org. The heart is a muscle that needs regular exercise in order to stay healthy. It's never too early or too late to start eating a healthy diet and getting enough exercise. (For more information, see Chapter 2, "Eating Well"; Chapter 3, "Alcohol, Tobacco, and Other Mood-Altering Drugs"; and Chapter 4, "Our Bodies in Motion.")

DIAGNOSTIC TESTS FOR CARDIOVASCULAR DISEASE

Diagnosis of heart disease presents a greater challenge in women than in men, for a variety of reasons. Our symptoms of angina or heart attack may be different from men's, and some of the tests health care providers use may be inappropriate for women or interpreted incorrectly. Some predictive tests for heart attacks may be

FACTORS IN CARDIOVASCULAR PROBLEMS YOU CAN'T CHANGE

NONMODIFIABLE FACTORS	HOW WOMEN'S RISK INCREASES	WHO IS AFFECTED
Age	Risk of CV death four times higher after menopause Higher risk of stroke Equal to men's risk by age 65	Women over 50
Family history	Mother, father, grandparent, or siblings with CVD, especially under 55 for men, under 65 for women	All ages, more over 50
Race/ethnicity	Increases with obesity,* hypertension, diabetes, and home stress	Black women, Mexican-Americans, First Nations, and Inuit (Canada)

* This chapter uses the term "obesity" because it is widely considered a risk factor for certain illnesses. However, many studies used to support the idea that people with a greater percentage of body fat are at higher risk for certain medical problems fail to differentiate between body weight and level of physical fitness. For example, some studies have suggested that fat people who exercise are at less risk of cardiovascular disease than thin sedentary people.

FACTORS IN CARDIOVASCULAR PROBLEMS YOU CAN CHANGE

MODIFIABLE FACTORS	HOW RISK CHANGES	WHO IS AFFECTED	HOW TO REDUCE RISK
Weight	Lower HDL levels, higher levels of LDL and triglycerides, leads to Type 2 diabetes and higher CVD risk	Overweight (BMI >25) or obese (BMI >30); excess fat around stomach	Diet, exercise Avoid salt (causes fluid retention) and caffeine (makes heart work harder)
Diet	Lower HDL levels, higher levels of LDL and triglycerides, leads to obesity, Type 2 diabetes, high BP, and vascular problems; higher risk of CVD	All of us	Minimize saturated and trans fats, lower carbs; eat more fruits and vegetables, fatty fish, omega-3 fatty acids, flaxseed, canola, and soybean oils, and walnuts; get antioxidants (esp. vitamin E)

MODIFIABLE FACTORS	HOW RISK CHANGES	WHO IS AFFECTED	HOW TO REDUCE RISK
Low Exercise Level	Risk of death from heart attack or stroke doubles; exercise can improve cholesterol levels and reduce chances of clot formation	Sedentary women	Aerobic exercise 30-60 min. 3-5 times weekly—walking, jogging or running, stairs, dancing, cycling, skating—strength training
Diabetes	Increases risk of CVD, which causes 50% of all deaths, and diabetes during pregnancy then Type 2 later	All with diabetes, women more than men	Control blood pressure, blood sugar, weight; diet, exercise, medication
Hypertension	Damages blood vessels; leads to heart attack and stroke, plus kidney and eye damage	Smokers, inactive, obese, diabetic	Control blood pressure with diet, exercise, medication
Smoking	Damages arterial linings, increases plaque, higher risk of hypertension, lowers oxygen, makes heart work harder, may lower "good" cholesterol levels	All women smokers	Don't smoke, or quit smoking
	Risk of death three times greater than for non-smokers, and higher when you take birth control pills	Premenopausal women	Stop using birth control pills; use barrier methods
Stress	Raises cholesterol levels and blood pressure	Most of us	See Chapter 6, "Emotional Well-Being"
Taking Hormones	Higher risk of CVD with conjugated equine estrogen	Women taking birth control pills or hormones for menopause	Stop taking hormones; reduce dose for menopause; use patch or cream, not pill; try other formulations
Socioeconomic Factors	Low income, high unemployment; poverty may lead to poor food choices	More black women, Mexican-American, Native American, First Nations and Inuit (Canada)	Avoid processed food and fast food with high fat, high salt
	Worse with alcohol and substance abuse, domestic violence		Campaign for better health programs and protection for women with low incomes

less accurate for women: Low levels of "good" cholesterol (HDL) in the blood appear to predict heart disease death in women better than in men under sixty-five,[18,19] and high triglyceride levels may be a particularly important risk factor in women and the elderly.[20] Also, "normal" reference ranges are based on data from white men, not from women or from different ethnic groups.[21]

Sex and race still tend to affect whether or not you get the right tests and diagnosis.[22,23,24] Fewer women than men are referred for angiograms, and black women are referred less often than white women, even with identical symptoms. Any woman who needs the following tests should have access to them.

- **Angiogram.** Contrast dye is injected into the bloodstream through a small plastic tube (catheter); then X rays record its passage in the heart. This brief procedure requires no anesthetic.
- **Echocardiogram** uses ultrasound to generate pictures of the heart. The procedure is noninvasive, risk-free, and painless, and takes about an hour. In *exercise echocardiography* (stress test), an echocardiogram is done while you walk on a treadmill. Every few minutes the speed and slope are increased until you feel you need to stop. The process is more accurate than exercise ECG for diagnosing coronary artery disease in both sexes, and less expensive than nuclear imaging (see below).
- **Electrocardiogram (ECG)** records the heart's electrical impulses through electrodes so your provider can evaluate your heart's rhythm, its size, and the position of the heart chambers; inflammation or damage to heart muscle; and how well cardiac nerves are working. It is noninvasive, risk-free, and painless, and it usually takes less than half an hour. Exercise electrocardiography *(stress ECG)* does the same thing on a treadmill. This test is readily available and less costly than MPI (see below),

but sometimes it is less helpful in women than in men. If you are out of shape, you may not be able to get your exercise heart rate up high enough. Hormone levels, heart size, and coronary artery function may also make a difference, and some age-associated illnesses can affect the usefulness of this test.

- **Nuclear imaging.** In this technique,[25] radioisotopes are injected into the body, then picked up on the image; it's somewhat invasive, but the risks are low. *Myocardial perfusion imaging* (MPI) is widely performed; it may be better than conventional exercise ECG testing and is particularly useful in identifying patients with more severe disease. Its accuracy in women has recently improved. False-positive results are more likely in younger women unless the technician has clinical experience and expertise in the method.

If it's over 80 percent likely that you have CAD, a stress test or angiogram will probably be suggested. In young, premenopausal women with chest pain but no risk factors for coronary artery disease, a stress test of any kind may yield false-positive results and should be avoided.

Researchers are trying to identify *biomarkers*—proteins in the blood—that indicate increased risk for a heart attack. One such indicator is C-reactive protein (CRP). However, testing for it is useful only in people over fifty with one or two other risk factors, not those at low risk or those already diagnosed with cardiovascular disease.

TREATMENTS FOR CARDIOVASCULAR DISEASE

Once we know we have CVD, there are various strategies for managing it so it doesn't get worse and cause a heart attack or stroke. The first line of treatment is a healthy diet and exercise. If these lifestyle changes are not enough, medication and surgery may improve cardiovascular health and prolong life expectancy. You will probably want to discuss all the options with your primary health care provider and a cardiologist.

Strength Training

While research has shown that weight training can increase strength and endurance in male cardiac patients, few studies have been done on its effect in women with heart disease; such studies are now beginning. Weight training can also reduce clinical depression, a CVD risk factor that's more common in women than in men.[26,27] Weight training is usually a component of cardiac rehab programs.

Cardiac Rehabilitation

These programs offer nonmedical, noninvasive treatment for individuals with cardiovascular disease. Women can benefit as much as men from them. They are usually tailored to the individual and include aerobic exercise, weight training, blood pressure monitoring, education on CVD-related topics, and ECGs at the beginning and end of the program to measure results.

In spite of the benefits, women are generally referred to cardiac rehab less often than men, particularly in rural areas or if there's a problem with payment. Even with referral, women participate less than men—sometimes because we are more out of shape, older when we start, more likely to have other illnesses, or less likely to have someone at home to take care of us. We may need active assistance to start rehab and stick with it, including information on community-based resources.

Medications

Medications for CVD range from simple *diuretics,* which help reduce the amount of water in the body and thus reduce blood pressure, to so-phisticated new drugs that are currently being heavily marketed. *Anticoagulants* such as aspirin help prevent clot formation. They do not dissolve clots that have already formed but may prevent them from getting larger. Many people take low-dose aspirin daily to prevent or control CVD. For this purpose, ibuprofen and acetaminophen are *not* substitutes for aspirin.

Angiotension-converting enzyme (ACE) inhibitors help relax blood vessels and increase the supply of blood and oxygen to the heart while reducing its workload. *Calcium channel blockers* work similarly to ACE inhibitors. *Beta-blockers* are most often used to control fast heart rate *(tachycardia).* All of these drugs may have side effects, depending on your age and other health factors, so you'll need to discuss them with your provider. If one drug doesn't work well for you, another drug or a different dose may be better.

Statins, such as Lipitor, Pravachol, and Mevacor, have been found most effective for lowering LDL cholesterol in the blood, a risk factor for CVD. However, most of the research on statins was done in older people with serious heart conditions, not in younger women or people without heart disease. There is no good evidence to support routine use of statin drugs to lower cholesterol in healthy people. Whether the benefit of statins might actually be due to their anti-inflammatory effects is uncertain. Statins may have negative effects on the liver and may cause muscle weakness, pain, and fatigue. There is some evidence that they may raise breast cancer risk. Patients taking statins have also reported memory loss, but this has not been studied in clinical trials, and the FDA has not acted on complaints. If you are taking statins, be sure to have regular blood tests to check your liver and muscle function. Women who are or may become pregnant or are nursing should not use statins. (For more information, see "Debate over Statins" [W73] on the companion website, www.ourbodiesourselves.org.)

Vitamins

Studies have shown little or no effect of antioxidant vitamins E and C in people who already had CVD, and smokers had a slightly higher risk of death from CVD if they took beta-carotene, which the body converts to vitamin A. If you take statin drugs, taking antioxidants may interfere with their ability to raise your "good" cholesterol. Studies of folate and B vitamins for risk reduction after angioplasty (see below) yielded contradictory results, so caution is suggested.

CARDIOVASCULAR SURGERY

Short of a heart transplant, less drastic surgical operations are now widely used to clear or bypass clogged coronary arteries. You may want to discuss with a cardiologist whether one of these procedures is appropriate for your condition and, if so, how urgent it may be to have it.

Angioplasty[28]

This relatively low-risk procedure widens blood vessels narrowed by plaque formation. It does not require opening the chest or the heart; rather, a catheter is inserted, usually in the groin, and snaked up through an artery to the heart. In *balloon angioplasty,* a balloon-tipped catheter pushes plaque back against the arterial wall to improve blood flow in the artery; the catheter is then removed. The procedure usually takes an hour or two and is done with local anesthesia after mild sedation. In another angioplasty technique, plaque is cut away from the arteries. After either type of angioplasty, a wire mesh tube *(stent)* can be installed to keep the artery open and reduce the chances of reclogging. Drug-coated stents that keep arteries open longer are now being more widely used.

Coronary Artery Bypass Graft (CABG)

CABG is a type of open-heart surgery done to reroute blood around a clogged coronary artery. A piece from a long vein in the leg or a piece of artery from the arm or chest wall is used as a graft and attached below the area of obstruction. In a *classic bypass* operation, the heart is stopped, and a heart-lung pump machine maintains blood flow to the body and brain. After the procedure, the heart is restarted and the incision closed. A newer type of bypass, called *off-pump surgery,* keeps the heart beating while the graft is put in; depending on the location of the clogged artery, it may be possible to insert the instruments through incisions the size of large peas and avoid cracking the breastbone to get at the heart. Recovery is faster with off-pump surgery, and the outcomes are about the same for both procedures.[29]

AVOIDING OR PREPARING FOR POSSIBLE EMERGENCIES

Ask your health care provider about the cardiovascular risks you face and the preventive measures you should take. Take time to write down the answers. If she or he doesn't know, contact one of the organizations in "Resources."

Have an annual medical exam, including blood pressure measurement. Learn as much as you can about your family history and report it to your doctor. If you are a caregiver for a family member with CVD, there is a greater chance that at least some of your lifestyle risk factors are the same or similar, so you, too, may be at risk of developing CVD. Take time to care for yourself as well as others.

If you have CVD or high blood pressure, speak to your doctor or pharmacist before taking decongestants for a cold. Most over-the-counter cold medications tend to raise blood pressure. Size, sex, and race can also influence how medications affect you. If you are taking any meds, be sure to monitor the dosages. Although women are generally smaller than men, physicians often prescribe the same dose for all. The results of studies done on white men are not necessarily applicable to women or to adults of different races.

Learn the symptoms of heart attack and stroke, and review them with your provider. Share your knowledge with your family and friends. You may be able to save your life and someone else's down the road. Find out how and where to get emergency help. Plan what to do in case you think you or someone close to you is having a heart attack, and review the plan with that person. If you or someone close to you is already on medication for CVD, keep a medical history and a list of the medications where they can be readily located if needed. Denial and/or fear often accompany a heart attack, so if you suspect a problem, it's better to call for help immediately.

COLORECTAL CANCER

Cancer of the colon (large intestine) and rectum is second only to lung cancer as a cause of cancer death, killing more than fifty-seven thousand people a year. The lifetime risk of getting it is about one in eighteen, but approximately 25 percent of adults have a higher risk because of personal or family history of colorectal polyps or cancer and/or certain other diseases. Almost all colorectal cancers develop from precancerous polyps, which are common in average-risk Americans over age fifty. The incidence of colorectal cancer is greater in African-American, Hispanic, and Ashkenazi Jewish populations.

Women with a history of cancer of the ovary, uterus, or breast are at a somewhat higher risk of developing colorectal cancer. Diets high in fat (especially animal fat); low in calcium, folate, and fiber; and very low in fruits and vegetables may increase the risk of colorectal cancer. Lack of physical activity may also increase risk. If you have a chronic condition that causes inflammation of the colon (such as ulcerative colitis or Crohn's disease), your risk of developing colorectal cancer is also higher. Smokers' risk is 50 percent higher.

Hereditary nonpolyposis colon cancer (HNPCC) is the most common type of genetic colorectal cancer, but it accounts for only about 2 percent of all colorectal cancer cases. About three out of four people with an inherited mutation of the HNPCC gene develop colon cancer.

Screening tests are the most important tools for preventing and curing colorectal cancer. When screening tests find pre-cancerous polyps in the colon or rectum, the polyps can be removed before they change into cancer. Cancers found during screening can be cured in over 90 percent of cases. When to begin screening for colorectal cancer depends on your family history and other risk factors. The usual recommendation is to start at age fifty, or forty if you are at special risk.

Fecal occult blood testing (FOBT or Hemoccult), the least invasive screening test, analyzes the stools for hidden blood as an indicator of growths in the colon. This test can be done once a year. You take the stool samples yourself with a thin, flat stick that comes with the kit; put them on a special card; and mail that directly to the doctor's office.

Colonoscopy uses a fiber-optic tube with a light at the end, inserted through the entire length of the bowel, to detect the benign growths called polyps. If a polyp is found, it is removed for biopsy. This test is usually done under sedation to minimize discomfort. You have to prepare for it beforehand by drinking lots of fluids and not eating after midnight the night before. You also have to drink special fluids that clean out your bowels. Somebody will have to pick you up at the hospital, because you're likely to be groggy afterward and may even forget things that happen on the way home. Many health care providers suggest having a colonoscopy every ten years, and more frequently if your risk for colon cancer is high. This test is much more likely to find growths than the FOBT, but because it can be uncomfortable and embarrassing, many people are reluctant to have it done. A "virtual colonoscopy" with a narrower tube, aided by a CT scan, can also be done, but this newer technology may be less accurate, and if polyps are found, they must still be removed by colonoscopy.

Sigmoidoscopy uses a shorter tube to explore only the rectum and lower third of the colon. It may miss cancers in the upper portion of the colon, which are more likely to occur with age; and it is done without sedation or anesthesia, which makes it more uncomfortable than colonoscopy.

Sometimes health care providers suggest a *double-contrast barium enema* with X rays to locate polyps. After an enema with a barium solution, air is pumped into the rectum. The barium and air outline the colon and rectum on the X rays.

PREVENTION AND REDUCING RISK

Besides regular screening, a healthy diet and an active lifestyle are important in reducing individual risk of colon and rectal cancer. High-fiber foods are still recommended, though studies haven't proved they actually prevent colon cancer. Reducing the amount of fat in your diet, especially animal fat, and cutting down on carbs also reduces colon cancer risk. Getting more calcium, drinking tea (especially green tea) regularly, and taking low-dose aspirin or ibuprofen may also be protective. Heavy alcohol use has been linked to colorectal cancer, especially in combination with smoking. Quitting smoking and limiting drinks to one a day are important risk reducers.

Regular physical activity has been shown to reduce both colon and breast cancer risk, independent of its effect on body weight. At least thirty minutes of moderate activity (such as a brisk walk) five days a week is good; forty-five minutes or more of moderate to vigorous activity is even better.

TREATMENT FOR CRC

Treatment for CRC involves surgery to remove the cancerous part of the colon and chemotherapy to keep the cancer from spreading or recurring.

DIABETES

Diabetes mellitus is a disease in which the body can't use sugar (glucose) properly. In good health, the pancreas, an organ near the stomach, makes *insulin* to help the body use and store glucose, keeping our blood sugar at normal levels. People with diabetes do not make enough insulin, can't use the insulin they make, or both.

- *Type 1 diabetes* (previously called insulin-dependent or juvenile diabetes) is caused by an autoimmune process in which the person's own immune system attacks and destroys the cells in the pancreas that produce insulin, causing a drop in insulin production that allows blood sugar to zoom out of control. It usually develops in children, but a small number of adults get it, too. It can affect people of any race or income level. Genetics may affect risk for Type 1 diabetes. Other factors, including viral infection and stress, are suspected as well, but the cause for any individual is never certain. About 5 percent of people with diabetes have this type.

- *Type 2 diabetes* (previously called adult-onset diabetes or non-insulin-dependent diabetes) is the most common form of the disease (95 percent of cases). In Type 2 diabetes, blood sugar goes up partly because tissues and organs don't react to the effects of insulin (insulin resistance) and partly because the pancreas doesn't make enough insulin. Risk factors for Type 2 diabetes are a family history of the disease, excess weight, lack of physical activity, and certain ethnicities (African-American, Asian-American, Latino, Native American, Pacific Islander).
- *Pre-diabetes* is a new term describing a tendency to have higher than normal blood sugar levels at certain times (after meals or after a set amount of glucose intake) but not yet full diabetes. Your blood sugar is normal when it's under 100 mg/dl; diabetes is defined by fasting blood sugar above 126 mg/dl on two occasions. Values between 100 and 126 suggest pre-diabetes. The 16 million Americans who have pre-diabetes are at high risk of developing Type 2 diabetes and heart attack or stroke.[30]
- *Gestational diabetes* is high blood sugar during pregnancy. Women are tested for it in weeks 26 to 28. You may be at risk for this condition if you are very overweight, have already had a baby weighing more than nine pounds at birth, or have close relatives with diabetes (family history). About 2.5 percent of pregnant women develop gestational diabetes. Women over 25 and most women of color (except Asian) in the United States are more likely to have it. Most women's blood sugar drops to normal after delivery, but women who had diabetes during pregnancy have a higher risk of developing Type 2 diabetes later in life. When women who have Type 1 diabetes get pregnant, it's not considered gestational. Controlling diabetes before pregnancy is crucial for women with Type 1, to prevent birth defects in the babies.

Symptoms

Children with Type 1 diabetes usually get very sick, with excess hunger, thirst, urination, and weight loss. Type 2 diabetes begins more slowly, with symptoms such as milder increases in thirst, urination, hunger, fatigue, skin infections, and yeast infections, but many people have no symptoms. One third of the adults with diabetes (about 5 million people in the United States) have Type 2 diabetes but don't know it.

WHO GETS DIABETES?

Obesity (see footnote on p. 674) defined as a body mass index (BMI) of 30 or above (not just being "overweight" compared to the skinny models in fashion magazines) is a risk factor for diabetes, and so is high blood pressure; both are part of a metabolic syndrome that's just starting to be understood. African-American, Hispanic, and Native American teenagers appear to be at greater risk of developing diabetes and heart disease from being overweight than white teens. In the United States, African-Americans, Mexican-Americans, Native Americans, and Alaska Natives are about twice as likely to develop diabetes as white adults. Men and women have similar rates of diabetes except among African-Americans (more black women than black men have it). People with lower incomes or less education and African-American women are more likely to develop diabetes than affluent, more educated white people, most likely because of less access to healthy foods, exercise facilities, information, and health insurance coverage. About 19 percent of people over age sixty have diabetes— you're more likely to get it as you get older.

DIABETES SCREENING

Screening can detect diabetes before it has progressed and may prevent complications. Because

diabetes is common and the symptoms may be subtle, screening is now recommended for people at high risk. The simplest screening test measures blood glucose from a sample drawn after fasting overnight *(fasting blood glucose)*. Blood tests after you fast overnight and then drink a measured amount of sugar can also be used *(oral glucose tolerance test)*. Measuring a chemical called *glycolysated hemoglobin* (HbAlc) can indicate how high your average blood sugar has been in the last three months. This is important because the risks from diabetes are related to overall exposure to high blood sugar, not just blood sugar level at any given moment.

PREVENTING DIABETES AND ITS COMPLICATIONS

Common complications of diabetes are kidney disease *(nephropathy)*, early heart attacks *(my-ocardial infarction)*, nerve injury *(neuropathy)*, blindness *(retinopathy)*, and amputations. Complications are more common when blood sugar levels and blood pressure are not controlled. To prevent and control diabetes, we need to change how we live. Access to healthy food, exercise, and medical care all affect how well a woman with diabetes can take care of herself. Diabetes poses a particular challenge for women because of the connection between diabetes and obesity. If we are heavy, we may already have plenty of experiences struggling with diets and exercise. There is much evidence that dieting to lose weight is ineffective: Under 5 percent of all dieters succeed in losing a significant amount of weight and maintaining that weight loss over a five-year period.[31] Rather than trying to lose weight, try choosing healthy foods and getting regular exercise. Eating well and exercising—along with not smoking—are the most important things you

- Age over 45
- First-degree relative (mother/father/sibling) with diabetes
- African-American, Latino, Native-American, Pacific Islander, Asian-American
- History of diabetes in pregnancy, or baby weighing over 9 pounds
- High blood pressure (hypertension)
- High cholesterol (hyperlipidemia)
- Obesity
- Polycystic ovarian syndrome (PCOS)
- History of impaired glucose tolerance or impaired fasting glucose
- History of vascular disease (disease affecting the arteries)
- Being in weeks 24 to 28 of pregnancy and either being over 25 or having other risk factors for diabetes

can do to prevent the onset of diabetes, slow it down, and limit its complications.

Food

The average American diet—with its large portions, high calories, too much sugar and salt, and trans fats—is part of the reason for the increase in diabetes. Eating well requires both information about what to eat and access to healthy food, such as fresh fruits and vegetables. If you can't get to a farmer's market or a supermarket, and you buy most foods at corner stores, your choices will be more limited. Also, a better diet costs more—low-fat sources of protein, fresh fruit, and vegetables are more expensive than hamburgers and canned foods, and milk costs more than soda.

Another problem is our relationship to food.

In many families, cooking and shopping remain women's work. If we put our family's preferences above our own health, we may end up cooking food that is popular but unhealthy, just to make others happy. Or we may try to cook the proper foods for our own or a family member's health, then find we can't control how others eat. And if food is a "reward" or a source of comfort for us, the idea of taking care of ourselves by restricting what we can eat may feel like a contradiction. On the other hand, when we make changes in our own diet to prevent or control diabetes, we can also reduce the risk of diabetes among others by switching the whole family to a healthier diet. Changing your diet can reverse or reduce the risks that go with diabetes, including obesity, high blood pressure, and high cholesterol.

The recommended diet in diabetes is a balance of complex carbohydrates (which break down into sugars), protein, and fat, with an emphasis on high fiber, less fat, and less salt. If you have diabetes, working with a nutritionist can help you understand how different foods affect your blood sugar so that you can develop a diet plan that works best for you. (For more about healthy eating, see Chapter 2, "Eating Well.")

Exercise

Exercise helps the body use insulin and decreases how much insulin the body needs. It can reverse pre-diabetes and is important in controlling blood sugar once diabetes has set in. Yet women are less likely to exercise for fun than men.[32] Many of us have no time or no place to leave our children, and many of us work at jobs that don't involve moving our bodies at all. We may have no safe place to exercise—the streets or parks may be dangerous, and joining a women's gym or health club may be too expensive. In some communities, it might not be acceptable for women to go out for physical exercise, apart from physical labor. And some of us may not be comfortable exercising in places where others will see us. The result is that exercise may be inaccessible, uncomfortable, or foreign to exactly those women who need it most—overweight women at risk of diabetes or already diabetic.

We need safe, comfortable ways to get exercise that fits into our lives. Just cutting back television watching to under ten hours a week and doing some more active things instead can reduce a woman's risk of diabetes, but we usually need support from others to make such changes. Finding one or two friends or family members to exercise with you can be a first step.

Moderate activity that involves sweating for thirty minutes, five days a week, slows the progression of Type 2 diabetes and helps prevent heart disease (see Chapter 4, "Our Bodies in Motion," and "Cardiovascular Problems" on p. 671). If you already have diabetes, talk to your doctor before starting an exercise program.

Smoking

Smoking speeds up the blood vessel damage that causes complications of diabetes, such as kidney disease, vision loss, and blindness. Smoking also increases the already high risk for heart attack, stroke, amputation, and death among people with diabetes. Quitting smoking is the best thing you can do for your overall health, especially if you already have diabetes (see Chapter 3, "Alcohol, Tobacco, and Other Mood-Altering Drugs").

PRE-DIABETES TREATMENT

Pre-diabetes can sometimes be reversed. Following a heart-healthy diet and exercising consistently for at least thirty minutes, five days a week, cuts the risk of diabetes in half within three years. In pre-diabetes, the early use of one medication, *metformin*, has been shown to prevent full diabetes from developing. As with diabetes itself, older people and people of color are more likely to have pre-diabetes.

MEDICAL TREATMENT FOR DIABETES

When diet and exercise are not enough to control blood sugar, medications become necessary; most people with diabetes take several. Some increase how much insulin the pancreas makes, while others help the body use insulin better. In addition, you may need to take medication to control your blood sugar, blood pressure, and cholesterol levels.

Insulin is absolutely necessary for people with Type 1 diabetes. It may be the best treatment (after diet) for gestational (pregnancy) diabetes, and it often becomes necessary in Type 2 diabetes as well. Metformin is helpful in opposing the insulin resistance of PCOS and pre-diabetes and can delay the development of diabetes in people with metabolic syndrome. It is not, however, as effective as exercise. People treated with insulin need to keep track of what we eat, watch how much we exercise, and carefully test our blood to avoid high and low blood sugar. Tight control of blood sugar helps prevent the long-term complications of blindness, kidney failure, and nerve damage in both Type 1 and Type 2 diabetes.

Some of these medications can be combined, but as diabetes progresses, it may not be possible to control blood sugar with just oral medications. Not everyone can take medications of every type. You will need to work with your diabetes team, including a pharmacist, to make sure which medications are safe for you. Ask your pharmacist to review your medicines with you every time you have a question or pick up a prescription.

At this point, you will probably need to begin checking your own blood sugar, using a test kit to take blood samples, and to learn the symptoms of a hypoglycemic (low blood sugar) at-

BLOOD SUGAR CONTROL

TYPE, DRUGS	HOW TAKEN	WHAT THEY DO	RISKS AND SIDE EFFECTS
Sulfonylureas: **glipizide,** **glyburide,** **glimepiride**	Pills	Increase insulin made by pancreas	Low blood sugar (hypoglycemia)
Metformin, **glitazones**	Pills	Help muscles use insulin better, keep liver from releasing sugar	Metformin–diarrhea, nausea, vomiting; cannot use if you have liver or kidney disease Glitazones–leg swelling, liver damage, worse heart disease
Acarbose	Pills	Keeps sugar from being absorbed by intestine	Abdominal pain, diarrhea, gas
Insulin	Daily injections or pump	Controls blood sugar	Severe hypoglycemia (test blood several times a day)
Secretagogues: **nateglinide,** **repaglinide**	Pills	Stimulate insulin release by pancreas	Low blood sugar (hypoglycemia)

tack. You may feel sweaty, shaky, hungry, and unable to concentrate. Keeping juice or hard candy with you at all times lets you manage these episodes yourself. Educating family and friends can be lifesaving, because an attack can lead to coma. A Glucagon kit can help family members treat your low blood sugar if you are too confused or sleepy to treat yourself. Wearing a Medic Alert bracelet (available at drugstores) lets people know in an emergency that you have diabetes.

Blood Pressure Control

People with diabetes need to keep blood pressure below 130/80 to reduce the risk of cardiovascular (heart and blood vessels) disease, particularly heart attack and stroke but also poor circulation that can lead to gangrene and, as a result, amputation. These complications can shorten your life. Once you have both diabetes and high blood pressure, blood pressure control has more effect on how long you live than control of blood sugar alone. Drugs called ACE-Is *(angiotensin converting enzyme inhibitors)* and ARBs *(angiotensin receptor blockers)* are often preferred for people with diabetes, because these medications can protect the kidney from further damage. It may take more than one medication to get your blood pressure reliably below 130/80. Sometimes blood pressure tests higher at a doctor's office than at home ("white-coat hypertension"), so checking your blood pressure at home or elsewhere can tell you whether it is under control between visits to your medical provider. Checking your own blood pressure is another way to take more control over your diabetes and over your health in general (see "Hypertension" on p. 671).

For those who are not allergic to it, aspirin is used to prevent heart attacks and strokes by thinning the blood. Because people with diabetes are at such high risk of these complications, doctors now put everyone with diabetes on aspirin unless there's a clear reason not to.

Cholesterol Lowering

The levels of cholesterol and several other fats (lipids) in the blood appear to be related to risk of heart disease, which is the most common cause of death among people with diabetes. The American Diabetes Association (ADA) now recommends keeping low-density lipoprotein (LDL, or "bad" cholesterol)—the type most closely associated with complications—under 100. People who do not have a physically strenuous life do not usually have LDL below 100. Statin drugs, the most effective option for rapidly lowering cholesterol and reducing the risk of a heart attack, are usually prescribed for most people with diabetes, to reduce LDL below 100.

Taking Medication

It may be hard to accept the idea that you need medications for something that you can't feel, like cholesterol or blood pressure, especially if you never previously needed to take any medicine at all. Because these drugs are also expensive, and drug companies make high profits on them, some people wonder whether we really need all those pills. Your doctor and pharmacist can help you understand what each medicine does and why it's important to your health. Ask whether any are optional, and whether less expensive versions are available and effective. Many of these medications have relatively rare serious side effects and require blood tests sev-

eral times a year to assure their continued safety for you.

Taking Control

It is important to understand how your body is affected by what you eat, what activities you do, and what medicines you take, so you can have as much control as possible of your diabetes. With today's technology, you can measure your own blood sugar regularly. Your physical sensations don't always tell you accurately whether blood sugar is high or low, so checking perceived symptoms with a glucometer gives you reliable information. You can monitor your own blood pressure, too. You can learn how stress, lack of sleep, and illness work on your body, as well as the healthful effects of exercise, meal spacing (when and how often you eat), meditation, or play. You may need to search until you find health care providers who will help you take charge of your own condition and make resources and information available.

WORKING WITH YOUR HEALTH CARE PROVIDER

Good control of diabetes requires a collaborative relationship with your health care provider and a team of people who are knowledgeable about the condition, often including a certified diabetes educator, a diabetes nurse, a nutritionist, and a pharmacist. You're the expert on your own body. This team will support you in maintaining the best diet and exercise plan for you, review your medications, and monitor you for possible complications.

Your practitioner should do a complete examination every year, including your heart, circulation, and nervous system. Once diabetes is diagnosed, you should also have a dilated exam of your eyes yearly, to look for any complications on your retina. Be sure to check your feet every day for skin breaks and infection; your doctor should examine your feet at every visit and perform a special test for sensation (filament testing) once a year. Many people with diabetes will need to be seen by a podiatrist for foot care. Your team should review your home glucose testing and suggest how to optimize your blood sugar results. Input from a pharmacy educator can help you manage all the medications you're taking for blood pressure, diabetes, cholesterol, and any other medical problems you may have.

MULTIPLE CHEMICAL SENSITIVITIES

As the environments in which we live and work have become more polluted, increasing numbers of people report developing a condition referred to as *multiple chemical sensitivity* or *multiple chemical sensitivities* (MCS); other terms for MCS include *environmental illness* and *chemical intolerance*. MCS is almost always expressed as symptoms that wax and wane—depending on current environmental exposure—typically affecting multiple organ systems (for example, respiratory, neurological, cardiovascular, musculoskeletal, immune, and digestive), either simultaneously or sequentially, in a particular person. Health care practitioners are beginning to recognize that MCS is a real physiological problem, although much remains to be learned about its various causes and treatments.

There has been insufficient scientifically sound research on this perplexing condition. Nevertheless, evidence from around the globe suggests that a wide variety of chemical exposures, including indoor and outdoor air pollutants, as well as a severe viral illness, can make those of us who are susceptible feel sick. Subsequently, we find that we can no longer tolerate everyday substances—those that don't bother most people and never bothered us before. Over time, our sensitivities seem to spread to common cleaning and remodeling products, foods, medications, alcoholic beverages, and caffeine, a process that has been called *toxicant-induced loss of tolerance,* or TILT.[33] Most of us suffer from long-term disabilities and lead restricted lives.

Once the condition develops, symptoms may be triggered by a wide variety of everyday exposures, including: pesticides, mothballs, and air fresheners; new construction and renovation materials, such as carpeting, plastics, fresh paint, particleboard, formaldehyde, and adhesives; release of chemicals from office equipment and supplies such as correction fluid, felt-tip markers, new computers, printers, and photocopy toners; incomplete combustion products from fuels such as gasoline, oil, and wood; scented cleaning and laundry products; fabric softeners; cosmetics containing fragrances; and hair spray, nail polish, and nail polish remover. These toxicants are ubiquitous, present in most indoor environments, where 90 percent of Americans spend 90 percent of each day. Different individuals describe being affected in different ways and to a different degree, depending upon genetic makeup and the extent to which we have been exposed to harmful substances in the past.

It appears that MCS is not simply an allergic response. Common symptoms include irritated eyes, nose, and throat; respiratory difficulties; fast or irregular heartbeat; digestive disturbances and adverse food reactions; joint pain; incapacitating exhaustion; drowsiness; headaches; dizziness; disorientation; impaired concentration and memory; and seizures. Hormonal differences may explain why more women than men report suffering from MCS, although both sexes are affected. Also, women and children may be more vulnerable to toxic exposures because of lower body weight or a higher proportion of body fat (certain toxic chemicals accumulate in fat).

Most health care providers know little about

MCS and may not yet recognize it as a legitimate physical illness. Hence, troubling multi-organ symptoms may go undiagnosed, and patients may be referred to psychiatrists as a last resort. It is important for health care providers to remain open-minded and respectful of a patient's ability to cope, and to offer healthier alternatives. Just because a woman reports so-called psychological symptoms—such as fatigue, depression, irritability, anxiety, or cognitive difficulties—does not mean that these symptoms are caused by her mind and emotions.

At the present time, no laboratory test is available for clearly diagnosing MCS, and there is no generally agreed-upon case definition used by doctors or researchers. However, those of us who suffer from MCS feel far different than we did before the toxic exposure—usually hyperreactive to substances we might ingest, breathe, or touch, often with the following response pattern: cognitive changes (sometimes experienced as "brain fog," brain fatigue, or a feeling of being drunk or spacey); heightened senses of taste and smell that trigger adverse reactions; irritation or burning of the mucous membranes of the eyes, nose, and throat; swelling or inflammation of tissue; and being hypersensitive to physical agents, such as light, sound, and touch.

Avoiding chemicals that trigger adverse reactions is the first line of defense for chemically sensitive individuals. Lifestyle changes (for example, moving to a different home or job, changing heating systems, or removing carpeting) can reduce exposure and lead to improved health and regaining of tolerance. On the other hand, these interventions can be costly and may not always have the desired effect. MCS can be draining physically, emotionally, and financially for all of us who experience it or are close to someone who has it. Both professional and self-help groups may serve as good sources of support and information (see "Resources").

Studies worldwide suggest that the number of people who report chemical intolerances is large—about 15 percent in the United States[34]—making this potentially one of the most prevalent environmentally induced illnesses. The problem appears to have grown rapidly since World War II, as exposures to synthetic chemicals have increased. New construction practices since the mid-1970s have led to tightly enclosed, energy-efficient homes, schools, and other buildings containing new materials that off-gas low levels of chemicals without sufficient dilution from outside (fresh) air. Reducing our exposures to toxic chemicals may well be the best way

COPING WITH MCS: WHAT HELPS

- Using water filters
- Avoiding plastic packaging and nonstick surfaces on pots and pans
- Eating organic foods to avoid the chemicals used in conventional agriculture
- Exercise and nutritional supplements
- Avoiding scented personal care and household cleaning products
- Asking friends to avoid scented products when we are around; some people with MCS are sensitive to cosmetic and personal care products even if used a day earlier
- Avoiding fabric softener, bleach, static removers, and gas dryers
- Reducing sources of mold, dust, animal dander, and mites (using air filters will help)
- Trying alternatives to sunblock and insect repellents
- Airing out new items for a while before wearing or installing them
- Using certain natural fibers rather than synthetics for clothes and home furnishings

to reverse the rise of MCS. This will require widespread education of health care providers and the public; major political and grassroots efforts; and enormous shifts in personal, community, and industry practices regarding chemical use—changes that involve every sphere of our lives.

SURGERY

Surgical operations may be performed by a surgeon, by a physician trained primarily as a surgeon (for example, a gynecologist), or by one who has special training in selected procedures. For example, some family practice physicians are trained to do cesarean sections or appendectomies. Two important predictors of any given doctor's competence are the number of procedures she or he has performed, and how frequently he or she currently performs them.

Because a great deal of unnecessary surgery has been performed on women, be careful when agreeing to an operation. In some regions, especially where there are many surgeons, unnecessary surgery continues to be a problem. The surgical mentality ("When in doubt, cut it out") still prevails in some places, so try to learn as much as you can about when surgery is and isn't necessary. Managed care programs generally have reduced the numbers of operations performed, in contrast to the fast-disappearing "fee-for-service" insurance plans, which gave doctors incentives to do more rather than less. Before giving your consent to surgery, you may want to take the following steps:

1. *Get a second or even third opinion,* preferably from a physician in a different specialty or one who is not one of your doctor's close colleagues. (Many insurance policies and BlueCross BlueShield programs will pay for the second opinion.) Try to find a doctor who is interested in helping you avoid surgery when possible. Internists may suggest nonsurgical (sometimes called *conservative*) alternatives not offered by obstetricians, gynecologists, and general surgeons. (See also "Our Rights as Patients," p. 702 in Chapter 30, "Navigating the Health Care System.")

2. *Ask whether research has shown improved outcomes* for the procedure in your case. For example, careful studies have shown that much coronary bypass surgery is futile and sometimes even shortens life; yet the popularity of this procedure is constantly increasing (see "Cardiovascular Problems," p. 671).

3. *Ask about potential risks and negative effects* of the surgical procedure. Ask how likely they are to occur in your case.

4. *Investigate other treatments,* medical and nonmedical, that you could try before or instead of surgery, in a self-help group or on your own.

5. *Ask how widely the procedure has been performed,* where, and on how many people; check with your insurer to see if it is known and reimbursable. Because there is no regulatory or legal authority anywhere that controls surgery, new experimental procedures are constantly being launched without adequate testing and evaluation.

6. *Ask about mortality (death) and morbidity (injury) rates* at the institution where the procedure will be performed (call your state department of public health). Some hospitals have more careful criteria and much better outcomes than others for certain procedures.

7. *Carefully investigate the training and affiliations of the surgeon* you are considering. Ask how often she or he performs the proposed procedure.

8. *Ask whether you can avoid* general anesthesia (a major risk of most surgical procedures) and hospitalization (a major source of postoperative infections) by having the surgery done as an outpatient or office procedure.

9. *Talk all this over* with your family and trusted friends.

10. *Take the time you need* to make a careful decision.

ANESTHESIA

Anesthesia can pose a greater risk than the surgical procedure itself. It is just as important to understand the type of anesthesia you will be getting as the type of surgery. Anesthesia capability varies from hospital to hospital as well as from one anesthesiologist or anesthetist to another, and not all facilities offer a choice.

Before surgery, you should be interviewed by the practitioner who will be administering the anesthesia. Be sure to ask:

- What type of anesthesia will be given
- Why she or he chose this type or combination
- How it will be given
- What are the possible risks and benefits of this type of anesthesia compared with others
- How you can expect to feel after the surgery

Be sure to tell the anesthesiologist about any allergies to medication, prior anesthesia reactions, and medications you're taking, and inform her or him about your past and current health.

Anesthesia works by blocking pain. There are three types: *general,* in which you are unconscious; *regional* or *conduction* (including spinal and epidural), in which you are awake but numb in a specific region, usually the lower half (or a zone) of your body; and *local,* in which you are awake and only the area being operated on is numbed. General anesthesia makes you unaware of pain by working on the part of the brain that recognizes pain. Conduction and local anesthesia block the signals sent to the spinal cord and brain from the area that is anesthetized. Another option for certain procedures is IV conscious sedation, where short-acting pain relievers and muscle relaxants are given intravenously (by needle, into a vein). Most types of anesthesia are administered after you get medication to help you relax, which makes the procedure easier for both you and the anesthesiologist.

General anesthesia is given intravenously, by inhalation, or a combination of both. Before intravenous anesthesia, you will probably get sodium pentothal to induce a condition resembling deep sleep.* Inhalation anesthesia is a gas going directly into the lungs via a tube inserted down your throat. You may experience nausea, confusion, or dizziness for several hours or days after general anesthesia. Rarely (about once in ten to twenty thousand cases), death or paralysis occurs as a direct result of general anesthesia.

Spinal anesthesia is injected into the spinal canal through the membrane that covers the spinal cord. It is most often used for surgery within the abdominal cavity. You will feel numb in the legs, in the pelvis, and possibly higher, depending on the operation. Anesthetic effects from spinals may last longer than those from general anesthesia. About one woman in twenty gets a post-op headache that may last for several days. Lying flat on your back for eight to sixteen hours after surgery, without lifting your head, may help relieve your symptoms.

Epidural or *caudal anesthesia,* frequently used in childbirth and sometimes for rectal and genital surgery, is injected continuously into the space near the base of the spinal column but

---

* However, you are not truly asleep, and you may hear or even remember conversations of those around you.

not into the canal itself. It works by bathing the nerve endings leading to large areas of the body with anesthetic solution. Always ask whether regional rather than general anesthesia is possible in your case, especially if you have respiratory problems. (For more information, see "Epidural Analgesia," p. 466.)

In *local anesthesia,* a solution or jelly that numbs the nerve endings is applied to the mucous membranes, followed by an injection that blocks specific nerves (such as lidocaine for dental work).

Before and after surgery, it's helpful to eat a diet high in protein, vitamins, and minerals to replenish the nutrients your body loses during the operation. You may also want to take supplements of vitamins A, B, C, and D as well as zinc and iron. Certain mind-body (relaxation and visualization) techniques may help you prepare for surgery and possibly lose less blood, use less pain medication, and heal faster.

TRICHOTILLOMANIA

Primarily a disorder of women, trichotillomania (TTM) is characterized by an overwhelming compulsion to pull out one's hair, most notably from the scalp, but also from the eyebrows, eyelashes, beard, pubic area, and elsewhere. It is classified as an impulse control disorder.[35] Current estimates indicate that 3.4 percent of all women will engage in clinically significant hairpulling at some point in our lives. TTM usually begins at about the age of twelve or thirteen, sometimes in conjunction with a traumatic event. Two common patterns of TTM include binge hair-pulling and more trancelike pulling when sedentary, such as when reading or watching television. TTM may result in scarring or permanent hair loss; it can involve eating the hair as well, resulting in a blocked intestinal tract that requires surgery.

The origins of TTM remain unknown. Although there are no definitive treatments, one or more of the following may be helpful: medications, cognitive-behavioral therapies, support groups, and alternative therapies such as acupuncture and acupressure. Women who develop TTM often function well in society, even while the secret hair-pulling continues to be a source of shame and embarrassment. Such shame and a fear of stigmatization may contribute to a reluctance to seek health care. Resources such as the Trichotillomania Learning Center (www.trich .org or 831-457-1004) are helping women cope more successfully with this disorder.

URINARY CONDITIONS

INTERSTITIAL CYSTITIS

Interstitial cystitis (IC) is a painful and debilitating inflammatory condition of the bladder wall that affects approximately 450,000 people in the United States, 90 percent of whom are women. It occurs in women of all ages, not only after menopause. The average age of onset is approximately forty, and 25 percent of women who have it are under thirty.

IC has symptoms similar to those of the common urinary tract infection known as cystitis. However, with IC, routine urine cultures come up negative, and there is usually no response to antibiotics. You may feel pelvic pain and pressure and an urgent need to urinate, sometimes as often as sixty to eighty times a day. You may also have vaginal and rectal pain. Pain during sexual intercourse is common. The symptoms can vary from mild to severe.

IC may be incorrectly diagnosed as urethral syndrome or *trigonitis,* or you may be told there's nothing wrong and that you have a "sensitive bladder." A complete battery of urologic tests typically produces negative results. Conditions that have similar symptoms include bladder infections, kidney problems, vaginal infections, endometriosis, and STIs. If you don't have an infection (urine cultures are negative) and no other disorder is identified, you should have a cystoscopy (an examination using an instrument inserted through the urethra, which allows the urologist to look directly inside the bladder). You'll get regional or general anesthesia for this procedure. A specimen is taken for biopsy to rule out bladder cancer.

There is no consistently effective treatment or cure for IC. However, the most commonly used remedies that may relieve symptoms are:

1. *Bladder distention,* stretching the bladder by filling it with water while you are under regional or general anesthesia.
2. *Pills,* including nonsteroidal anti-inflammatory drugs, antispasmodics, and antihistamines.
3. *Antidepressants,* which appear to have anti-pain properties.
4. *Diet,* eliminating caffeinated beverages, alcohol, artificial sweeteners, spicy foods, citrus fruits, and tomatoes.
5. *Dimethyl sulfoxide* (DMSO, Rimso-50), an anti-inflammatory medication instilled directly into the bladder.
6. *Sodium pentosan polysulfate* (Elmiron), an oral medication that protects the bladder from irritants in the urine.
7. *Oxychlorosene sodium* (Clorpactin), placed directly into the bladder; regional or general anesthesia may be necessary for this.
8. *Transcutaneous electrical nerve stimulation* (TENS) to block pain, using a small portable unit worn on the body.
9. *Surgery* (partial or complete removal of the bladder, or of certain nerves leading to the bladder). Surgery poses a substantial risk of complications and should be done only as a last resort.

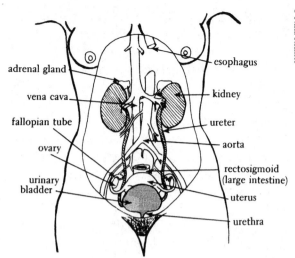

© Nina Reimer

The Interstitial Cystitis Association (ICA), a patient advocacy group, provides information, education, and support to people with IC and our families. It also raises funds for research (see "Resources").

URINARY TRACT INFECTIONS

Urinary tract infections (UTIs) are so common that most of us get at least one at some point in our lives. They are usually caused by bacteria, such as *E. coli,* that get into the urethra and bladder (and occasionally the kidneys) from the colon. Trichomoniasis and chlamydia can also cause UTIs. Low resistance, poor diet, stress, and damage to the urethra from childbirth, surgery, catheterization, and so on can predispose you to getting them. A sudden increase in sexual activity can trigger symptoms ("honeymoon cystitis"). Pregnant women are especially susceptible, as pressure of the growing fetus keeps some urine in the bladder and ureters (the tubes carrying urine from the kidneys to the bladder), allowing bacteria to grow.

Postmenopausal women are also susceptible because of hormonal changes. Occasionally, UTIs are caused by a congenital anatomical abnormality or a prolapsed (fallen) urethra or bladder, mostly in older women or women who have had many children.

Cystitis (inflammation or infection of the bladder) is by far the most common UTI in women. While the symptoms can be frightening, cystitis in itself is not usually serious. If you suddenly have to urinate every few minutes and it burns like crazy even though almost nothing comes out, you probably have cystitis. There may also be blood and/or pus in the urine. You may have pain just above your pubic bone, and sometimes there is a peculiar, heavy odor when you first urinate in the morning.

It's also possible to get mild temporary symptoms (such as peeing frequently) without actually having an infection, simply because of drinking too much coffee or tea (both are diuretics), premenstrual syndrome, food allergies, vaginitis, anxiety, or irritation to the area from bubble baths, soaps, or douches. As long as you are in good health and not pregnant, you can usually treat mild symptoms yourself for twenty-four hours before consulting a practitioner.

Cystitis often disappears without treatment. If it persists over forty-eight hours, recurs frequently, or is ever accompanied by chills, fever, vomiting, or pain in the kidneys (near the middle of the back), see a doctor. These symptoms suggest that infection has spread to the kidneys, resulting in *pyelonephritis,* a serious problem that requires medical treatment. Also see your provider if you have blood or pus in the urine; pain on urination during pregnancy; diabetes or chronic illness; or a history of kidney infection or diseases or abnormalities of the urinary tract. Untreated chronic infections can lead to serious complications, such as high blood pressure, or premature births (if they occur during pregnancy).

Diagnosis

When cystitis does not respond to self-help treatments within twenty-four hours or it recurs frequently, get a urine test. Make sure your provider takes a clean voided specimen* and does a pelvic exam to rule out other infections. Your urine should be examined for evidence of blood and pus, then cultured. Sometimes, even when you have symptoms, the culture may come back negative (not show a cause of the infection). False-negative cultures may be due to mishandling or too-dilute urine; you may also get a false-negative report if your cystitis is caused by something other than bacterial infection. White blood cells in the urine plus a negative culture (acute urethral syndrome) may indicate a chlamydia infection (see Chapter 15, "Sexually Transmitted Infections"). Some women have bacteria in the urine without symptoms; especially in pregnant women, this should be treated with antibiotics to prevent kidney infection and other complications.

Treatments

For symptoms that are severe or indicate a kidney infection, medications are usually started immediately. For milder infections, many health care providers prefer to wait for culture results before prescribing a drug.

Most UTIs respond rapidly to a variety of antibiotics. Drugs commonly used include antibiotics such as ampicillin, nitrofurantoin, tetracycline, sulfonamides (Gantrisin), or Bactrim. (Women who have a deficiency of glucose-6-phosphate dehydrogenase should not take sulfonamides; see "Hereditary and Other Types of Anemia," p. 660.) You may get a single large dose or several spread out over three to ten days. If

---

* Wash the area carefully, urinate a little, then collect the rest of your urine in a sterile jar.

PREVENTING UTIS AND AVOIDING REINFECTION

1. *Drink lots of fluids every day.* Try to drink a glass of water every two or three hours. For an active infection, drink enough so you can pour out a good stream of urine every hour. It really helps.

2. *Urinate frequently* and try to empty your bladder completely each time. Never try to hold your urine once your bladder feels full.

3. *Wipe from front to back* after urinating or having a bowel movement, to keep the bacteria in your bowels and anus away from your urethra. Wash your genitals from front to back with plain water or very mild soap at least once a day.

4. *Wash your hands and genitals before sex,* and after contact with the anal area before touching the vagina or urethra. That goes for your partner(s), too. Any sexual activity that irritates the urethra, puts pressure on the bladder, or spreads bacteria from the anus to the vagina or urethra can contribute to cystitis. *To prevent irritation, avoid pressure* on the urethral area or prolonged direct clitoral stimulation during sex or masturbation. Make sure your vagina is well lubricated before penetration of any kind. Rear-entry positions and prolonged vigorous intercourse tend to put additional stress on the urethra and bladder. Emptying your bladder before and immediately after sex is a good idea; so is having a glass of water. If you tend to get cystitis after sex despite these precautions, you may want to ask your medical practitioner for preventive drugs (sulfa, ampicillin, nitrofurantoin); a single tablet after sex can prevent infections and usually doesn't have the same negative effects as taking antibiotics for a longer time.

5. *Try changing your birth control method.* Women taking oral contraceptives have a higher rate of cystitis than those who don't take them. Some diaphragm users find that the rim pressing against the urethra can contribute to infection. (A different-size diaphragm or one with a different rim may solve this problem.) Contraceptive foams or vaginal suppositories may irritate the urethra. Dry condoms may put pressure on the urethra, or the dyes or lubricants may cause irritation.

6. *Change sanitary napkins often,* because the blood on the pad provides a bridge for bacteria from your anus to your urethra. Wash your genitals twice a day during your period. Some women also find that tampons or sponges put pressure on the urethra.

7. *Wear loose clothing and drink extra water when doing sports.* Tight jeans, bicycling, or horseback riding may cause trauma to the urethra.

8. *Drink less or no caffeine and alcohol*—both irritate the bladder. Drink enough water to dilute them if you use them.

9. *Acidify your urine.* Some women find that unsweetened cranberry juice, cranberry concentrate supplements, or vitamin C every day makes urine more acidic and helps prevent UTIs. The hippuric acid in cranberry juice also helps prevent bacteria from sticking to the bladder lining (mucosa). If you have an infection, try combining 500 milligrams of vitamin C with cranberry juice four times a day; or have half a cup of fresh cranberries in plain, live-culture yogurt instead. Whole grains, meats, nuts, and many fruits also help to acidify the urine. Avoid strong spices such as curry, cayenne, chili, and black pepper.

10. *Avoid refined (white) sugars and starches* (white flour, white rice, ordinary pasta)—they may facilitate urinary tract infections by feeding bacteria.

11. *Herbal remedies* are widely used for UTIs. Drinking teas made of uva ursi, horsetail or shavegrass, barberry, echinacea, cornsilk, cleavers, lemon balm, or goldenseal may be beneficial to the bladder. You may want to consult an herbalist about them.

12. *Keep up your resistance* by eating and resting well and by finding ways to reduce stress in your life as much as possible.

13. *Vitamin B$_6$ and magnesium-calcium* supplements help to relieve spasm of the urethra that can predispose you to cystitis.

symptoms persist longer than two days after you start taking drugs, see your health care provider again. The organisms you have may be resistant to the antibiotics you are using. Eating plain, unsweetened, live-culture yogurt or taking acidophilus in capsule, liquid, or granule form may help to prevent diarrhea or yeast infection by replacing the normal bacteria in your intestines that were killed by the drugs.

Acetaminophen may relieve pain from UTIs. Some practitioners recommend a prescription drug called Pyridium, a local anesthetic that relieves pain but does not treat the infection itself. (Pyridium dyes the urine a bright orange, which will permanently stain clothing. It also can cause nausea, dizziness, and possibly allergic reactions.)

Surgery is often recommended to correct a prolapsed bladder or urethra, which can be connected with chronic UTIs. Kegel exercises (see p. 235 in Chapter 13, "Sexual Anatomy, Reproduction, and the Menstrual Cycle"), can forestall the need for this operation and help prevent future infections. Your doctor may recommend other surgical procedures, such as stretching the urethral opening and/or making a slit in the urethra to help drainage (internal urethrotomy). Ask for documentation showing how effective these procedures are.

Even with drugs and/or surgery, many women continue to have recurrent urinary tract infections. Sometimes it helps to treat chronic infections with long-term, low-dose medications.

VON WILLEBRAND DISEASE: A BLEEDING DISORDER

The underlying cause of very heavy periods may be von Willebrand disease (VWD), the world's most common inherited bleeding disorder. It's a deficiency in the amount or quality of a protein that is required for blood to clot. VWD affects about 1 percent of people of all racial and ethnic backgrounds. Both men and women can inherit it from either parent. Because of our monthly periods, VWD affects females more regularly than males, but health care providers don't always realize that is what's wrong. The bleeding can range from being simply annoying to interfering with school, work, sleep, and mood. The most common symptoms are heavy or prolonged periods, easy bruising, prolonged nosebleeds, and prolonged bleeding following surgery, injury, dentistry, and childbirth. VWD may result in miscarriage and unnecessary surgery, including D&C, uterine ablations, and hysterectomy at a young age.

VWD bleeding can be described as "oozing and bruising." Bleeding typically occurs in the mucous membranes. Other signs include gastrointestinal bleeding and bleeding into the joints and urine. Affected family members can have different bleeding patterns, as can people with the same type of VWD. Absence of bleeding does not rule out the disease. People with severe VWD have the same level of joint damage as do those with moderate hemophilia.

There is no cure for VWD, but there are effective treatments. Treatment varies according to how severe your condition is. It may include hormones, a synthetic nasal spray, or medication that is injected under the skin or infused into a vein. You may need a VWD specialist for accurate diagnosis and appropriate treatment.

The American College of Obstetricians and Gynecologists (ACOG) recommends screening all women with severe uterine bleeding for VWD. If you are told hysterectomy or endometrial ablation is required for your bleeding, get a second and even a third opinion to check the diagnosis, including one from a federally supported hemophilia treatment center, before deciding whether to have one of these procedures. (For information on federally supported U.S. hemophilia treatment centers, see "Resources.")

NOTES

1. J. M. Wright, "The Double-Edged Sword of COX-2 Selective NSAIDs," *Canadian Medical Association Journal* 167, no. 10 (November 2002): 1131–37.
2. L. Klareskog et al., "Therapeutic Effect of the Combination of Etanercept and Methotrexate Compared with Each Treatment Alone in Patients with Rheumatoid Arthritis: Double-Blind Randomized Controlled Trial," *Lancet* 363, no. 9410 (February 28, 2004): 675–81.
3. D. A. Sullivan, A. Belanger, J. M. Cermak, et al., "Are Women with Sjögren's Syndrome Androgen-Deficient?," *Journal of Rheumatology* 30, no. 11 (November 2003): 2413–19.
4. W. Reeves, Department of Health and Human Services Chronic Fatigue Syndrome Coordinating Committee meeting, Boston, October 13, 1998.
5. L. A. Jason, J. A. Richman, A. W. Rademaker, et al., "A Community-Based Study of Chronic Fatigue Syndrome," *Archives of Internal Medicine* 159, no. 18 (October 11, 1999): 2129–37.
6. O. Gureje, M. Von Koff, G. Simon, and P. Gater, "Persistent Pain and Well-Being: A World Health Organization Study in Primary Care," *Journal of the American Medical Association* 280, no. 2 (July 8, 1998): 147–51.
7. J. Burns, B. Glenn, et al., "Cognitive Factors Influence Outcome Following Multidisciplinary Chronic Pain Treatment: A Replication and Extension of a Cross-Lagged Panel Analysis," *Behavioral Research and Therapy* 41, no. 10 (October 2003): 1163–82. See also H. Picavet, J. Vlaeyen, and J. Schouten, "Pain Catastrophizing and Kinesiophobia: Predictors of Chronic Low Back Pain," *American Journal of Epidemiology* 156, no. 11 (December 1, 2002): 1028–34; R. Severeijns, et al., "Pain Catastrophizing Predicts Pain Intensity, Disability, and Psychological Distress Independent of the Level

of Physical Impairment," *Clinical Journal of Pain* 17, no. 2 (June 2001): 165–72; J. Turner, M. Jensen, et al., "Blinding Effectiveness and Association of Pretreatment Expectations with Pain Improvement in a Double-Blind Randomized Controlled Trial," *Pain* 99, no. 1–2 (September 2002): 91–99; and I. Viane, G. Crombez, et al., "Acceptance of Pain Is an Independent Predictor of Mental Well-Being in Patients with Chronic Pain: Empirical Evidence and Reappraisal," *Pain* 106, no. 1–2 (November 2003): 65–72.

8. American Chronic Pain Association, "Chronic Pain," accessed at www.acpa.org. See also American Pain Foundation, accessed at www.apf.org.

9. P. Creamer, B. Singh, et al., "Sustained Improvement Produced by Non-pharmacologic Intervention in Fibromyalgia: Results of a Pilot Study," *Arthritis Care Research* 13, no. 4 (August 2000): 198–204. See also H. Taggart et al., "Effects of T'ai Chi Exercise on Fibromyalgia Symptoms and Health-Related Quality of Life," *Orthopedic Nursing* 22, no. 5 (September–October 2003): 353–60.

10. AHA, "Facts About Women and Cardiovascular Diseases," accessed at www.americanheart.org/presenter .jhtml?identifier=2876, on December 5, 2003.

11. C. D. Naylor and P. M. Slaughter, eds., *Cardiovascular Health and Services in Ontario: An ICES Atlas* (Toronto: Institute for Clinical Evaluative Studies, 1999).

12. P. M. Slaughter and S. J. Bondy, "Differences in Access to Care," Canadian Cardiovascular Society, 2000 Consensus Conference, accessed at www.ccs.ca/society/confer ences/archives/2000/2000coneng-10.asp on November 8, 2004.

13. E. Lonn, "Epidemiology of Ischemic Heart Disease in Women," Canadian Cardiovascular Society, 2000 Consensus Conference, accessed at www.ccs.ca/society/ conferences/archives/2000/2000coneng-03.asp on November 8, 2004.

14. Canadian Women's Health Network, 2001 (updated 2003), "Women and Heart Disease," accessed at www .cwhn.ca/resources/faq/womenhd.html.

15. Health Canada, "Women and Heart Health," accessed at www.hc-sc.gc.ca/english/women/facts_issues/facts_ heart.htm on November 8, 2004.

16. CWHN, "Women and Heart Disease."

17. Centers for Disease Control and Prevention, "Heart Disease Burden," *Chronic Disease Notes and Reports* 17, no. 1 (Fall 2004): 4–7, accessed at www.cdc.gov/need php/cdnr/CDNR fall04.pdf on November 8, 2004.

18. AHA, "Facts About Women and Cardiovascular Disease."

19. B. Abramson, "Risk Factors and Primary Prevention of Ischemic Heart Disease in Women," Canadian Cardiovascular Society, 2000 Consensus Conference, accessed at www.ccs.ca/society/conferences/archives/2000/2000 coneng-04.asp on November 8, 2004.

20. AHA, "Facts About Women and Cardiovascular Diseases."

21. M. R. Buchanan and S. J. Brister, "Sex-Related Differences in the Pathophysiology of Cardiovascular Disease," Canadian Cardiovascular Society, 2000 Consensus Conference, accessed at www.ccs.ca/society/ conferences/archives/2000/2000coneng-02.asp on November 8, 2004.

22. K. A. Schulman, J. A. Berlin, W. Harless, et al., "The Effect of Race and Sex on Physicians' Recommendations for Cardiac Catheterization," *New England Journal of Medicine* 340 (February 25, 1999): 618–26.

23. S. B. Jaglal, P. M. Slaughter, R. S. Baigrie, C. D. Morgan, and C. D. Naylor, "Good Judgement or Sex Bias in the Referral of Patients for the Diagnosis of Coronary Artery Disease? An Exploratory Study," *Canadian Medical Association Journal* 152, no. 6 (March 15, 1995): 873–80.

24. L. J. Shaw, D. D. Miller, J. C. Romeis, D. Kargl, L. T. Younis, and B. R. Chaitman, "Gender Differences in Noninvasive Evaluation and Management of Patients with Suspected Coronary Artery Disease," *Annals of Internal Medicine* 120, no. 7 (April 1, 1994): 559–66.

25. D. Isaac and A. Walling, "Clinical Evaluation of Women with Ischemic Heart Disease: Diagnosis and Noninvasive Testing," Canadian Cardiovascular Society, 2000 Consensus Conference, accessed at www.ccs.ca/society/ conferences/archives/2000/2000coneng-06.asp on November 8, 2004.

26. H. Arthur, "Rehabilitation," Canadian Cardiovascular Society, 2000 Consensus Conference, accessed at www .ccs.ca/society/conferences/archives/2000/2000coneng-09.asp on November 8, 2004.

27. Heart and Stroke Foundation of Canada, "News: Women Heart Attack Survivors Can Get a 'Lift' Out of Weight Training," September 4, 2003, accessed at http:// ww2.heartandstrokeon.ca/Page.asp?PageID=740&Rec ordID=2564&Src=news&Language=English&Category ID=20&SubcategoryID=96 on November 8, 2004.

28. A. D. Michael and K. Chatterjee, "Angioplasty vs. Bypass Surgery for Coronary Artery Disease," *Circulation* 106, no. 23 (December 3, 2002): e187.

29. J. D. Puskas et al., "Off-pump vs. Conventional Coronary Artery Bypass Grafting: Early and 1-Year Graft Patency, Cost, and Quality-of-Life Outcomes," *Journal of the American Medical Association* 291, no. 15 (April 21, 2004): 1841–49. See also R. Cartier, S. Brann, F. Dagen-

nairs, R. Martineau, A. Couturier, "Systemic Off-pump Coronary Artery Revascularization in Multivessel Disease: An Experience with 300 Cases," *Journal of Thoracic and Cardiovascular Surgery* 119, no. 2 (February 2000): 221–29; J. C. Cleveland, A. L. W. Shroyer, A. Y. Chen, E. Peterson, E. L. Grover, "Off-pump Coronary Artery Bypass Grafting Decreases Risk-Adjusted Mortality and Morbidity," *Annals of Thoracic Surgery* 72, no. 4 (October 2001): 1282–89; M. E. Plomondon, J. K. Cleveland, S. T. Ludwig, et al., "Off-pump Coronary Artery Bypass Is Associated with Improved Risk-Adjusted Outcomes," *Annals of Thoracic Surgery* 72, no. 1 (July 2001): 114–19; and J. D. Puskas, V. H. Thourani, J. J. Marshall, et al., "Clinical Outcomes, Angiographic Patency and Resource Utilization in 200 Consecutive Off-pump Coronary Bypass Patients," *Annals of Thoracic Surgery* 71, no. 5 (May 2001): 1477–84.

30. B. C. Choi and F. Shi, "Risk Factors for Diabetes Mellitus by Age and Sex: Results of the National Population Health Survey," *Diabetologia,* 44, no. 10 (2001): 1221–31. See also R. B. Lipton, Y. Liao, G. Cao, R. S. Cooper, and D. McGee, "Determinants of Incident Non-Insulin-Dependent Diabetes Mellitus Among Blacks and Whites in a National Sample: The NHANES I Epidemiologic Follow-up Study," (erratum appears in *American Journal of Epidemiology* 139, no. 9 May 1, 1994) *American Journal of Epidemiology* 138, no. 10

(1993): 826–39; J. M. Robbins, V. Vaccarino, H. Zhang, and S. V. Kasl, "Socioeconomic Status and Type 2 Diabetes in African American and Non-Hispanic White Women and Men: Evidence from the Third National Health and Nutrition Examination Survery," *American Journal of Public Health* 91, no. 1 (2001): 76–83; and S. K. West, B. Munoz, R. Klein, A. T. Broman, R. Sanchez, J. Rodriguez, and R. Snyder, "Risk Factors for Type II Diabetes and Diabetic Retinopathy in a Mexican-American Population: Proyecto VER," *American Journal of Ophthalmology* 134, no. 3 (2002): 390–98.

31. See *Tufts Health and Nutrition Letter,* 22, no. 5 (July 2004) for a good discussion of diet and weight loss.

32. Centers for Disease Control and Prevention, "Prevalence of No Leisure-Time Physical Activity—35 States and the District of Columbia, 1988–2002," *Mortality and Morbidity Weekly Report* 53, no. 4 (February 6, 2004): 82–86.

33. For more information, see Nicholas Ashford and Claudia Miller, *Chemical Exposures: Low Levels and High Stakes* (New York: John Wiley and Sons, 1998).

34. National Research Council, *Multiple Chemical Sensitivities: Addendum to Biologic Markers in Immunotoxicology* (Washington, DC: National Academy Press, 1992).

35. *Diagnostic and Statistical Manual of Mental Disorders,* 4th ed. (Washington, DC: American Psychiatric Association, 2000).

Knowledge Is Power

Unlike most developed countries, the United States does not have an integrated health care system that ensures access to health care and related services for everyone. As the maze we call our health care system becomes more complex and social policies change, we must learn a great deal in order to get appropriate care, assess its quality, and advocate for change.

I, extremely well informed, well connected, verbally aggressive, have had to summon all my resources to get what I wanted in my treatment for breast cancer: medical care that was consistent with the findings of the latest literature and that took into account my needs as a woman.

This chapter provides some of the information you will need to navigate the health care system as it currently exists. As you become better informed, you are more likely to stand up for your rights, to be heard, to obtain the care you need, and to avoid abuse and harmful or unnecessary treatment. Still, there are many limits to what any one of us can do individually to get quality health care. Ultimately, the entire system needs to be reformed in major ways. Many nurses—who are the backbone of much of our health care system—and doctors are now working with lay people and nonmedical organizations to create these major reforms. (For more information, see Chapter 31, "The Politics of Women's Health.")

OUR RIGHTS AS PATIENTS

A number of specific rights protect you in your daily life and as a user of health care services. In any health care setting, your most important right is the right to control what happens to your body, including the right to decide about treatment alternatives. All competent adults have the right to refuse any treatment, even if refusing means you will likely get sicker or even die. You also have the right to privacy regarding your medical conditions and treatments.

INFORMED CONSENT AND INFORMED DECISION MAKING

The doctrine of informed consent is founded on two fundamental propositions:

- It is your body, and you should be able to decide what is done to it.
- You are likely to make a better decision about your care if you are provided with information on which to base a rational decision.

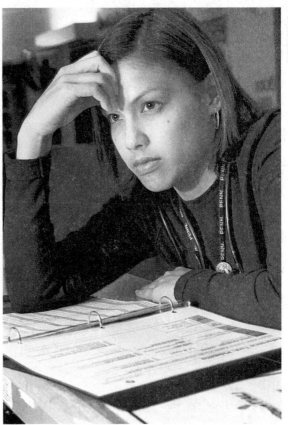

© Paula Lerner

No one can treat or even touch you until you make an informed decision to accept or reject treatment. When health care providers and patients take informed consent seriously, you can have a true partnership with your caregivers, with shared authority, decision making, and responsibility.

Providers must describe thoroughly:

- The recommended treatment or procedure
- The risks and benefits of the recommended treatment or procedure, with a special emphasis on the risk of death or serious disability
- Medically reasonable alternative treatments and procedures, together with the risks and benefits of each
- Likely results if you refuse any treatment

- Probability of success, and what the physician means by "success" (for example, will the treatment cure the condition, or will it only alleviate symptoms?)
- Major problems anticipated in recuperation, including how long it will be until you can resume your normal activities
- Any other information that patients in your situation generally receive, such as cost and how much of the cost your health plan will cover

Informed consent is a process, not just a written sheet to be signed. For consent to be informed, you must also understand all that is being explained. It is not enough for a physician or other practitioner to catalog the risks and benefits in a hasty or complicated manner, to do so when you are under the effects of medication, or to speak to you in English if it is a language you do not understand. The consent form itself can be used as evidence of consent, so do not sign it if you do not understand and agree with what is written in it. You may cross out, reword, or otherwise amend a prepared form before signing it. Insist on getting a second opinion if you have any unanswered questions about proposed treatment or surgery.

You also have a right to know if a medication is being used for a purpose not approved by the U.S. Food and Drug Administration (FDA). Check the *Physicians' Desk Reference* (found in local libraries), online sources, or the medication's package insert for the approved purposes. Because many routinely used obstetric drugs, many hormonal preparations, and some psychiatric drugs are given for purposes not specifically FDA-approved, it is especially important for women to ask about such off-label use.

Informed consent is particularly important when the treatment offered is part of a clinical trial or research program. In research settings, where you may be given an unproven or experimental drug or other therapy, practitioners must follow federal regulations that govern such research. The researcher must give you a copy of any informed consent form that you sign, as well as the name of a person who can provide you with additional information. You are *never* obligated to participate in research. Even if you decide to, you can change your mind at any time.

If the research project that you are asked to participate in includes diagnostic tests, it is important to ask whether the institution conducting the study will provide and pay for treatment for conditions that may be found by the tests.

SOURCES OF HEALTH INFORMATION

In order to exercise your right of informed consent, you need accurate information about your body and the health care system. To begin with, it is important to listen to and trust what your body tells you. Changes in yourself and those you care for are often the first and most important indicators of illness. Health care providers are likely to learn the most about you from what you tell them, even when they may not appreciate the value of your self-knowledge. Your relatives, friends, and coworkers can also teach you a great deal.

Health care providers are one important source of information. Most of us learned while growing up to turn to doctors for health information, yet there are many limits to what they can or will tell us. The information we get from doctors and other health care providers may be constrained by:

- Limited time to diagnose and teach patients
- Financial incentives not to recommend certain care if it costs the managed care plan more money
- Pressures from drug company representatives to push certain medications

- Their mistrust of our ability to understand or make good use of complex information
- The sexism, racism, homophobia, and class bias of their training
- Their not keeping up with the latest research or their inability to evaluate it
- Their lack of knowledge about prevention, self-care, less invasive procedures, nonmedical alternatives, and holistic healing traditions
- Their desire to appear "sure" and "dependable," which creates an unwillingness to admit to uncertainty or controversy

Consult your health care providers for their advice and information, but also turn to other sources. No one person or institution is likely to be aware of all the health information relevant to your condition or situation.*

In giving up our unquestioning trust of the information we get from doctors and other health care providers, we also give up the comfort that comes from their reassurance. Learning more about alternative approaches and treatments may mean living without the kind of certainty or hope that can come with this unquestioning trust. In addition, you and your providers may have to make decisions without complete information, because not even the "experts" know enough about certain problems to recommend one approach over another. Often what's most needed is courage in the face of uncertainty.

We get our information about health from a variety of sources: books, magazines, newspapers, television, the Internet. Often the problem is not *lack* of information—health information is abundant—but lack of *quality* information. Some sources do not always present accurate information or recommendations supported by good research. Since not all material is trustworthy, it is crucial to check that your sources are both accurate and independent and to evaluate the material from technical, public interest, user, and feminist perspectives. The best information describes practices that are supported by research that uses rigorous scientific methods to evaluate medical care and that is free of commercial and professional biases. (For more information on scientific research, see "Evidence-Based Practice and the Cochrane Collaboration" [W74] on the companion website, www.ourbodiesourselves.org.)

HOW TO EVALUATE HEALTH INFORMATION ON THE INTERNET

The Internet can be a great resource for those of us seeking information about and support for our health concerns. Through a computer with Internet access, a woman entering menopause can find self-help information; a pregnant lesbian can discuss parenting with other lesbian moms; a woman on welfare can find organizations that may help her advocate for the assistance she needs; and a woman with heart disease can research the latest medical treatments.

But while the amount of material available on the Internet is vast, the quality of the information varies greatly. When you visit a website, it's important to consider the source of the information and to view critically any material you find. Remember that anyone can create a site and put up any content he or she wants. Some sites push dubious medicine, both conventional and alternative; some are concerned only with selling you their products; and some sites (as well as research studies) are biased by the drug compa-

---

* One valuable tool that can improve health care is the powerful Problem-Knowledge Coupler system, developed by Lawrence Weed, M.D., and colleagues. Rather than depending upon how much an individual provider may know, the PKC system guides the user through the collection of relevant information regarding his or her overall health or a specific problem, then couples that information with timely, researched knowledge. The result is an individually tailored list of options regarding prevention, diagnosis, and treatment, all cited to authoritative sources. For more discussion of this approach, see www.pkc.com.

nies, professional societies, and other advertisers who support them.

Separating questionable or misleading information from accurate and reliable material can sometimes be daunting. Below are some questions to ask yourself to help evaluate the quality of online health information.

- *Who developed and maintains the site?* Any good health-related site should make it easy for you to learn who is responsible for the site and its content. One way to tell is to look at the site's URL (which is usually listed in a box labeled "address" near the top part of your screen): the name or initials of the organization are often part of the URL, as is a two- or three-letter "root domain" designation that tells you the nature of the organization. Some common designations are "edu" for educational institution, "org" for nonprofit organization, "gov" for government agency, "com" for commercial company, "net" for network, "ca" for Canada, and "uk" for Great Britain. For example, by looking at the URL www.cdc.gov, you can figure out that you are at a site created by a government agency (gov) whose initials are probably cdc (they are: the Centers for Disease Control).

   To find additional information about who runs the site, look for a link that says "Who We Are" or "About . . ." If there is no information available about who owns the site or develops the content, be wary.

- *Who pays for the site?* It costs money to run a website. Although some sites are labors of love, most have outside sources of funding, and this should be clearly presented on the site. How does the site pay for its existence? Does it sell advertising? Does it sell products or services? Is it sponsored by a drug company? Is it funded through grants or donations? The source of funding can affect what content is presented, how the content is presented, and what the site owners want to accomplish on the site. For example, drug-company-sponsored information tends to downgrade or ignore nonmedical or non-pharmacological approaches, and is slow to present innovative alternatives or preventive treatments. Try to figure out if the author(s) or site owner(s) have a financial interest or anything else to gain from proposing one particular point of view over another.

- *Who is the author of the particular material you're reading?* The authors and contributors of all content should be clearly identified. Often information posted is collected from other websites or from offline sources. If the person or organization in charge of the site did not create the information, the original source should be clearly labeled.

- *What is the basis of the information on the site?* In addition to the authorship of the material you are reading, the evidence that material is based on should be provided. Medical facts and figures should have references, and opinions or advice should be clearly labeled as such and set apart from information that is evidence-based (that is, based on research results).

- *When was the material written or compiled?* All content should have a date on it, so you can tell when the material was written, when it was posted, and when it was last revised.

- *Does the information sound too good to be true?* Be wary of "cures" for incurable diseases. Question sites that credit themselves as the sole source of information on a topic as well as sites that disparage other sources of knowledge.

- *Does the site ask you for personal information?* If so, read its privacy statement to find out if your information will be shared by others without your permission.

- *Is there a way to contact the site?* There should be a way for you to contact the site owners with problems, feedback, and questions, and someone should respond to your messages in a timely way. If the site hosts chat rooms or other online discussion areas, it should tell visitors what the terms of using this service

SUPPORT, SELF-CARE, AND SELF-HELP GROUPS

There are a few different types of groups that women can join to learn about and share information on different health topics and aspects of health care. These groups help because they give us a chance to talk with other people in our situation, to trade ideas, to feel less alone, and maybe to learn some skills.

Some physicians, medical centers, and hospitals offer groups or classes on a wide variety of health topics. These groups often emphasize self-care, activities that we can do to manage our care in conjunction with our providers. Local support groups are also often offered by voluntary health organizations such as the American Cancer Society and the American Heart Association.

We sometimes form our own self-help groups. Often these groups are organized without formal leaders and reflect early women's health movement values about inclusivity and the sharing of information. Implicit in these groups is the belief that we all can understand medical information, that it belongs rightfully to us, and that we need to feel empowered by it. Because these groups are independent of health care institutions and professionals, they can freely question, challenge, and evaluate accepted medical treatments and explore nonmedical therapies and providers. If the group you seek does not already exist in your area, consider starting one of your own.

are. If a site is moderated, you should be able to find out who the moderator is and how he or she was chosen.

THE RIGHT TO REFUSE TREATMENT

You have a legal right to refuse any medical treatment at any time, even if you agreed to it previously. This right applies to all competent adults and mature minors—those who can understand and appreciate the information necessary to give informed consent. Simply disagreeing with your provider's recommendation does not mean that you are incompetent. In life-or-death matters involving decisions for others who are unable to decide for themselves, individual providers and hospitals may try to resist your choice to refuse treatment on behalf of them. All states have passed laws that, through the use of a living will or health care proxy, allow competent people to authorize the withholding or withdrawal of medical treatment, even though such an order may lead to their death after they become incompetent. Remember, too, that accepting one part of a treatment plan does not mean that you must accept the whole thing. You always have the right to leave the hospital if your wishes are not respected (with the exception, in some cases, of a psychiatric facility). Enlisting the support of a family member or other advocate may be particularly helpful in such situations. (For more information about refusing treatment, see *The Rights of Patients* by George Annas in "Resources.")

REPRODUCTIVE AUTONOMY

The right to refuse treatment is of particular importance to women regarding our reproductive autonomy. While it is generally recognized that people have a right to bodily integrity and informed consent, both legal and political action increasingly suggest that upon becoming pregnant, women lose these rights. Examples of such actions include laws restricting access to abortion services, court orders forcing women to undergo cesarean sections, and medical tests performed without consent. In several cases, pregnant women who have refused a recommended cesarean section or who have used drugs have been arrested and charged with endangering fetal health.

In 2001 the U.S. Supreme Court ruled that "drug testing of pregnant women for the purpose of criminal investigation may not be conducted without a warrant or explicit consent, even when justified by the benign purposes of protecting fetuses and promoting drug treatment."[1] In such states as South Carolina, where being addicted to drugs during pregnancy has essentially been criminalized, many women face enormous challenges to seeking medical care without being prosecuted.

National Advocates for Pregnant Women (NAPW) is a national nonprofit organization that advocates on behalf of all women, especially those who are most marginalized and most likely to be targeted for these punitive actions: women of color, low-income women, and women who use drugs. NAPW uses a variety of strategies, from litigation and public education to organizing on the local and national level, to ensure that we do not lose our constitutional and human rights as a result of pregnancy or under the guise of "fetal rights," children's rights, or family protection.

(For more information about NAPW, see www.advocatesforpregnantwomen.org.)

THE RIGHT TO RECEIVE CARE IN EMERGENCIES

An emergency—a sudden injury or illness—can cause serious harm or death if it is not treated right away. In an emergency situation, you have a legal right to treatment. The physician's role is central. He or she has a duty to determine whether an emergency exists. If it does, law and medical ethics require the physician to treat you or to find someone who can. If either transfer or discharge from an emergency department will threaten or adversely affect your condition, then treatment must be given, regardless of your ability to pay. This does not mean that the treatment is free: The hospital will bill you or your insurance company, and the bill may be sent to a collection agency if you do not pay.

Emergency department care is expensive. Emergency departments are not the most appropriate places for primary care problems such as sore throats, sprained ankles, and urinary tract infections. Patients are seen in order of the severity of the problem, not in the order in which they arrive. Managed care plans tend to limit emergency department visits. However, go to the hospital if you believe that you have a medical emergency. Most health plans have now adopted the "reasonable layperson" standard as the basis for making a decision about going to the emergency department. There are many circumstances, too numerous to list here, that should prompt an emergency department visit. The emergency department is also appropriate for some less serious conditions, such as broken bones, high fevers, and cuts that require stitches. For help in deciding whether to go to an emergency department, call your primary care provider (PCP).

Other than emergency care, we have no legal right to health care. A few entitlement programs exist for pregnant women, people with low incomes, the elderly, and people with disabilities— for example, Medicare, Medicaid, and Social Security payments for those who are disabled regardless of age. However, even with these programs—some of which are being cut back— many of us receive either inadequate care or no care at all.

Some health care providers and policy makers have accused lower-income Americans of using emergency room facilities inappropriately for basic primary care. However, until other kinds of health care facilities are available that accept all patients regardless of ability to pay, emergency rooms may be the only option for some of us.

RIGHTS REGARDING MEDICAL RECORDS

You have a legal right to see, obtain, or have access to your hospital and medical records. Since 2003, this right has been backed by federal law, the HIPAA (Health Insurance Privacy and Accountability Act) legislation and regulations. You will receive a written statement of your rights regarding your medical record when you see a health care provider or are admitted to the hospital. Your right to see your medical records includes all hospital and individual provider records about you, except for psychotherapy records. They are after all, *your* medical records, not your provider's. It is advisable to keep copies of records from all health care encounters for future reference and make sure they are accurate.

BARRIERS TO GETTING HEALTH CARE

FINANCIAL BARRIERS

For many years, employment-based health insurance has been seen as the usual way for Americans to obtain health care. In recent years, however, increasing numbers of Americans of all races and classes have had to scrape by for months or years without employment-based health insurance. And even those of us who do have private insurance are now required to pay more out of pocket for health care than in previous years, in the form of higher insurance premiums, increased co-payments, and payments for prescription drugs. Medical debt has become a leading cause of personal bankruptcy in the United States. In 1999, "nearly half of all bankruptcies involved a medical problem, and certain groups—particularly women heads of household and the elderly—were even more likely to report a health-related bankruptcy."[2]

In 2003 more than 45 million Americans did not have health coverage for some time during the year. People of color and people with low incomes were the least likely to have stable health insurance coverage. One third of low-income women lack health insurance, compared to 9 percent of higher-income women. Low-income women are two times more likely than higher-income women to lack a regular source of care, not have seen a physician in the last year, lack timely Pap smears or clinical breast examinations, and go without prescribed medication.[3] Other women who are particularly likely to lack health insurance include those of us who are divorced; who work in service jobs such as waitressing; who work part-time or as temps; or who provide full-time caregiving for our children, aging parents, or ill family members.

There is no safety net to serve the millions of Americans who do not have health insurance. Medicaid covers only a small portion of those without private health insurance. Many counties and cities run some type of public clinic with a sliding scale for fees, but these clinics are underfunded and typically are so overwhelmed with patients that the wait for an appointment can be several months. Nonprofit hospitals are required to offer charity programs, but often fail to inform patients that these programs exist. Some communities have volunteer-run clinics. However, these clinics generally are open only one evening a week or month and are limited in their ability to provide free or low-cost medication to patients. Emergency departments are required to stabilize a patient's condition regardless of ability to pay, but they are not required to provide any further treatment. In addition, they bill uninsured patients for the care provided.

Those of us without health insurance, and those of us who are underinsured or sporadically insured, or who have insurance that does not cover all of our medical expenses, need to make the most of these sparse, disorganized, and inadequate resources and services. Keep in mind these two key strategies: (1) health care costs may be more negotiable than they seem, and (2) keeping careful, written track of your needs and treatments will better enable you to patch together services from various agencies.

The following are additional options that have worked for some women.

To Control the Cost of Care

- Hospitals and health care providers (including labs) often quote higher fees to uninsured patients than the insurance companies have negotiated. You can call the billing department of the institution or provider and ask what their best rate is. Then (in a separate conversation) tell the person billing you that you are willing to pay only that rate.
- In some communities, Planned Parenthood offers low-cost or free reproductive health care to uninsured women. Their services may include family planning, breast and cervical cancer screening, mammograms, and sexually transmitted infection testing, counseling, and treatment.
- Sometimes you can save the cost of a trip to a specialist if your primary care provider will

agree to call the specialist and discuss your case on the phone. Do not hesitate to ask your provider to do this for you; it is a reasonable part of his or her job.

- Many doctors work in more than one facility, with different rates at each. A few phone calls often will help you discover the least expensive way to see your provider.
- In some settings, a nurse practitioner, physician assistant, or nurse midwife may provide the same services as a doctor at a lower cost.
- You may be able to avoid repeating blood and other laboratory tests by keeping copies of the results.
- Hospital social workers often develop expertise in navigating the health care system. If you are hospitalized, ask to see a social worker.
- People living near the Mexican border or near the Canadian border find that medical and dental care cost less outside the United States. Others with ties to European countries (such as Ireland) find that it is more economical to purchase a plane ticket and obtain medical care abroad than to pay for the care at home.
- Low-cost dental care is particularly difficult to find, and even many of us with medical insurance do not have dental coverage. Many dental schools offer free or low-cost programs where dental students are supervised by more experienced dentists. Some schools even offer low-cost orthodontia.

Addressing Medicaid Issues

- If you are receiving public assistance (financial assistance from a government program) and get a job, you may no longer qualify for Medicaid. If this is your situation, try contacting your congressperson and your caseworker. They may be able to find a way to extend Medicaid for you. When the Welfare Reform Act of 1996 was passed, lawmakers promised that women would not lose Medicaid after leaving public assistance for jobs.

Obtaining Drugs as Cheaply as Possible

- Pharmaceutical companies have patient assistance programs (PAPs) to distribute a limited amount of free and discounted medication. The downside is that the application is too complex for most people. However, in many communities, charitable organizations (such as Catholic Charities) employ someone to help people fill out and submit this kind of application.
- Doctors and nurses can sometimes guide you toward more economical ways to manage your medication. For example, in some cases medicine can be ordered at a higher dose for the same cost and the pills can be cut in half to provide the desired dose. This is a much better alternative than taking partial doses or skipping days or weeks, which can be more dangerous than not taking the medication at all.
- You can ask your provider if a generic or over-the-counter drug may be a cheaper but effective alternative to a brand-name prescription drug.
- You can order prescription drugs more cheaply from Canada via the Internet. Some states, such as Minnesota, have established procedures to help people buy medicine from Canada.
- If you are insured by Medicare, check current medication benefits. Local senior centers or agencies on aging can be helpful.

(For more sources of assistance, see "Resources.")

RACISM AND PREJUDICE

Racism, prejudice, and bias create especially severe barriers to obtaining health care. For example, blacks and Latinos are less likely than whites to receive the standard treatment for heart disease, medications for HIV, pain medication for broken bones, surgery for lung cancer, or preventive services, even when we have health insurance.[4]

Women of color are less likely to get prompt, adequate follow-up for abnormal cancer screening tests such as mammograms. This may contribute to the higher rates of death from breast cancer among black women compared to white women. Similarly, even though those of us who are women of color are more likely than white women to report being in fair or poor health, we are less likely to have a regular health care provider, less likely to have health insurance, and less likely to see a doctor when we are ill.[5]

Women with low incomes and women of color receive abusive and damaging care more often than other women. If you do not speak fluent English, some providers may treat you as if you are stupid. Low-income and less well-informed women are more likely to be used as "teaching material" in hospitals where residents (physicians training in a particular area of medicine) are learning and refining their skills.[6] Some practitioners stereotype women, offering different diagnoses and treatment to women of color and low-income women, even when our symptoms are identical to those of middle-class women.

It often makes a positive difference when we have access to caregivers with race, class, and ethnic backgrounds similar to our own. To make this more possible, we need to support affirmative action programs in medical schools as well as hospital staffing practices that emphasize diversity.

BIAS AGAINST SUBSTANCE USERS

Women who have current drug and alcohol problems and women who have histories of such problems may also experience discrimination. For example, women who are believed to be drug users may be denied pain medication during labor, because of misinformation and prejudice about drug use. Such women often report extremely hostile comments from medical staff, and some have been turned over to the police rather than offered appropriate confidential medical care. Those of us receiving methadone treatment, a federally approved treatment for opiate addiction, may be treated as if we are using an illegal drug. Despite laws prohibiting discrimination, drug-using women often face extensive barriers to accessing appropriate drug treatment.[7]

I wish that health care was a lot more accessible for women in this country. . . . The people in hospitals, doctors and nurses, just treat drug addicts really badly. I think it's really unfair. . . . I can't go into a doctor's office and say, "Look, I'm a heroin addict," to tell them everything that I need to tell them about what I've done to my body and health. I don't think there is a doctor in this city that I can go to and be comfortable with and they can be comfortable with me and treat me totally equal as anybody else, you know?[8]

LANGUAGE AND CULTURAL DIFFERENCES

Receiving appropriate health care can be complicated by differences between the patient and provider in language and culture. The majority of health care providers in the U.S. are white and were born in this country. Women of color and immigrant women may be at a disadvantage, since many providers do not understand the health beliefs and practices of each specific culture, including issues such as women's physical and sexual modesty around male health care providers. Interpreters may not be available for women who do not speak English. Even though Title VI of the Civil Rights Act states that individuals cannot be discriminated against based on language, and every individual with limited English skills is entitled to care in her language, an interpreter may not always be available.

If an interpreter is not available in a hospital,

you might want to ask for the chaplain or social worker. While neither may be able to translate, these professionals are usually trained to work with people of many different backgrounds and may be able to help you track down someone in the community who can help interpret.

Smaller clinics and offices are unlikely to have interpreters on-site. Face-to-face communication is better, but you can also get help from an interpreter over the phone. It is helpful to request an interpreter in advance, when you make an appointment, if it is not an emergency visit.

Most states offer health assessments to refugees soon after arrival, but the sites, type of services available, and time frames vary between states. Refugees are eligible for Refugee Medical Assistance, a federally funded, state-administered program with benefits similar to Medicaid, for the first eight months in the United States. Families with minor children are eligible for Medicaid. After eight months, refugees are subject to the same limitations in access to health care as other Americans. Finding and maintaining employment is a priority for refugees, but the employment available may not carry health benefits and may also lead to loss of eligibility for Medicaid benefits. Mental health and reproductive health services are increasingly recognized as important to offer to refugees, but traditionally, there has been an emphasis on screening refugees only for infectious diseases such as tuberculosis.

DISABILITY ISSUES

People with physical and mental disabilities and chronic illnesses may experience many barriers to receiving health care, including lack of accessible transportation, limited income and insurance coverage, and inaccessible practitioners' offices. Even when women can enter the office, there may be additional barriers, such as exami-

nation tables that do not adjust, which may mean that those of us who cannot stand up cannot safely get onto a table.

Providers are not always knowledgeable about particular disabilities or conditions. Because of their lack of experience with people with disabilities and social stigmas about disabilities, they may be uncomfortable interacting with us. We may have to provide them with medical information and educate them about our disability. It is often difficult to be a "teacher" and advocate for ourselves at a time when we are vulnerable and need medical care.

HOMOPHOBIA, TRANSPHOBIA, AND HETEROSEXISM*

Some lesbian, gay, bisexual, or transgender (LGBT) people experience financial, personal, and cultural barriers to getting appropriate health care.[9] Sometimes we do not seek health care because we believe or are told that certain services are not necessary. For example, you may incorrectly think that if you have sex with women, you are not vulnerable to sexually transmitted infections or do not need regular preventive care.

A good health care provider should take a thorough health and family history. Such a conversation provides an opportunity to disclose the intimate or family relationship we live in. Questions about sexual activity should be gender-inclusive and open-ended, such as "Do you practice safer sex?" rather than "What kind of birth control do you use?"

Even practitioners who are lesbian or bisexual themselves may not understand or be sensitive to the needs of women who have a different racial and/or cultural background than their own, work as sex workers, or use drugs.

* For definitions and further information on these terms, see Chapter 9, "Gender Identity and Sexual Orientation."

Those of us who are butch and trans women and men, intersexed people, and others whose gender presentation may be different from our biological sex might encounter health care practitioners who do not know how to treat us. If we do not identify as male or female, the "male" or "female" box on intake forms can create anxiety.

In addition, LGBT people who have partners are often unable to get health insurance through them, because many employers and insurance companies will not provide spousal benefits to unmarried couples. Fortunately, that is changing.

Here are a few suggestions to help lesbian, bisexual, and transgender people find health care providers who are attentive to our needs, create a safe environment, and are educated about our lives.

- Ask other lesbian, gay, bisexual, and transgender (LGBT) friends and acquaintances if they have a health care provider whom they like and with whom they can talk easily.
- Find out if there is a health center near you that specializes in care for LGBT people.
- Search for a doctor on the Gay and Lesbian Medical Association's website (www.glma.org/programs/prp/index.html).
- Contact your local LGBT community center for information and referrals.
- When calling to schedule an appointment, ask, "Can you recommend a provider who is experienced in LGBT health care?"

IMBALANCE OF POWER IN THE DOCTOR-PATIENT RELATIONSHIP

The doctor-patient relationship is often one of inequality, an exaggeration of the power imbalances inherent in many client-professional relationships in our society. This is more likely to be true in a male physician/female patient relationship, but it can also be true of female physician/female patient encounters. Racial and social class differences can also aggravate the power imbalance.

There may always be something about needing help or being a patient that calls up the child in us and makes us feel dependent, especially when we are in pain or are afraid. When you raise real, matter-of-fact questions, a doctor may say, "What's the matter, don't you trust me?" or "I can't take care of you if you don't believe in my advice." Some physicians will seek to contradict and replace your own knowledge and sense of yourself and your problem with their own convictions about what is "really" going on.

Today the problem of doctor-patient communication is even more serious than before. In most health systems, primary care visits are limited to fifteen minutes—insufficient time to raise, let alone resolve, the most pressing issues we need to discuss. Some health plans penalize doctors who take more time with their patients, and offer bonuses if doctors utilize fewer resources, resources that may turn out to be medically necessary. Thus, doctors generally have less control than they did before the era of managed care.

As in any relationship in which we lack power, we tend to evaluate what happens during a medical encounter in terms of our own behavior rather than the doctor's. For example, if you do not understand something, you may feel inadequate or intimidated. You may find it hard to admit your feelings, and fail to ask for a clearer explanation. Does a doctor's superior education, training, experience, and/or age automatically produce infallible judgment?

It is crucial to make whatever efforts we can to improve doctor visits. *It can make a big difference to bring along an advocate—a family member, or a friend* whose presence will reduce any hostile or surprised reactions to your questioning. Try not to let any negative reactions prevent you from persisting.

If you encounter problems with your practi-

MAKING THE MOST OF YOUR HEALTH CARE VISIT

You can do a number of things to help ensure that you get what you need. Those of us who are more active in determining our care and more assertive with our providers tend to be more satisfied and achieve better outcomes.

• Ask for written information about how the practice or clinic works. This should include hours of operation, evening and weekend coverage, what to do in an emergency, and numbers to call for appointments, prescriptions, and referrals. Find out what hospitals the practice uses and who will care for you if you need to be in the hospital.

• Bring someone you trust to your appointments. It is often helpful to have another pair of eyes and ears to "record" what happens at visits.

• Keep a diary or journal of your health information, and bring it with you to visits. Practitioners often do not recall the details of your specific case, so they will benefit from this important information about your previous experience. If possible, research relevant issues before your visit, and discuss what you find with your health care provider.

• Bring to the visit any medicines, herbal preparations, or over-the-counter preparations you are taking to make sure you do not receive duplicate medications or medications that cross-react. Ask your provider to write down how to take any new medications or any changes in your existing medications.

• Ask your provider for an explanation of anything you do not understand. If necessary, ask for pictures or diagrams that explain your condition. Ask for a written statement of the treatment plan in order to monitor your care or in case you choose to seek a second opinion later. When no medical emergency exists, take as much time as you need to think about any decisions.

• List all of your questions and make sure that they are addressed. Take into account that insurance companies allow doctors to spend only relatively short amounts of time with you, so ask the most pressing questions first.

• If you need more time for the visit, ask for another appointment. You can also ask to schedule longer visits. If you have tests, make sure you get test results, an explanation of any abnormal findings, and recommendations for follow-up. Request a printed copy of the results, since it may show additional helpful information. Since some providers do not call if test results are normal, call and ask to be sent the information if you do not hear about your results within two weeks.

tioner, let her or him know that a problem exists. If he or she does not address the problem or change his or her behavior, find someone else, if possible. If the problem is really significant, you may want to submit a formal complaint (see "Complaint Mechanisms," p. 717).

Friends now marvel at my close relationship with my current doctor and my ability to talk back, question, and disagree with him and his colleagues. He respects me and trusts me to tell him what is going on, and I, in turn, trust him to listen, make suggestions, and consult with me before any action is taken. When I don't want a procedure done or feel the psychological burden of making yet another trip to the lab or to his office is just too much for me on an occasion, I will tell him and he understands me most of the time.

It is particularly important to choose a primary care provider (PCP) whose approach to health care, and to you as a person, suits your needs. Primary care refers to a general form of care that emphasizes first contact with the health care system, prevention, and health promotion. Most managed care plans require members to choose a PCP to coordinate care and make referrals to specialists. Good PCPs are trained to give well-person care and checkups. Your primary care provider should also provide high-quality, comprehensive care over the long term, and coordinate complex treatment given by multiple providers.

Three main types of physicians serve as PCPs: family medicine physicians, primary care internists, and some obstetrician-gynecologists (OB-GYNs). However, PCPs do not have to be physicians; they can also be osteopaths, nurse practitioners, or physician assistants. (For descriptions of these PCPs, see "Types of Primary Care Providers" [W76] on the companion website, www.ourbodiesourselves.org.)

A FEMALE OR MALE PROVIDER?

Women often say that we prefer to be cared for by a woman rather than a man. We hope, and often believe, that female physicians and other health care providers will be different from their male colleagues, in that they will listen better

CHOOSING A HEALTH CARE PROVIDER

Here are some issues you may want to consider in choosing a primary care provider (PCP):

- If you have insurance coverage, does it cover the PCP you are considering?
- What is his or her training and experience?
- Is the provider female or male, and how important is that to you?
- Is she or he familiar with any special health problems you have?
- Will she or he take the time to explain health issues to you?
- Is she or he attentive to needs related to your culture, race, or sexual orientation?
- Will she or he speak your language or provide a medical interpreter?
- Will she or he support your use of complementary, alternative, and traditional medicine?
- Is the office accessible for your disability?
- Is the office in a convenient location?

and be more understanding, sensitive, and caring.[10] Unfortunately, however, female providers emerge from the same stressful and dehumanizing medical training process that affects all doctors. Sometimes their anticipation of prestige, money, and position interferes with providing good care. Once in practice, female physicians face the same financial and time constraints as male physicians and thus may disappoint us in similar ways.

At the medical plan I belong to, I chose one of the two women doctors because I believed a woman would be less likely to push drugs and surgery, and would look with me first for the less invasive nonmedical alternatives. In the first visit, she suggested not only thyroid medication but also a routine X ray; she talked crisply, rapidly, coolly, with many complicated medical terms. I felt as if I were sitting across from a medical school curriculum.

Although we cannot assume that a female physician will be better than a male physician, studies have shown some relevant differences. Female physicians generally see fewer patients than male physicians do in a given time period and thus spend more time with each individual.[11] Female physicians may be more successful communicators than male physicians because they listen better, tell you more, ask you more questions, elicit more patient disclosure, facilitate more patient participation, establish a dialogue, and are more empathetic.[12] Female physicians are more likely to advise and offer preventive services such as Pap smears, clinical breast examinations, and mammograms.[13] Research on the effect of gender among other types of providers is limited, perhaps because of the small number of men in fields such as nursing and midwifery.

SEXUAL ABUSE

One of the consequences of the imbalance in the doctor-patient relationship is that some doctors abuse their power. Women have reported increasing numbers of cases of sexual assault by and sexual relations with doctors over the past ten years. Doctors explain their behavior by saying they believed such relations to be either harmless or actually beneficial and "therapeutic" to the women involved. Sometimes a woman agrees to "consensual" sex with a doctor, perhaps believing that the doctor has fallen in love with her. This is sexual abuse as well as unethical professional behavior on the part of the doctor, and

not the woman's fault. Because of the broken trust involved, sexual abuse by health care providers can be severely damaging.

Only a few cases of sexual abuse reach state boards of registration in medicine. They frequently drag on for months and are often resolved with inadequate controls on future abuse. Institutions are required to report physicians who lose their hospital privileges or are otherwise disciplined to a national central registry. Hospitals hiring or granting privileges to a new doctor must check this registry first.

ENFORCING OUR RIGHTS

Our rights as patients mean little if they cannot be effectively enforced. The method of enforcement we use will depend on state laws and the right involved. Some of the most common ways to exercise and enforce our rights are listed below. You can obtain further information and possible assistance by contacting women's health groups, consumer groups, or legal services organizations (see "Resources").

PATIENT ADVOCACY

Probably the best way to safeguard your rights is to bring someone as an advocate to all your health care appointments. Before your medical visit, discuss with your advocate what you want and expect to happen. Make sure you both understand the kinds of diagnostic tests, treatments, or surgical procedures being proposed. Ask your advocate to keep a record of events that occur when you are unable to be aware of them. Anticipate situations that may make you feel powerless or inadequately informed. Make a list of your questions. If more than one provider is involved, your advocate can help coordinate your care. If the health care staff raises questions about your emotional or psychiatric stability (thereafter dismissing your concerns and complaints), your advocate can speak up for you. No good hospital (or individual provider) should object to patients having an advocate, and many actively encourage it.

Large hospitals and health plans may employ patient advocates or representatives who can be helpful in cutting through red tape. Yet because they represent the hospital, these people may not be free to represent your interests if they conflict with the interests of the hospital or provider. Even so, some patient advocates do an excellent job. To find out if the hospital has a patient advocate program, ask a nurse or call the hospital switchboard.

COMPLAINT MECHANISMS

Complaints are important because they alert health care providers to potential problems that, if corrected, can improve care for everyone. If you are unhappy with the results of a medical encounter or experience any inappropriate behavior on the part of the provider, do not hesitate to complain. Write down the events as soon as they occur, and draft a letter that clearly states what happened and when. If friends or family members have firsthand knowledge of what happened, ask them to record their thoughts and observations right away. If your complaint is lodged against a licensed health professional, send it to the appropriate licensing board, and send a copy to the relevant county and state professional societies. You can also contact a local women's health group for assistance and encouragement. Especially in the case of sexually inappropriate behavior, consider discussing your experience with a reliable lawyer or women's law group.

When complaining about a state-licensed facility (hospital, nursing home, clinic, etc.), contact the appropriate licensing agency as well as the consumer protection division of the attorney general's office. If you think you have received an experimental drug, or if you experience a strong drug reaction, report it to the U.S. Food and Drug Administration (FDA) MedWatch program at 1-800-332-1088 or www.fda.gov/medwatch.

Consider sending a letter of complaint to the following people or organizations: the individual provider involved; the provider who referred you; the administrator or director of the clinic, hospital, or managed care organization; the local medical society; the organization that will pay for your visit or treatment, if different from the organization providing care (such as your union, insurance plan, or Medicare); the local health department; your neighborhood health council or community board; community agencies; local women's groups, women's centers, magazines, and newspapers.

It is sometimes useful to discuss your intentions with your practitioner before actually lodging any complaints, since this may provide the incentive necessary to improve the situation. Make certain that all your medical records and supporting materials are together before you discuss the matter with your provider, as she or he may become defensive or try to manipulate the information included in your record after that point.

When we are sick or in pain, we may be reluctant to complain about our treatment out of fear of alienating our health care providers. However, many of us find that giving voice to our concerns not only improves the care we receive, but also contributes to our own sense of well-being.

NOTES

1. Lisa H. Harris and Lynn Paltrow, "The Status of Pregnant Women and Fetuses in U.S. Criminal Law," *Journal of the American Medical Association* 289, no. 13 (April 2, 2003): 1697.
2. M. B. Jacoby, T. A. Sullivan, and E. Warren, "Rethinking

the Debates over Health Care Financing: Evidence from the Bankruptcy Courts," *New York University Law Review* 26, no. 2 (May 2001): 3.

3. Henry J. Kaiser Family Foundation, "Issue Brief: Health Coverage and Access, Challenges for Low-Income Women," findings from the 2001 Kaiser Women's Health Survey.

4. Brian Smedley et al., *Unequal Treatment* (Washington, DC: National Academy Press, 2003).

5. Kaiser Family Foundation, "Racial and Ethnic Disparities in Women's Health Coverage and Access to Care: Findings from the 2001 Kaiser Women's Health Survey," Publication #7018, March 2004, accessed at www.kff.org/womenshealth/7018.cfm on November 3, 2004.

6. Diana Scully, *Men Who Control Women's Health: The Miseducation of Obstetrician-Gynecologists* (New York: Teachers College Press, 1994).

7. The Harm Reduction Coalition, "The Need for Harm Reduction," www.harmreduction.org/prince.html.

8. Interview from *Pregnant Women on Drugs: Combating Stereotypes and Stigma* by Sheigla Murphy and Marsha Rosenbaum (New Brunswick, NJ: Rutgers University Press, 1999). See also Wendy Choukin, "Cocaine and Pregnancy: Time to Look at the Evidence," *Journal of the American Medical Association* 285 (2001): 1626.

9. Institute of Medicine, *Lesbian Health: Current Assessment and Directions for the Future* (Washington, DC: National Academy Press, 1999).

10. Michelle Harrison, *A Woman in Residence* (New York: Fawcett Book Group, 1993).

11. Lucy Candib, "The Gender of the Doctor: What Is the Difference in Practice?," Cabot Series Primary Care Lecture, Harvard Medical School, December 12, 1996.

12. D. L. Roter and J. A. Hall, "Examining Gender Specific Issues in Patient-Physician Communication," Women's Health and Primary Care: A Workshop to Build a Research and Policy Agenda (Washington, DC: George Washington University Center for Health Policy Research, 1994).

13. N. Lurie, J. Slater, P. McGovern, et al., "Preventive Services for Women: Does the Sex of the Physician Matter?," *New England Journal of Medicine* 329 (1993): 478–82.

CHAPTER 31

Just after dawn on April 25, 2004, close to three dozen immigrant women boarded a bus in Brooklyn and left New York, many of them for the first time since coming to the United States. They were headed to the March for Women's Lives in Washington, D.C.

Fabiola Peña and the others who rode from New York to Washington said they had seen the devastating consequences of outlawing abortion in their native countries: botched abortions; families larger than intended; neglected children. In some ways, they said, these real-life experiences speak louder than the abstract though powerful anti-abortion belief system in which they were raised.

"One has to respect a person's freedom and rights," said

Daniela Taveras, forty, from the Dominican Republic.[1]

A selling point for these Latinas was the idea that they would march not just for abortion rights but for a range of issues that affect immigrant women, including the need for better prenatal health care, medical insurance, and access to birth control.

"I'm not doing this for me, because I'm old," said Estrella Flores, sixty-four. When she immigrated to Brooklyn in April 1993, she recalled, bilingual services were scarce at hospitals and social service agencies. Now, when she goes to see a doctor anywhere in the area, interpreters are easily found, she said, adding, "If there hadn't been protests, that help wouldn't exist."[2]

More than 1 million people, mostly women, attended the March for Women's Lives; a third of the crowd was under age twenty-five. Women of all ages need government policies to provide for healthy lives and communities and to regulate health care systems. We need policies that respect and value women's rights, including the right to equal treatment and to make decisions about our bodies. We also need policies and programs that provide broad access to vital human and social services that no individual can establish alone, including health care, education, water, and sanitation. For decades, though, U.S. policies have threatened to intrude on women's rights to reproductive choice, while shrinking financial support for social programs we depend on.

Public policies can influence, and are influenced by, the nature and distribution of economic wealth and power, social values, and ideologies. Women benefit from policies that encourage economic and social equality. While we have made progress, we still face significant obstacles to equality by gender, as well as by race, ethnicity, class, age, health status, sexual orientation, and gender identity.

This chapter explores the effect of political developments in the United States and internationally on women's health. Advances in transportation, communications, and other technologies have set the stage for an increasing volume and pace of cross-border trade in goods, services, and money. The Internet provides women and health advocates around the globe with access to information and to one another. Increased economic activity could increase standards of living globally. However, the growth of corporate power and the resulting concentration of wealth are global trends that may have negative consequences for women. In the past, businesses anchored in particular countries perceived a benefit in providing financial support for education, public health, a safe environment, and roads and other infrastructure. As businesses circle the globe seeking the lowest wages and the least restrictive governments, this "social contract" is under fire, as are public funding and public accountability for services.

THE POLITICS OF WOMEN'S HEALTH IN THE UNITED STATES

The politics of women's health in the United States has been shaped by serious challenges, including growing corporate influence over government policy and global economic inequality and uncertainty. Ideological opposition to women's rights, including the right to reproductive choice, has played a more prominent role in recent years, increasing sharply after President George W. Bush took office in 2001.

Control over conception, including access to legal abortions, has freed women from disability and death due to illegal abortions. This fundamental advance has been eroded by organized opposition, including acts of violence, and by restrictive state and federal laws. A declining number of doctors and other health professionals receive training in abortions and provide them in their practices, particularly in rural areas where community opposition may have more of a deterring effect. Though there is a high level of popular support for women's rights, anti-choice legislation continues to be enacted at both state and national levels.

Economically, the income gap between the richest and poorest has grown since the late 1970s. The real average after-tax income of the top 1 percent of the population rose by $576,000, or 201 percent, in the 1980s and 1990s, while the average income of those in the middle of the income scale rose $5,500, or 15 percent.[3] While women have made gains in income equality, a report by the Institute for Women's Policy Research found that in 2002 women overall were paid 68 cents on average for every dollar paid to white men. Asian-American women were paid the most, 75 cents on the dollar, and white women were paid 70 cents. African-American women were paid 63 cents, Native American women 58 cents, and Hispanic women 53 cents.[4]

By many measures, women's health has improved significantly over the last fifty years. Women in the United States have a life expectancy at birth of eighty years, compared with seventy-four for men, ranking the United States twenty-first for women and twenty-fourth for men among other countries. Nations with a higher life expectancy for women include some with lower average incomes than the United States, such as Spain and Greece, as well as high-income countries that provide universal health care, such as Japan, Norway, and Canada.[5] While both women and men in the United States are living longer, there were more than 3 million women over age eighty-five in 2001, compared with 1.3 million men.[6] There were 1.5 million nursing home residents in 1999, more than half over eighty-five years old, and three quarters female.[7] Yet by critical measures such as infant mortality, the United States lags behind many other developed countries. Research now acknowledges that women have unique health needs, which should be pursued with more studies and funding. Our race, ethnicity, and economic status can greatly affect our health and the quality of treatment we receive.

DISPARITIES IN HEALTH

Women are the majority of health care users and health care givers. But when it comes to health and health care, women have unique problems that often go unrecognized. A number of health conditions strike women at a higher rate than men, and some strike groups of women disproportionately based on attributes such as race and ethnicity, income, education, or age. In some cases, it is known that the differences are due largely to biological factors, such as conditions related to older age. In many other cases, the reasons for the differences are complex, reflecting inequalities in social and economic status and in power, which can in turn affect the health of communities and health-related behaviors, as well as poorer access to adequate health care. Researchers refer to differences related to these inequalities as *disparities*. Awareness of disparities has led to calls for policies and programs that can alleviate them. Ongoing research is exploring the relationships among social, environmental, physical, and emotional health. The following examples highlight some important disparities that may be preventable.

Health Disparities Between Women and Men

Heart disease is the leading cause of death for women, but our symptoms are less often recognized or treated appropriately by physicians than those of men. About a quarter of women and men have hypertension (high blood pressure), but it is increasing among women faster than among men, in every age group.[8] The rate of hypertension increases as we get older. But even comparing women and men of the same age, it is appearing at a faster rate in women. Because women now live longer, we often require services that are poorly provided in our fragmented health care system, ranging from coordinated psychosocial and medical treatment to home health and long-term care for chronic conditions, including cancer and Alzheimer's disease.

My doctor for many years always asked the standard questions about my health, but he didn't go beyond that. Being of an older generation, neither did I. Most of the time, I didn't even know what to ask.

I happened to go to a free testing for osteoporosis, and it was recommended that I seek further testing. By this point, my doctor had retired. My new doctor arranged the test, and the results showed I had already lost 50 percent of my bone mass. She immediately put me on Fosamax and Evista, plus calcium. She keeps me updated and informs me about new studies and recommends tests appropriate to my age. It seems to me if my first doctor had checked me when menopause began or alerted me to the possibility that bone loss was something to consider at my age, I might have prevented this condition.

Health Disparities Among Women by Race and Ethnicity

Life expectancy for U.S. women varies by race; white women can expect to live approximately 80.2 years, compared to only 75.5 years for black women.[9] Infant mortality is highest among blacks, at 13.6 per 1,000 births, and lowest for women of Chinese descent, at 3.5 per 1,000.[10] Maternal mortality for women over 35 is 71 per 100,000 births for blacks, and 11.4 for whites.[11]

The incidence of breast cancer is higher among white women, but black women are diagnosed at later stages, and five-year survival is 15 percent lower for blacks than for whites.[12] Latinas living in the U.S. have twice the incidence of cervical cancer as do non-Latina white women, and their death rate is 40 percent higher.[13] Sixty-nine percent of American Indian women receive prenatal care, compared with 90 percent of Japanese-Americans.[14] AIDS cases per 100,000 women are 2.3 for whites, 11.8 for Latinos, and 50 for blacks.[15]

Health Disparities Among Women by Income

Women with higher incomes are more likely to have health insurance and better access to health care. For example, 72 percent of women defined as poor by federal standards had preventive Pap smears in 2000, compared with 84 percent of non-poor women.[16] Poor women are hospitalized twice as often as the non-poor (168 per 1,000 population, compared to 87 per 1,000), which indicates lack of access to timely preventive care.

Health Disparities Among Women by Education

Mortality is twice as high among infants born to white women with less than a high school education as it is among infants born to white women with high school education or greater.[17]

THE U.S. HEALTH CARE SYSTEM

An uninsured white emergency room nurse in Mississippi says:

Florence Nightingale . . . believed that hospitals just cannot be kept clean enough over the long term, so that every 20 years, they just need to be burned down and rebuilt, so that there can be a clean and healthy facility. And that's what I say about the health care system. It needs to be burned down and rebuilt.

Health is recognized as a basic human right under international law. In most countries, the government is responsible for setting health goals and funding health and medical services. Although medical care and insurance systems are becoming increasingly mixed between the public and private sectors, the responsibility for organization lies with government. However, that is not the case in the United States, which relies to a great extent on the private sector for financing and providing medical care. Commercial industries, in turn, have had a growing influence over the way health care is managed and delivered.

The United States is the only industrialized country without universal coverage for health care services. Seventeen percent of U.S. residents under age sixty-five, more than 44 million people, are uninsured at any time. The rate varies by state and by race and ethnicity; about 39 percent of Mexican-Americans are uninsured, compared with 12 percent of non-Hispanic whites. Forty-three percent of uninsured workers earn under $7 per hour.[18] People without insurance are less likely to seek needed health care and, consequently, suffer from poor health.

The United States spends more than any country on health care, about 14.9 percent of gross domestic product in 2002. About 44 percent of personal health expenditures are covered by public programs, 36 percent are covered by private insurance, and 16 percent by out-of-pocket payments. The spiraling cost of health care is attributable to the 25 percent increases in administrative costs of private insurance, compared with 3 percent in the federal Medicare program, and to 15 percent annual increases in prescription drug charges and increasing charges for hospital care.[19]

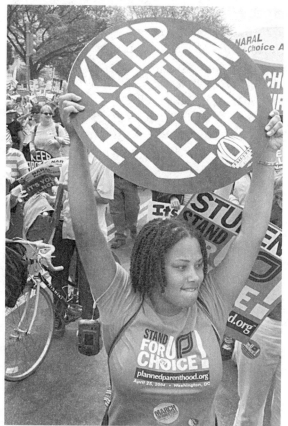

The March for Women's Lives brought more than 1 million people to Washington, D.C., on April 25, 2004, to show support for women's reproductive rights and health.

Our medical culture also puts a premium on high-tech equipment and testing, along with surgical procedures and expensive prescription drugs. While many of these are necessary and useful, treatments that may be less expensive in the long run, including preventative and some alternative health practices and care by nurse practitioners and nurse midwives, are often dismissed or overlooked.

I lived in Berlin, Germany, between 2000 and 2002. Once, when I suffered a severe back injury, I went to the doctor, and she recommended acupuncture. I was worried that an "experimen-

tal" treatment would not be covered. She chuckled at the suggestion that it was experimental and assured me that it would definitely be covered, as would regular visits to the "krankengymnast," a sort of chiropractor. She made me feel comfortable, and I was feeling well.

However, on a visit to the States over Christmas, I injured my back again. It was Christmas Eve, so I had to go to the emergency room. They immediately gave me a shot of Demerol in the thigh to "break the cycle of pain," they said. I left the ER with a prescription for Vicodin (sixty pills) and a refill option. I was also given a strong muscle relaxant. The difference in attitude has always fascinated me.

Publicly paid health programs include Medicare, the federal health insurance program for the elderly, and Medicaid, the federal/state program for some of the very poor and disabled. Both programs are undergoing radical changes in financing and organization.

Most people who have private health insurance receive it through an employer. Women are less likely than men to have jobs that offer employment-based private health insurance. This means, for example, that middle-aged women who are single, divorced or widowed, and not yet old enough for Medicare are often uninsured. And even under Medicare, the long-term care that many women require is not covered.

Women are more likely to be covered by Medicaid than men, due to certain improvements in eligibility during pregnancy, but the coverage frequently does not continue after birth. And in states where Medicaid funding is low, many providers may not take Medicaid patients.

CORPORATE POWER AND THE FREE MARKET ECONOMY

Shifts in the U.S. economy help to explain the dramatic changes in the health care system in the late twentieth century. Beginning in the 1980s, conservative political policies in the U.S. increasingly shifted power to the states and to corporations. Today we are told that a free market economy, in which corporations are successfully creating profits and thus wealth, benefits the society as a whole by trickling down the wealth to poorer people. Yet in recent years, we have seen corporations downsize, laying off thousands of employees. Worker benefits, especially health care, have shrunk. Salaries for most workers have remained stagnant, while the salary and benefit packages of CEOs have exploded. This is especially true within the health industry, where the nonprofit principle itself is under systematic attack.

HEALTH CARE AND PROFITS

When health care is turned over to private enterprise, the driving motive in providing care is profit, just as in any other industry. The need to reduce costs, and even to optimize profits, competes with a commitment to optimum health care, despite industry rhetoric and the many conscientious practitioners who care about their patients. For this reason, most women's health activists have long opposed the profit motive in health and medical care systems.

Like many other citizens, most women's health activists believe in the principle of the public good and the public interest. Many services are provided by governments that benefit the community as a whole: police, firefighting, land conservation, education, roads and bridges, to name a few. Similarly, health should be considered a public good, not a commodity to be sold in the marketplace like a car. There are many social needs that a free market cannot possibly fulfill effectively, and health care is one of them.

Most providers—hospitals, health centers, and clinics—are private. Although the majority of hospitals are private not-for-profit institutions, a growing number of for-profit hospitals are dominating small markets, particularly in rural areas and smaller urban areas. In the past, most big cities and counties had public hospitals and clinics for the poor; these are increasingly being closed down or privatized.

The two public health services are the Indian Health Service, which is being privatized and turned over to tribes, and the Veterans Administration (VA), which is downsizing its hospitals and programs. The VA system, while suffering from budget cuts and other serious problems, has kept administrative costs down and effectively implemented many reforms that have reduced medication errors in hospitals.

In contrast, the fragmented organization of the U.S. health care system obstructs access to high-quality care for women with complex medical conditions such as breast cancer. We may find that we are passed among a series of specialists who do not coordinate with one another regarding diagnosis or treatment plans. The burden of arranging separate appointments with doctors, laboratories, and diagnostic centers can be overwhelming when we are sick. Without a common system to manage or administer care, it is difficult to get doctors to agree on standards for high-quality care, and to practice to those standards. In short, there is no accountable authority, in the public or private sector, effectively encouraging standards of care.

PRIVATIZATION OF MEDICARE

For over thirty-eight years, the Medicare program has successfully provided basic, nearly universal health coverage to Americans who are over age sixty-five or disabled. Because women live longer, the majority of Medicare beneficiaries are women. Medicare's success derives from its social insurance model, under which nearly all working Americans and all beneficiaries contribute toward a national pool that shares both risks and resources. That is why Medicare can provide a guaranteed standard of health care to the nation's highest consumers of care at an administrative cost far lower than that of the private insurance that covers younger and healthier Americans.

The Medicare Prescription Drug Improvement and Modernization Act, passed in 2003, represents a major restructuring of Medicare. It began the segmentation of the strong national risk pool of more than 40 million individuals into smaller regional groups. The law provides subsidies to convince private companies to offer a complex array of plans whose benefits and costs are not specified in the law. The program is designed to entice or even force seniors out of Medicare as we know it and into competing private health insurance plans. In the past, similar private health plans have lost money on Medicare enrollees and eventually dropped the insurance plans.

The program took political cover from the demands of busloads of U.S. seniors crossing the border to buy affordable prescription drugs in Canada. In the past, Medicare did not cover most drugs. Beneficiaries could buy private supplemental plans, but even these became unaffordable for many as drug prices skyrocketed. In 1997 relaxed regulations allowed drug companies to advertise directly to consumers, which helped inflate drug prices. A well-financed army of drug company lobbyists saw to it that the 2003 Medicare law did not threaten the windfall.

The new Medicare benefit for prescription drugs is scheduled to begin in 2006. While it may offer some improvements for low-income seniors, the benefits, cost, and access are not guaranteed in the law. The benefit has a complex and confusing structure, containing provisions such as holes in coverage and new types of private prescription-drug-only plans. Most critically, it directs billions in federal subsidies to pharmaceutical companies while expressly prohibiting effective cost-control measures. Drug reimportation from lower-cost countries such as Canada is unlikely under the bill. The federal government is specifically banned from negotiating for lower prices with the pharmaceutical companies, as do other federal agencies, such as the VA. Those of us who are seniors could end up paying more than we do today for medications.

For the first time, the part of Medicare that pays for doctor visits and other outpatient care (Part B) will be means-tested: People will pay a premium based on income beginning in 2007. This will erode the equitable nature of the program. It will also allow health plans to cherry-pick wealthier—and hence, likely healthier—enrollees.

Finally, the law sets an artificial and arbitrary cap on Medicare financing. Once this limit is hit, which is considered inevitable, an "emergency" will be artificially created, and seniors will be forced to accept large benefit cuts or cost increases.

(For a detailed summary of the law and more information concerning its prescription drug benefits and Medicare costs, see "The Medicare Prescription Drug Improvement and Modernization Act" [W77] on the companion website, www.ourbodiesourselves.org.)

REFORM OF THE U.S. HEALTH CARE SYSTEM

Across the country, consumer and government efforts encouraging reform have been met with great resistance. As corporate managed care fails to control the cost of medical care, private-sector interests actively—and so far successfully—have blocked even popular reforms such as controlling the cost of prescription drugs.

In the absence of prospects for universal coverage, Congress passed an incremental reform, the State Children's Health Insurance Program (SCHIP) in 1997. Created under Title XXI of the Social Security Act, the program expands health coverage to uninsured children whose families

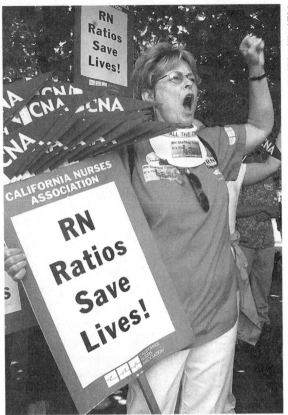

Charlene Arrington, a registered nurse, joined more than two hundred other nurses and supporters to voice their enthusiasm for a law requiring a higher nurse-per-patient ratio in California hospitals.

earn too much for Medicaid but too little to afford private coverage. Like Medicaid, the program is financed using state and federal funds and is administered by the states. Some states have reached out to communities and reduced the rate of uninsured children, while others have done relatively little.

In states such as California, where a growing immigrant population is increasingly demanding and winning civic rights, some county- and state-level programs have extended coverage to children in families with undocumented workers. However, cuts in funding for these incremental programs threaten to erode gains in coverage.

During the 1990s, federal proposals for expanding access to comprehensive health coverage gained serious attention. The criteria developed then by women's health advocates remain vital guideposts for a health care system that meets women's needs for patient-responsive, coordinated, evidence-based, and equitable care. Many women's health activists, for instance, believe that all health plans should include an emphasis on readily accessible, coordinated primary care for women that emphasizes prevention and is based on ongoing relationships over time with providers, including midwives, nurses, and other midlevel practitioners.

In addition to these building blocks, many women have concluded that broader reforms in the financing, organization, and delivery of U.S. health and social service systems are necessary to assure that health care is affordable and effective for women. These policies also recognize that public health services, economic security, and social justice are important determinants of women's health. Expanding parental leave benefits and child care services, for example, would greatly improve women's working conditions.

Local, state, and federal legislators continue to propose single-payer bills that would be financed like traditional Medicare, through a single government payer instead of through multiple private insurance schemes. Numerous studies have documented that this would make it possible to control administrative expenses and eliminate profits, to cover everyone in the U.S. at an affordable cost, and to improve care. The single-payer approach has faced fierce and effective opposition from the private health insurance industry.

These single-payer bills would cover all residents, a feature referred to as universal coverage. Because the program would be publicly financed, people would not have to depend on a workplace for health insurance. This would en-sure that we have continuous access to health care, even when we change jobs, work for small businesses that traditionally have not provided insurance, or are unemployed.

I am a nurse practitioner who works in a community health clinic that provides care to an underserved, primarily African-American female population. Nearly half of our patients are 200 percent below poverty level. Recently, a Catholic hospital took over the community hospital, limiting access to reproductive care. Services that were routine, like discussing birth control options or performing tubal ligation following delivery of a baby, were eliminated, and patients from primary care clinics associated with the hospital now come to our clinic for birth control.

As the primary care provider, I spent 15 minutes in a new-patient interview for an appointment that could have been five minutes with a nurse had the patient been able to go to her regular clinic. Women who choose a tubal ligation now have to be transferred to another hospital. Again, the women are being shuffled around to adapt to the limitations of a system, one that limits the options and health care of women.

Many other countries explicitly track and address the social, economic, and environmental determinants of health through their public health systems. U.S. Representative Barbara Lee (D-CA) has set a tradition of introducing House Resolution 3000 in every session of Congress. This bill would create a universal health service in which the public sector both finances and operates the health care delivery system. It was originally drafted by Lee's predecessor in Congress, Representative Ron Dellums, in collaboration with activists in women's and community-based health movements. This updated proposal takes advantage of the United States' vast capability to harness information technology to improve medical care, while creating accountable entities at the community and national government levels that are responsible for health. This and similar proposals would provide coordinated medical care services and would also give women a needed voice in our health and health care. These proposals call for:

- Affordability: financing the health care system through a single government payer to achieve universal coverage and to control costs through streamlined administration, elimination of profits, and control over fraud and advertising.
  - Implementation of fair cost-control mechanisms that restrain health care providers' ability to raise prices excessively. For example, some countries successfully set global budgets as annual expenditure targets for hospitals.
  - Reducing the exorbitant prices of prescription drugs and focusing drug industry research on new treatments instead of profitable copies of existing drugs.
- Fair treatment: eliminating discrimination in insurance coverage and all aspects of care against women and all populations confronting geographic, physical, cultural, language, and other nonfinancial barriers to service.
- Accountability: involving health care users, women, and communities in the governance and policy decision making of health care systems, including measures that assure provider accountability and the right of redress.
  - Assuring that medical records are confidential.
  - Establishing an individual's right of ownership over her or his genetic material as well as control over who has access to her or his genetic information.
- Comprehensive benefits: providing comprehensive benefit packages that are responsive to women's needs.

- Including coverage for reproductive/gynecological health, occupational and environmental health, prescription drugs, mental, dental, and long-term care.
- Effective planning: ensuring ongoing evaluation and planning of the delivery of health services, with consumer and provider participation.
  - Monitoring health status and providing weighted funding to address the needs of vulnerable populations (the young, the elderly, rural areas, and areas with a high density of health problems such as disabilities and AIDS).
- Support for public health: improving the investment in and recognition of public health programs.
- High quality of care: improving the quality of medical care.
  - Training health professionals in the economic, cultural, psychological, and social (race/gender/age) determinants of health and effective caregiving for different populations.
  - Developing and implementing clinical practice standards, with participation and review by health care users and teams of health care providers, including consumer- and community-based research on appropriate elements of primary care for women.
  - Assessing and evaluating technology, with results publicly available.
  - Providing access to high-quality, unbiased women's health information.
- Support for health care workers: supporting education, training, employment, and promotion of professional and nonprofessional health care workers, to assure pay equity, the advancement of women workers, clinicians who represent their communities, and the provision of high-quality care.
- Social/economic policies: directing health

institutes to research and implement social and economic policies that would improve women's health, including protection of occupational safety and health.

(For more information about reforms needed to meet women's needs, see "Women and Health Care Reform" [W78] on the companion website, www.ourbodiesourselves.org.)

DIRECT-TO-CONSUMER DRUG ADS: A NEW BATTLEGROUND

In 1997 the Food and Drug Administration relaxed its regulations so that radio and TV ads[20] for prescription drugs have to mention only the major side effects. The new rules opened the floodgates to drug advertising aimed at consumers. Industry spending on such ads increased from $791 million in 1997 to $2.6 billion in 2002.[21] The prevalence of drug ads in popular media has sparked debates about the effects of drug advertising on inappropriate drug use and on rising spending on drugs.

Direct-to-consumer advertising concentrates on a small number of relatively new, expensive drugs for common, chronic conditions.[22] One example is Pfizer's heavily promoted drug Aricept, which British researchers concluded has "disappointingly little overall benefit"[23] for Alzheimer's patients. Campaigns aimed at women often medicalize ordinary experience. Eli Lilly repackaged the antidepressant Prozac as Sarafem to treat "premenstrual dysphoric disorder" (see "The Truth About Sarafem," p. 91). SmithKline Beecham (now Glaxo-SmithKline) promoted a previously rare psychiatric diagnosis as "social anxiety disorder" and then marketed Paxil, its antidepressant, as a treatment.[24]

In May 2001, a watchdog coalition of health advocacy groups called the Preven-

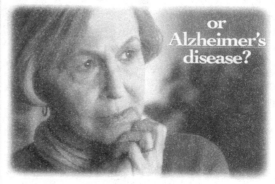

Pfizer's ad for the drug Aricept plays on our fears of serious mental deterioration. You wouldn't guess from this ad, however, that independent assessments consistently find the drug's benefits in fighting Alzheimer's disease to be modest. About ten of every hundred patients experience small, short-lived improvements in cognitive function,[25] but these don't translate into improved quality of life.[26] For a guide to reading drug ads critically, see "How to Read a Drug Ad," prepared by the Center for Medical Consumers in New York.[27] The guide is available online at www.medicalconsumers.org/pages/newsletter_articles.html#howtoreadadrugad.

tion First Coalition testified before the FDA that "far too often, [direct-to-consumer] ads mislead in a way that presents a threat to the public health."[28] Prevention First urged the FDA to ban ads promoting prescription drugs to consumers, something every other country except New Zealand has done. The industry argues that the ads inform and empower consumers. But ads don't provide the balanced information consumers need to make informed decisions. Prevention First filed complaints to the FDA that AstraZeneca's promotion of the breast cancer drug Nolvadex (tamoxifen) overstated the drug's benefits and downplayed its risks. The FDA agreed and forced AstraZeneca to withdraw its ads, but the process took over a year.[29]

Drug advertisements play on viewers' insecurities, on our natural desire for good health, and on our trust in medicine. Ultimately, advocacy is needed to stop the onslaught of half-truths: Consumer complaints to the FDA about an offensive campaign might help to trigger an investigation. Groups like Prevention First hope to eventually get misleading drug promotions off our screens for good. In the meantime, it is important to view these ads critically. (For more information, see "Direct-to-Consumer Advertising" [W79] on the companion website, www.ourbodiesourselves.org.)

EMERGING BIOTECHNOLOGIES

EMBRYO STEM CELL RESEARCH AND EMBRYO CLONING

In recent years, some biotechnology companies and researchers have made dramatic claims about the medical potential of human embryonic stem cells, promising treatments and cures for a wide range of chronic, degenerative, and acute diseases, including diabetes, Parkinson's disease, cancer, and Alzheimer's disease. Their predictions have won impassioned support from many patient advocacy groups and stirred hopes in all who want to alleviate the suffering that these diseases inflict.

Thus far, embryo stem cell research in nonhuman animals has produced only limited therapeutic results. Some of the claims made by the biotech industry are exaggerated. But many researchers believe that significant breakthroughs are close at hand.

Embryo stem cell research has also generated heated controversy. The critical voices most often heard are those with strong moral objections to all embryo stem cell work on the grounds that it uses and then destroys embryos for the sole purpose of harvesting stem cells. Although not reflected in most media coverage, there are strong pro-choice advocates who support most embryo stem cell research while remaining critical of one type of this research—embryo cloning (also called somatic cell nuclear transfer, research cloning, and therapeutic cloning).* However, some of these advocates remain relatively silent, because they are concerned that any criticism of embryo stem cell research will be used by anti-choice advocates to elevate the legal and moral status of embryos.

Many critics of embryo cloning do support embryo stem cell research, if such research uses embryos initially produced in IVF clinics to help women become pregnant and are subsequently donated, with informed consent, by the women who no longer intend to use them for reproduc-

---

* The organization Our Bodies Ourselves is one of these pro-choice voices.

tive purposes. But because the crucial distinction between embryo stem cell research and embryo cloning is often blurred in the public debate, it is not widely understood that support for embryo stem cell research can and often does coexist with deep wariness about embryo cloning.

Feminist and Social Justice Concerns About Embryo (Research) Cloning

Why are many people who are concerned with social justice wary of embryo cloning?

First, the envisioned treatments would require (at least initially) thousands of donated eggs, which means that many women would be subjected to the substantial risks of the drugs and surgical procedures involved. Although women already undergo these procedures in infertility clinics, the risks—even as inadequately defined as they are—may be justified because there is a demonstrated possibility that a baby will result. It is premature to ask women to undergo these risks for purposes of research alone until embryo stem cell research that does not require such egg donations has better demonstrated its potential. There also must be better data on the risks, so that women involved in this research would be able to provide true informed consent.

Second, many women's health advocates are concerned about the creation of a large market in human eggs, since women donating eggs in IVF clinics already receive reimbursement that ranges from $4,000 to $10,000 (some ads on college campuses have offered as much as $50,000 to $60,000). It is unlikely that many women will donate eggs without reimbursement, and it is economically disadvantaged and young women who are most vulnerable to such incentives.

Third, the production of cloned embryos would provide a key component needed for the

EMBRYO STEM CELL RESEARCH VS. EMBRYO CLONING

Embryonic stem cells are derived from early-stage embryos. To date, almost all have been derived from already existing embryos that were donated by people who no longer needed them as part of infertility treatment. Such embryos are developed in vitro in the "traditional" way: by the union of an egg and sperm. Another way to create embryo stem cells is through embryo cloning, an asexual method of developing embryos that uses no sperm and involves transferring the nucleus of a cell from one person's body into a human egg (from another person) that has had its nucleus removed.

engineering of inheritable genetic modifications (see "Genetic Modification of Future Generations," next page). Whether for purposes of medical therapy or for producing other non-medical enhancements (often referred to as creating "designer babies," with characteristics chosen by the parents), such inheritable modifications would be passed on to future generations with potential harmful effects that are impossible to predict regardless of how much previous research is conducted.

Fourth, in many countries, including the United States, there is no existing agency or policy that would provide effective regulation or monitoring of embryo cloning. This increases the likelihood that the "rogue" physicians and researchers now attempting to clone a baby (human reproductive cloning) might succeed, especially since the U.S. and a number of other countries have not yet passed national laws prohibiting such cloning.

Finally, as acknowledged by some prominent

figures in the biotech industry, treatments based on embryo cloning, if they ever prove feasible, are likely to be prohibitively expensive in the foreseeable future. Currently, there are no meaningful controls on private patents, so that companies may charge exorbitant fees and create enormous access problems.

GENETIC MODIFICATION OF FUTURE GENERATIONS

A disturbing number of influential scientists, biotechnology entrepreneurs, and others are openly promoting not only medical therapies that would use inheritable genetic modifications but also the idea of human genetic enhancements (in such characteristics as looks, talents, and intelligence). Based on what we currently know about genetics, however, it seems unlikely that it will be possible to make changes in a human embryo that can *predictably* produce a single healthy child.

Some proponents of human genetic enhancement say they look forward to the day when parents quite literally assemble their children from genes listed in a catalog. Others have a grand vision of seizing control of human evolution and altering the human species to create "post-humans" or "transhumans."

Dr. Gregory Pence, a professor of philosophy at the University of Alabama, is one such advocate. He has written, "Many people love their retrievers and their sunny dispositions around children and adults. Could people be chosen in the same way? Would it be so terrible to allow parents to at least aim for a certain type, in the same way that great breeders . . . try to match a breed of dog to the needs of a family?"[30]

Nobel laureate James Watson, famous for his role in figuring out the molecular structure of DNA, also advocates redesigning the genes of future generations. "People say it would be terrible if we made all girls pretty," he has said in one of many such statements. "I think it would be great."[31]

Princeton University biologist Lee Silver envisions the possibility that inheritable genetic modification will eventually lead to the emergence of genetic castes and human sub-species. "The GenRich class and the Natural class will become . . . entirely separate species," he has written, "with no ability to cross-breed, and with as much romantic interest in each other as a current human would have for a chimpanzee."[32]

As George Annas, chair of the Department of Health Law, Bioethics and Human Rights at Boston University School of Public Health, has noted, to the extent that there is any possibility of this vision actually becoming a reality such a class division of the human species is a sufficient argument not to pursue inheritable genetic modification at all in humans. The history of humans teaches us that it is more likely than not that these two "post-human" species would view each other as so different that one would either enslave or destroy the other—and it is this potential for either slavery or "genetic genocide" that makes pursuit of this technology a potential crime against humanity. Even if one finds this argument far-fetched, the potential impact on the entire species of such genetic modifications means that no individual scientist, corporation, or country has the moral warrant to make the decision to use such technology; only an accountable and democratic worldwide body should be able to authorize its use.

Many early discussions of inheritable genetic modification proposed drawing a line between its use for the treatment of disease and its use for "enhancement" of traits, such as height, eye color, strength, coordination, and intelligence. Increasingly, it is clear that this is not a workable approach, since people often disagree about what constitutes an enhancement and what constitutes a necessary medical intervention. In addition, some potential "modifications" would fall somewhere between treatment and enhancement—strengthening the immune system, for example, or increasing general alertness. And we have already seen many procedures, such as plastic surgery, that were introduced for medical purposes but soon became commercialized for clearly nonmedical use.

It is also important to keep in mind that researchers have no reliable way of predicting the effects of adding or changing a gene or the interaction of genes with each other. It is one thing to produce genetically modified plants or animals; it is quite another to experiment on human beings. If inheritable genetic modification were to be used on people, its consequences (intended and unintended, beneficial or detrimental) would be passed to all future generations. Thus, it is unethical research.

Inevitably, women will be subject to pressures to produce the "perfect baby." Genetic modification is likely to bring on new forms of discrimination and prejudice based on genetics and could fuel the resurgence of a powerful new eugenics movement. Some advocates of inheritable genetic modification (and of reproductive cloning and social sex selection) are attempting to appropriate the language of choice, claiming that these high-tech procedures are extensions of individual privacy rights. This sort of claim blurs the difference between the right for which women have fought for so many years—the right to terminate an unwanted pregnancy—and a very different thing: the right of individuals (parents) to exercise unfettered choice in the genetic manipulation and design of a future child. Women's health advocates need to challenge this cooptation of the language of choice in the public debate on many biotechnology issues.

Media coverage and popular culture have imbued biotechnologies with a mystique, power, and inevitability that make critical assessment and public discourse difficult. All of us want to find ways to treat illness and alleviate suffering,

so we may become excited each time we hear about a new research finding. However, predictions of medical breakthrough are often largely speculative, and media reports do not necessarily reflect the areas of research demonstrating the most promise.

We often hear genetic explanations for complex medical and social conditions. Assertions that our genes hold the key to shyness or sexual orientation or even our lifelong tendency to be optimistic or pessimistic are simplistic at best and often misleading. Given the far-reaching consequences of these technologies, we owe it to ourselves, our children, and future generations to think carefully about which ones we can responsibly and beneficially use as a society. The key question is where and how we would draw the line.

(For more information about research cloning, human reproductive cloning, gene patents, legislation, eugenics, and human rights issues, see "Emerging Biotechnologies" [W80] on the companion website, www.ourbodiesourselves.org.)

WOMEN'S HEALTH AROUND THE GLOBE

Discussing the politics of health and medicine around the world presents a few challenges:

- Health policies are reflections of a country's economy and resources, culture, and political system.
- Policies change over time, and not necessarily in an evolutionary way.
- Generalizations about regions, hemispheres, or other groupings of nations tend to be inaccurate.

In addition, the discussion of women's health presents other dilemmas:

- Women's roles in society are not uniform, despite other political, societal, economic, religious or cultural similarities among countries.
- Women's political movements vary from nation to nation, not just in their reach and power, but also in the priority given to different elements of health.

Notwithstanding these differences, and regardless of wealth or level of industrial development, certain characteristics commonly affect women's health in every society.

RELATIONSHIP AMONG ECONOMICS, EDUCATION, AND WOMEN'S HEALTH

Women's health status varies greatly depending on economic class, race, ethnicity, education, and home country. The same, of course, can be said of men. Women, however, are less likely to have educational opportunities and often lack decision-making power within communities—both of which affect our health status.

A woman's life expectancy in the United States is 80 years, as compared to 85 in Japan, 73 in Saudi Arabia, 63 in India, 53 in Haiti, and 47 in Ethiopia.[33] The great variation in life expectancy is strongly related to the wealth of each country and how evenly that wealth is distributed across the population. Life expectancy is also related to whether economic resources have been used to provide basic public health services, such as safe, clean food and water; basic or primary-level health care, including immunizations and well-child programs; and enough education to ensure literacy.

There is also a wide variation in life expectancy within countries. According to data from 2001, in the United States, for example, life expectancy among white women was 80.2 as compared to 75.5 among black women.[34] Al-though there is some evidence that race and ethnicity affect health status, the strong relationship between minority status and poverty clouds the issue. Women with low incomes in all countries have a lower life expectancy than women in the middle and upper classes. Poor women often have limited access to nourishing food and quality health care and may be exposed to more occupational and environmental hazards.

Throughout the world, those of us with access to education are more likely to believe we can control many aspects of our lives, including whether and when to have children. Women with more education will have fewer children than women with less education, even if both groups of women have equal economic status. We may also have more egalitarian relationships with our husbands (if we are married) and more decision-making power.[35] Education alone, however, does not guarantee this. Religious or racial oppression, for example, can make educational gains irrelevant for women in certain communities. In other words, knowledge is power only when we're given the opportunity to use it.

Policies that stimulate economic growth, promote a reasonably equitable distribution of wealth, and provide basic health care and education are essential for improving women's health throughout the world. Policies that promote the education of girls and women often lead to reductions in the birth rate, as well as improved health for women and for the community as a whole.

In the United States, women deliver an average of two children each, although this varies by ethnic group. (White women have an average of 1.8 children, compared to 2.1 for black women and Asian/Pacific Islanders, and 3.1 for Latinas.)[36] Women have an average of 1.3 children in Italy, Spain, and Romania; 4.4 in Guatemala; 5.0 in Iraq; and 7.1 in Somalia.[37] In developing countries, many of these children die before the age of five. In poor societies where women do not have enough nutritious food and do not receive adequate health care, bearing children can be dangerous to one's health. Women who deliver more children have higher rates of anemia and other nutritional deficiencies and suffer more frequent complications of pregnancy and childbirth, including death. In the United States, there are 11 maternal deaths per 100,000 live births. In Austria, there are 4 maternal deaths; in Denmark, there are 5; in Mexico, there are 83; and in Haiti, there are 680.[38] Many maternal deaths could be averted if societies had more resources for health care services, or if more resources were put toward quality maternity care. This would require making maternal health a high priority.

In Afghanistan, where internal and external conflicts have ravaged the health system, a 2002 survey found 1,600 maternal deaths per 100,000 live births. The most common causes of maternal death were hemorrhage and obstructed delivery, which often could have been averted or managed if the woman had been attended by a skilled health care practitioner. Women did not receive appropriate care for several reasons. In many cases, a woman and her family did not recognize that the pregnancy and delivery were not proceeding normally. In other cases, the woman did not have the decision-making power to seek care. Some families could not afford medical care or did not have the transportation to reach the health care facility, and in some situations the quality of care received was too poor or the care came too late to save the woman's life. As a postscript to the tragedy of maternal mortality, the study found that the infant of the deceased mother had only a one-in-four chance of surviving to its first birthday.[39]

Improving life expectancy and reducing maternal mortality require a sufficient investment in the accessibility and quality of health care—both primary health care and emergency obstetric care—basic health education, women's empowerment, and availability and accessibility of quality family planning services.

PROMOTION OF ECONOMIC EQUALITY

According to the International Labour Organization (ILO), more women are actively employed than ever before. In 2003, of the 2.8 billion people who worked, 1.1 billion were women. This varies greatly throughout the world. In the Middle East, North Africa, and South Asia, only forty women are counted as economically active for every hundred men in the labor force. Throughout the world, women are less likely to be regular wage or salaried employees and typically earn less than men for the same type of work.[40]

Also, women do an enormous amount of domestic work, as well as work in the agricultural sector, that is unpaid and thus not included in the employment figures. This is particularly true for rural women, who provide most of the labor for farming, from soil preparation to harvest. Rural women are generally responsible for preparing family meals, which involves finding fuel for cooking or heating and obtaining water for domestic use. These are very time-consuming tasks in many countries. On a global scale, women produce over half the food, up to 80 percent in Africa and 50 percent in Asia.[41] Nevertheless, women own only 2 percent of the land[42] and receive only 1 percent of all agricultural credit.[43]

A potentially successful model of empowering women economically is to provide access to credit and capital for micro-enterprises. Women are given loans to start small businesses, such as making clothing or household items, selling food, or providing other common goods and services. These lending programs are often associated with literacy and business training. In countries as diverse as India, Nepal, Nicaragua,

THE INTERNATIONAL MOVEMENT TO PROMOTE GENDER EQUALITY

Four world conferences have been held since 1975 to address the issue of gender equality. The first world conference, held in Mexico in 1975, was organized by the United Nations General Assembly with three objectives: to promote full gender equality; to integrate women in development; and to increase women's contribution in strengthening world peace. The second world conference, held in Copenhagen in 1980, in part called for stronger national measures to ensure women's ownership and control of property as well as improvements in women's rights to inheritance and child custody. The third world conference was held in Nairobi in 1985. Responding to UN data that showed little improvement in gender equality over the past decade, the delegates were given the mandate to seek new ways to promote gender equality and the integration of women in development and peace initiatives. The Nairobi conference declared all issues to be women's issues and asserted that women's participation in all decision making was not only our legitimate right but a social and political necessity.

In 1995 the Fourth World Conference on Women, held in Beijing, was the largest such gathering of government and NGO representatives to date, with seventeen thousand in attendance. The NGO Forum held parallel to the conference brought the combined number of participants to more than forty-seven thousand. The Beijing conference shifted the focus from women to the concept of gender, defined by the entire structure of society and all relations between women and men. The platform for action addressed twelve topics, including poverty, education, health, and violence.[44]

In September 2000, the member states of the United Nations participated in the Millennium Summit. Its purpose was to develop a process for reviewing the challenges facing the United Nations in the new century. Following consultations among international agencies—including the World Bank, the International Monetary Fund (IMF), the Organization for Economic Cooperation and Development (OECD), and specialized UN agencies—the General Assembly recognized eight goals as essential. The third goal is to "Promote gender equality and empower women."[45] The four target indicators[46] are:

- Ratio of girls to boys in primary, secondary, and tertiary education
- Ratio of women to men among literate 15-to-24-year-olds
- Share of women in wage employment in the nonagricultural sector
- Proportion of seats held by women in national parliaments

Some women's advocates have criticized these goals as being too weak. However, to the extent that such education, literacy, and participation goals are met, women will have stronger roles within the family and, therefore, better health.

Vietnam, and Yemen, women have participated in micro-enterprise loan programs, starting successful businesses, repaying the loans, and thus financing loans for other women.[47]

Although it is difficult to measure the impact of micro-enterprise programs on women's lives, studies suggest that they can improve a woman's income and self-confidence and boost her status within the family.[48] Other studies find a negative effect on women's lives, such as increased workloads and greater social pressure to repay the loans.[49] In India, there is a growing concern about micro-credits; critics say they are used as a means to get the poor to finance increasing medical care costs.

GENDER ROLES AND WOMEN'S HEALTH

The extent to which a culture allows women to make autonomous decisions has a great impact on women's health. Gender roles may make it impossible for women to refuse sex or negotiate condom use, which leaves women vulnerable to sexually transmitted infections, including HIV/AIDS. Some countries grant men full control and custody of children in case of divorce. In such circumstances, women may feel unable to leave unhappy or abusive marriages.

In communities where having a large family is a woman's only way to improve her social status, and where being childless is grounds for divorce or abandonment, women may feel pressured to have many, closely spaced children. In some societies where entire families are suffering from undernourishment, women may be affected even more because community expectations dictate that husbands and children be fed first.

FAMILY PLANNING AND ABORTION

The use of contraceptives has increased worldwide, particularly in developing countries. In the 1960s, only 9 percent of married women used modern methods of contraception, as compared to about 60 percent of married women in 2000. In spite of this increase, more than 120 million married couples in the developing world have an unmet need for family planning, either for limiting or for spacing births.[50]

According to the World Health Organization, there are 19 million unsafe abortions each year. Unsafe abortions account for 68,000 deaths, or approximately 13 percent of the estimated 529,000 maternal deaths worldwide. African women suffer the consequences of illegal and unsafe abortions more than women in any other region of the world. Women in Africa represent 44 percent of all women globally who die from abortion-related causes every year. This tragedy is further compounded by the fact that unsafe abortion is preventable. The tools, knowledge, and resources to address the problem exist, but they are not being adequately implemented.

The global gag rule disqualifies foreign nongovernmental organizations (NGOs) from receiving U.S. family planning funds if they provide legal abortion services, provide counseling and referral for abortion, or lobby to make abortion legal or more available in their country. The rule prohibits health care organizations from counseling women about abortion, even when it is legal within that country (for example, to protect the woman's health). This policy was introduced by President Ronald Reagan and remained in place until 1993, when it was rescinded by President Bill Clinton. It was reinstated by President George W. Bush in 2001, on his first business day in office.

The global gag rule requires NGOs to choose between continuing their non-U.S.-funded efforts to change public policy around abortion in their own countries and receiving U.S. family planning funds. Ironically, reductions in family planning services lead to more abortions.[51]

There is some confusion about whether the global gag rule precludes counseling women about emergency contraception—which involves taking a high dose of birth control pills within seventy-two hours of unprotected intercourse. Some organizations don't discuss emergency contraception because they fear losing U.S. funds.

REFUGEE WOMEN'S HEALTH

Worldwide, more than 20 million people were classified as refugees, asylum seekers, and internally displaced persons in 2002. Approximately 50 percent were women. A refugee is an immigrant who leaves her country of origin because of persecution for reasons of race, religion, nationality, political opinion, or membership in a particular social group.

Many refugee women have experienced significant trauma as a result of civil unrest such as war, or persecution based on politics, ethnicity, or gender. This trauma may include arrest, detention, and torture, including rape. Refugees may have witnessed the deaths of family members. Sometimes the goal of persecution is not to kill but to destroy the physical well-being of individuals and entire communities. According to Amnesty International, there were more than 150 countries worldwide practicing torture in 2003. In addition, the difficulty of leaving home, family, and friends to start over in a foreign culture where the climate, language, food, and social customs often are different can produce a particular kind of emotional pain known as refugee trauma.

As a result of these experiences, many refugee women suffer from post-traumatic stress disorder, depression, anxiety, substance abuse, and sleep disorders. In addition, refugee women have often lost the ability to trust, and building a therapeutic bond with anyone may be difficult. These burdens can complicate the already difficult task of adjusting to a new environment and should be identified and treated.

Many refugee women face other risks. In families under stress, women may become victims of domestic violence, including emotional and physical abuse, as well as sexual and reproductive abuse. Often refugee women find it difficult or impossible to negotiate for contraception with partners. This may increase the risk of unwanted pregnancy and childbearing, and of sexually transmitted infections, including HIV. Last, many refugees of both sexes are subject to dangerous, exploitive, and underpaid work, which can have a serious impact on health. For those with undocumented status, employment benefits are few.

Other important health issues for refugee women from many parts of the world include tuberculosis, HIV, and illnesses related to lack of immunizations, such as measles. All refugee women should undergo tuberculosis screening with a purified protein derivative (PPD) and treatment for latent tuberculosis, if recommended. In addition, all refugee women from areas where HIV is prevalent, or who otherwise might be at risk, should undergo testing for HIV. Risk factors for HIV include unprotected sexual intercourse and exposure to blood through transfusion or needles or instruments that have not been sterilized. Often the stigma and fear associated with this disease are overwhelming; the process of counseling and testing requires extra time to provide education about HIV and treatment. Women should also be screened for parasitic diseases and hepatitis. Many women will have complex dental needs due to lack of prior preventative services and/or previous trauma. Women will need to receive immunizations for or document immunity to measles, mumps, rubella, and varicella. A tetanus series may be necessary, as well as a polio series in some cases.

Refugee women have specialized health needs and should seek care from professionals who have knowledge about and experience in addressing these needs. Specialized centers for treatment of refugee trauma exist in the United States.

SEXUAL EXPLOITATION OF WOMEN

In developing countries, poor women and women with little or no formal education have few means of support. These women's traditional work—such as caring for family members, producing food, and transporting water—is unpaid. Economic need drives some women to become commercial sex workers. Others, particularly undocumented immigrants to other developing and industrialized nations, are forced into the sex trade. All of these women are at exceptionally high risk of a host of sexually transmitted infections, including syphilis, gonorrhea, hepatitis, chlamydia, and HIV/AIDS, as well as violence inflicted by clients and others who market and profit from the women's sexual services.

According to the International Labour Organization (ILO), surveys of workers in massage parlors and brothels in Thailand confirm that most of the women entered the sex industry to provide financial support to families. Brothel workers often reported becoming prostitutes to earn money to support children, while women in massage parlors were often supporting parents.[52]

In addition to providing financial support for families, commercial sex workers have become an important part of the economic base of entire countries. For example, the commercial sex industry in Southeast Asia has grown into a key economic sector that accounts for anywhere between 2 and 14 percent of the gross domestic product, according to a new study by the ILO. The number of Southeast Asians earning a living directly or indirectly from prostitution—including waitresses, security guards, and employees of escort services and tour agencies—could easily be several million.[53]

The debate over legalizing and regulating prostitution frequently focuses on protecting the sex worker and her clients from sexually transmitted infections and providing treatment for her when she becomes infected. Although such practices may protect the health and safety of sex workers and clients, they ignore the fact that many of these women are sex workers because it is the best-paying choice. Many sex workers would gladly assume other types of employment if they paid well enough; commercial sex is predominantly a consequence of poverty. It is easier for a society to legalize and regulate commercial sex work than to provide economic support, job training, and adequate employment for women. The clients of commercial sex workers may prefer that society place emphasis on reducing the transmission of infections rather than on creating economic alternatives for women.

Decriminalizing the sex industry and ensuring that sex workers are protected against abuse are essential for fulfilling all women's human rights. (For more on the distinction between decriminalizing and legalizing prostitution, see "Prostitution and Sex Trafficking," p. 134 in Chapter 8, "Violence and Abuse.") Commercial sex workers also benefit from policies that support alternative employment.

Child prostitution is a particularly heinous aspect of the commercial sex industry. UNICEF estimates that approximately 1 million children (mainly girls) enter the multibillion-dollar com-

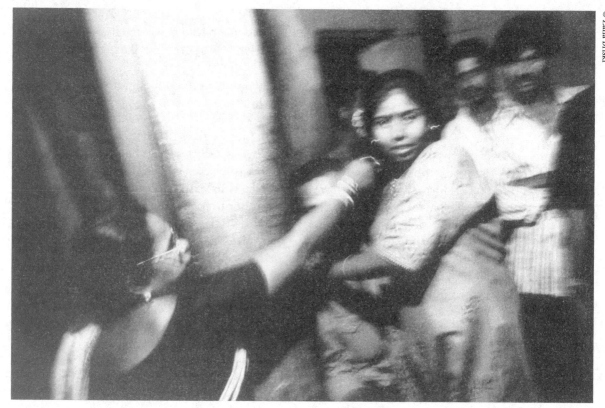

A madam pulls the braid of a prostitute during an argument in Calcutta, India, 2001.

mercial sex trade every year. There are many reasons children enter the sex trade: Parental abuse and neglect cause children to run away from home; homeless children may be sold to commercial sex organizations; the trade might seem to offer a chance for a lot of money; in an environment of armed conflict, children who become separated from their parents may seek protection from the military in return for sex; AIDS orphans may end up in the commercial sex industry.[54]

In some societies, children may be sold by their families to sex traffickers. The majority of customers for child sex in every country are local men, but foreign tourists, businessmen, and even peacekeeping forces are also involved.[55] Customers might prefer a child prostitute because they think she is less likely to carry a sexually transmitted infection or because they want to have sex with a virgin.

Child prostitution must be prohibited in all countries, and these prohibitions must be enforced. Children must be provided with safe and secure housing, economic support, and education.

HIV/AIDS

HIV/AIDS was first identified among a few subpopulations in the United States and Europe—gay men, intravenous drug users, and hemophiliacs. But almost immediately, the "wasting disease" of sub-Saharan Africa was recognized as HIV/AIDS. Because of the disease's initial identification in the United States with gay men, transmission through heterosexual contact to women was ignored, and U.S. education and outreach programs did not target women. This regional anomaly at first hindered comprehensive AIDS education programs in other parts of the world. Within ten years of the virus being identified, its transmission was understood, as was the range of at-risk populations; this influenced AIDS programs of international organizations. Women who have sex with men are at significant risk, particularly if the men have multiple partners.

The extent of the danger of the AIDS virus is finally being realized by international bodies, financial institutions, health organizations, and global funders, after two decades of learning. But in those two decades, the epidemic has devastated entire populations and continues to threaten the economic and cultural survival of many regions. For instance, HIV/AIDS is a critical factor in declining life expectancy in much of sub-Saharan Africa. In some countries, the life expectancy will be cut in half by AIDS unless antiretroviral drugs become available on a massive scale, a vaccine is found, or prevention becomes universal.

Lifesaving antiretroviral drugs are widely available in developed nations, at high prices. However, they are not being sold at an affordable price to developing nations in desperate need. The U.S. pharmaceutical industry has relied on international trade agreements that maintain patents for over twenty years to keep prices high and has prevented generic manufacturers in India and Brazil from exporting their own AIDS drugs to other nations.

The transmission of HIV/AIDS to women during heterosexual intercourse could be prevented *if* there were a safe and effective microbicide that could be introduced into the vagina or rectum just prior to intercourse, to kill the AIDS virus and other STIs. The microbicide might also serve as a spermicide. This option may be more acceptable to a male partner than a condom and would give women more power to protect ourselves. Efforts to develop such a microbicide are under way, and there is growing recognition of the need for greater funding in this field. (For more information, see "Future Prevention Methods," p. 271 in Chapter 14, "Safer Sex.")

VIOLENCE AGAINST WOMEN

In many societies, it is not only legal for men to abuse their wives, it is often expected because of patriarchal values. Most countries have histories and patterns of violence against women. Men may perceive that they have the right to dominate their wives physically, and the cultural and legal environment supports that perception.

Studies in more than three dozen countries have found that from one tenth to over one half of women have been beaten by a male partner.[56] In many countries, there is no protection against domestic violence for women—no legal action, no shelters, and no option for divorce. In those countries where these protections exist, often they are in insufficient supply. In some societies, women are blamed, punished, or even killed for being the victim of sexual violence. Without the economic means and the cultural support to live independently of men, women cannot leave abusive situations.

Although most violence against women is inflicted by a husband or a family member (domestic violence), there is growing concern about violence targeted at women in association with political or military conflicts—particularly soldiers raping women in countries such as Sierra Leone, Rwanda, Zimbabwe, Sudan, and Bosnia. In some circumstances, sexual violence is condoned by the government.[57]

U.S. foreign policy should require or at least encourage trade partners and recipients of aid to protect women from domestic violence, and there can be no tolerance for sexual violence perpetrated by the military.

FEMALE GENITAL CUTTING

Female genital cutting (FGC), also known as female genital mutilation or circumcision, is a traditional practice that involves cutting or altering the female genitalia as a rite of passage or for other sociocultural reasons. It usually involves excising the clitoris and may include removal of the labia and suturing the vagina, leaving a small opening for menstrual flow. The practice can have serious health consequences, including hemorrhage, shock, pain, infection, difficulties during childbirth, and psychological and sexual problems[58] (for more information, see p. 643).

FGC exists mainly in sub-Saharan and northeastern Africa, but it has spread to other regions of the world through migration. It is practiced by people from all educational levels and social classes, among urban and rural residents, and among many different religious and ethnic groups.

The national prevalence of FGC ranges from nearly universal (90 percent or more) in Egypt, Eritrea, Mali, and Sudan, to 18 percent in Tanzania. In Burkina Faso, Central African Republic, Eritrea, Kenya, and Tanzania, there has been some decline in the practice among younger women. On the other hand, in Egypt, Mali, and Sudan, there has been virtually no change over the past twenty years.[59] Egypt and Senegal have passed legislation prohibiting FGC, though to be effective, these laws need to be accompanied by cultural changes, such as implementing alternative rite-of-passage ceremonies and helping women whose income is dependent on being cutters.

In order to reduce the occurrence of FGC, there is an effort to promote a symbolic cutting (such as a nick in the clitoris) rather than clitoridectomy or more severe alteration of the vulva. This may be a more realistic policy option than trying to eradicate the practice entirely. For example, in Singapore's small Muslim community, female circumcision involves nicking the prepuce, the skin covering the clitoris. This is viewed as a more modern symbol of the tradition.[60]

In several countries, women have been recognized as refugees under the 1951 UN Convention Relating to the Status of Refugees (Geneva Refugee Convention) on the grounds that they would be at risk of FGC if they returned to their country. However, there are still only a tiny number of such cases. In the United States, the Immigration and Naturalization Service and international laws and treaties recognize gender-based violence as a human rights violation. Still, women are often denied asylum in the United States because the definition of a refugee entitled to protection is too narrow.

U.S. FOREIGN POLICY AND THE INTERNATIONAL MONETARY FUND AND WORLD BANK

During the 1970s, U.S. banks made loans to developing countries throughout Latin America, Asia, and Africa. The colonized countries had been left pauperized numerous times. Many of these loans are now believed to have been made irresponsibly, without considering how the debtor countries would repay the loan. Comparisons have been made to credit card companies that entice people to charge beyond their means, leaving the debtor burdened with heavy payments and tied to the lender forever. By the end of 1980, U.S. banks were charging 21.5 percent interest on all loans to developing countries. World prices for many of the major products exported by developing countries fell in the 1980s. This drastically reduced their ability to repay loans and made further borrowing necessary.[61]

Many developing countries now must choose between repaying their loans or funding needed domestic priorities, such as building roads and providing health care and education programs. The International Monetary Fund (IMF) has pressured debtor countries to reduce spending, and discourages price controls and government subsidies, even on essential items such as food, fuel, and water. The IMF and the World Bank encourage the privatization of state-run industries, which results in massive layoffs. The position of the IMF and the World Bank is based on several goals: to ensure that developing countries do not default on their loans; to combat inflation; to shift from a public-sector to a private-sector economy; and to increase the efficiency of private industry. Arguments can be made that these are worthy goals, although economists and development experts are far from unanimous.

IMF and World Bank policies, at least in the short run, can lead to higher prices for food and fuel, less government spending on education and health, and layoffs. This can cause widespread discontent and political instability.[62]

It is essential to recognize and balance the trade-off between many economic goals. Economic policies seek to make credit available for economic development, to ensure the stability of the international monetary system, to discourage defaulting on loans, and to protect basic economic security and political stability. Some economic policies have unfortunately led to irresponsible lending practices that have created serious problems for the debtor countries. Many global activists encourage loan forgiveness, with standards of economic development and democratic growth, though it's questionable whether donor and lending nations can reach suitable agreements.

Policy makers debate whether the United States should withhold foreign aid or impose trade sanctions against countries that do not protect human rights. The debate focuses on whether such activities help or hurt the victims of human rights abuses. Some U.S. policy makers argue that the best means of promoting freedom and human rights remains economic and moral engagement. This is sometimes but not always true.

The subject of human rights must always be raised in association with foreign aid and trade agreements, and each case should be analyzed to determine the best course of action to improve human rights. We also must ensure that donor countries scrutinize and address their own record on human rights.

THE WORLD TRADE ORGANIZATION

The World Trade Organization (WTO), established in 1995, has grown from setting the rules for trade in commodities to imposing IMF– and World Bank–style policies on developed and developing countries. A series of WTO agreements addresses trade in services. The service sector now accounts for most jobs in the developed world. These services include health care, education, water and sanitation, and energy.

Public health rules often conflict with the demands and interests of corporations, and local and national officials have the authority to balance those interests, with the presumption that people's health takes priority. However, trade rules assert that local and national governments can enforce laws that protect health, labor standards, and the environment only to the extent that these laws do not present unnecessary barriers to international trade by private corporations. The WTO facilitates international commerce, which can create wealth and raise living standards.

Critics contend that WTO policies favor countries and businesses that are already wealthy, and that these policies are thus at odds with the public's health and well-being. Many also question whether it is legitimate or beneficial for an international financial institution to limit countries' rights to regulate vital services such as health care and education. Women and communities are not consulted in trade negotiations, which are conducted secretly, even though we are vitally affected by the results. Trade agreements prohibit local drug companies from manufacturing lifesaving drugs at an affordable cost, if international drug companies hold patents on those drugs. This effectively maintains very high drug prices in both developed and developing nations, and has increased the impact of the HIV/AIDS epidemic in Africa.

Some European countries sought to prohibit the importation of beef treated with artificial hormones. The WTO noted studies that strongly suggested these products posed a real health risk, but found that the evidence was not yet conclusive. The WTO concluded that the ban was a trade barrier, and imposed financial sanctions.

The WTO has pressured countries to increase the influence of market forces in the provision of health care services and health insurance. This policy can be harmful if it results in the reduction of affordable health care services. Involving private or nongovernmental organizations can lead to an improvement in the quality and availability of services if governments provide appropriate oversight. However, WTO rules that remove governments' authority over decisions to privatize do not build their capacity for accountability.

A growing number of women's groups and health care organizations are demanding democratic participation in setting international trade rules, to assure that the benefits of global economic activity are widely realized by women and communities and not only by corporations.[63]

Increasingly, effective women's health activism is requiring that we take both a global and a local perspective and that we link our struggles across national borders.

NOTES

1. Andrea Elliot, "Against Abortion but in Favor of Choice," *New York Times,* April 26, 2004, A15.
2. Ibid.
3. Robert Greenstein and Isaac Shapiro, "The New, Definitive CBO Data on Income and Tax Trends," Center on Budget and Policy Priorities, September 23, 2003, accessed at www.cbpp.org/9-23-03tax.pdf.
4. Amy Caiazza, April Shaw, and Misha Werschkul, "The Status of Women in the States: Women's Economic Status in the States: Wide Disparities by Race, Ethnicity, and Region," Institute for Women's Policy Research, accessed at www.iwpr.org/pdf/R260.pdf on November 2, 2004.
5. National Center for Health Statistics, "Table 26: Life Expectancy at Birth and Age 65," *Health, United States, 2003,* pp. 131–32, accessed at www.cdc.gov/nchs/data/hus/tables/2003/03hus026.pdf on November 2, 2004.
6. National Center for Health Statistics, "Table 1: Resident Population, According to Age, Sex, Race and Hispanic Origin: United States, Selected Years 1950–2001," *Health, United States, 2003,* pp. 95–96, accessed at www.cdc.gov/nchs/data/hus/tables/2003/03hus001.pdf on November 2, 2004.
7. National Center for Health Statistics, "Highlights," *Health, United States, 2003,* p. 8, accessed at www.cdc.gov/nchs/data/hus/hus03.pdf on November 2, 2004.
8. National Center for Health Statistics, "Table 66: Hypertension Among Persons 20 Years of Age and Over, According to Sex, Age, Race and Hispanic Origin: United States, 1988–94 and 1999–2000," *Health, United States, 2003,* p. 227, accessed at www.cdc.gov/nchs/data/hus/tables/2003/03hus066.pdf on November 2, 2004.
9. National Center for Health Statistics, "Table 27: Life Expectancy at Birth, at 65 Years of Age, and at 75 Years of Age, According to Race and Sex: United States, Selected Years 1900–2001," *Health, United States, 2003,* p. 133, accessed at www.cdc.gov/nchs/data/hus/03hus027.pdf on November 2, 2004.
10. National Center for Health Statistics, "Highlights," *Health, United States, 2003,* p. 6, accessed at www.cdc.gov/nchs/data/hus/hus03.pdf on November 2, 2004.
11. National Center for Health Statistics, "Table 43: Maternal Mortality for Complications of Pregnancy, Childbirth, and the Puerperium, According to Race, Hispanic Origin, and Age: United States, Selected Years 1995–2001," *Health, United States, 2003,* p. 179, accessed at www.cdc.gov/nchs/data/hus/tables/2003/03hus043.pdf on November 2, 2004.

12. National Center for Health Statistics, "Highlights," *Health, United States, 2003*, p. 7, accessed at www.cdc.gov/nchs/data/hus/hus03.pdf on November 2, 2004.

13. American Cancer Society, "Cancer Facts and Figures for Hispanics/Latinos 2003–2005," accessed at www.cancer.org/downloads/STT/CAFF2003HispPWSecured.pdf on November 2, 2004.

14. National Center for Health Statistics. "Highlights," *Health, United States, 2003*, p. 8, accessed at www.cdc.gov/nchs/data/hus/hus03.pdf on November 2, 2004.

15. National Center for Health Statistics, "Table 53: Acquired Immunodeficiency Syndrome (AIDS) Cases, According to Age at Diagnosis, Sex, Detailed Race, and Hispanic Origin: United States, Selected Years 1985–2002," *Health, United States, 2003*, p. 200, accessed at www.cdc.gov/nchs/data/hus/tables/2003/03hus053.pdf on November 2, 2004.

16. National Center for Health Statistics, "Highlights," *Health, United States, 2003*, p. 9, accessed at www.cdc.gov/nchs/data/hus/hus03.pdf on November 2, 2004.

17. National Center for Health Statistics, "Highlights," *Health, United States, 2003*, p. 6, accessed at www.cdc.gov/nchs/data/hus/hus03.pdf on November 2, 2004.

18. Susan Starr Sered and Rushika Fernandopulle, *Uninsured in America: Life and Death in the Land of Opportunity* (Berkeley, CA: University of California Press, 2005), citing 1999 Current Population Survey.

19. National Center for Health Statistics, "Highlights," *Health, United States, 2003*, accessed at www.cdc.gov/nchs/data/hus/hus03.pdf on November 2, 2004.

20. The 1997 revisions did not affect print ads. In early 2004, however, the FDA began a process of revising its guidelines for print advertisements. This process was still in progress when this book went to press.

21. IMS Health, "Total U.S. Promotional Spending by Type: 1996–2002," accessed at www.imshealth.com/ims/portal/front/articleC/0,2777,6652_44304752_44889690,00.html, on November 2, 2004.

22. United States General Accounting Office, "Prescription Drugs: FDA Oversight of Direct-to-Consumer Advertising Has Limitations," Washington, DC: USGAO, October 2002, pp. 1–34, accessed at www.gao.gov/new.items/d03177.pdf on November 2, 2004.

23. AD2000 Collaborative Group, "Long-Term Donepezil Treatment," *Lancet* 363 (June 26, 2004): 2114.

24. Joseph Glenmullen, M.D., *Prozac Backlash* (New York: Simon & Schuster, 2000): 229–30.

25. "Anticholinesterases in Alzheimer's Disease: A Modest Effect on Moderately Severe Disease," *Prescrire International* 68, no. 12 (December 2003): 230–31.

26. AD2000 Collaborative Group, "Long-Term Donepezil Treatment in 565 Patients with Alzheimer's Disease: Randomized Double-Blind Trial," *Lancet* 363 (June 26, 2004), 2105–15.

27. Maryann Napoli, "How to Read a Drug Ad," Center for Medical Consumers, December 2001, accessed at www.medicalconsumers.org/pages/newsletter_articles.html#howtoreadadrugad on November 2, 2004.

28. Member groups are the Boston Women's Health Book Collective, Breast Cancer Action, Breast Cancer Action Montreal, the Center for Medical Consumers, DES Action, Massachusetts Breast Cancer Coalition, National Women's Health Network, Women's Community Cancer Project, and Women and Health Protection (Canada). See "Prevention First—FDA Testimony, May 23, 2001," accessed at www.bcaction.org/Pages/LearnAboutUs/PreventionFirst.html on November 2, 2004.

29. Food and Drug Administration, Department of Health and Human Services, "Memo re Nolvadex (tamoxifen citrate)," July 20, 2000, accessed at www.fda.gov/cder/warn/july2000/dd9075.pdf on November 2, 2004.

30. Gregory Pence, *Who's Afraid of Human Cloning?* (Lanham, MD: Rowman & Littlefield, 1998), 168.

31. Shaoni Bhattacharya, "Stupidity Should Be Cured, Says DNA Discoverer," *NewScientist.com* 18:13 (February 28, 2003), accessed at www.newscientist.com/news/news.jsp?id=ns99993451 on October 29, 2004.

32. Lee Silver, *Remaking Eden: Cloning and Beyond in a Brave New World* (New York: Avon Books, 1997), 4–7, 11.

33. Population Reference Bureau, "2004 World Population Data Sheet," accessed at www.prb.org/pdf04/04WorldDataSheet_Eng.pdf on November 2, 2004.

34. Elizabeth Arias, "United States Life Tables 2001," *National Vital Statistics Reports* 52, no. 14 (February 18, 2004): 1–39, accessed at www.cdc.gov/nchs/data/nvsr/nvsr52/nvsr52_14.pdf on November 2, 2004.

35. Teresa Castro Martin and Fatima Juarez, "The Impact of Women's Education on Fertility in Latin America: Searching for Explanations," *Family Planning Perspectives*, June 1995, accessed at www.agi-usa.org/pubs/journals/2105295.html on November 2, 2004.

36. Population Resource Center, "Motherhood in the U.S.," accessed at www.prcdc.org.

37. Population Reference Bureau, "2004 World Population Data Sheet," accessed at www.prb.org/pdf04/04WorldDataSheet_Eng.pdf on November 2, 2004.

38. Maternal Mortality in 2000, estimates developed by WHO, UNICEF, and UNFPA, accessed at www.unfpa.org/upload/lib_pub_file/237_filename_maternal_mortality_2000.pdf, on November 5, 2004.

39. "Maternal Mortality in Afghanistan: Magnitude, Causes, Risk Factors, and Preventability," UNICEF, CDC, Afghan Ministry of Health, accessed at www.afghana.com/Articles/maternalmortalityafghanistan.doc on November 5, 2004.

40. "Global Employment Trends for Women, 2004," International Labour Organization, accessed at http://kilm.ilo.org/GET2004/DOWNLOAD/trendsw.pdf on November 3, 2004.

41. "Women's Contributions to Agricultural Production and Food Security: Current Status and Perspectives," Food and Agriculture Organization of the United Nations, accessed at www.fao.org/docrep/X0198E/x0198e02.htm#P166_12601 on November 3, 2004.

42. Eve Crowley, "Women's Right to Land and Natural Resources: Some Implications for a Human Rights–Based Approach," Food and Agriculture Organization of the United Nations, posted in 1999, accessed at www.fao.org/sd/LTdirect/LTan0025.htm on November 3, 2004.

43. Jacques du Guerny, "Gender, Land and Fertility—Women's Access to Land and Security of Tenure," Food and Agriculture Organization of the United Nations, March 1996, accessed at www.fao.org/sd/wpdirect/wpan0001.htm on November 3, 2004.

44. "The Four Global Women's Conferences 1975–1995: Historical Perspective," Division for the Advancement of Women, United Nations, May 2000, accessed at www.un.org/womenwatch/daw/followup/session/presskit/hist.htm on November 3, 2004.

45. Millennium Development Goals, accessed at www.developmentgoals.com/Gender_Equality.htm on November 3, 2004.

46. United Nations Statistics Division, May 2004, accessed at http://unstats.un.org/unsd/mi/mi_goals.asp on November 3, 2004.

47. "Working to Empower Women, Women and the Economy," United Nations Population Fund, accessed at www.unfpa.org/intercenter/beijing/economy.htm on November 3, 2004.

48. International Labour Organization, "Women in the Informal Sector and Their Access to Microfinance," April 1998, accessed at www.ilo.org/public/english/employment/ent/papers/women.htm on November 3, 2004.

49. Ibid.

50. WHO Reproductive Health Plan of Work 2002–2003, accessed at www.who.int/reproductive-health/hrp/plan_of_work/fplanning.en.html.

51. "Breaking the Silence: The Global Gag Rule's Impact on Unsafe Abortions," Center for Reproductive Rights, 2003, accessed at www.crtp.org/pdf/pdf_GGR_impact_1003B.pdf on November 3, 2004.

52. International Labour Organization, "Sex Industry Assuming Massive Proportions in Southeast Asia: Economic Incentives and Hardships Fuel the Growth of the Sex Sector," August 1999, accessed at www.walnet.org/csis/reports/ilo-98-31.html on November 3, 2004.

53. "South-East Asia: Sex Industry Thrives, But States Look Away," InterPress News Service, August 19, 1998, accessed at www.aegis.com/news/ips/1998/IP980803.html on November 3, 2004.

54. "End Child Prostitution, Child Pornography and Trafficking of Children for Sexual Purposes (ECPAT)," accessed at www.ecpat.net/eng/index.asp on November 3, 2004.

55. Liz Kelly and June Kane, "Taking Stock: Progress in Europe and Central Asia Since the First World Congress Against Commercial Sexual Exploitation of Children (Stockholm 1996)," UNICEF Draft Paper in preparation for UNICEF 2nd World Congress Against Sexual Exploitation of Children (November 2001), accessed at www.unicef.org/events/yokohama/summary-csec-europe-centralasia.html on November 5, 2004.

56. "Gender and Sexual Health: Overview and Lessons Learned," Reproductive Health Outlook, accessed at www.rho.org/html/gsh_overview.htm on November 5, 2004.

57. Amnesty International, "Zimbabwe: Assault and Sexual Violence by Militia," April 5, 2002, accessed at www.amnestyusa.org/library/Index/ENGAFR460322002?open&of-ENG-ZWE.htm l on November 5, 2004. See also Amnesty International, "Sierra Leone: Rape and Other Forms of Sexual Violence Against Girls and Women," June 30, 2000, accessed at www.amnestyusa.org/library/Index/ENGAFR510482000?open&of-ENG-SLE on November 5, 2004; and Amnesty International, "Marked for Death: Rape Survivors Living with HIV/AIDS in Rwanda," April 6, 2004, accessed at www.amnestyusa.org/library/index/engafr470072004 on November 5, 2004.

58. "Female Genital Mutilation," World Health Organization, June 2000, accessed at www.who.int/mediacentre/factsheets/fs241/en/ on November 5, 2004.

59. "Abandoning Female Genital Cutting: Prevalence, Attitudes, and Efforts to End the Practice," Population Reference Bureau, accessed at www.prb.org/pdf/AbandoningFGC_Eng.pdf on November 5, 2004.

60. Gillian Wee, "Muslim Rite Is Modernized," *Toronto Star,* November 16, 2002, LI2. Accessed at http://static_highbeam.com/+/thetorontostar/november162002/muslimriteismodernized/index.html on November 3, 2004.

61. Dragoslaw Avramovic, "Occasional Paper 3: Developing Countries in the International Economic System.

Part I: International Financial Market, Poor Countries, and Poor People," *Human Development Report,* 1992, accessed at http://hdr.undp.org/docs/publications/ocational_papers/oc3a.htm on November 5, 2004.

62. The International Monetary Fund Global Policy Forum, accessed at www.globalpolicy.org/socecon/bwi-wto/imfind.htm on November 5, 2004.

63. See the Center for Policy Analysis on Trade and Health, www.cpath.org.

CHAPTER 32 ▪ ▪ ▪ ▪ ▪ ▪ ▪ ▪ ▪ ▪ ▪ ▪ ▪ ▪ ▪ ▪ ▪

For years, a San Francisco Bay area woman with breast cancer sought information about the causes and treatment of her disease. She consistently encountered unresponsive government agencies and other organizations that provided inadequate, superficial information, rather than hard data. She grew angry and shared that anger with other women in her breast cancer support group. In the summer of 1990, they formed Breast Cancer Action (BCA), a grassroots organization of breast cancer survivors and their supporters.

The woman's name was Elenore Pred, and Breast Cancer Action, the organization she helped to found, now has more than eleven thousand supporters across the country. It has received national media attention for being at the forefront of the breast cancer activist movement. BCA is a classic example of organizing that started with one woman and grew to be part of a strong movement. Its motto, "Do Something Besides Worry," could be the motto for any individual or group ready to take action.

We are usually motivated by something that affects us personally. We may be concerned about our own health or that of our family and friends. We may be concerned about our neighborhoods, schools, libraries, or environment. Women in positions of power are not the only ones able to create change. Women in prison, older women, and low-income women have all been able to make an impact through organizing. While working for social justice can be difficult in an era when conservative political forces wield much influence and financial resources are scarce, working together on a common issue can give us power and enable us to be effective.

Community organizing does not take experts or a lot of money. What it does take is a committed group of individuals willing to invest time and energy to work together toward a common goal. Can one woman make a difference? Yes! In fact, a far-reaching campaign is often started by just one person taking action. Activism can be writing a letter, making a phone call, or sending an e-mail. It is amazing how empowering these simple steps can be. However, creating change on a larger level takes many voices. Sometimes, after we have taken a few steps on our own, we may go on to get involved with groups working for change.

GETTING TOGETHER

Once a group starts to meet, the need for information and taking effective action generates its own energy and fuels enthusiasm. Many questions come up about how to proceed. Here are some questions that may be helpful to ask:

- Can we clearly define our issue?
- What do we already know about the issue? What don't we know? What research has already been done? By whom?
- What will be the scope of our work? Do we have enough people to manage the work we want to do?
- Are there organizations or individuals already working on the problem? If so, how can we work together?
- How many women are affected? Are the women most affected involved in efforts to create solutions?
- Who and what are the opposition? How are they supported/funded?
- What approaches to the problem are we considering? What resources are needed to accomplish them? Where will we find the needed resources?
- How will our group be organized? What will be our group norms on inclusiveness, diversity, decision making, and logistics?

The answers to these questions will help you formulate your plan. Think of a specific goal; for example, that the insurance company agrees to change its practices on covering certain procedures. You may use various methods to try to reach that goal: for example, using the media, contacting policy makers, or organizing consumer boycotts.

PRINCIPLES OF SUCCESSFUL ORGANIZING

Many models of organizing exist, but most contain common elements. Toxics Action Center (www.toxicsaction.org), an organization in New England that works with community groups to fight toxic pollution in their communities, has outlined six principles for successful organizing:

1. **Set achievable goals.** Make sure the group agrees on its goals. When setting achievable goals, differentiate your long-term goals from your short-term goals. Long-term goals are what you ultimately want to achieve; short-term goals are smaller steps along the way that will ultimately lead to your overall, long-term goals. Sometimes achieving a smaller goal that is more doable can be important for creating group identity internally and in the public eye.

2. **Secure the support of the community.** Democracy still works. When the community is on your side, you are more likely to be successful. As you work to gain support of the many people in your neighborhood, town, or other group, consider both quantity (demonstrating a large amount of public support) and quality (demonstrating support of specific influential people in your community).

3. **Build your group as you run your campaign.** A strong group lends legitimacy to your project and provides more resources to implement your tactics. Use opportunities along the way to bring in new people and build leadership. Your group should be stronger at the end of your project than it was when you started. Trust and support your new members in taking on tasks. Some groups have a core of activists that becomes hard to enter, and new people do not feel welcome or able to get involved. Avoid this common pitfall.

4. **Escalate your campaign over time.** Begin your project with simple steps and then build momentum over time. A letter to the editor of the local newspaper or a community meeting at the local library can generate new ideas and supporters. The next step may be a meeting with a local policy maker to gain his or her support and insight into ways to make change. Each opportunity will create new energy and broaden your support.

5. **Craft a message using the four C's.** In order to be successful, you will need to tell your story in such a way that any reasonable person has only one choice—to side with you. Your story should have a *c*oncise, *c*ompelling, and *c*onsistent message that *c*ontrols the issue.

6. **Evaluate.** Take time to step back and evaluate your plan periodically. Are you still on the right track to achieve your goals? Do you need to switch targets or change tactics? For example, has your opposition addressed some of your concerns but not all of them? Have you found another group challenging the same opposition? The evaluation process is an important opportunity for your group to talk through your responses to these questions and what they mean for your effort, and to formulate the best way to move ahead.*

You can adapt this or a similar model to fit your specific organizing effort.

RESOURCES AND TACTICS

Many grassroots change efforts share common tactics: getting publicity through media, using the Internet, contacting people inside government and health institutions, direct lobbying, coalition building, and fund-raising.

THE MEDIA

Knowing when and how to get media publicity when we need it is essential to our efforts to bring about change, since most people get information from TV, radio, the Internet, newspapers, and magazines. The media can be an effective tool for gaining public support, recruiting new members, and pressuring decision makers to listen to our concerns.

* Text adapted with permission from training materials produced by Toxics Action Center entitled "Campaign Planning."

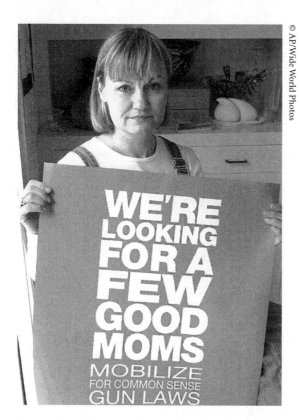

Donna Dees-Thomases, the driving force behind the Million Mom March, holds a poster for the gun control event at her home in Short Hills, New Jersey. The march was intended to pressure Congress to enact tougher gun control laws.

In our group, very few women had experience speaking publicly to or before the media. So we set aside some meetings to role-play, to practice speaking before a group, and to learn how to say the most important things in the least amount of time. We also practiced saying the things we wanted people to hear, even if they were not related to the interviewer's question. Doing all this is a great way to break through shyness and stage fright.

Marketing experts say that people need to see or hear a message seven times before it is clearly taken in and understood. Make sure you put out a consistent message and plan the num-

ber of times various people in your community will have the opportunity to see and hear it; for example, once from a poster, twice in a public service announcement, twice in the local newspaper, and twice via e-mail alerts.

THE INTERNET

The Internet has rapidly become a key tool in organizing. Never before have we had such a simple and quick way to connect people with similar interests and concerns. Many resources are available for creating free websites, sending e-mail petitions, and posting notices. An excellent example of organizing over the Internet is MoveOn.org, an electronic advocacy group that claims more than 2 million online activists. Your group may start small.

E-mail has been a powerful tool for community building in Boston. I have a list geared toward queer women. . . . We send information about queer and progressive political actions, benefit parties, and cultural events. We also provide space for roommate, job, and creative classifieds. My goal is to create linkages between political, artistic, and social communities and to assist them with outreach. . . . My advice to organizers is to have a clearly defined mission and to make participation as easy as possible ([while] requiring as few keystrokes as possible).

ALLIES INSIDE GOVERNMENT AND HEALTH INSTITUTIONS

Those working within the establishment can be useful sources of information about upcoming meetings, new legislation or policy making, proposals for new technologies, or studies and can help us develop strategies for achieving specific goals. Sometimes these contacts can offer invaluable advice about how to best approach a key official. By offering assistance from the "in-

GET YOUR MESSAGE OUT

This list, adapted with permission from the *Citizen's Handbook* (2003) by the Vancouver Citizen's Committee, outlines simple steps for getting your message out to the general public.

- **Find the media professionals in your community.** Seek help from the people in your community who work for newspapers, radio, and television stations. Seek advice from groups you think have been successful in using the media for their cause.

- **Define your objective and then your messages.** Use your objective to create a clear message. For example, if your objective is to prevent further erosion of reproductive rights at the state legislature, your message might be "I'm pro-choice, and I vote."

- **Make actions newsworthy.** To get media attention, you need to tell a good, current story with a human focus.

- **Link actions to other news events.** Your actions are more likely to get covered if they tie in to other events in the news, such as government announcements, holidays, local conferences, world events, and hot issues.

- **Send out news releases.** Send out a news release if you have fresh information you wish to publicize. Follow-up calls to the media after sending a news release are critical to getting the media to cover your story.

- **Aim at TV.** Some of the most effective citizens' groups get TV coverage by staging events that provide action and good pictures.

- **Practice your message.** Practice what you want to say before the event. Make it short, catchy, and memorable.

- **Don't forget radio.** If you can get on a live radio show, you will not be edited as you would on TV or in the newspaper.

- **Write a letter to the editor.** Writing a letter to the editor of a community newspaper is an easy way to get publicity. To improve the chances that your letter will be published, check the newspaper's guidelines for letters.

- **Consider other kinds of announcements.** Community bulletin boards run by radio and some cable stations can announce your event. Public service announcements on radio and TV offer another opportunity.

- **Consider alternative media.** Consider using printed T-shirts, buttons, window signs, posters, bumper stickers, flyers, e-mail networks, and the newsletters of other groups.

(For more information, see the *Citizen's Handbook* at www.vcn.bc.ca/citizens-handbook.)

side," these women and men can make significant contributions to our causes.

LOBBYING

Contacting legislators and key officials about specific legislation, institutional policies, and regulatory proposals, either in person or through letter writing, is an effective way to influence change. Contact policy makers as a group or as private individuals, and point out why your position is in the best interests of the official's constituents. Be persistent in trying to reach these busy people. Sometimes you have to start by speaking with a legislative aide or an assistant who will facilitate reaching the official. It is also important to thank officials for their efforts on your behalf. A letter to the editor of your local newspaper will both publicly achieve that purpose and get your message out to the community.

FORMING COALITIONS

By forming coalitions so that more groups and individuals support and work together on the same cause, you can increase public influence as well as establish stronger bonds for future collaboration. Coalitions can provide an excellent means of exchanging new information and ideas, comparing different strategies for change, and even creating a larger organization or movement. It is critical for a coalition to clarify its focus, establish decision-making guidelines, and maintain open lines of communication among its members.

FUND-RAISING

Many of us are uncomfortable asking for money. However, money is one of the resources we need to create positive social change in our communities. Our issues are important and deserve resources.

An increasing number of small foundations and grant-making organizations are recognizing the need to support grassroots organizing. In other words, you do not have to be an established nonprofit organization to get funding for a project. Securing grant money for your project can cover costs involved in printing, faxing, mailings, and holding meetings. Get to know your local community foundations. Research foundations with an interest in your issue at your local library, at a foundation center, or on the Internet. In-kind contributions from community groups, faith-based organizations, and labor unions that care about your issue are another option.

EXAMPLES OF ORGANIZING FOR CHANGE

Other groups that are organizing for change can offer ideas for your group. The following are some examples of recent organizing efforts, each with its own challenges and successes.

YOUNG WOMEN ORGANIZING

For many activists, our first experience with organizing was when we were teenagers or even younger. Attending a march or rally, running for student government, or joining a club may have been our initial opportunity to work together for change.

For those of us who continue education after high school, whether at community colleges or at universities, there are numerous opportunities to get involved in change projects. Many of us are inspired to take the idea of equality beyond women's studies or political science classrooms and into our campus communities.

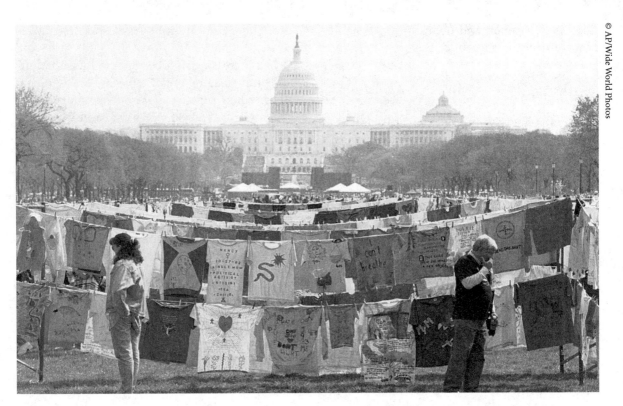

T-shirts hang on the Mall in Washington, D.C., as part of the Clothesline Project's campaign to break the silence about violence against women. Each shirt bears artwork or a personal story by a woman who experienced domestic abuse, rape, incest, or other act of violence.

One of the most effective ways to build a feminist campus environment is to get support from established national organizations. The Feminist Majority's Feminist Majority Leadership Alliance, Planned Parenthood's Vox: Voices for Planned Parenthood, and NARAL Pro-Choice America's campus chapters have all dramatically increased the level of college activism in recent years. These groups provide a chance for students to connect with larger movements and to build on the efforts of women before us. Students can also take advantage of internships that such organizations offer.

Whether or not students choose to start a chapter of a national organization or an independent local group, much can be done. Meaningful issues at the college level include emergency contraception availability, body image, voter registration, violence against women, and reproductive rights. We can coordinate candlelight vigils, speak-outs, and consciousness-raising groups, and develop forums for discussion. As with all organizing, people are the most valuable resource. Other campus groups, faculty, and alumni can also be allies.

A recent college graduate reflects on her experiences organizing on campus:

As one of the first women's colleges in the country, my college prides itself on cultivating strong female leaders committed to building a better world. Yet when the school's housekeepers, most of whom are women, started organizing a union to improve their working conditions and demand

*respect and dignity, this same college opposed
their campaign.*

*As part of the Student Coalition for Action, I
helped support the housekeepers' union drive.
Our group knew the administration would feel
more pressure with student support behind the
housekeepers. We worked hard to educate students
and faculty about low-wage women's work and
the right to organize. In 2001 the housekeepers
voted in favor of a union and won their first
contract.*

*Since then, students and other workers have
established a passionate campus dialogue about
fair labor standards and the values of our college.
Four of the housekeepers who are now members of
the union wrote in a statement: "Why do we have
to continually fight . . . to get respect and dignity
and fair treatment? This should be a given at a
progressive women's college."*

*Working with the housekeepers and getting to
know them personally has shaped my feminism as
much as any class or theory. After they told me
about their negative experiences as women working on a very feminist-oriented college campus, I
realized that even institutions driven by a vision
of social justice need policies and checks and bal-
ances to ensure that their practices really match
their message. We must be constantly striving to
make our own actions and institutions more re-
flective of the values we hold.*

Although college campuses provide a unique
setting for easy access to others with similar interests and a desire to get involved, there are
many other ways for young women to initiate or
join in organizing efforts. Those of us who work
or have other obligations after leaving formal
schooling may be able to get involved in organizing through community groups, workplaces,
and church groups.

CHALLENGING MAINSTREAM SCIENCE AND INDUSTRY: BREAST CANCER ACTION

Breast cancer is a growing epidemic; one in
seven of us will have breast cancer at some point
in our lives. In the last several years, the fight
against breast cancer has become a popular
cause. Walks, runs, and fund-raisers exist in
every major city in the U.S. Breast Cancer Action
(BCA), described at the beginning of this chapter, has been successful because it has used this
growing public interest to challenge the cancer
industry—that is, hospitals, pharmaceutical
companies, research institutes, and other organizations—and insist on increased focus on prevention.

In the past, women often were not empowered to ask questions, particularly when it came
to challenging physicians and scientists. Now
there are more forums in which we can ask questions about our health. For example, through organizations like BCA, we are encouraged to ask
questions about scientific studies based on existing evidence, how a study is designed, and who is
paying for the research. Women may also choose
to get a second opinion or seek out alternative
care options for ourselves and our families.

An increasing number of groups are starting
to ask questions about the environmental links
to diseases such as cancer and asthma and problems with infertility. We are taking a closer look
at industry and government regulations, to see
what is safe for our food, water, and air. Another
example of challenging the mainstream is seen
in one coalition of breast cancer organizations,
Follow the Money: An Alliance for Accountability in Breast Cancer. Follow the Money asks people to question where our money goes when we
support a breast cancer event. How much of the
money raised actually goes to supporting breast
cancer organizations? Does the sponsor of the
event consult the local community about the

distribution of money raised through the event? Does the sponsor have good environmental practices, so as not to benefit from promoting the fight against breast cancer while at the same time possibly contributing to the problem? (For example, do a cosmetics company's products contain toxins that may be linked to breast cancer?)

Asking such questions and getting involved in efforts to find the answers are helpful for some of us who are struggling with our own illnesses. One fifty-five-year-old recalls how meeting and working with other women transformed her experience:

I was first diagnosed with breast cancer in September of 1991 at the age of 42. I was angry, depressed and hopelessly paralyzed. I was certain that I would die—never to see my children grow up. Within two months, I found a small group of women who were meeting at a coffee shop in my neighborhood. What began as a support group turned into a call to action. I recall bringing homemade petitions to the group and asking people to sign letters to senators, representatives and even the president of the United States asking for more money for research. We found women in other support groups who were also wanting to mobilize—to channel our anger and our energy. We started to talk about things like environmental exposures and prevention. . . . As I think back to those first years, I remember clearly the faces of the women in those groups. Some are still alive, many are not. Now, it is clear to me how much becoming active in a movement was a vital piece of my getting through treatment and getting well again. For this I am eternally grateful.

For more information, visit Breast Cancer Action at www.bcaction.org.

WOMEN OF COLOR: SISTERLOVE, INC.

SisterLove, Inc., was founded by an African-American woman in her late twenties in July 1989. It started as a volunteer group of women interested in educating Atlanta, Georgia, and especially Atlanta's women of color, about AIDS prevention, self-help, and safer-sex techniques. Today SisterLove runs health education, advocacy, housing, and support services in metropolitan Atlanta. Since 1999, SisterLove also has been working in South Africa to combat the spread of HIV/AIDS.

SisterLove's Bridge Leadership Program tries to integrate the issues of HIV/AIDS, sexual and reproductive health, and human rights. Through both formal and informal collaboration, SisterLove provides opportunities to network, share training, and develop culturally appropriate programs at the grassroots level.

SisterLove founder Dázon Dixon Diallo, now forty-three, reflects on her work:

After over 18 years in the AIDS and reproductive health movements I am still humbled by the people who step forward, who make a personal commitment to make a difference in our communities. They remind me of my own choice and the reasons why I began, and continue, this important work. . . . We must work together and not give in to those who would rather see us fight amongst ourselves and compete for dwindling dollars and resources. We must look beyond our own backyard and understand the larger picture, the greater implication and meaning of human struggles everywhere. . . . Our struggle is part of THE struggle for human dignity and quality of life.

WOMEN IN PRISON: CHICAGO LEGAL ADVOCACY FOR INCARCERATED MOTHERS

When Joanne Archibald was a pregnant college student, she was arrested on drug charges. She remained out on bail until her son was seven months old, and was then sent to federal prison for a year. Even though she was one of the lucky few allowed brief visits with her children while incarcerated, the separation was devastating.

Today, nineteen years later, Joanne Archibald directs the Advocacy Project at Chicago Legal Advocacy for Incarcerated Mothers (CLAIM). One program of the Advocacy Project is Visible Voices, a support and empowerment group run by and for formerly incarcerated women. In support groups, women tell their stories, learn from one another, and shed the invisibility of former and current women prisoners.

The Advocacy Project believes that incarcerating women is an inappropriate and ineffective response to profound social problems such as poverty, racism, childhood sexual abuse, and mental illness. The project works to change laws and policies regarding family preservation and reproductive rights, and it advocates for alternatives to incarceration. In 2000 it convinced the Illinois legislature to prohibit the shackling of women prisoners while in labor.

The Advocacy Project recently collaborated with Beyondmedia Education to produce two videos on the experiences of women in prison. *What We Leave Behind*, which was created entirely by formerly incarcerated women, and *Voices in Time* are available from Beyondmedia Education (www.beyondmedia.org/vv.html).

INTERNATIONAL ORGANIZING: MADRE

In 1983 a group of female activists, poets, teachers, artists, and health professionals traveled to Nicaragua to witness the impact of the U.S.-sponsored contra war. They saw day care centers, schools, and clinics that had been bombed by contras supported by the U.S. government. The experience horrified and angered them. These women returned to the U.S. with a mandate from the women of Nicaragua: to bring the stories of Nicaraguan women and children to the attention of the U.S. public and to mobilize people to demand a change in U.S. government policy.

MADRE's founding director, Kathy Engel, and the women she brought together had a vision of a women-led, women-run organization, dedicated to informing people in the U.S. about the effects of American policies on communities around the world. MADRE resolved to build real alternatives to war and violence by supporting the priorities of like-minded organizations and linking them to the needs of women and families in the U.S. through a people-to-people exchange of direct relief and understanding.

Today MADRE is an international women's rights organization that works in partnership with women's community-based groups in conflict areas worldwide. Its programs address issues of sustainable development, community improvement, and women's health; violence and war; discrimination and racism; self-determination and collective rights; women's leadership development; and human rights education. MADRE provides resources and training to enable organizations to meet immediate needs in their communities and develop long-term solutions to crises. Since it began, MADRE has delivered over $20 million worth of support to community-based women's groups in Latin America, the Caribbean, the Middle East, Africa, the countries of the former Yugoslavia, and the United States. (For more information see MADRE's website, www.madre.org.)

MOVING FORWARD

Each of the well-established organizations described above started with one or two people acting on their concerns. Many such efforts remain small and grassroots, but every effort offers the potential for successes, both small and large.

Feminist activists have become known for organizing with a vision for fundamental social change. Not only are we concerned about the immediate problems having to do with our health, neighborhoods, or environment, but we also work to change perceptions, stereotypes, power structures, and patriarchal traditions. We share a common vision of a future of fairness and equality. To make this vision a reality, we must create change by working together.

Why do I keep at it year after year, when progress seems so slow? . . . Knowing what I know about the injustices pervading our society and seeing how racism and sexism ruin the lives of so many, especially women, how could I not contribute at least some of my time and energy to efforts that might change the status quo? It seems immoral not to do so. As long as I don't push myself too much or forget about my own and my family's day-to-day needs, the work I do enriches my whole life.

Absorptiometry = a technique that measures the density or mass of a material (bone or fat) by comparing the amounts of x-radiation of two different energies that it absorbs

Acute effect = a severe immediate reaction, usually after a single, large exposure, such as nausea and dizziness from pesticide poisoning or blistering of air sacs in the lungs from toxic gases such as ammonia or chlorine

Adenosis = abnormal proliferation or occurrence of glandular tissue

Androgen = a hormone that produces male secondary sexual characteristics (such as hair growth, deep voice, and development of the penis)

Anemia = lack of red blood cells

Antibodies = proteins produced by the immune system that build resistance to antigens

Anticholinergics = drugs that block the action of certain substances in nerve fibers

Antigens = foreign substances inside the body that provoke attack by the immune system

Antihistamines = drugs that relieve certain symptoms of allergic reactions and colds

Antioxidant = a substance that inhibits combining with oxygen (oxidation, which can cause damage)

Asphyxiant = a substance or gas that cuts off breathing

Bartholin's glands = glands that secrete a lubricating mucus, located on either side of the lower part of the vagina

Biodegradable = able to break down into harmless substances by the action of living things

Bioethical = related to the ethical implications of biology and medicine

Bisphosphonates = a class of drugs that prevents bone breakdown

Carcinogen = a substance or agent that causes cancer, a condition characterized by usually rapidly spreading abnormal cell growth

Cardiovascular = concerning the heart and blood vessels

Cerclage = surgical treatment to keep the cervix closed after cone biopsy has weakened it

Cervix = the base of the uterus, located at the upper end of the vagina

Chlamydia = a sexually transmitted microorganism that can cause pelvic inflammatory disease

Cholesterol = a type of fat in the blood; combines with a protein to form lipoproteins that carry the fat to cells; high-density lipoprotein

(HDL) is the "good" cholesterol, and low-density lipoprotein (LDL) is the "bad" cholesterol that clogs arteries

Chronic effect = a recurrent or constant reaction, usually occurring after repeated smaller exposures; chronic effects can take years to develop or be detected, such as lung disease caused by asbestos; most cancers and progressive liver diseases are found fifteen to forty years after exposure

Circumcision = surgical removal of the prepuce (foreskin) of the penis or hood of the clitoris

Clitoris = the most sensitive spot in female genital area; swells during arousal

Collagen = a fibrous protein in connective tissue, including skin

Contagious = catching (as a disease), passed from one person to another

Contraceptive = a substance or device that prevents conception (birth control)

Diaphragm = a rubber cap inserted in the vagina to cover the cervix and keep sperm out, for birth control

Dams, dental = thin rubber squares used as a barrier against body fluids

Ectopic = outside its normal location, as an ectopic (tubal) pregnancy outside the uterus

Emphysema = a lung disease affecting the air spaces inside the lungs; causes shortness of breath

Endometrial = related to the lining of the uterus

Endometritis = inflammation of the uterine lining

Endometrium = lining of the uterus

Epidemic = an outbreak of disease among a large number of individuals within a population, community, or region at the same time

Epididymis = the structure on the testicle that stores sperm

Epithelium = the upper tissue layer of the skin or an internal organ

Estrogen = a hormone that regulates development of sexual organs, characteristics, and function

Fibrocystic = a catchall term for noncancerous lumps of fibro-glandular breast tissue; may be used to describe different types of lumps

Fibroids = benign growths, usually in, on, or around the uterus

Gastrointestinal = concerning the digestive tract (especially the stomach and intestines)

Hematocrit = a lab test to count red blood cells

Hormone = a substance in the body that sends messages to distant cells

Hyperthyroidism = overactivity of the thyroid

Hypothalamus = the structure in the brain that controls or regulates automatic functions such as sleep/wakefulness, body temperature, and water balance

Hypothyroidism = underactivity of the thyroid

Incarceration = imprisonment

Infibulation = sewing the lips of the vulva together

Lactobacilli = a type of bacteria living normally in the intestines; a bacteria used to start yogurt cultures

Lesions = wounds, injuries to skin or organs

Ligaments = tissues that connect and support bones and organs

Lipoprotein = a complex of protein and fat; carries fat through the blood to the cells

Lubrication = the process of reducing friction, making a surface slippery

Lymphedema = swelling of lymph nodes

Melatonin = a hormone that regulates concentration of pigment (color) in skin; also affects sleep

Microorganisms = living things too small to see except under a microscope

Mutagen = a substance or agent that causes mutations in the genetic material of living cells; when a mutation occurs in the egg or sperm, it can be passed on to future generations, and because genetic material controls the growth of cells, mutagens may cause abnormal cell growth that becomes cancer—either immediately or later

Neurotransmitters = substances that carry messages to and from the nerves

Nutrients = substances that nourish the body; found in food and supplements

Ob-gyn = abbreviation of obstetrician-gynecologist, a doctor specializing in female organs, pregnancy, and childbirth

Ombudsman = an official who receives, investigates, and settles complaints

Organic compound = a mixture based on carbon; derived from living things

Organic food (produce) = food grown or made without any chemicals added to it, to the soil it grows in, or to animal feed

Orphan drug = a drug produced with U.S. government support to treat a rare disease

Osteoporosis = condition of thin, brittle bones

Pessary = a rubber cap, inserted in the vagina to cover the cervix

pH = balance of acidity and alkalinity, expressed by a numerical scale

Pituitary = the gland in the brain that controls growth

PMS = premenstrual syndrome, caused by hormone changes; may include mood swings, irritability, insomnia, depression, headache, bloated feeling, cramps

Polyps = benign intestinal growths

Postpartum = after childbirth

Progestin/progestagen = a substance (natural or synthetic) that acts like progesterone

Progesterone = the female sex hormone that prepares the uterus for pregnancy

Prolapse = a condition in which the uterus or bladder drops from the pelvis into the vagina

Prostaglandins = substances that function like hormones to control certain processes in the body

Prophylactic = preventive

Pyelonephritis = infection of the kidneys resulting from bladder infection

Resveratrol = a substance in some plants, fruits, and seeds that may reduce risk of cancer and coronary artery disease

SERMs = selective estrogen receptor modulators, a class of drugs that change or block the action of estrogen in some parts of the body

Skene's glands = small glands in the female urethra, near its opening

Solvent = a liquid in which another substance dissolves

Specimen = sample

Speculum = a metal or plastic instrument used to hold the vagina open during pelvic examination

Spermicide = a substance that kills sperm

Sphincter = muscles that keep the anus closed

Steroids = a class of chemical compounds that includes hormones and effects various changes in the tissues and organs

Synovium = the membrane that lines and lubricates a joint

Teratogen = a substance or agent that can cross the placenta of a pregnant woman and cause a spontaneous abortion or birth disabilities and developmental anomalies in the fetus; all carcinogens are mutagens, most mutagens are carcinogens, and many mutagens are also teratogens

Topical = used on a small area, as when cream is applied to the skin

Toxins = harmful substances (poisons, contaminants)

Tubal ligation = the surgery that ties a woman's fallopian tubes, to prevent pregnancy

Urethra = the tube that carries urine away from the bladder

Urology = the medical specialty concerned with the urinary mechanisms and organs

Sources

Berkow, R, ed. *Merck Manual of Medical Information* (New York: Pocket Books, 1997).

Merriam Webster's Collegiate Dictionary, 10th ed. (Springfield, MA: Merriam-Webster, 1994).

The National Library of Medicine, MedLinePlus online medical dictionary, www.nlm.nih.gov/medlineplus/mplusdictionary.html.

RESOURCES

CHAPTER 1: BODY IMAGE

For a longer list, please see the companion website, www.ourbodiesourselves.org.

Books

Brumberg, Joan Jacobs. *The Body Project: An Intimate History of American Girls.* New York: Vintage, 1998.

Fraser, Laura. *Losing It: False Hopes and Fat Profits in the Diet Industry.* New York: Plume, 1998.

Odes, Rebecca, Esther Drill, and Heather McDonald. *The Looks Book: A Whole New Approach to Beauty, Body Image, and Style.* New York: Penguin, 2002.

Peiss, Kathy. *Hope in a Jar: The Making of America's Beauty Culture.* New York: Metropolitan Books, 1998.

Periodicals

Bitch
1611 Telegraph Avenue, Suite 515, Oakland, CA 94612
877-21-BITCH
www.bitchmagazine.com

Teen Voices
888-882-TEEN
www.teenvoices.com

Organizations

About-Face
P.O. Box 77665, San Francisco, CA 94107
415-436-0212
www.about-face.org

Girls, Incorporated
120 Wall Street, New York, NY 10005
800-374-4475
www.girlsinc.org

Websites

Adios Barbie
www.adiosbarbie.com

Jean Kilbourne
www.jeankilbourne.com

CHAPTER 2: EATING WELL

For a longer list, please see the companion website, www.ourbodiesourselves.org.

Books

Nestle, Marion. *Food Politics: How the Food Industry Influences Nutrition and Health.* Berkeley, CA: University of California Press, 2002.

Richardson, Brenda Lane, and Elane Rehr. *101 Ways to Help Your Daughter Love Her Body.* New York: Harper-Collins, 2001.

Willett, Walter. *Eat, Drink, and Be Healthy.* New York: Simon & Schuster, 2001.

Wood, Rebecca. *The New Whole Foods Encyclopedia.* New York: Penguin, 1999.

Organizations

National Association of Nutrition Professionals
P.O. Box 971, Veradale, WA 99037-0971
800-342-8037
www.certifiednutritionist.com

National Eating Disorders Association
603 Stewart Street, Suite 803, Seattle, WA 98101
206-382-3587
www.nationaleatingdisorders.org

The Vegetarian Resource Group
P.O. Box 1463, Baltimore, MD 21203
410-366-8343
www.vrg.org

Organic Consumers Association
6101 Cliff Estate Road, Little Marais, MN 55614
218-226-4164
www.organicconsumers.org

Websites

Arbor Nutrition Guide
www.arborcom.com

The Food Allergy Network
www.foodallergy.org

CHAPTER 3: ALCOHOL, TOBACCO, AND OTHER MOOD-ALTERING DRUGS

For a longer list, please see the companion website, www.ourbodiesourselves.org.

Books

Action on Women's Addictions—Research and Education (AWARE). *Give and Take: A Booklet for Pregnant Women About Alcohol and Other Drugs.* Kingston, ON: AWARE, 1996. Available from www.aware.on.ca/frames.htm.

Covington, S. *A Woman's Way Through the Twelve Steps.* Center City, Minnesota: Hazelden Educational Materials, 1994. Available from www.hazelden.org.

National Institutes of Health. *Clearing the Air: How to Quit Smoking.* Washington, DC: National Cancer Institute, 1995. Available free from the National Cancer Institute, 800-422-6237.

Audiovisual Materials

Spin the Bottle: Sex, Lies and Alcohol, by Jean Kilbourne (45 minutes), 2004. Videocassette and DVD. Available from the Media Education Foundation, www.mediaed.org.

Organizations

Drug Policy Alliance
70 West 36th Street, 16th Floor, New York, NY 10018
212-613-8020
wwwdrugpolicy.org/communities/women/

National Institute on Drug Abuse, National Institutes of Health
6001 Executive Boulevard, Room 5213, Bethesda, MD 20892-9561
301-443-1124
www.drugabuse.gov/Infofax/treatwomen.html

Websites

Quitnet.com: Helping Smokers Quit
www.quitnet.com/q_corp/helpingsmokers.html

Center for Substance Abuse Treatment
800-487-4889 (TDD); 877-767-8432 (Spanish)
http://findtreatment.samhsa.gov

Benzodiazepine Addiction, Withdrawal and Recovery
www.benzo.org.uk

In the Mix (PBS television series for and by teens; episode on Ecstasy)
www.pbs.org/inthemix/ecstasy_index.html

CHAPTER 4: OUR BODIES IN MOTION

For a longer list, please see the companion website, www.ourbodiesourselves.org.

Books

Betancourt, Marian, and Nancy Lieberman-Cline. *Playing Like a Girl: Transforming Our Lives Through Team Sports.* New York: McGraw-Hill, 2002.

Griffin, Pat. *Strong Women, Deep Closets: Lesbians and Homophobia in Sports.* Champaign, IL: Human Kinetics, 1998.

Gottesman, Jane. *Game Face: What Does a Female Athlete Look Like?* New York: Random House, 2001.

Heywood, Leslie, Shari Dworkin, and Julie Foudy. *Built to Win: The Female Athlete as Cultural Icon.* Minneapolis, MN: University of Minnesota Press, 2003.

Organizations

National Black Women's Heath Imperative
600 Pennsylvania Avenue, S.E., Suite 310, Washington, DC 20003
202-548-4000
www.blackwomenshealth.org/site/PageServer?pagename=WFW Pledge

Stroller Strides
1531 Crescent Place, San Marcos, CA 92078
866-FIT-4-MOM
www.strollerstrides.com

Women's Sports Foundation
Eisenhower Park, East Meadow, NY 11554
800-227-3988
www.womenssportsfoundation.org

Adaptive Sports Organizations

Adaptive Sports Association
P.O. Box 1884, Durango, CO 81302
970-259-0374
www.asadurango.org

Special Olympics
1325 G Street, N.W., Suite 500, Washington, DC 20005
202-628-3630
www.specialolympics.org

Websites

Melpomene Institute
www.melpomene.org

CHAPTER 5: COMPLEMENTARY HEALTH PRACTICES

For a longer list, please see the companion website, www.ourbodiesourselves.org.

Books

Blumenthal, Mark, ed. *The ABC Clinical Guide to Herbs.* Austin, TX: American Botanical Council, 2003.

Domar, Alice, and Henry Dreher. *Healing Mind, Healthy Woman: Take Control of Your Well-Being Using the Mind-Body Connection.* New York: Henry Holt, 1996.

Frawley, David. *Ayurvedic Healing: A Comprehensive Guide.* Twin Lakes, WI: Lotus Press, 2000.

Fugh-Berman, Adriane. *Alternative Medicine: What Works.* Philadelphia: Lippincott, Williams and Wilkins, 1997.

Kaptchuk, Ted. *The Web That Has No Weaver: Understanding Chinese Medicine.* 2nd ed. New York: McGraw-Hill, 2000.

Lansky, Amy L. *The Promise of Homeopathy.* Portola Valley, CA: R. L. Ranch Press, 2003.

Reichenberg-Ullman, Judyth. *Whole Woman Homeopathy.* Roseville, CA: Prima Publishing, 2000.

CHAPTER 6: EMOTIONAL WELL-BEING

For a longer list, please see the companion website, www.ourbodiesourselves.org.

Books

Caplan, Paula, and Lisa Cosgrove. *Bias in Psychiatric Diagnosis.* Livingston, NJ: Jason Aronson, 2004.

Chesler, Phyllis. *Women and Madness.* Garden City, NY: Doubleday, 1972.

Glenmullen, Joseph. *Prozac Backlash: Overcoming the Dangers of Prozac, Zoloft, Paxil, and Other Antidepressants with Safe, Effective Alternatives.* New York: Simon & Schuster, 2001.

Herman, Judith. *Trauma and Recovery.* New York: Basic Books, 1992.

Johnstone, Lucy. *Users and Abusers of Psychiatry: A Critical Look at Psychiatric Practice.* London and Philadelphia: Brunner-Routledge/Taylor & Francis Group, 2000.

Jordan, Judith V., Maureen Walker, and Linda M. Hartling, eds. *The Complexity of Connection: Writings from the*

Jean Baker Miller Training Institute. New York: The Guilford Press, 2004.

Medawar, Charles, and Anita Hardon. *Medicines Out of Control? Antidepressants and the Conspiracy of Goodwill.* Amsterdam: Aksant Academic Publishers, 2004.

Miller, Jean Baker. *Toward a New Psychology of Women.* Boston: Beacon Press, 1986.

Unger, R. K., ed. *Handbook of the Psychology of Women and Gender.* New York: John Wiley & Sons, 2001.

Whitaker, Robert. *Mad in America: Bad Science, Bad Medicine, and the Enduring Mistreatment of the Mentally Ill.* Cambridge, MA: Perseus Books, 2002.

CHAPTER 7: ENVIRONMENTAL AND OCCUPATIONAL HEALTH

For a longer list, please see the companion website, www.ourbodiesourselves.org.

Books

Schettler, Ted, Gina Solomon, Marian Valenti, and Annette Huddle. *Generations at Risk: Reproductive Health and the Environment.* Cambridge, MA: MIT Press, 2000.

Steingraber, Sandra. *Having Faith: An Ecologist's Journey to Motherhood.* Cambridge, MA: Perseus, 2001.

Periodicals

New Solutions: A Journal of Environmental and Occupational Health Policy
New Solutions
P.O. Box 281200, Lakewood, CO 80228

Audiovisual Materials

Blue Vinyl, Judith Helfand, 2002. A video journey from home to workplace to corporate headquarters, to understand the impacts of polyvinylchloride on environmental health. Available from www.bluevinyl.org.

Organizations

Association of Occupational and Environmental Clinics
1010 Vermont Avenue, N.W. #513, Washington, DC 20005
202-347-4976 or 888-347-2632
www.aoec.org

Center for Health, Environment and Justice
P.O. Box 6806, Falls Church, VA 22040
703-237-2249
www.chej.org

Rachel's Environment and Health News, Environmental Research Foundation
P.O. Box 160, New Brunswick, NJ 08903-0160
732-828-9995 or 888-272-2435
www.rachel.org

Silent Spring Institute
29 Crafts Street, Newton, MA 02458
617-332-4288
www.silentspring.org

Women's Environment and Development Organization
355 Lexington Avenue, 3rd Floor, New York, NY 10017-6603
212-973-0325
www.wedo.org

Websites

National Council for Occupational Safety and Health (COSH)
www.coshnetwork.org

CHAPTER 8: VIOLENCE AND ABUSE

For a longer list, please see the companion website, www.ourbodiesourselves.org.

Books

Renzetti, Claire, Jeffrey Edleson, and Raquel Kennedy Bergen, eds. *Sourcebook on Violence Against Women.* Thousand Oaks, CA: Sage Publications, 2000.

Farley, Melissa, ed. *Prostitution, Trafficking, and Traumatic Stress.* Binghamton, NY: Haworth Press, 2003.

White, Evelyn. *Chain Change: For Black Women in Abusive Relationships.* Seattle: Seal Press, 1994.

Audiovisual Materials

Defending Our Lives, 1993. Oscar-winning documentary on domestic violence. Available from Cambridge Documentary Films, P.O. Box 390385, Cambridge, MA 02139; 617-484-3993; www.cambridgedocumentaryfilms.org.

No!, Aishah Shahidah Simmons, 2004. Documentary about

rape in the African-American community. Available from P.O. Box 58085, Philadelphia, PA 19102-8085; 215-557-8154; www.echosoul.com/aishah.htm.

Rape Is, 2002. A comprehensive look at rape. Distributed by Cambridge Documentary Films, P.O. Box 390385, Cambridge, MA 02139; 617-484-3993; www.cambridgedocumentaryfilms.org; accompanied by resource website www.rapeis.org.

Organizations

National Domestic Violence Hotline
P.O. Box 161810, Austin, TX 78716
800-799-7233 (SAFE) or 800-787-3224 (TTY)
www.ndvh.org/

Rape, Abuse & Incest National Network (RAINN)
Hotline for survivors of sexual assault: 800-656-HOPE
www.rainn.org

U.S. Department of Justice, Office on Violence Against Women
810 7th Street, N.W., Washington, DC 20531
202-307-6026 or 202-307-2277 (TTY)
www.ojp.usdoj.gov/vawo/

Websites

Coalition Against Violence Network
www.cavnet.org/

CHAPTERS 9-12: GENDER IDENTITY AND SEXUAL ORIENTATION, RELATIONSHIPS WITH MEN, RELATIONSHIPS WITH WOMEN, AND SEXUALITY

For a longer list, please see the companion website, www.ourbodiesourselves.org.

Gender Identity

Bornstein, Kate. *My Gender Workbook: How to Become a Real Man, a Real Woman, the Real You, or Something Else Entirely.* New York: Routledge, 1998.

Transgender

Israel, Gianna E., and Donald E. Tarvel. *Transgender Care: Recommended Guidelines, Practical Information and Personal Accounts.* Philadelphia: Temple University Press, 1997.

General Relationships

hooks, bell. *Communion: The Female Search for Love.* New York: William Morrow, 2002.

Rubin, Lillian. *Intimate Strangers: Men and Women Together.* New York: HarperCollins, 1983.

Schnarch, David. *Passionate Marriage: Love, Sex, and Intimacy in Emotionally Committed Relationships.* New York: Owl Books, 1998.

Marriage (to Men)

Carter, Betty, and Joan Peters. *Love, Honor, and Negotiate: Making Your Marriage Work.* New York: Pocket Books, 1996.

Maushart, Susan. *Wifework: What Marriage Really Means for Women.* New York and London: Bloomsbury, 2001.

Divorce (from Men)

Ahrons, Constance. *The Good Divorce: Keeping Your Family Together When Your Marriage Falls Apart.* New York: HarperCollins, 1995.

LBTQI Nonfiction

Berzon, Betty. *Permanent Partners: Building Gay and Lesbian Relationships That Last.* New York: NAL–Dutton, 1997.

Clunis, Marilee D., and G. Dorsey Green. *Lesbian Couples: A Guide to Creating Healthy Relationships.* Seattle: Seal Press, 2000.

Nestle, Joan, et al. *Genderqueer: Voices from Beyond the Sexual Binary.* Los Angeles: Alyson Publications, 2002.

Ochs, Robyn, ed. *Getting Bi: The Bisexual Resource Guide.* Cambridge, MA: Bisexual Resource Center, 2004. (To order, send $13.95 postage-paid to Bisexual Resource Center, P.O. Box 400639, Cambridge, MA 02140; 617-424-9595.)

Sonnie, Amy, ed. *Revolutionary Voices: A Multicultural Queer Youth Anthology.* Los Angeles: Alyson Publications, 2000.

LGBT Organizations (Youth)

Lavender Youth Recreation and Information Center (LYRIC)
127 Collingwood Street, San Francisco, CA 94114
Talkline: 800-246-PRIDE
www.lyric.org

Gay, Lesbian, Straight Education Network (GLSEN)
121 West 27th Street, Suite 804, New York, NY 10001
212-727-0135
www.glsen.org

LGBT Organizations (General)

Gay and Lesbian National Hotline
888-THE-GLNH
www.glnh.org

Human Rights Campaign
1640 Rhode Island Avenue, N.W., Washington, DC 20036
800-777-4723
www.hrc.org

National Association of LGBT Community Centers
(NALGBTCC)
www.lgbtcenters.org

Parents, Families, and Friends of Lesbians and Gays
(P-FLAG)
1726 M Street, N.W., Suite 400, Washington, DC 20036
202-467-8180
www.pflag.org

LGBT Organizations (Legal)

Gay & Lesbian Advocates & Defenders (GLAD)
30 Winter Street, Suite 800, Boston, MA 02108
617-426-1350
www.glad.org

Lambda Legal Defense and Educational Fund (LLDEF)
120 Wall Street, Suite 1500, New York, NY 10005
212-809-8585
www.lambdalegal.org

National Center for Lesbian Rights Headquarters
870 Market Street, Suite 570, San Francisco, CA 94102
415-392-6257
www.nclrights.org

Sylvia Rivera Law Project (on gender identity and
expression)
www.srlp.org

General Sexuality

Ellison, Carol Rinkleib. *Women's Sexualities: Generations of Women Share Intimate Secrets of Sexual Self-Acceptance.* Oakland, CA: New Harbinger, 2000.

Tiefer, Leonore, and Ellyn Kaschak, eds. *A New View of Women's Sexual Problems.* Binghamton, NY: Haworth Press, 2001.

Winks, Cathy, and Anne Semans. *The Good Vibrations Guide to Sex: The Most Complete Sex Manual Ever Written,* 3rd ed. San Francisco: Cleis Press, 2002.

Sexuality-Related Organizations

American Association of Sex Educators, Counselors,
and Therapists (AASECT)
P.O. Box 238, Mount Vernon, IA 52314
319-895-8407
www.aasect.org

Sexuality Information and Education Council of the
United States (SIECUS)
130 West 42nd Street, Suite 2500, New York, NY 10036-7802
212-819-9770
www.siecus.org

Masturbation, Orgasm, and Female Ejaculation

Barbach, Lonnie G. *For Yourself: The Fulfillment of Female Sexuality.* New York: Signet, 2000.

Sundahl, Deborah. *Female Ejaculation and the G-Spot: Not Your Mother's Orgasm Book!* Alameda, CA: Hunter House, 2003.

Erotica

Bright, Susie, Mary Sheiner, et al. *Herotica 1–7.* New York: Plume Books.

Disability

Kaufman, Miriam, M. D., Cory Silverberg, and Fran Odette. *The Ultimate Guide to Sex and Disability.* San Francisco, CA: Cleis Press, Inc., 2003.

Kroll, K., and E. L. Klein. *Enabling Romance: A Guide to Love, Sex, and Relationships for the Disabled.* Horsham, PA: No Limits Communications, 2001.

Teens and Sexuality

Bell, Ruth. *Changing Bodies, Changing Lives: A Book Every Teenager Should Have,* 3rd ed. New York: Three Rivers Press, 1998.

Levy, Barrie. *Dating Violence: Young Women in Danger.* Seattle: Seal Press. 1991.

Tolman, Deborah L. *Dilemmas of Desire: Teenage Girls Talk About Sexuality.* Cambridge, MA: Harvard University Press, 2002.

Periodicals

Teen Voices
Women Express, Inc.
P.O. Box 120-027, Boston, MA 02112-0027
www.teenvoices.com

CHAPTER 13: SEXUAL ANATOMY, REPRODUCTION, AND THE MENSTRUAL CYCLE

For a longer list, please see the companion website, www .ourbodiesourselves.org.

Books

Houppert, Karen. *The Curse: Confronting the Last Unmentionable Taboo: Menstruation.* New York: Farrar, Straus & Giroux, 1999.

Love, Susan M. *Dr. Susan Love's Breast Book.* Cambridge, MA: Perseus Publishing, 2000.

Martin, Emily. *The Woman in the Body: A Cultural Analysis of Reproduction.* Boston: Beacon Press, 2001.

Singer, Katie. *The Garden of Fertility: A Guide to Charting Your Fertility Signals to Prevent or Achieve Pregnancy— Naturally—and to Gauge Your Reproductive Health.* New York: Avery/Penguin, 2004. Available from www .GardenofFertility.com.

Stewart, Elizabeth Gunther, and Paula Spencer. *The V Book: A Doctor's Guide to Complete Vulvovaginal Health.* New York: Bantam Books, 2002.

Weschler, Toni. *Taking Charge of Your Fertility: The Definitive Guide to Natural Birth Control, Pregnancy Achievement, and Reproductive Health.* New York: HarperCollins, 2002. Available from www.TCOYF.com.

Audiovisual Materials

(Period): The End of Menstruation, Giovanna Chesler. A documentary. Available from www.gopictures.com,

858-534-7027; or UCSD Department of Communication, 9500 Gilman Drive, 503, La Jolla, CA 92093-0503.

Websites

Feminist Women's Health Center (on menstruation)
www.fwhc.org/health/moon.htm

Intersex Society of North America
www.isna.org

Museum of Menstruation & Women's Health
www.mum.org

Scarleteen's Sexual Anatomy tour
www.scarleteen.com/body/female_anatomy.html

CHAPTER 14: SAFER SEX

For a longer list, please see the companion website, www .ourbodiesourselves.org.

Books

Foley, Sallie, et al. *Sex Matters for Women: A Complete Guide to Taking Care of Your Sexual Self.* New York: The Guilford Press, 2002.

Fulbright, Yvonne. *The Hot Guide to Safer Sex.* Alameda, CA: Hunter House, 2003. (Tailored to straight twenty-somethings.)

Joannides, Paul, and Daerick Gross. *The Guide to Getting It On!: The Universe's Coolest and Most Informative Book About Sex,* 4th ed. West Hollywood, CA: Goofy Foot Press, 2004.

Winks, Cathy, and Anne Semans. *The Good Vibrations Guide to Sex: The Most Complete Sex Manual Ever Written,* 3rd ed. San Francisco: Cleis Press, 2002.

Organizations

Coalition for Positive Sexuality
P.O. Box 77212, Washington, DC 20013
773-604-1654
www.positive.org/www/JustSayYes/safesex.htm

Planned Parenthood Federation of America (PPFA)
434 West 33rd Street, New York, NY 10001
212-541-7800
Hotline: 877-4ME-ASK
www.ppfa.org/sti

Websites

About Sexuality: Safer Sex Practices and Guidelines
http://sexuality.about.com/od/saferse1/

EngenderHealth: Preventing STIs
www.engenderhealth.org/wh/inf/dprev.html

HIV InSite: Safer Sex Methods
http://hivinsite.ucsf.edu/InSite?page-pr-r-08&doc-kb-07-
02-02

Talking About Safer Sex
www.itsyoursexlife.com/com_sub2.html

CHAPTER 15: SEXUALLY TRANSMITTED INFECTIONS

For a longer list, please see the companion website, www
.ourbodiesourselves.org.

Organizations

American Social Health Association (ASHA)
P.O. Box 13827, Research Triangle Park, NC 27709
919-361-8400
www.ashastd.org/stdfaqs/index.html

Planned Parenthood Federation of America (PPFA)
434 West 33rd Street, New York, NY 10001
800-230-7526; Hotline: 877-4ME-ASK
www.ppfa.org/sti

Websites

Centers for Disease Control and Prevention
National Center for HIV, STD and TB Prevention;
    Division of Sexually Transmitted Diseases
www.cdc.gov/std

International Herpes Alliance
www.herpesalliance.org

Lesbian STD
www.lesbianstd.com

The STD World of Resources Network
www.sworn.org/main.html

Hotlines

STD Hotline
800-227-8922

National Herpes Hotline
800-230-6039

CHAPTER 16: HIV AND AIDS

For a longer list, please see the companion website, www
.ourbodiesourselves.org.

Periodicals

WORLD Newsletter
Women Organized to Respond to Life Threatening
    Diseases (WORLD)
3958 Webster Street, Oakland, CA 94609
510-658-6930

Hotlines

Centers for Disease Control and Prevention National
    AIDS Hotline
800-342-2437, 24 hours a day, 365 days a year
Spanish: 800-344-7432, 7 days a week, 8 A.M.–2 P.M. EST
TTY: 800-243-7889, Monday–Friday, 10 A.M.–10 P.M. EST
www.ashastd.org/nah/index.html

Teens and AIDS Hotline
800-234-TEEN

Treatment

Project Inform
1965 Market Street, San Francisco, CA 94103
415-558-8669
Treatment hotline: 800-822-7422
www.projinf.org

Legal Issues

American Civil Liberties Union AIDS Project
132 West 43rd Street, New York, NY 10036
212-944-9800, ext. 545
E-mail: aidsinfo@aol.com
www.aclu.org/HIVAIDS/HIVAIDSMain.cfm

Websites

HIV Positive: Women and Children
www.hivpositive.com/f-Women/WoChildMenu.html

National Center for HIV, STD, and TB Prevention,
    Divisions of HIV/AIDS Prevention
www.cdc.gov/hiv/dhap.htm

AVERT.org
www.avert.org/womstata.htm

The Body: An AIDS and HIV Information Resource
www.thebody.com

CHAPTER 17: CONSIDERING PARENTING

For a longer list, please see the companion website, www
.ourbodiesourselves.org.

Books

Cain, Madelyn. *The Childless Revolution: What It Means to
Be Childless Today.* Cambridge, MA: Perseus, 2001.

Douglas, Susan, and Meredith Michaels. *The Mommy
Myth: The Idealization of Motherhood and How It Has
Undermined Women.* New York: Free Press, 2004.

Mattes, Jane. *Single Mothers by Choice.* New York: Times
Books, 1994.

Pavao, Joyce Maguire. *The Family of Adoption.* Boston: Beacon Press, 1999.

Roberts, Dorothy. *Shattered Bonds: The Color of Child Welfare.* New York: Basic Books, 2003.

Squire, Susan. *For Better or Worse: A Candid Chronicle of
Five Couples Adjusting to Parenthood.* Garden City, NY:
Doubleday, 1993.

Varon, Lee. *Adopting on Your Own.* New York: Farrar, Straus
& Giroux, 2000.

Vissing, Yvonne Marie. *Women Without Children: Nurturing Lives.* New Brunswick, NJ: Rutgers University Press,
2002.

Organizations

National Adoption Information Clearinghouse
330 C Street S.W., Washington, DC 20447
888-251-0075
http://naic.acf.hhs.gov/

Websites

Childfree Resources
www.fred.net/turtle/kids/resources

CHAPTER 18: BIRTH CONTROL

For a longer list, please see the companion website, www
.ourbodiesourselves.org.

Books

Harrison, Polly F., and Allan Rosenfield, eds. *Contraceptive
Research, Introduction, and Use: Lessons from Norplant.*
Washington, DC: National Academies Press, 1998.

Hatcher, Robert, and James Trussell, et al. *Contraceptive
Technology,* 18th ed. New York: Ardent Media, 2004.

Periodicals

Journal of Family Planning and Reproductive Health Care
27 Sussex Place, Regent's Park, London NW1 4RG, England
020-7724-5681
www.ffprhc.org.uk/the_journal/
www.ingenta.com/journals/browse/ffp/jfp

Organizations, Hotlines, Websites

Cervical Barrier Advancement Society
P.O. Box 382031, Cambridge, MA 02238-2031
617-349-0025
www.cervicalbarriers.org

CONRAD Program
Eastern Virginia Medical School
1611 North Kent Street, Suite 806, Arlington, VA 22209
703-524-4744
www.CONRAD.org

Feminist Women's Health Center
www.fwhc.org/birth-control/index.htm

The Fertility Awareness Network
P.O. Box 1190, New York, NY 10009
800-597-6267 or 212-475-4490
www.FertAware.com

Nationwide EC Hotline
888-NOT-2-LATE, 24 hours a day, 365 days a year, in
English and Spanish
www.rhtp.org/ec/ec_hotline.htm
www.not-2-late.com (has information in English, Spanish,
French, and Arabic)

Planned Parenthood Federation of America (PPFA)
434 West 33rd Street, New York, NY 10001
212-541-7800
www.ppfa.org/bc

CHAPTER 19: UNEXPECTED PREGNANCY

For a longer list, please see the companion website, www
.ourbodies.ourselves.org.

Books

Ludtke, Melissa. *On Our Own: Unmarried Motherhood in
America.* New York: Random House, 1997.
Simpson, Carolyn. *Coping with an Unplanned Pregnancy.*
New York: Rosen Publishing Group, 1996.

Pamphlets and Articles

Hoffman, Saul D. "Teenage Childbearing Is Not So Bad
After All . . . Or Is It? A Review of the New Literature."
Family Planning Perspectives 30, no. 5, 1998.
National Abortion Federation. "Unsure About Your Preg-
nancy: A Guide to Making the Right Decision for You."
Available at www.prochoice.org/Pregnant/Choices/
UnsureGuide.htm.
Seiler, Naomi. "Is Teen Marriage a Solution?" Available at
www.clasp.org/publications/teenmariage02-20.pdf.
Planned Parenthood Federation of America. *"What If I'm
Pregnant?"* Available at www.ppfa.org/womenshealth/
WhatifPregnant.html.

Organizations

National Adoption Information Clearinghouse
330 C Street, S.W., Washington, DC 20447
703-352-3488 or 888-251-0075
http://naic.acf.hhs.gov/

National Guardianship Association, Inc.
1604 North Country Club Road, Tucson, AZ 85716-
3102
520-881-6561
www.guardianship.org

Planned Parenthood Federation of America (PPFA)
434 West 33rd Street, New York, NY 10001
800-230-PLAN or 212-541-7800
www.ppfa.org

CHAPTER 20: ABORTION

For a longer list, please see the companion website, www
.ourbodiesourselves.org.

Organizations

Abortion Access Project (AAP)
552 Massachusetts Avenue, Suite 215, Cambridge, MA
02139
617-661-1161
www.abortionaccess.org

Alan Guttmacher Institute (AGI)
1301 Connecticut Avenue, N.W., Suite 700, Washington,
DC 20036
202-296-4012
www.agi-usa.org/sections/abortion.html

The Center for Reproductive Rights (CRR; formerly
Center for Reproductive Law and Policy, CRLP)
120 Wall Street, 18th Floor, New York, NY 10005
917-637-3600
www.reproductiverights.org

Choice USA
1010 Wisconsin Avenue, N.W., Suite 410, Washington,
DC 20007
888-784-4494 or 202-965-7700
www.choiceusa.org

Ipas USA
300 Market Street, Suite 200, Chapel Hill, NC 27516
919-967-7052 or 800-334-8446
www.ipas.org

NARAL Pro-Choice America
1156 15th Street, N.W., Suite 700, Washington, DC
20005
202-973-3000
www.naral.org

The National Abortion Federation (NAF)
1755 Massachusetts Avenue, N.W., Suite 600, Washington,
DC 20036
202-667-5881
Hotline: 800-772-9100, Monday–Friday 8 A.M.–10 P.M.
EST
Saturday–Sunday 9 A.M.–5 P.M.
www.prochoice.org

National Network of Abortion Funds (NNAF)
c/o CLPP, Hampshire College, Amherst, MA 01002-
5001
413-559-5645
www.nnaf.org

Planned Parenthood Federation of America (PPFA)
434 West 33rd Street, New York, NY 10001
212-541-7800
www.ppfa.org/abortion

The Religious Coalition for Reproductive Choice
    (RCRC)
1025 Vermont Avenue, N.W., Suite 1130, Washington,
    DC 20005
202-628-7700
www.rcrc.org

Sistersong Women of Color Reproductive Health
    Collective
P.O. Box 311020, Atlanta, GA 31131
www.sistersong.net/index.html

CHAPTERS 21 AND 22: PREGNANCY AND CHILDBIRTH

For a longer list, please see the companion website, www
.ourbodiesourselves.org.

Books

Balaskas, Janet. *Active Birth: The New Approach to Giving Birth Naturally.* Boston: Harvard Common Press, 1992.
Davis-Floyd, Robbie E. *Birth as an American Rite of Passage.* Berkeley, CA: University of California Press, 1992.
Gaskin, Ina May. *Ina May's Guide to Childbirth.* New York: Bantam Books, 2003. Also see Ina May Gaskin, *Spiritual Midwifery,* 4th ed. Summertown, TN: The Book Publishing Company, 2002.
Goer, Henci. *The Thinking Woman's Guide to a Better Birth.* New York: Perigee, 1999.
Kitzinger, Sheila. *Rediscovering Birth.* New York: Pocket Books, 2001.
Harper, Barbara. *Gentle Birth Choices: A Guide to Making Informed Decisions.* Rochester, VT: Healing Arts Press, 1994.
McCutcheon, Susan. *Natural Childbirth the Bradley Way.* New York: Plume, 1996.
Perkins, Barbara. *The Medical Delivery Business: Health Reform, Childbirth and the Economic Order.* New Brunswick, NJ: Rutgers University Press, 2003.
Pincus, Jane. "Critique of Childbearing Advice Books," Available at www.ourbodiesourselves.org/advice.htm.
Simkin, Penny, Janet Whalley, and Ann Keppler. *Pregnancy, Childbirth and the Newborn: The Complete Guide.* Minnetonka, MN: Meadowbrook Press, 2001.
Wertz, Richard W., and Dorothy C. Wertz. *Lying-In: A History of Childbirth in America.* New Haven: Yale University Press, 1989.

Periodicals

Midwifery Today
541-344-7438; toll-free from the U. S. and Canada (orders
    only): 800-743-0974
www.midwiferytoday.com

Mothering
800-984-8116
www.mothering.com

Organizations and Websites

Association of Labor Assistants and Childbirth Educators
    (ALACE)
P.O. Box 390436, Cambridge, MA 02139
617-441-2500 or 888-222-5223
www.alace.org

Childbirth.org
www.childbirth.org

Doulas of North America (DONA)
P.O. Box 626, Jasper, IN 47547
888-788-DONA (3662)
www.dona.org

International Cesarean Awareness Network (ICAN,
    formerly Cesarean Prevention Movement)
1304 Kingsdale Avenue, Redondo Beach, CA 90278
310-542-6400 or 800-686-ICAN
www.ican-online.org

International Childbirth Education Association (ICEA)
P.O. Box 20048, Minneapolis, MN 54420
952-854-8660
www.icea.org

Lamaze Institute for Normal Birth
2025 M Street N.W., Suite 800, Washington, DC 20036-3309
202-367-1128 or 800-368-4404
http://normalbirth.lamaze.org/institute/

Maternity Center Association
281 Park Avenue South, 5th Floor, New York, NY 10010
212-777-5000
www.maternitywise.org

National Association of Childbearing Centers (NACC)
3123 Gottschall Road, Perkiomenville, PA 18074
215-234-8068
www.birthcenters.org

CHAPTER 23: THE FIRST YEAR OF PARENTING

For a longer list, please see the companion website, www.ourbodiesourselves.org.

Breast-feeding Organizations

La Leche League USA
800-LALECHE or 847-519-7730
www.lllusa.org

Office on Women's Health
U.S. Department of Health and Human Services Helpline
(in English and Spanish)
800-994-WOMAN (9662)
www.4woman.gov/owh/breastfeeding.htm

International Lactation Consultants' Association
(ILCA)
919-861-5577
www.ilca.org

Audiovisual Materials

In Your Hands: The Best Start for Your Breastfed Baby. Available from the Breastfeeding Center, Boston Medical Center, 850 Harrison Avenue ACC5, Boston, MA 02118-2393, 617-414-MILK (6455).

Books (Postpartum and New Parenting)

Jordan, Pamela L., Scott M. Stanley, and Howard J. Markman. *Becoming Parents: How to Strengthen Your Marriage as Your Family Grows.* San Francisco: Jossey-Bass, 1999.

Lim, Robin. *After the Baby's Birth: A Woman's Way to Wellness, a Complete Guide for Postpartum Women.* Berkeley, CA: Celestial Arts, 2001.

Placksin, Sally. *Mothering the New Mother: Women's Feelings and Needs After Childbirth, a Support and Resource Guide.* New York: Newmarket Press, 2000.

Semans, Anne, and Cathy Winks. *The Mother's Guide to Sex: Enjoying Your Sexuality Through All Stages of Motherhood.* New York: Three Rivers Press, 2001.

Websites

ParentsPlace.com
www.parentsplace.com

www.ppdsupportpage.com
(online postpartum depression support page)

CHAPTER 24: CHILDBEARING LOSS

For a longer list, please see the companion website, www.ourbodiesourselves.org.

Books and Articles

Cecil, Rosanne, ed. *The Anthropology of Pregnancy Loss: Comparative Studies in Miscarriage, Stillbirth and Neonatal Death.* Oxford: Berg Publishers, 1996.

Cote-Arsenault, Denise, and R. Marshall. "One Foot In— One Foot Out: Weathering the Storm of Pregnancy After Perinatal Loss." *Research in Nursing & Health* 23, no. 6 (December 2000): 473–85.

Kluger-Bell, Kim. *Unspeakable Losses: Understanding the Experience of Pregnancy Loss, Miscarriage, and Abortion.* New York: Norton, 1998.

Layne, Linda L. *Motherhood Lost: A Feminist Account of Pregnancy Loss in America.* New York: Routledge, 2003.

Resources for Planning Rituals

Cardin, Nina Beth. *Tears of Sorrow, Seeds of Hope: A Jewish Spiritual Companion for Infertility and Pregnancy Loss.* Woodstock, VT: Jewish Lights Publishing, 1999.

Lamb, Sister Jane Marie. *Bittersweet . . . hellogoodbye: A Resource in Planning Farewell Rituals When a Baby Dies.* Belleville, IL: Charis Communications, 1989.

Organizations

Wisconsin Stillbirth Service Program (WiSSP); (medical evaluation of stillborn infants) www.wisc.edu/wissp

Hygeia Foundation, Inc., and Institute for Perinatal Loss and Bereavement
P.O. Box 3943, New Haven, CT 06525
www.hygeia.org

SHARE Pregnancy Loss and Infant Support, Inc.
St. Joseph Health Center
300 First Capitol Drive, St. Charles, MO 63301-2893
636-947-6164 or 800-821-6819
www.nationalshareoffice.com

The MISS Foundation
P.O. Box 5333, Peoria, AZ 85385-5333
623-979-1000
www.missfoundation.org

CHAPTER 25: INFERTILITY AND ASSISTED REPRODUCTION

For a longer list, please see the companion website, www
.ourbodiesourselves.org.

Books

Bercollone, Carol Frost, Heidi Moss, and Robert Moss. *Helping the Stork: The Choices and Challenges of Donor Insemination.* New York: Macmillan, 1997.

Cooper, Susan, and Ellen Glazer. *Choosing Assisted Reproduction: Social, Emotional and Ethical Considerations.* Indianapolis: Perspective Press, 1999.

Frisch, Rose. *Female Fertility and the Body Fat Connection.* Chicago: University of Chicago Press, 2002.

Johnston, Patricia. *Taking Charge of Infertility.* Indianapolis: Perspective Press, 1995.

Organizations

American Fertility Association
666 Fifth Avenue, Suite 278, New York, NY 10103
888-917-3777
www.theafa.org

American Society for Reproductive Medicine
1209 Montgomery Highway, Birmingham, AL 35216-2809
205-978-5000
www.asrm.org

Council for Responsible Genetics
5 Upland Road, Suite 3, Cambridge, MA 02140
617-868-0870
www.gene-watch.org

Infertility Network
160 Pickering Street, Toronto, ON M4E 3J7 Canada
416-691-3611
www.infertilitynetwork.org

International Council on Infertility Information Dissemination (INCIID)
P.O. Box 6836, Arlington, VA 22206-0836
703-379-9178
www.inciid.org

RESOLVE, Inc.
1310 Broadway, Somerville, MA 02144-1731
617-623-1156 or 888-623-0744
www.resolve.org/

CHAPTERS 26 AND 27: MIDLIFE AND MENOPAUSE AND OUR LATER YEARS

For a longer list, please see the companion website, www
.ourbodiesourselves.org.

Books (General)

Bauer-Maglin, N. and A. Radosh, eds. *Women Confronting Retirement: A Nontraditional Guide.* New Brunswick, NJ: Rutgers University Press, 2003.

Cruikshank, Margaret. *Learning to Be Old.* Lanham, MD: Rowman and Littlefield, 2001.

Doress-Worters, Paula B., and Diana Laskin Segal, in cooperation with the Bostom Women's Health Book Collective. *The New Ourselves, Growing Older: Women Aging with Knowledge and Power.* New York: Simon & Schuster, 1994.

Gullette, Margaret Morganroth. *Aged by Culture.* Chicago: University of Chicago Press, 2004.

Caregiving

Lieberman, T. *Consumer Reports Complete Guide to Health Services for Seniors: What Your Family Needs to Know About Finding and Financing Medicare, Assisted Living, Nursing Homes, Home Care and Adult Day Care.* New York: Three Rivers Press, 2000.

McLeod, Beth W., ed. *And Thou Shalt Honor.* Emmaus, PA: Rodale Press, 2002.

Memory Loss

Doty, L., K. M. Heilman, J. T. Stewart, D. Bowers, and L. J. G. Rothi. *Helping People with Progressive Memory Disorders,* 3rd ed. Gainesville, FL: University of Florida and Shands HealthCare, 2005.

McKhann, G. M., and M. Albert. *Keep Your Brain Young: The Complete Guide to Physical and Emotional Health and Longevity.* New York: John Wiley & Sons, 2002.

Menopause and Hormones

Benson, Herbert, Leslee Kagan, and Bruce Kessel. *Mind Over Menopause: The Complete Mind/Body Approach to Coping with Menopause.* New York: Free Press, 2004.

Love, Susan M., and Karen Lindsey. *Dr. Susan Love's Menopause and Hormone Book: Making Informed Choices.* New York: Three Rivers Press, 2003.

National Women's Health Network. *The Truth About Hormone Replacement Therapy: How to Break Free from the Medical Myths of Menopause.* Roseville, CA: Prima Publishing, 2002.

Seaman, Barbara. *The Greatest Experiment Ever Performed on Women: Exploding the Estrogen Myth.* New York: Hyperion, 2003.

Sex

Butler, R. N., and M. I. Lewis. *The New Love and Sex After 60.* New York: Ballantine, 2002.

Kaschak, E., and L. Tiefer, eds. *A New View of Women's Sexual Problems.* Binghamton, NY: Haworth, 2001.

Organizations

Alzheimer's Association
225 N. Michigan Avenue, 17th Floor, Chicago, IL 60601
800-272-3900
www.alz.org

Eldercare Locator
800-677-1116, Monday–Friday 9 A.M.–8 P.M. EST
www.eldercare.gov

Gray Panthers
733 15th Street, N.W., Suite 437, Washington, DC, 20005
800-280-5362 or 202-737-6637
www.graypanthers.org

National Family Caregivers Association
10400 Connecticut Avenue, Suite 500, Kensington, MD 20895
800-896-3650
www.thefamilycaregiver.org

National Hispanic Council on Aging
2713 Ontario Road, N.W., Washington, DC 20009
202-265-1288
www.nhcoa.org

OWL: Older Women's League, The Voice of Midlife and Older Women
1750 New York Avenue N.W., Suite 350, Washington, DC 20006
800-825-3695 or 202-783-6686
www.owl-national.org

Senior Action in a Gay Environment (SAGE)
305 7th Avenue, New York, NY 10001
212-741-2247
www.sageusa.org

CHAPTERS 28 AND 29: UNIQUE TO WOMEN AND SPECIAL CONCERNS FOR WOMEN

For a longer list, please see the companion website, www.ourbodiesourselves.org.

Books (General)

Fugh-Berman, Adriane. *The 5-Minute Herb and Dietary Supplement Consult.* New York: Lippincott Williams & Wilkins, 2003.

Organizations

Center for Medical Consumers
130 MacDougal Street, New York, NY 10012
212-674-7105
www.medicalconsumers.org

Arthritis

The Arthritis Foundation
P.O. Box 7669, Atlanta, GA 30357-0669
800-283-7800
www.arthritis.org

Chronic Fatigue Syndrome

CFIDS Association of America, Inc.
P.O. Box 220398, Charlotte, NC 28222-0398
704-365-2343 or 800-442-3437
www.cfids.org

Fibromyalgia

Fibromyalgia Network
P.O. Box 31750, Tucson, AZ 85751-1750
800-853-2929
www.fmnetnews.com/

Graves' Disease

EndocrineWeb.com
www.endocrineweb.com/hyper4.html

Lupus

Lupus Foundation of America
2000 L Street, N.W., Suite 710, Washington, DC 20036
202-349-1155 or 800-558-0121
www.lupus.org/

Scleroderma

American College of Rheumatology
1800 Century Place, Suite 250, Atlanta, GA 30345-4300
404-633-3777
www.rheumatology.org/public/factsheets/scler.asp

Sjögren's Syndrome

Sjögren's Syndrome Foundation
8120 Woodmont Avenue, Bethesda, MD 20814
800-475-6473
www.sjogrens.org

Cancer

National Cancer Institute. "What Are Clinical Trials All About?" Available from the National Cancer Institute, Office of Cancer Communications, 31 Center Drive, MSC 2580, Bethesda, MD 20892-2580; 800-4-CANCER. See also www.cancer.gov.

Love, Dr. Susan. *Dr. Susan Love's Breast Book.* Reading, MA: Addison-Wesley, 1995.

McTiernan, Anne. *Breast Fitness: An Optimal Exercise and Health Plan for Reducing Your Risk of Breast Cancer.* New York: St. Martin's Press, 2001.

Breast Cancer Action
55 New Montgomery Street, Suite 323, San Francisco, CA 94105
415-243-9301 or 877-278-6722
www.bcaction.org/index.html

Chemical Injury and Multiple Chemical Sensitivity (MCS)

Rachel's Environment and Health News, Environmental Research Foundation
P.O. Box 160, New Brunswick, NJ 08903-0160
732-828-9995 or 888-272-2435
www.rachel.org

DES

DES Action
610 16th Street, Suite 301, Oakland, CA 94612
800-DES-9288
www.desaction.org

Endometriosis

Ballweg, Mary Lou, and the Endometriosis Association. *Endometriosis: The Complete Reference for Taking Charge of Your Health.* Chicago: Contemporary Books, 2003. Also see www.endometriosisassn.org.

Female Genital Cutting

Research, Action and Information Network for the Bodily Integrity of Women (RAINBO)
915 Broadway, Suite 1109, New York, NY 10010-7108
212-477-3318
www.rainbo.org/

Heart Disease, Heart Attack, Hypertension, and Stroke

American Heart Association
7272 Greenville Avenue, Dallas, TX 75231
800-242-8721
www.americanheart.org

American Stroke Association
7272 Greenville Avenue, Dallas, TX 75231
888-478-7653
www.strokeassociation.org

Canadian Cardiovascular Society
222 rue Queen/Queen Street, Suite/Pièce 1403, Ottawa, Ontario K1P 5V9, Canada
613-569-3407 or 877-569-3407
www.ccs.ca

Urinary Tract Infections/Disorders and Interstitial Cystitis

Interstitial Cystitis Association (ICA)
110 North Washington Street, Suite 340, Rockville, MD 20850
301-610-5300 or 800-HELP-ICA
www.ichelp.com

Hysterectomy and Oophorectomy

Hysterectomy Educational Resources and Services (HERS)
422 Bryn Mawr Avenue, Bala Cynwyd, PA 19004
610-667-7757 or 888-750-4377
www.hersfoundation.com/facts.html

PCOS

Polycystic Ovarian Syndrome Association
P.O. Box 3403, Englewood, CO 80111
877-775-PCOS
www.pcossupport.org

Vulvodynia

National Vulvodynia Association
P.O. Box 4491, Silver Spring, MD 20914-4491
301-299-0775
www.nva.org

CHAPTER 30: NAVIGATING THE HEALTH CARE SYSTEM

For a longer list, please see the companion website, www
.ourbodiesourselves.org.

Books

Annas, George J. *The Rights of Patients: The Authoritative ACLU Guide to the Rights of Patients,* 3rd ed. Carbondale, IL: Southern Illinois University Press, 2004.
Kasper, Anne S., and Susan Ferguson, eds. *Breast Cancer: Society Shapes an Epidemic.* New York: St. Martin's Press, 2000.

Organizations

National Health Law Program (NHeLP)
2639 South La Cienega Boulevard, Los Angeles, CA 90034
310-404-6010
www.healthlaw.org/consumer.shtml

National Women's Health Network
514 10th Street, N.W., Suite 400, Washington, DC 20004
202-628-7814 (for health information) or 202-347-1140 (office)
www.nwhn.org/publications/fact.php

Agency for Healthcare Research and Quality
Executive Office Center
540 Gaither Road, Rockville, MD 20850
800-358-9295
www.ahrq.gov/consumer

National Women's Health Information Center
8550 Arlington Boulevard, Suite 300, Fairfax, VA 22031
800-994-9662 (TTY) or 888-220-5446
www.4woman.gov

National Women's Health Resource Center
157 Broad Street, Suite 315, Red Bank, NJ 07701
877-986-9472
www.healthywomen.org/

Resources for the Uninsured and Underinsured

Covering Kids and Families is an initiative in forty-five states and Washington, DC, that helps eligible children and adults sign up for public health insurance coverage: http://coveringkidsandfamilies.org/

To find free or low-cost health care:
- For the nearest Community Health Center (which will see all patients regardless of ability to pay, and charge based on a sliding scale): http://ask.hrsa.gov/pc/.
- For a free clinic near you: www.freeclinic.net.

For assistance in finding programs that provide free or low-cost medications to those who cannot afford them: www.needymeds.com and www.rxassist.org.

CHAPTER 31: THE POLITICS OF WOMEN'S HEALTH

For a longer list, please see the companion website, www
.ourbodiesourselves.org.

Books

Alvarez Martínez, Luz. *Homenaje a Nuestras Curanderas: Honoring Our Healers.* Oakland, CA: Latina Press, 1997.
Angell, Marcia. *The Truth About the Drug Companies: How They Deceive Us and What to Do About It.* New York: Random House, 2004.
Doyal, Lesley. *What Makes Women Sick: Gender and the Political Economy of Health.* New Brunswick, NJ: Rutgers University Press, 1995.

Institute of Medicine Committee on the Consequences of Uninsurance. *Insuring America's Health: Principles and Recommendations.* Washington, DC: National Academies Press, 2004.

Krieger, Nancy, ed. *Embodying Inequality: Epidemiologic Perspectives.* Amityville, NY: Baywood Publishing Company, 2004.

Medawar, Charles, and Anita Hardon. *Medicines Out of Control?: Antidepressants and the Conspiracy of Goodwill.* Amsterdam: Askant Academic Publishers, 2004.

Ruzek, Sheryl Burt, et al., eds. *Women's Health: Complexities and Differences.* Columbus, OH: Ohio State University Press, 1997.

Sered, Susan, and Rushika Fernandopulle. *Uninsured in America: Life and Death in the Land of Opportunity.* Berkeley, CA: University of California Press, 2005.

Silliman, Jael, Marlene Gerber Fried, Loretta Ross, and Elena Gutierrez. *Undivided Rights: Women of Color Organize for Reproductive Justice.* Cambridge, MA: South End Press, 2004.

Worcester, Nancy, and Mariamne H. Whatley, eds. *Women's Health: Readings on Social, Economic, and Political Issues,* 4th ed. Dubuque, IA: Kendall/Hunt Publishing, 2004.

Article

Leigh, Wilhelmina A. "The Health of Women: Minority/Diversity Perspective, an American Perspective," presented at the Canada/USA Women's Health Forum, August 1996. Available at www.hc-sc.gc.ca/canusa/papers/usa/english/minority.htm

CHAPTER 32: ORGANIZING FOR CHANGE

For a longer list, please see the companion website, www.ourbodiesourselves.org.

Books

Alinksy, Saul D. *Rules for Radicals: A Practical Primer for Realistic Radicals.* New York: Vintage Publishing, 1989.

Baumgardner, Jennifer, and Amy Richard: *Grassroots: A Field Guide for Feminist Activism.* New York: Farrar, Straus & Giroux, 2005.

Kaufman, Cynthia. *Ideas for Action: Relevant Theory for Radical Change.* Boston: South End Press, 2003.

Minkler, Meredith, ed. *Community Organizing and Community Building for Health,* 2nd ed. New Brunswick, NJ: Rutgers University Press, 2004.

MoveOn.org. *MoveOn's 50 Ways to Love Your Country: How to Find Your Political Voice and Become a Catalyst for Change.* Maui, HI: Inner Ocean Publishing, 2004.

Sen, Rinku, and Kim Klein. *Stir It Up: Lessons in Community Organizing and Advocacy.* San Francisco: Jossey-Bass, 2003.

Organizations

National Organization for Women
733 15th Street, N.W., 2nd Floor, Washington, DC 20005
202-628-8NOW
www.now.org

National Women Health Network
514 10th Street, N.W., Suite 400, Washington, DC 20004
202-347-1140
www.nwhn.org

Public Interest Research Groups
www.pirg.org

Third Wave Foundation
511 West 25th Street, Suite 301, New York, NY 10001
212-675-0700
www.thirdwavefoundation.org

THE PRODUCTION TEAM FOR *OUR BODIES, OURSELVES* 2005

Editorial Team: Judy Norsigian, Heather Stephenson, and Kiki Zeldes

Managing Editor: Heather Stephenson

Companion Website Editor: Kiki Zeldes

Photo Editor: Sarai Walker

Tone and Voice Editor: Zobeida Bonilla

Interns: Meghan Killian, Laura Subramanian, Stephanie Feuer-Beck, Katherine L. Burchell, and Jennifer O'Donnell

Volunteers: Esther Dairiam and Jennifer Gariepy

Staff and Consultants: Sally Whelan, Amanda Matos, Pam McCarthy, and Marianne McPherson

Authors of the OBOS Update Manual: Sally Whelan and Wendy Sanford, with Marianne McPherson

At Simon & Schuster: Doris Cooper, Sara Schapiro, Caroline Sutton, Christina Duffy, Marcia Burch, Ellen Silberman, Sue Fleming, Debbie Model, Lisa Healy, Mark Gompertz, Chris Lloreda, and Trish Todd

Our Bodies Ourselves board members: Jayne Carvelli-Sheehan, Dharma Cortes, Elizabeth Daake-Kelly, Sally Deane, Vilunya Diskin, Nancy Forsyth, Ileana Jimenez Garcia, Teresa Harrison, Mary (Bebe) Poor, Penelope Riseborough, Patricia Roche, Bonnie Shepard, Fiona Smith, Donna Soodalter-Toman, Amanda Buck Varella, and Rachel A. Wilson

Founders of the Boston Women's Health Book Collective: Ruth Bell-Alexander, Pamela Berger, Vilunya Diskin, Joan Ditzion, Paula Doress-Worters, Nancy Miriam Hawley, Elizabeth MacMahon-Herrera, Pamela Morgan, Judy Norsigian, Jane Pincus, Esther Rome (1945–1995), Wendy C. Sanford, Norma Swenson, and Sally Whelan

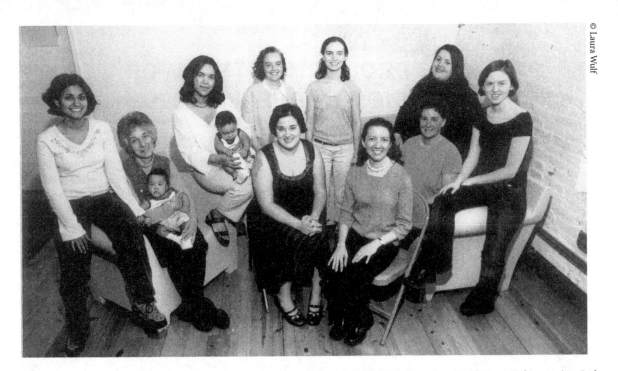

The staff, consultants, and interns who worked on the 2005 edition of *Our Bodies, Ourselves*: (L-R) Laura Subramanian; Judy Norsigian; Zobeida Bonilla; Sally Whelan (standing); Meghan Killian (sitting); Marianne McPherson (standing); Heather Stephenson (sitting); Kiki Zeldes (sitting); Sarai Walker; Jennifer O'Donnell. The babies are Zobeida Bonilla's twin sons, Benjamin and Fernando. Not pictured: Stephanie Feuer-Beck and Katherine L. Burchell.

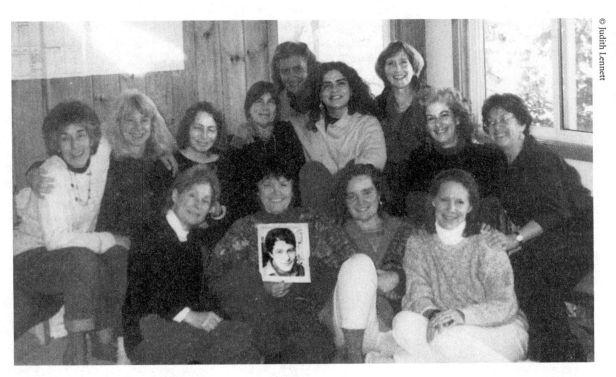

Founders of the Boston Women's Health Book Collective in 1996.

AUTHORSHIP AND ACKNOWLEDGMENTS

Taking Care of Ourselves

1: Body Image

By Sarai Walker, with Lori Tharps (African-American women's hair).

Edited by Alison Amoroso and the Editorial Team.

Thanks for help on this edition to: Elizabeth Bastos, Ann Sexton Foye, Dinah Herlands, Jin In, Lisa Jervis, Eugenia SunHee Kim, Liz Massie, Emily Pilowa, Catherine Steiner-Adair, and Rose Weitz.

Contributors to earlier editions: Demetria Iazzetto, Linda King, Jennifer Yanco, Allison Abner, Deborah Levine, Marsha Sexton, Judith Stein, Becky Thompson, Linda Villarosa, Kiki Zeldes, Wendy Sanford, the women of Boston Self-Help, Frances Deloatch, Mary Fitzgerald, Jean Gillespie, Nancy Miriam Hawley, Janna Zwerner, Joan Lastovica, Oce, Rosemarie Ouilette, Jane Pincus, Esther Rome, Marsha Saxton, Judith Stein, and Jill Wolhandler.

2: Eating Well

By Emily Bender, with Kami-Leigh Agard (eating disorders) and Sarai Walker (dieting).

Edited by Cara Feinberg and the Editorial Team.

Thanks for help on this edition to: Mary Barger, Hannah Doress, Lori Lipinski, Julie Matthews, Zoe Nierenberg, Susie Reel, Michael Reel, Gigi Shames, Jan Smith, Catherine Steiner-Adair, Becky Thompson, Walter Willett, and Allen Worters.

Contributors to earlier editions: Maria Bettencourt, Christina Economos, Trisha Brown, Patricia Cooper, Marilyn Figueroa, Bonnie Gage, Deb Levine, Bonnie Liebman, Ruth Palombo, Caterina Rocha, Judith Stein, Margo N. Woods, Esther Rome, Judy Norsigian, Marsha Butman, Tricia Copeland, Demetria Iazzetto, Vivian Mayer, and Christine Rugen.

3: Alcohol, Tobacco, and Other Mood-Altering Drugs

By Nancy Poole (alcohol and other drugs), Deborah McLellan (tobacco), and Victoria Almquist (tobacco).

Edited by Nancy Adess and the Editorial Team.

Thanks for help on this edition to: Ruth Bell Alexander, Paula Caplan, Marcia Gordon, Elizabeth Hakas, Abigail Halperin, Cheryl Healton, Carolyn Howard, Corinne Husten, Melissa Ostrow, Jodi Sperber, and Alan Trachtenberg.

Contributors to earlier editions: Norma

Finkelstein, Cheryl Kennedy, Janet Smeltz, Caryn Kauffman, Denise Bergman, Archie Brodsky, Suzy Bird Gulliver, Deborah McLellan, Wendy Sanford, Amy Rubin, Jennifer Yanco, Marian Sandmaier, Martha Wood, Nancy Miriam Hawley, Judy Norsigian, and Yvonne Rushin.

4: Our Bodies in Motion

By Suzanne Bremer.

Edited by Angelina Malhotra-Singh and the Editorial Team.

Thanks for help on this edition to: Kami-Leigh Agard, Diane Dahm, Jennifer Hastings, Moira Heiges, Leslie Heywood, Amelia Glynn Hornick, Roberta Lenard, Miranda Lutyens, Erin O'Donnell, Rajinder Kaur Singh, Maria Skinner, and Sarai Walker.

Contributors to earlier editions: Janet Jones; Maureen Ferrera and Cindy Higgins of Boston Self-Help; Lynn Jaffee of Melpomene Institute; Karen Kahn; Jennifer Yanco; Wendy Zinn; Pat Lyga; Carol McEldowney; Mary Lee Slettehaugh; and Judith Stein.

5: Complementary Health Practices

By Adriane Fugh-Berman.

Edited by Jennie Goode and the Editorial Team.

Thanks for help on this edition to: Amy Bollinger, Ted Chapman, Savitri Clarke, Leilani Doty, Ellen Fineberg, Maureen Flannery, Wendy Garling, Lisa Handwerker, Ellen Silver Highfield, Bonnie S. Hillsberg, Amelia Glynn Hornick, Ellen Langer, Miranda Lutyens, Richard Moskowitz, Rita Raj, Susan Sered, Laura Subramanian, Carmen Tamayo, Ariana Vora, and Youko Yeracarif.

Contributors to earlier editions: April Taylor, Claire M. Cassidy, Ellen Fineberg, Pamela Berger, Nancy Miriam Hawley, Adriane Fugh-Berman, Savitri Clarke, Rose Dubosz, Mary Fillmore, Jon Kabat-Zinn, Pamela Pacelli, Jane Pincus, Billie Pivnik, Lori Ponge, Susan Reverby, and Linnie Smith.

6: Emotional Well-Being

By Paula J. Caplan, with Amy Agigian and Judi Chamberlin.

Edited by the Editorial Team.

Thanks for help on this edition to: Amy Banks, Bette Begleiter, Courtney Bell, Jan Brin, Nikki Gerard, Jill M. Goldstein, David Healy, Elizabeth MacMahon-Herrera, Carolyn Howard, Ellen Langer, Hala Najjar, Eli Newberger, Malkah Tolpin Notman, Deborah Raptopoulos, Rachel Josefowitz Siegal, Nada Stotland, Anita Taylor, Sara Walz, and Sally Whelan.

Contributors to earlier editions: Nancy Miriam Hawley, Cassandra Clay, Nancy and Lani Keyes, Jeffrey McIn-

tyre, Susan Yanow, Judith Herman, Rachel Lanzerotti, Judy Norsigian, Catherine Riessman, Wendy Sanford, and Norma Swenson.

7: Environmental and Occupational Health

By Lin Nelson (environmental health) and Barbara Sattler (occupational health).

Edited by Jacqueline Lapidus and the Editorial Team.

Thanks for help on this edition to: Cathy Amoroso, Elizabeth Blackburn, Julia Brody, Richard Clapp, Nancy Evans, Gen Howe, Lina Lander, Dina Nasser, Melissa Perry, Laura Punnett, Judith Schreiber, Sandra Steingraber, Joel Tickner, Donna Vivio, and Heidi Worley.

Contributors to earlier editions: Patricia Logan, Regina H. Kenen, MassCOSH Women's Committee: Letitia Davis, Marian Marbury, Laura Punnett, Margaret Quinn, Cathy Schwartz, and Susan Woskie, Carol Dansereau, Maureen Gorman, Norma Grier, Elizabeth Gullette, Pat Hynes, Kristin Lacijan of NCAMP; Jacqueline Lapidus, Cheri Lucas-Jennings, Karen McDonell, Manju Mehta, Vernice Miller, Cydney Pullman, Dorothy Wigmore, Susan O'Brien, Ngazi Oleru, Judy Norsigian, the Shalan Foundation, Joan Bertin, Katsi Cook, and Maureen Paul.

8: Violence and Abuse

By Margaret Lazarus.

Edited by Laurie Rosenblum and the Editorial Team.

Thanks for help on this edition to: Lunden Abelson, Alison Byers, Lucy Candib, Judith L. Herman, Trina Jackson, Jackson Katz, Leslye Orloff, Pat Paluzzi, Emily Pitt, Penny Saunders, Shauna Shames, and Jessica Xavier.

Contributors to earlier editions: Marianne Winters, Dina Carbonell, Lois Glass, Suzanne Gosselin, Carol Mamber, Jill Stanzler, Alice Friedman, Margaret Lazarus, Lynn Rubinett, Lena Sorensen, Denise Wells, Nancy Wilbur, Terrie Antico, Wendy Sanford, Jackie Herskovitz, Judith Lennett, Laura Tandara, Gene Bishop, Andrea Fischgrund, Roxanne Hynek, Janet Jones, Freada Klein, Rachel Lanzerotti, Carol McEldowney, and Judy Norsigian.

Relationships and Sexuality

9: Gender Identity and Sexual Orientation

By Elizabeth Sarah Lindsey.

Edited by Jennie Goode and the Editorial Team.

Thanks for help on this edition to: Shannon Berning, Suzanne Bremer, Diane Ellaborn, Loraine Hutchins, Karen Kubby, Taryn Levitt, Gordene MacKenzie, Suneel(a) Mubayi, Nancy Nangeroni, Ashli Owen-Smith, Wendy Sanford, Stephanie Simard, and Gunner Scott.

Contributors to earlier editions: Wendy Sanford, Loraine Hutchins, and Rebecca Rabinowitz.

10: Relationships with Men

By Kristin Bloomer with Jill Maio (resources).

Edited by Rachel Fudge and the Editorial Team.

Thanks for help on this edition to: JoAnne Fischer, Leah Freij, Gardner Harris, Jennifer Hirsch, Loraine Hutchins, Zoe Nierenberg, Melissa Ostrow, Juli Parker, Emily Pilowa, Lynn Rosenbaum, and Heather Stephenson.

Contributors to earlier editions: Sara Burke, Denise Bergman, Paula B. Doress-Worters, Peggy Nelson Wegman, Maria Baez, Donna Bright, Mayra Canetti, Leah Dishkin, Cheryl Majeed, Charlotte Mayerson, Catherine Kohler Riessman, Rose Wright, Nancy Miriam Hawley, Elizabeth Matz, Catherine Cobb Morocco, and Sandy Rosenthal.

11: Relationships with Women

By Shannon Berning.

Edited by Angela Watrous and the Editorial Team.

Thanks for help on this edition to: Diane Anderson-Minshall, Suzanne Bremer, Celina De Leon, Nancy Forsyth, Jennifer Hartung, Loraine Hutchins, Meghan Kilian, Elizabeth Sarah Lindsey, Juli Parker, Wendy Sanford, Judith Sansone, and Heather Stephenson.

Contributors to earlier editions: Emily Bender, Anoosh Jorjorian, Peggy Lynch, Amelia Craig Cramer, Barbara A. Burg, Loly Carillo, Sasha Curran, J. W. Duncan, Buffy Dunker, Deanna Forist, D. Hamer, B. J. Louison, Judy Norris, Gwendolyn Parker, Mariana Romo-Carmona, Wendy Sanford, Lynn Scott, Ann Shepardson, Judy Brewer, Gilda Bruckman, Loly Carillo, Hannah Doress, Karen Kahn, Connie Panzarino, Lisa Rankow, Amy Alpern, Mary Bowe, Brenda Reeb, Holly Ellison, the Lesbian Mothers group at the Cambridge Women's Center, Jill Wolhandler, a Boston Gay Collective (who wrote the original chapter, titled "In Amerika They Call Us Dykes"), and others who remain anonymous.

12: Sexuality

By Lynn Rosenbaum, with Janna Zwerner (sexuality and disability).

Edited by Wendy Sanford and the Editorial Team.

Thanks for help on this edition to: Peg Anderson, Ani Colt, Anne Finger, Debra Haffner, Becca Heller-Steinberg and the staff at Grand Opening!, Jennifer Hirsch, Ana Jimenez-Bautista, Kristi Kirschner, Wanda Larrabee, Judith Levine, Elizabeth Sarah Lindsey, Linda Long, Gina Ogden, Judy Panko-Reis, Cindy Purcell, Monica Rodriguez, Marsha Saxton, Rose Weitz, Cindy Wentz, and Sheri Winston.

Contributors to earlier editions: Wendy Sanford, Nancy

Miriam Hawley, Elizabeth McGee, Gina Ogden, Linda King, Judy Brewer, Denise Bergman, Eithne Johnson, Curdina Hill, Amy Alpern, Diana Chase, Francis Deloatch, Paula Doress-Worters, Bonnie Engelhardt, Mary Fitzgerald, Jean Gillespie, Ginger Goldner, Shere Hite, Janice Irvine, Nancy London, Jenny Mansbridge, Oce, Rosemarie Ouilette, Jane Pincus, Brenda Reeb, Marsha Saxton, and Jean Lastovica.

Sexual Health

13: Sexual Anatomy, Reproduction, and the Menstrual Cycle

By Marianne McPherson, with Toni Weschler (fertility awareness method), Monica Casper, Cheryl Chase, Alice Dreger, and Esther M. Leidolf (intersex) and Chris Bobel (menstrual activism).

Edited by Marianne McPherson, Lauren Korfine, and the Editorial Team.

Thanks for help on this edition to: Amy Allina, Chris Bobel, Lisa Handwerker, Geneva Kachman, Claudia Morrissey, Kathleen O'Grady, Nancy Reame, Ilene Richman, Katie Singer, Laura Subramanian, Sheri Winston, Summer Wood, and Nancy Woods.

Contributors to earlier editions: Esther Rome, Nancy Reame, Wendy Sanford, Abby Schwartz, Katherine Saldutti, Cindy Irvine, Nancy Woods, Leah Diskin, Nancy Miriam Hawley, Barbara Perkins, and Roni Randall.

14: Safer Sex

By Laura Subramanian, Christie Burke, and Amelia Glynn Hornick.

Edited by Jennifer Block, Jacqueline Lapidus, and the Editorial Team.

Thanks for help on this edition to: Court Cline and all the people who worked on Chapter 15, "Sexually Transmitted Infections," and Chapter 16, "HIV and AIDS" (see below).

Contributors to earlier editions: listed under "Sexually Transmitted Infections" and "HIV and AIDS" chapters (see below).

15: Sexually Transmitted Infections

By Christie Burke.

Edited by Jacqueline Lapidus and the Editorial Team.

Thanks for help on this edition to: Jennifer Baumgardner, Shannon Berning, August Burns, Ann Duerr, Amelia Glynn Hornick, Ana Jimenez-Bautista, Ashli Owen-Smith, Sylvie Ratelle, Marianne Scharbo-Dehaan, Jill E. Tabbutt-Henry, and Sheri Winston.

Contributors to earlier editions: Christie Burke, Sylvie

Ratelle, Mary Crowe, Judy Norsigian, Katherine M. Stone of the Centers for Disease Control and Prevention, Catherine Liu of the American Social Health Association, Esther Rome, Fran Ansley, Hilde Armour, William McCormick, Michelle Topal, Pam White, and Paul Wiesner.

16: HIV and AIDS

By Deborah Anderson, Amelia Glynn Hornick, and Laura Subramanian.

Edited by Jennifer Block and the Editorial Team.

Thanks for help on this edition to: Terry Allen, Marge Cohen, Marlene Diaz, Ann C. Duerr, Anne Eckman, Jerry Feuer, Jill Gay, Ana Jimenez-Bautista, Sue Rochman, Jihad Slim, Mitchell Warren, and Leslie Wolfe.

Contributors to earlier editions: Michele Russell, Wendy Sanford, Maria Jobin-Leeds, Mary Ide, Wanda Allen, the Women of Color AIDS Council (especially Karen McManus, Malkia Kendricks, and Charlotte, Colleen, Jackie, Shirley, and Yohani), Patricia O. Loftman, Peggy Lynch, Lucia Ortiz-Ortiz, Belynda Dunn, Anna Forbes, Sophie Godley, Mary Guinan, Laura Whitehorn, Amy Alpern, Marion Banzhaf, Laurie Cotter of ACT UP New York, Deborah Cotton, Risa Denenberg, Liz Galst, Jenny Keller, Vicky Legion, the Chicago Women and AIDS Project, Patricia O. Loftman, Janet L. Mitchell, Jamie Penney, Lindsey Rosen, and Susan Rosenberg.

Reproductive Choices

17: Considering Parenting

By Merle Bombardieri, Meredith W. Michaels, Rachel Gaillard Smook, and Merryl Pisha (resources).

Edited by Nancy Adess and the Editorial Team.

Thanks for help on this edition to: Terry Allen, Adrienne Asch, Denise Bergman, Hope Bryer, Liz Coolidge, Natalie Dunlop, Rachel Gingold, Lynn Gordon, Lisa Handwerker, Susan Izumo, Monica Lange, June Lapidus, Linda Layne, Carolyn Libelo, Nancy Matthews, Amy Martyn, Jennifer O'Donnell, Cindy Purcell, Susan J. Roll, Katie Singer, Teresa Rust Smith, Kim Smith-Potts, Amy Waldman, and Toni Weschler.

Contributors to earlier editions: Joan Ditzion, Mary Howell Raugust, Denise Bergman, Norma Swenson, Joan Rachlin, Joyce Maguire Pavao, and Corinne Rayburn of the Center for Family Connection.

18: Birth Control

By August Burns, Michelle Martelle, Maura Graff, Melanie Steeves, Emma Ottolenghi, Elaine Lissner (male sterilization), Kirsten Thompson (experimental male contraceptives), David Sokal (Essure), and Toni Weschler (Fertility Awareness Method).

Edited by Penelope Riseborough and the Editorial Team.

Thanks for help on this edition to: Amy Allina, Susan Bell, Kathryn Clancy, Sunny Daly, Teresa Harrison, John Snow, Inc., Elaine Lissner, Christine Mauck, Kavita Nanda, Ilene Richman, Misty Romero, Barbara Seaman, Jill Schwartz, Katie Singer, Felicia H. Stewart, Mitchell Warren, and Carolyn Westhoff.

Contributors to earlier editions: Susan Bell, Lauren Wise, Suzannah Cooper-Doyle, Judy Norsigian, Felice Apter, Charon Asetoyer, Sara Dickey, Anne Kelsey, Sophie Martin, Ava Moskin, Cindy Pearson, Linda Potter, Judith Richter, James Trussell, Kevin Whaley, Susan Wood, Ruth Bell, Pamela Berger, Jennifer S. Edwards, Charlotte Ellertson, Philip Hart, Nancy Miriam Hawley, Rachel Lanzerotti, Ken Legins, Pamela Morgan, Barbara Perkins, Susan Reverby, Wendy Sanford, Abby Schwarz, Felicia Stewart, Alice Steinhardt, James Trussell, and Beverly Winikoff.

19: Unexpected Pregnancy

By Judith Winkler and Alison Amoroso.

Edited by Alison Amoroso and the Editorial Team.

Thanks for help on this edition to: Adrienne Asch, Euna August, Dorothy Berting, Miranda Lutyens, Carla Ortique, Monica Romanko, Laureen Tews, and Francine Thompson.

Contributors to earlier editions: Catherine Harris-Vincent, Jennifer Yanco, Linda King, Jane Pincus, Jill Wolhandler, Denise Bergman, Paula Harris-Vincent, Joyce Maguire Pavao, Carolyn Rudin, Kay Schlozman, and Dianne Weiss.

20: Abortion

By Marlene Gerber Fried, Maureen Paul, and Laureen Tews.

Edited by Jennifer Block and the Editorial Team.

Thanks for help on this edition to: Nina Carroll, Wendy Chavkin, Kathleen Dean, Diana Dukhanova, Annelise Galdes, Carol Joffe, Martha Katz, Lydie Ky, Linda Layne, Laury Oaks, Darrah Sipe, A'yen Tran, and Judith Winkler.

Contributors to earlier editions: Jill Wolhandler, Trude Bennett, Ruth Weber, Dana Gallagher, Centre de Santé des Femmes de Montréal, Carol Franzblau, Suzanne Hendrick, Luita Spangler, Laurie Williams, Vickie Alexander, Diane Balser, Pamela Berger, Sarah Buttenwieser, Helen Caulton, Concord Feminist Health Center, Terry Courtney, Debra Drassner, Carol Driscoll, Margie Fine, Marlene Gerber Fried, Linda Gordon, Nancy Miriam Hawley, Liz Hill, Debra Krassner, Elizabeth McGee, Judy Norsigian, Ana Ortiz, Jane Pincus, Stephanie Poggi, Loretta Ross, Wendy Sanford, Kira Sarpard, Meredith Tax, and Susan Yanow.

Childbearing

21: Pregnancy

By Tekoa King, with Maria Iorillo, Judith Bishop, Lisa Paine, and Carol Sakala.

Edited by Leslie Miller and the Editorial Team.

Thanks for help on this edition to: Adrienne Asch, Nancy Bardacke, Denise Bergman, Eugene Declercq, Esther Entin, Joanna Gaunt, Timothy Johnson, Kathryn Kravetz, Linda Layne, Judy Luce, Julie Mottl-Santiago, Lynn Paltrow, Jane Pincus, Cindy Purcell, Marcie Richardson, Marsha Saxton, and Deanne Williams.

Contributors to earlier editions: Jane Pincus, Judy Luce, Audrey Levine, Robin J. Blatt, Linda Holmes, Marsha Saxton, Carol Sakala, Denise Bergman, Esther Entin, Ruth Bell, Robin Blatt, Jenny Fleming, Linda Holmes, Judy Luce, Mary (Bebe) Poor, Judi Rogers, Becky Sarah, and Norma Swenson.

22: Childbirth

By Tekoa King, Maria Iorillo, Judy Luce, and Jane Pincus, with Judith Bishop and Carol Sakala.

Edited by Leslie Miller and the Editorial Team.

Thanks for help on this edition to: Nancy Bardacke, Mary Barger, Victoria Budson, Eugene Declercq, Jeffrey Ecker, Abby Kinne, Linda Layne, Ellice Lieberman, Lisa Paine, Marcie Richardson, Rachel Gaillard Smook, and Deanne Williams.

Contributors to earlier editions: Judy Luce, Jane Pincus, Audrey Levine, Norma Swenson, Carol Sakala, Ruth Bell, Jenny Fleming, Nancy Miriam Hawley, Linda Holmes, Becky Sarah, and Gail Sullivan.

Chapter 23: The First Year of Parenting

By Deborah Issokson and Alice LoCicero, with Anne Merewood (breast-feeding), Barbara L. Philipp (breast-feeding), and Tekoa King (formula).

Edited by Wendy Garling and the Editorial Team.

Thanks for help on this edition to: Cathy Amoroso, Mary Barger, Kathryn Clancy, Maureen Corry, Kathleen Kendall-Tackett, Polly Kornblith, Linda Layne, Karen Ledbetter, Harriet McCarthy, Elizabeth Noble, Shelley Page, Carol Sakala, Katie Singer, Jan Smith, Sandra Steingraber, Mary Rose Tully, Amanda Varella, Jan Weingrad-Smith, and Deane Williams.

Contributors to earlier editions: Alice LoCicero, Deborah Issokson, Dennie Wolf, Mary Crowe, Laurie Williams, Helen Armstrong, Jane Honikman, Gail Levy, Veronica Miletsky, Carol Sakala, Dianne Weiss, Paula Doress-Worters, Esther Rome, Vilunya Diskin, Marty Reudi, and Robbie Pfeufer Kahn.

Chapter 24: Childbearing Loss

By Linda L. Layne.

Edited by Wendy Garling and the Editorial Team.

Thanks for help on this edition to: Adrienne Asch, Mary Atkinson, Susan Bell, Deb Blizzard, Diane Clapp, Catherine Clute, Tamar Gordan, Lisa Handwerker, Mary Hinton, Tekoa King, Harvey Kliman, Carolyn Libelo, Stella Ng, Catherine Romeo, Renee Samelson, Katie Singer, Kim Smith-Potts, Dorothy Tischler, and Susan Wood.

Contributors to earlier editions: Catherine Romeo, Jane Pincus, and Ellen Glazer.

Chapter 25: Infertility and Assisted Reproduction

By Nancy King Reame, with Rachel Gaillard Smook (donor insemination).

Edited by Abby Lippman and the Editorial Team.

Thanks for help on this edition to: Adrienne Asch, Diane Allen, Lori Andrews, Jean Benward, Diane Clapp, Catherine Clute, Lynn Gordon, Katie Grames, Lisa Handwerker, Francie Hornstein, Harvey Kliman, Linda Layne, Lynne Millican, Marsha Saxton, Katie Singer, Jeanie Ungerleider, Rose Weitz, and Sally Whelan.

Contributors to earlier editions: Diane Clapp, Ruth Hubbard, Ami Jaeger, Wendy Sanford, Gena Corea, Ellen Glazer, Barbara Eck Menning, Marcie Richardson, Ester Shapiro, Lori Andrews, Geri Ferber, Nancy Reame, Barbara Katz Rothman, and Resolve, Inc.

Growing Older

26: Midlife and Menopause

By Joan Ditzion, with Nancy Fleming (menopause), Amy Allina (hormone therapy), Diana Siegal (urinary incontinence), and Lisa Begg and Loretta Finnegan (eating well).

Edited by Jacqueline Lapidus and the Editorial Team.

Thanks for help on this edition to: Peggy Brick, Kate Clancy, Leilani Doty, Elaine Lissner, Margaret Morganroth Gullette, Kathleen O'Grady, Ruth Palombo, Betsy Peterson, Jane Pincus, Elizabeth Plourde, Nancy Reame, Marcie Richardson, and Abby Schwarz.

Contributors to earlier editions: Paula Doress-Worters (formerly Paula Brown Doress), Joan Ditzion, Norma Meras Swenson, Diana Laskin Siegal, Robin Cohen, Mickey Troub Friedman, Lois Harris, Kathleen MacPherson, Denise Bergman, Janine O'Leary Cobb, Linda King, Susan M. Love, Cindy Pearson of the National Women's Health Network, Jane Pincus, Lynn Rosenberg, Wendy Sanford, Stephanie Studentski, Mary Yeaton, Louise Corbett, Tish Anisimov, Lorraine Doherty, Ruth Hubbard, Audrey Michaud, Pamela Berger, Irene Davidson, Meg Hickey, Judy

Norsigian, Josephine Polk-Matthews, Ruth Hubbard, Edith Fletcher, Barbara Krentzman, Lucile Longview Schuck, Anna Schenke, Anne Smith, and Marian Saunders.

27: Our Later Years

By Joan Ditzion, with Diana Siegal (osteoporosis and memory loss) and Leilani Doty (memory loss).

Edited by Jacqueline Lapidus and the Editorial Team.

Thanks for help on this edition to: Judy Simmons; see also acknowledgments under Chapter 26, "Midlife and Menopause."

Medical Problems and Procedures

28: Unique to Women

By Julia Brody (breast cancer), Barbara Brenner (breast cancer testing), and Susan Troyan (breast cancer); Mary Lou Ballweg (endometriosis); Monica Casper, Adele E. Clarke, Martha Ellen Katz, Mitchell Levine, and Marcie Richardson (cervix, uterus, and ovaries); Kristina Graff (obstetric fistula); RAINBO (FGC); Monica Casper and Adele E. Clarke (cervix); and Marianne McPherson (vulvitis/vulvodynia).

Edited by Jacqueline Lapidus and the Editorial Team.

Thanks for help on this edition to: Terry Allen, Robin Barnett, Marlies Bosch, Lucy Candib, Karen Carlson, Mary Costanza, Paula Johnson, Paula Kamen, Anne Kasper, Martha Katz, Mitchell Levine, Susan Love, Maryann Napoli, JoDean Nicolette, and Nawal Nour.

Contributors to earlier editions: Judy Norsigian, Susan Troyan, Cathie Ragovin, Judi Hirshfield-Bartek, Adele Clarke, Monica Casper, Carmen Tamayo, Anne Kahn, Mimi Secor, Selma Mirsky, Lisa Whiteside, Kath Doyle, Nahid Toubia, RAINBO, Carol Englender, Mitchell Levine, Mary Lou Ballweg, Endometriosis Association, Mary Crowe, Margaret Lee Braun, Pat Cody, DES Action, Dorothy Reider, Esther Rome, Debi Milligan, Kristina Graff, and Women's Dignity Project.

29: Special Concerns for Women

By Kim O'Connor, with Emily Wong (autoimmune disorders); Lori Clovis, Pat Fero, Jean Harrison, Mary Schweitzer, Malcolm Hooper, and Meghan Shannon (CFIDS/ME); Mickey Spencer, with Marilyn Hoffman and Claudia S. Miller (multiple chemical sensitivity); Abby Schwarz (cardiovascular diseases); Jacqueline Lapidus (chronic pain); Ernestine Hambrick (colon and rectal cancer); Genevieve Pagalilauan, Emily Wong, and Lucy Candib (diabetes); Vicki Ratner (interstitial cystitis); Susan Boughn (trichotillomania); Martha Katz (urinary tract infections); and Judith Baker (von Willebrand disease).

Edited by Jacqueline Lapidus and the Editorial Team.

Thanks for help on this edition to: Paula Devitt, Ellen Fineberg, Paula Johnson, JoDean Nicolette, Jennifer Potter, and Karen Wolf.

Contributors to earlier editions: Judy Norsigian, Carol Englender, Wendy Sanford, Laurel Berger, Rebecca Rabinowitz, Pamela Berger, Beverly Richstone, Barbara White, Barbara Henry, Barbara Horgan, Kathleen Quinlan, Mary Crowe, Judy Spear, Joanne Palmisano, Ruth Thomasian, Sheryle Ruzek, Paula Johnson, JoAnne Manson, and Vicki Ratner.

Knowledge Is Power

30: Navigating the Health Care System

By Judy Ann Bigby, Susan Sered, George Annas (patients' rights), Shannon Berning (LBT issues), Laurie Rosenblum (disability), and Kiki Zeldes (evaluating health information).

Edited by Laurie Rosenblum and the Editorial Team.

Thanks for help on this edition to: Robyn Duran, Anne Kasper, Valerie Leiter, Melissa Ostrow, Lynn Paltrow, Jane Pincus, Ellen Shaffer, J. Jina Shah, Eliza Shulman, Nancy Stoller, and Karen Wolf.

Contributors to earlier editions: Norma Meras Swenson, Wendy Sanford, Judy Norsigian, and George Annas.

31: The Politics of Women's Health

By Ellen Shaffer (U.S. politics) and Gail Price-Wise (international politics), with Marcy Darnovsky (genetic technologies), Elizabeth J. Rourke, Sondra Crosby, and Michael Grodin (refugee women), Sharon Batt (direct-to-consumer advertising), and Cindy Young (Medicare).

Edited by Christine Cupaiuolo and the Editorial Team.

Thanks for help on this edition to: Lori Andrews, George Annas, Jane Cottingham, May Haddad, Betsy Hartmann, Camara Phyllis Jones, Anne Kasper, Wendy Kline, Nancy Krieger, Judith Kurland, Marsha Lillie-Blanton, Sathya Mala, Marian McDonald, Wilhelmine Miller, Stuart Newman, Melissa Ostrow, Robin Roth, Alan Sager, Susan Sered, J. Jina Shah, Deborah Socolar, Joan Stieber, Nancy Stoller, Sally Whelan, and Karen Wolf.

Contributors to earlier editions: Norma Meras Swenson, Wendy Sanford, Judy Norsigian, Carol Sakala, Nalini Visvanathan, Vilunya Diskin, Hilary Salk, Judith Dickson Luce, Nancy Krieger, Anne Kasper, Ellen Shaffer, Steffi Woolhandler, Karen Kahn, Jacqueline Lapidus, Arnold Relman, Philip R. Lee, Roz Feldberg, Julie Friesen, Anne-Emmanuelle Birn, Nancy Worcester, Mariamne Whatley, Gabriela Canepa, Marilen Danguilan, Betsy Hartmann, Jennifer Yanco, Anita Anand, Asoka Bandarage, Elizabeth

Coit, Jane Cottingham, H. Patrica Hynes, Marilee Karl, Una MacLean, Annie Street, Amy Alpern, David Banta, Gene Bishop, Robin Blatt, Lucy Candib, David Clarke, Mary Fillmore, Mary Howell, Sherry Leibowitz, Barbara Perkins, Joan Rachlin, Sheryl Ruzek, Kathy Simmonds, Mary Stern, Nancy Todd, and Karen Wolf.

32: Organizing for Change

By Susan J. Roll, with Victoria Passarella (young women) and Ellen Miller-Mack (women in prison).

Edited by Laurie Rosenblum and the Editorial Team.

Thanks for help on this edition to: Hannah Hafter, Amelia Glynn Hornick, Anne Kasper, Karen Kubby, Paula Johnson, and Nancy Stoller.

Contributors to earlier editions: Eugenia Acuna, Judy Norsigian, Jane Pincus, Caty Laignel, Meizhu Lui, Suzanne Nam, Norma Meras Swenson, and Rachel Lanzerotti.

ABOUT THE CONTRIBUTORS

EDITORIAL TEAM

Judy Norsigian is executive director of Our Bodies Ourselves. A cofounder of the Boston Women's Health Book Collective and coauthor of all Simon & Schuster editions of *Our Bodies, Ourselves,* she is a renowned speaker and writer on women's health.

Heather Stephenson is a program manager for Our Bodies Ourselves. An award-winning writer, she holds degrees from Princeton and Harvard. She thanks all the people who worked on this book and dedicates her own efforts in memory of her mother.

Kiki Zeldes manages the Our Bodies Ourselves website. Passionate about women's health, she has worked for Our Bodies Ourselves since 1997.

TONE AND VOICE EDITOR

Zobeida Bonilla is the Latina Health Initiative program manager for Our Bodies Ourselves.

She holds a doctorate in medical anthropology from the University of Florida and a master's degree in public health from Boston University School of Public Health.

PHOTO EDITOR

Sarai Walker, MA, MFA, is an associate editor at Our Bodies Ourselves. Thanks to a groundbreaking yet little-known affirmative action program for "plus-size" women, she once worked for several high-profile teenage fashion magazines. She is now writing a novel.

CONTRIBUTORS

Amany Abouzeid is programs manager at RAINBO, an African-led international nongovernmental organization working on issues of women's empowerment, gender, reproductive health, sexual autonomy, and freedom from violence. RAINBO focuses on eliminating the practice of female circumcision/female genital mutilation.

Nancy Adess, MA, is a freelance editor specializing in health education and evaluation, social change, and non-profit functioning. She is also the editor of the Kim Klein Chardon Press series for Jossey-Bass Publishers and the *Grassroots Fundraising Journal*(naedit@horizoncable.com).

Kami-Leigh Agard is a journalist who has reported extensively in the United States and British press on global body image and women with eating disorders. She earned her journalism degree at Northeastern University in Boston.

Amy Allina is program director of the National Women's Health Network, a nonprofit organization based in Washington, DC. She is also an author of *The Truth About Hormone Replacement Therapy: How to Break Free from the Medical Myths of Menopause.*

Victoria Almquist is the manager of outreach at the Campaign for Tobacco-Free Kids in Washington, DC. She heads the campaign's initiative on women, girls, and smoking and is the North American representative for the International Network of Women Against Tobacco.

Alison Amoroso is an editorial, publishing, and nonprofit consultant, and a nationally recognized presenter and advocate of women's issues. She has been a print and online magazine founder, editor in chief, and publisher. She holds degrees from Duke and Harvard.

Deborah Anderson, Ph.D., directs a research laboratory and teaches at Harvard Medical School, where she studies vaginal immunology and HIV transmission. She is the mother of a thirteen-year-old boy, with whom she raises funds and awareness for AIDS orphans.

Judith R. Baker, MHSA, is administrative director for the Federal Hemophilia Treatment Centers in Region IX. She earned her master's degree in health services from the University of Michigan and has been a women's health advocate for thirty years.

Maggie Bangser is the director of the Women's Dignity Project in Tanzania, an organization that mobilizes action on obstetric fistula and health equity. She holds a master's degree from Yale University and has published works on reproductive health and health rights.

Sharon Batt is the author of *Patient No More: The Politics of Breast Cancer* (Gynergy Books, 1994). She is a member of the feminist health coalition Prevention First and is currently in a Ph.D. program at Dalhousie University in Halifax, Nova Scotia, Canada.

Jennifer Baumgardner writes articles for *The Nation, Harper's, Glamour, Elle,* and *Ms.* and commentaries for NPR. She is the coauthor (with Amy Richards) of *Manifesta: Young Women, Feminism, and the Future* and *Grassroots: A Field Guide for Feminist Activism.*

Lisa Begg, DrPH, RN, educated at Boston College, University of California, San Francisco, University of California, Los Angeles, and University of Pittsburgh, has experience in cancer and women's health research. She works at the National Institutes of Health, U.S. Department of Health and Human Services.

Emily Bender, MA, NC, is a nutrition consultant who specializes in women's health and fertility. In addition to her nutrition certification, she holds a master's degree in art from San Francisco State University and a bachelor's degree from Oberlin College.

Shannon Berning is an editor working for an independent book publisher. She was formerly managing editor of *Teen Voices,* a national magazine written by, for, and about teenage women. She lives in Brooklyn, New York.

JudyAnn Bigby, M.D., serves as the medical director of Community Health Programs at Brigham and Women's Hospital and as associate professor of medicine at Harvard Medical School. She also directs Harvard Medical School's Center of Excellence in Women's Health.

Jennifer Block is a freelance journalist based in New York. Her articles have appeared in *The Village Voice, The Nation, POZ,* and *Ms.,* where she was an associate editor, and in the 2004 anthology *The W Effect: Bush's War on Women.*

Kristin Bloomer is a Ph.D. candidate at the University of Chicago. Her work has appeared in *The Boston Globe, San Francisco Chronicle, In These Times, Quarterly West, Cambridge-Oxford Short Story Anthology,* and *All This Was Meant to Burn,* a chapbook.

Merle Ann Bombardieri is a clinical social worker, hypnotherapist, and life coach in Lexington, MA. She is the author of *The Baby Decision,* articles in *The Boston Globe, Bride's, Glamour,* and *Self,* and a novel about two sisters' surrogate pregnancy.

Suzanne Bremer is a writer, librarian, and webmaster. A world-class competitor in the slow jog, she has completed scores of road races and fun runs.

Julia Brody, Ph.D., is executive director of Silent Spring Institute, a scientific research group studying the environment and women's health. She is the principal investigator for the Cape Cod Breast Cancer and Environment Study.

Christie Burke, LICSW, MPH, has worked in women's health for fifteen years, including a stint as director of education and planning in STD prevention at the Massachusetts Department of Public Health. She thanks Diana Laskin Siegal and Dr. Paul Etkind.

August Burns, PA, CM, MPH, has been a women's health provider for the past twenty-six years. She consults internationally on issues of reproductive health and is coauthor of *Where Women Have No Doctor.* She is currently working on a documentary.

Paula J. Caplan, Ph.D., is a clinical and research psychologist and author of twelve books, including *The Myth of Women's Masochism, Don't Blame Mother,* and *They Say You're Crazy.* She is a visiting scholar at Brown University and American University.

Monica J. Casper, a sociologist, is author of *The Making of the Unborn Patient: A Social Anatomy of Fetal Surgery.* She is currently director of women's studies and associate professor of sociology and women's studies at Vanderbilt University.

Adele E. Clarke, Ph.D., is professor of sociology and history of medicine at University of California at San Francisco. She is coeditor of *Women's Health: Differences and Complexities* (Ohio State University Press, 1997) and *Revisioning Women, Health and Healing* (Routledge, 1999).

Sondra S. Crosby, M.D., is the director of medical services for the Boston Center for Refugee Health and Human Rights at Boston University and Boston Medical Center.

Christine Cupaiuolo is the online editor of *Ms.* and author of "ms. musings," the magazine's daily weblog on women, media, and popular culture. She is also the editor and founder of PopPolitics.com.

Marcy Darnovsky, Ph.D., is associate executive director at the Center for Genetics and Society (www.genetics-and-society.org), a public affairs organization working to encourage responsible uses and effective societal governance of new reproductive and genetic technologies.

Joan Ditzion is a founder of the Boston Women's Health Book Collective and coauthor of all editions of *Our Bodies,*

Ourselves. A geriatric social worker and educator, she appreciates the support of her husband, her two sons, and her eighty-nine-year-old mother.

Leilani Doty, Ph.D., is an associate scientist in the Department of Neurology, University of Florida, and has led its Memory Disorder Clinic since 1988. Her interests include neuro-behavioral geriatrics, progressive memory disorders, women's health, leadership training, and academic professional development.

Cara Feinberg is a freelance writer and editor living in Boston. Her articles have appeared in *The Boston Globe, The American Prospect Magazine, The Atlantic Monthly* online, and *Ed. Magazine,* where she was a senior writer.

Pat Fero holds a master's degree in education. In 1988 she went on medical leave due to chronic fatigue syndrome and later went on disability. A writer, she is currently the executive director of the Wisconsin CFS Association.

Nancy Fleming is a certified nurse-midwife who prepared at Stanford University (BS), the University of California at San Francisco (MS), and the University of Illinois at Chicago (Ph.D.). She has a small clinical practice and teaches nurse-midwifery at UIC.

Marlene Gerber Fried is a professor at Hampshire College, director of the Civil Liberties and Public Policy Program, and founding president of the National Network of Abortion Funds. She recently coauthored *Undivided Rights: Women of Color Organizing for Reproductive Justice.*

Rachel Fudge is a freelance editor and writer based in San Francisco. She is also the senior editor of *Bitch: Feminist Response to Pop Culture.*

Adriane Fugh-Berman, M.D., is associate professor, Department of Physiology, Georgetown University School of Medicine, author of *The 5-Minute Herb and Dietary Supplement Clinical Consult,* and coauthor of the National Women's Health Network's *The Truth About Hormone Replacement Therapy.*

Wendy Garling, MA, is a writer and editor specializing in health care and women's issues. She earned her master's in Sanskrit at University of California at Berkeley and teaches in the women's spirituality program at the Women's Well in Concord, Massachusetts, www.womenswell.org.

Jennie Goode works as a freelance editor and writer in Seattle. She is cofounder of the magazine *Push: Queer Fem-*

inist *Subversions* and editor of *Drive: Women's True Stories from the Open Road* (Seal Press).

Kristina Graff is a master of public affairs candidate at Princeton University's Woodrow Wilson School. Her previous publications include *Counseling the Postabortion Client* for EngenderHealth and *Faces of Dignity* for the Women's Dignity Project.

Michael A. Grodin, M.D., is the codirector of the Boston Center for Refugee Health and Human Rights at Boston University and Boston Medical Center and director of the Human Rights, Advocacy and Education Program.

Ernestine Hambrick, M.D., trained at the University of Illinois College of Medicine in Chicago and at Cook County Hospital. The nation's first female board-certified colon and rectal surgeon, she promotes screening and healthy lifestyles to eradicate colorectal cancer.

Jean Harrison, a 1974 graduate of Wellesley College, trained in London as an oil painting conservator. In December 1994 she had to stop work when ME/CFS, an illness that had been hampering her in a mild form, became severe.

Maria Iorillo is a licensed midwife in a home birth practice in San Francisco. She is a former chairwoman of the California Association of Midwives and a former board member of the Midwives Alliance of North America. She has two children.

Deborah Issokson is a licensed psychologist specializing in perinatal mental health. In addition to her private practice in Watertown, Massachusetts, she teaches in the Nurse-Midwifery Education Program of Boston University School of Public Health's Department of Maternal and Child Health.

Lisa Jervis is the publisher and founding editor of *Bitch: Feminist Response to Pop Culture*. She has written for *Ms.,* the *San Francisco Chronicle, Utne Reader, Mother Jones, Women's Review of Books, Bust,* and others. She lives in Oakland, California.

Martha Katz, M.D., has practiced medicine with a focus on women's health for over twenty years. She practices at Children's Hospital, Brigham and Women's Hospital, and Harvard University Health Services, and teaches at Harvard Medical School.

Eugenia SunHee Kim, MFA, is a writer, teacher, and graphic designer in Washington, D.C.

Tekoa L. King, CNM, MPH, is editor in chief of the *Journal of Midwifery & Women's Health* and an associate professor in the Department of Obstetrics, Gynecology and Reproductive Sciences at the University of California at San Francisco.

Jacqueline Lapidus is an editorial consultant with extensive experience in the fields of health care, business, and travel; she is also a poet and essayist. She teaches the writing component of "Current Topics in Medicine" at Harvard Extension School.

Linda Layne completed her doctorate at Princeton in 1986, the year she had the first of seven miscarriages. She is author of *Motherhood Lost: A Feminist Account of Pregnancy Loss in America* (2003) and a professor at Rensselaer Polytechnic Institute.

Margaret Lazarus is an Academy Award–winning documentary filmmaker who has spent most of her adult life working on issues of social justice and as an activist in the anti-violence movement. She has contributed to earlier editions of this book.

Elizabeth Sarah Lindsey, a 2002 graduate of Swarthmore College, works in the nonprofit world and fights for queer people of color liberation. Her other passions include grassroots fund-raising and sexual health education. She thanks her loved ones for their support.

Abby Lippman, Ph.D., is a professor in McGill University's Faculty of Medicine and cochair of the Canadian Women's Health Network. She is a feminist researcher and activist interested in the social justice and human rights implications of reproductive and genetic technologies.

Elaine Lissner is director of the Male Contraception Information Project and author of *Frontiers in Nonhormonal Male Contraception: A Call for Research.* Her work has appeared in *Issues in Reproductive Technology* and in *Ms.* She lives in San Francisco.

Alice LoCicero is a clinical psychologist who practices in Cambridge, Massachusetts, and teaches at Suffolk University and the Center for Multicultural Mental Health in Boston. She is the mother of two young adults and has studied birth and family transitions.

Judy Luce, MA, LM-CPM, a home birth midwife since 1975 and a hospice volunteer, has written about home birth, home dying, and midwifery. She is a mother, grandmother, and teacher and promotes the culture, practice, and status of Mayan midwives in Guatemala.

Jill Maio is a writer and visual artist who, as a grateful and wide-eyed child, read every single word of *Our Bodies, Ourselves.*

Angelina Malhotra-Singh has worked as a print and photo journalist for fifteen years. She has produced prizewinning investigative stories for *Girlfriends, Frontline,* and *India Today.* She holds a master's degree in journalism from Columbia University and thanks her husband, Romy.

Deborah McLellan works at the Dana-Farber Cancer Institute and is a founding mother and past president of the International Network of Women Against Tobacco. She is an author of the 2001 U.S. Surgeon General's Report on Women and Smoking.

Marianne McPherson, BA, lives in Boston and attends the Harvard School of Public Health. Her undergraduate research in psychology and women's studies concerns women's menstrual experiences, attitudes, and behaviors from menarche through young adulthood. She thanks her wonderful family and friends.

Anne Merewood, MA, IBCLC, a former journalist, is director of research at the Breastfeeding Center, Boston Medical Center, and an instructor of pediatrics at Boston University School of Medicine. She is studying for her master's degree in public health.

Meredith W. Michaels is a research associate in the Smith College philosophy department. Her books include *The Mommy Myth: The Idealization of Motherhood and How It Harms Women* (2004) with Susan Douglas, and *Fetal Subjects/Feminist Positions* (1999) with Lynn Morgan.

Leslie Miller is senior editor at Seal Press, an independent feminist publisher. Before earning her master's degree in English, she worked in public health. She is also the editor of the collection *Women Who Eat.*

Lin Nelson teaches in the Environmental Studies Program at the Evergreen State College in Olympia, WA. She has been a board member of the Washington Toxics Coalition and is active with a number of community-based environmental organizations.

Kim O'Connor, M.D., is an acting instructor in the Department of General Internal Medicine at the University of Washington in Seattle. She earned her medical degree at the same university. She thanks her mother, Dede, for her support and encouragement.

Genevieve Pagalilauan, M.D., is ambulatory chief resident of internal medicine at University of Washington Medical Center in Seattle. She earned her medical degree at the University of Washington. She thanks her husband, Alberto Arriola, Jr., and her mentor, Emily Wong, M.D.

Lisa L. Paine, CNM, DrPH, has held numerous clinical, research, and policy positions in women's health, including academic appointments at Johns Hopkins and Boston Universities. She currently directs the Hutchinson Dyer Group, a women's health consultation service based in Cambridge, Massachusetts.

Victoria Passarella is a women's studies major at the State University of New York at New Paltz. She is a cofounder of the New Paltz Feminist Majority Leadership Alliance and coordinator of Take Back the Night, and has interned with NARAL/NY.

Maureen Paul, M.D., MPH, is medical director at Planned Parenthood Golden Gate and associate clinical professor in the Department of Obstetrics, Gynecology, and Reproductive Sciences at the University of California, San Francisco. She is chief editor of *A Clinician's Guide to Medical and Surgical Abortion.*

Barbara L. Philipp, M.D., FAAP, is associate professor of pediatrics at Boston University School of Medicine and a practicing pediatrician at Boston Medical Center. She is a coauthor of *Breastfeeding: Conditions and Diseases.* Jessie and Abby, you go, girls.

Jane Pincus, a cofounder of the Boston Women's Health Book Collective, has participated in writing and editing every edition of *Our Bodies, Ourselves.* Her two children, grandson, and husband, horse, art, and health work are the joys of her life.

Nancy Poole currently works as a research consultant on women and substance use issues with the British Columbia Centre of Excellence for Women's Health and BC Women's Hospital in Vancouver, British Columbia, Canada.

Gail Price-Wise works for Management Sciences for Health, an international health agency, where she focuses on reducing racial and ethnic health disparities. She holds a master's degree in health policy and management from the Harvard School of Public Health.

Vicki Ratner, M.D., a former orthopedic surgeon, is founder and president of the Interstitial Cystitis Association, a nonprofit women's health organization that, since 1984, has been dedicated to promoting advocacy, education, and research for interstitial cystitis, a painful bladder disorder.

Nancy King Reame, a nursing professor and scientist at the University of Michigan, has studied women's fertility and menstrual cycles for twenty-five years. She thanks the Boston Women's Health Book Collective for teaching her everything she knows about the politics of women's health.

Penelope Riseborough is director of communications for John Snow, Inc., and World Education, Inc. She edited *PocketGuide for Family Planning Service Providers* (JHPIEGO, 1994); *Norplant Guidelines for Family Planning Service Providers* (1995); and *JHPIEGO International Family Planning Guide* (JHPIEGO, 1995).

Susan J. Roll, MSW, is associate executive director of the Massachusetts Breast Cancer Coalition. She has a bachelor's degree in political science from the University of Rochester and a master's degree in social work from Arizona State University. Thanks, Mom and Dad.

Lynn Rosenbaum, MA, is an educator and performing artist in Arlington, Massachusetts, who has taught sociology and sexual communication. Currently, she spends her time singing, dancing, and meditating and is perhaps best known for her original song "Rejection."

Laurie B. Rosenblum, MPH, is a health writer and editor at the Education Development Center, Inc., and also a freelancer. She has worked on increasing access to health and disability information and services as an educator and project coordinator.

Elizabeth J. Rourke, M.D., is a primary care physician at the Boston Center for Refugee Health and Human Rights at Boston University and Boston Medical Center.

Carol Sakala, Ph.D., MSPH, is director of programs at the Maternity Center Association, where she leads Maternity Wise, a national program promoting safe, effective, and satisfying maternity care (www.maternitywise.org). She has been an advocate, researcher, and educator for two decades.

Wendy Sanford is a cofounder of the Boston Women's Health Book Collective and longtime coauthor/editor of previous editions of *Our Bodies, Ourselves.* Editing Lynn Rosenbaum's careful work on Chapter 12, "Sexuality," was a pleasure.

Barbara Sattler, RN, DrPH, FAAN, is director of the Environmental Health Education Center and associate professor at the University of Maryland School of Nursing. She coauthored *Environmental Health and Nursing Practice* and directs an environmental health nursing program. See www.enviRN.umaryland.edu.

Abby Schwarz, Ph.D., is a behavioral biologist at Langara College, Vancouver, BC, Canada. She was an originator of *Our Bodies, Ourselves* in 1969 and cofounded the Society for Canadian Women in Science and Technology. She thanks Anka, Tina, and Rob.

Susan Starr Sered, Ph.D., directs research at Harvard's Center for the Study of World Religions. Her books include *Uninsured in America: Life and Death in the Land of Opportunity* and *What Makes Women Sick?: Maternity, Modesty and Militarism in Israeli Society.*

Ellen R. Shaffer is a director of the Center for Policy Analysis, which conducts policy research on access to health care and on economic globalization and health. She is an assistant professor at the University of California at San Francisco.

Meghan-Morgan Shannon has been working for women's health and awareness for twenty years. She left her careers in health care and education in 1983 due to illness. She received a master's degree in multicultural education and marriage/family therapy in 1988.

Diana Laskin Siegal is the coauthor of *Ourselves, Growing Older: Women Aging with Knowledge and Power.* She worked in public health for over thirty years, retiring as director of elder health services in the Massachusetts Department of Public Health.

Judy Dothard Simmons, writer, poet, and former *Ms.* and *Essence* editor, has published in *33 Things Every Girl Should Know About Women's History, Wild Women Don't Wear No Blues,* national periodicals, and *Decent Intentions* (Blind Beggar Press).

Rachel Gaillard Smook, Psy.D., earned her doctorate in clinical psychology and focuses her work around young adulthood and perinatal health. She is a writer, psychotherapist, mother, and breast-feeding/midwifery advocate. She thanks the I.F. group and her daughter, Abigail.

David C. Sokal, M.D., based at Family Health International, has been conducting research on both male and female sterilization methods since 1992. Before joining FHI, he worked for CDC, Atlanta, and spent five years living in West Africa working in public health.

Laura Subramanian is a graduate student at the Harvard School of Public Health, studying women's health and reproductive health. She holds a degree in biology and sociology from Brandeis. She thanks her family and friends for their continued support.

Laureen Tews, MPH, graduated from Colgate University and Temple University's master of public health program. She worked four years as a family planning counselor at Planned Parenthood and has been a program director at the National Abortion Federation since 1997.

Lori Tharps is a mother, writer, and editor based in Brooklyn, New York. She is the coauthor of *Hair Story: Untangling the Roots of Black Hair in America* (St. Martin's Press).

Kirsten Thompson is the director of the Male Contraceptives Information Center and creator of MaleContraceptives .org. She got her biology degree from Bryn Mawr College and her feminism from her mother.

A'yen Tran is a recent graduate of Columbia University, where she developed and coordinated an abortion clinic escorting program. She coordinates volunteers with Downtown for Democracy and works at Chat the Planet, a youth activism TV show.

Susan Troyan, M.D., is the surgical director of the Breast-Care Center at Boston's Beth Israel Deaconess Medical Center and is on the faculty at Harvard Medical School. She earned her medical degree at the University of Miami School of Medicine.

Angela Watrous is the editor of *Bare Your Soul: The Thinking Girl's Guide to Enlightenment,* and the coauthor of *Talk to Me, After the Breakup,* and *Love Tune-ups.* She writes the PlanetOut.com advice column "Kiss and Tell." Find her at www.AngelaWatrous.com.

Toni Weschler, MPH, is the author of the best-selling book *Taking Charge of Your Fertility.* A women's health educator with a master's degree in public health, she is a frequent guest on television, radio, and websites. Her website is www.TCOYF.com.

Judith Winkler is a consultant and former executive vice president for Ipas. She is an expert in communications, education, and health, and an advocate in support of women's health and rights worldwide.

Janna Zwerner, MRC, CRC, is the chief of staff for the Massachusetts Rehabilitation Commission. She formerly led several nonprofits. She thanks Irv Zola for inspiring her to work on disability issues and the disability community for teaching her so much.

anemia, 439, 659–60
  birth control and, 347, 349,
    352, 355, 358, 360
  from chemo, 615
  see also specific types of anemia
anesthesia:
  for abortion, 397, 398, 401, 402
  allergies and, 690
  epidural, 402
  fetal risk and, 465
  types of, 690–91
angiogram, 676
angioplasty, 678
anorexia nervosa, 38–39, 40, 259
anovulatory cycles, 244, 259
antianxiety agents, 48
antibiotics, 363
  abortion and, 402, 405, 406
  STIs and, 274, 275, 648
antibody test, HIV, 298, 300
anti-choice groups, 374, 390,
  392–93, 403, 409
anticoagulants, 677
antidepressants, 48, 53, 89–92,
  200, *222*
  see also selective serotonin
    reuptake inhibitors
antigens, 661
antihistamines, 246
antihypertensives, *222*
antioxidants, 22, 26, 567
antiretrovirals, 302–3, 304
antiseizure medications, *222*
anus, 228, *229*, 229, 274, 275, *339*
  stimulation of, 199, 210–11
  see also anal sex
anxiety, 49, 52, 91, 133–34, 504
appendectomy, infertility and,
  511
appetite, changes in, 83, 296, 358,
  382
areola, 231, *239*, 239
ArginMax, 202
Aricept, 729–30, *729*
aromatase inhibitors, 617
aromatherapy, 72
arthritis, 563, 660–61

artificial insemination, 304, 316,
  522
artificially ruptured membranes,
  421, 463, 464
asexual person, 147
Asian-American women, 40, 158,
  177–78, 188
aspirin, 436, 661, 677
assisted living, 574–75
assisted reproductive
  technologies (ARTs), 519–23
  see also in vitro fertilization
asthma, 48, 103, 115, 303
Astroglide, *233*, 264, 267, 335
atherosclerosis, 671
Ativan (lorazepam), 616
atmosphere, hazards to, *101*
atypical ductal lumps, 603–4
augmentation, of labor, 464
autoimmune disorders, 512, 613,
  661–64
auxillary lymph nodes, 611–12
ayurvedic medicine, 67, 72

baby blues, *see* postpartum blues
back pain, 83, 358
  complementary health
    practices and, 72, 74
  occupational hazards and,
    106–7
baclofen, *222*
bacterial vaginosis (BV), 268,
  273, 281, *286*, 655
balloon angioplasty, 678
balloon catheter techniques, 516
barrier methods of birth control,
  332–45
Bartholin's glands, *see* vestibular
  glands
basal body temperature, *see*
  waking or basal body
  temperature
bathing, after vaginal birth, 77
battered women, *see* abuse;
  physical abuse; sexual abuse;
  violence
beans, 25, *27*, 31, 41

benzodiazepines, 48–49
bereavement, 496, 555–56, 580,
  581
beta-carotene, 23
Bethesda System SIL, 623
bikini waxing, 4
Billings (ovulation) method, *370*
binge-eating disorder (BED), 39
biomarkers, 618
biopsies, 515, 592–94, 601, 602–4,
  625–26
  see also specific types of biopsies
biotechnologies, 730–33
birth control, ix, 155, 161, 201,
  322–80
  advocacy for vs. backlash
    against, 323
  after abortion, 346, 353, 354,
    357, 395–96, 402–3, *403*
  barrier type, 332–45; *see*
    specific barrier methods
  breast-feeding as, 371–73, *379*
  after child birth, 486
  combined with other drugs,
    222, 350, 352, 358
  comparison of methods of,
    378–79
  disabilities and, *218–22*, 325,
    340–41
  dual protection and, 329–30,
    332
  effectiveness and safety of,
    331–32
  in emergencies, *see* emergency
    contraception
  fertility awareness method
    and, 241, 245, 247, 369–71,
    370, 379
  hormonal methods of, 201,
    345–65; *see specific hormonal*
    methods
  infertility and, 509, 512
  lack of, 309
  men and, 326–27, 367–68, 373,
    379
  movement for, 406
  myths vs. reality about, 331

birth control (*cont.*)

natural methods of, 369–71, *370*

obstacles to getting and using of, 324–25

personal considerations about, 328–29

pregnancy despite, 332, 350, 351, 357, 364, 367

protection of women's interests and, 325–26

selection of method of, 328–29

side effects of, *see specific methods*

sterilization as, *see* tubal ligation; vasectomy

teenagers and, 324, 329

websites about, 323*n*, 329, 330, 332*n*, 356, 374

withdrawal as, 373–74, *379*

woman-controlled methods of, 330–31, 338

birth control pills, 259, 327, 328, 345–50, 357, *378*, 620, 622

after abortion, *403*, 405

cervical fluid and, 246–47, 346, 350

DES daughters and, 627

disabilities and, *218–22*

drug interactions with, 350

dual protection and, 330

effectiveness of, 331, 346

as emergency contraception, 350, 374, 375

estrogen in, *218, 222*, 345–46, 347

health concerns for, 349–50

how to use, 346–48

menstrual suppression and, 255, 346, 348–49

in midlife, 543

PCOS and, 633

pregnancy after use of, 350

progesterone in, *218*, 345–46

safer sex and, 262, 268

safety of, 332, 338, 347

St. John's wort and, 68, 70

sexuality and, 188, *218–22*

side effects of, 349

skipped periods and, 331, 348

smoking and, 47, 48, 329, 349

social effects of, 322–23

switching to Vaginal Ring after, 354

UTIs and, 694

see also progestin-only pills

birth defects, 439

abortion and, 396, 398

alcohol use and, 47

environmental hazards and, 96, 102, 104

vitamin A and, 32

see also fetal impairments

birthing centers, 423, 425, 426, 428, 429, 444

birth plan, 444

bisexuality, bisexuals, 143, 146–52, 162, 188, 264

see also relationships with women

bisphosphonates, 539, 564

black men, HIV/AIDS and, 293, 297

black women, 115

abortion and, 413–14

body image of, 5, 7, 11–12, *11*, 14, 39

cancer screenings and, 711

childbearing loss in, 496, 502

complementary health practices of, 68, 77

diabetes in, 60, 681

eating disorders of, 38, 39–40

endometriosis in, 629

environmental and occupational hazards of, 99, 100, 106, 560

frequency of fibroids in, 639

frequency of hysterectomy in, 639

grandparents raising grandchildren among, 530

hair of, 5, 7, 11, *11*

heart disease in, 58

HIV/AIDS and, 292–93

hypertension in, 47

LBTQ relationships and, 177

lupus symptoms in, 663

menopause in, 531

as mothers, 310–11

occurrence of SIDS in, 502

racial barriers to health care and, 710–11

sex and gender of, 149–50

sexuality of, 188

sickle-cell anemia in, 660

bladder, 235, 275, 327, *339*

bladder catheters, 421

bladder control, 430, 432, 442, 535–36

bladder infections, *222*, 341, 366

see also cystitis; urethritis

"blame the victim" attitude, 80

blepharoplasty, 8

bloating, 91, 247, 256, *257*, 358, 382, 405

blood, bleeding:

abortion and, 396, 397, 398, 400, 402–5

birth control and, 255, 331, 345–46, 349, 351, 353, 355–63

HIV and, 294

and perimenopausal changes, 537–38

Rh positive vs. Rh negative, 394*n*

safer sex and, 264

STIs and, 273, 281, 288

see also menstrual cycle; von Willebrand disease

blood clots:

abortion and, 396, 405

birth control pills and, 347, 349

estrogen and, *220, 222*

blood pressure, 511, 545, 685–86

blood sugar, controlling, *685*

blood type, 499

boarding care, 574

body burden, 101

body image, 3–18, 38–41
    exercise and, 63–66, *65*
    sexuality and, 187–88
body language, sex and, 214
body mass index, 37
body position, during childbirth, 455–56, 461, 464
Body Revisited, *12*
bodywork, 72–74
bondage and discipline (B&D), 212–13, 266
bone density, bone loss, 303, 546–47
    decline in, 564
    hormones and, 540
    prevention of, 547
    testing for, 546–47
    treatments and supplements for, 539, 546–47
    see also osteoporosis
bone spurs, 563
borderline personality disorder (BPD), 93
bottle feeding, *see* formula
bowels, bowel movements, diet and, 23, 339
bowel transit time (BTT), 23
boycotts, consumer, 112
Bradley Method, 438
brain injuries, sex and, 215–16, *218–19*
Braxton-Hicks contractions, 443, 452
bread, 25, *27, 28,* 35
breakfast, 29, 35
breakups, 183, 203
breast cancer, 47, 58, 74, 599
    abortion and, 406
    biologic and targeted therapies for, 617–18
    birth control and, 329, 347, 349, 351, 359, 363
    carcinoma in situ, 608–9
    chemo and, 607, 610, 614, 615–17
    in DES daughters, 627
    endocrine therapy for, 617

environmental factors in, ix, 98, 102, 106
future promise for prognosis of, 618
genetic testing and risks of, 605–6
inflammatory, 610
invasive, 608
lumpectomy vs. mastectomy, 611
myths of, 598
politics of research funding for, ix
reducing risk of, 605
removal of lymph nodes, 611–12
risk of, 604–7
screening for, 597–99
smoking and, 48
stages of, 608, *608*
survival rates of, 611, 614
systemic therapy and, 614–18
treatment of, 607–18
Breast Cancer Action (BCA), 748–49, 755–76
breast-feeding, 255, 259, 444, 478–83
    alcohol and, 51
    as birth control, 371–73, *379*
    breast changes and, 240
    after breast surgery, 482–83
    challenges in, 480–83
    diet and, 24, 31
    environmental hazards and, 97, 98, 104–5, 106
    food allergies and, 37
    formula as alternative to, 484
    health benefits of, 478
    HIV transmission and, 294, 304
    hormonal birth control and, 350, 353, 354, 359, 361, 363
    immediately after childbirth, 458
    latch and positioning in, 480–81
    oxytocin and, 458, 479

preparations and first days of, 444, 479–80
in public, 482, *482*
after returning to workplace, 482
sexuality and, 201, 208
sleep disruption and, 485
supply and demand of, 479–80
supply supplementation and, 483
taking medications during, 489
breast implants, 5, 7, 613
breast pumps, 480–81
breast reconstruction surgery, 612–14
breasts, 199, 238, 240
    anatomy of, 231, *239, 239–40*
    benign conditions of, 595–97
    biopsies of, 601, 602–4
    changes over time to, 596–97
    clinical examination of, 599–602
    diagnostic imaging of, 602
    examination of, 238
    fibrocystic changes in, 346, 350
    infection in, 481–82
    lumps in, 597, 598, 599–604
    media images of, 10
    medical evaluation of problems in, 602
    menstrual cycle and, 238, 247, 253, 256, *257*
    self-examination of, 597–98
    size of, 5, 238, 240
    soreness from breast-feeding of, 481–82
    structure of, *596*
    tail of, 240
    tenderness of, 247, 256, *257,* 349, 353, 355, 358, 382, 405
    see also nipples
breast ultrasound, 602
breathing, breath:
    conscious, 85
    relaxation techniques and, 462
    shortness of, 350
    techniques, 438

baby's breathing and
appearance at, 457
baby's position during, 456
birth control after, 354, 357,
362
body position during, 455–56,
461, 464
celibacy after, 203
choice of place for, 420, 425,
429–30
climate of doubt and, 422–23
contractions during, 455
by C-section, *see* cesarean
sections
disappointment with
experience of, 476
environment during, 421
heightened emotions after,
487–88
HIV and, 294
IV medications during, 421–22
Kegel exercises and, 235
looking back on experience of,
471–72
mechanical assistance for,
467–68
medical complications during,
459
medical interventions during,
463–65
meeting the challenges of,
459–63
mismanagement during, 209
os and, 234
painful childhood memories
and, 311
pain relief during, 465–67
physical recovery from, 476–78
planning of, 444
postpartum health and, 421
premature, 48, 74, 104, 289,
363
relaxation techniques for,
438–39
restrictions on patients during,
421
sexuality after, 486

standardization of, 421–23
support system during, 463
unnecessary procedures
during, 422
see also pregnancy
childbirth classes, 438–39
child care, exercise and, 61–62
child-free people, 312, 313, 315
childhood, sexuality shaped in,
187
children:
abuse of, 84, 93, 119, 121,
132–35, 189
developmental delays in, 98,
104
diet of, 24, 31, 33–34
environmental hazards and,
97, 98, 102, 104
exercising with, 62
food allergies of, 36, 37
HIV/AIDS and, 292, 294, 297,
305
impact of intimate-partner
violence on, 124–25
loss of custody of, 51, 89*n*
number of, 313–14
pros and cons of, 311–12
prostitution of, 739–40, *740*
secondhand smoke and, 48
see also adolescent girls; infants
chills, 396
Chinese medicine, 67, 68, 70–71,
72, 79, 303, 616
chiropractic, 68, 71–72
chlamydia, 262, 273–76, 281, *282*,
288, 289, 377, 621, 624, 647
infertility and, 511
protection against, 328, 331,
334, 338
reporting of, 281
cholesterol, 303, 686
choline, 25
chorionic villi sampling (CVS),
439, 599
chromosomal anomolies,
miscarriage and, 499
chromosomes, abnormal, 259

chronic cervicitis, 594
chronic fatigue syndrome
(CFIDS), 90, 665–68
chronic illness, 446–48, 558
chronic pain conditions, 668–71;
see also pain management
Cialis (tadalafil), 202
cigarettes, 47, 50, *50*
circumcision:
female, *see* clitoridectomy
male, 268
civil unions, 169, 184
class action lawsuits, 114
class discrimination, 99
classic bypass, 678
classism, personal power and, 159
clear-cell adenocarcinoma,
626–27
climax stage, 194
clinical trials, informed consent
and, 703
clitoridectomy, 195, 209, 277,
643–46
clitoris, 193–96, 643, 645
anatomy of, 231, *235, 236*
female condom and, 337
intersex and, 232
masturbation and, 199
orgasm and, 188, 205, *234*
vagina-to-penis intercourse
and, 205, 207
Clomid, 633
clomiphene citrate, 633
clothes, body image and, 15, 16
Clothesline Project, *754*
clotrimazole, 655
coalitions, 113
COBRA, 557
cocaine, 46, 55, 294, 435
cocktails, drug, 301, 303
coenzyme Q10, 41
cognitive disabilities, *218–19*
cognitive therapy, 304
coitus interruptus, 373–74, *379*
cold and respiratory symptoms,
70
cold sores, 83, 288

cough medicine, 246
Coumadin, 435
counselors, *see* health care providers; therapy, therapists
Cowper's gland, *327*
COX-2 inhibitors, 563, 661
crabs, 275, *286*
cramp bark, dried, *70*
cramps, 52, 288
  abortion and, 396, 397, 400–403, 405
  diaphragm and, 341
  IUD and, 361–62
  menstrual, 70, 245, 253–56, 258–59, *258*, 349, 352, 355, 358, 360, 362, 363
  pregnancy and, 382
cranberry juice, 68, 654, 695
creams and jellies, spermicide, 345
creative activities, 83, 159, 192, 253, 256
creative tension, 168
Crohn's disease, 41, 69
crura, 231, *235*, *236*
cryosurgery, 621
cryotherapy, 594, 625
cultural differences:
  as barrier to health care, 711–12
  as barrier to intimacy, 160–61
cunnilingus, 209
curanderismo, 69, 77
curettage, *see* dilation and curettage
cyclophosphamide and adriamycin (CA), 615
cystic fibrosis, 440
cystitis, 210, 275, 281, 341, 693
cysts, 259, 597, 598, 599
  ovarian, 209, 346, 350, 351
cytobrush, 591
cytomegalovirus (CMV), 288

dairy products, 24, 25, *27*, 28, *28*, 30, 32, 111–12

Dalkon Shield, 361
danazol, 620
dance and movement therapies, 77
D&C, *see* dilation and curettage
dating, 157, 161, 170–76, 542
DDT, 98, 114
death, planning and support for, 580, 581
Declaration of Sexual Rights, 191
defensive medicine, 453, 469
deinfibulation, 209
dementia, 70, 567
  see also Alzheimer's disease
dental care, 710
dental dams, 189, 210–11, 263, 265–66, *265*, 268, 269, 274
Depo-Provera, 201, 255, 332, 346, 354, 356–58, *378*, 411
  after abortion, *403*
  health concerns for, 357–58
  lasting effects of, 512
depression, 273, 639, 642–43
  aging and, 565
  biological basis of, 89
  birth control and, 188, 346, 349, 353, 357, 364
  diet and, 25, 26, 36, 40
  exercise and, 58
  in midlife, 537
  mood-altering drugs and, 47, 49, 51, 52, 89–92
  postpartum, 487–88, *490–91*
  premenstrual, 256, *258*
  STIs and, 278
  symptoms of, 90
  treatment for, 70, 84–85, 89–92
  weight and, 39
Depression After Delivery, 489
DES (diethylstilbestrol), 626–28
  daughters, 626–27, 653
  exams for, 626–28
  exposure rates to, 626
desire, sexual, 187, 188, 191–93
  hormones and, 200–201, 202
  medications and, 200

negative attitudes toward, 324
  variations in, 191–93
developing countries:
  birth control in, 325
  breast-feeding in, 478–79
  politics and women's health in, 734–35
diabetes, 303, 459, 465, 560, 566, 680–87
  birth control and, 349, 363
  breast cancer and, 614
  complications of, 682–83
  diet and, 21, 26, 36, 37
  exercise and, 58, 59–60
  food choices and, 683
  gestational, 442
  PCOS and, 633
  during pregnancy, 442, 445
  prevention of, 682–83
  risk factors for, 683
  screening for, 681–82
  sex and, *219*
  symptoms of, 681
  taking control of, 686
  testing for, 442
  treatment of, 684–86
  Type 2, 58, 59–60
  types of, 680–81
diabetic retinopathy, 562
diagnostic tests:
  for abnormal uterine bleeding, 619
  in basic physical exam, 592–95
  for CVD, 673, 676
  D&C as, 592, 637
  during pregnancy, 436
diapers, 250, 253
diaphragms, 207, 208, *325*, *339*, 338–41, *338*, *378*
  after abortion, *403*
  advantages of, 339, 625
  disabilities and, *222*, 340–41
  menstrual flow and, *249*, 250, 251
  safer sex and, 262, 268, 269, 331, 338

risks and complications of, 639
safer sex and, 263
and sexuality, 639–40
when called for, 638, 649
hystereoscopic exam, 619, 638
hysterosalpingogram (hsg),
514–15

ibuprofen, 436
imagery and mantras, 462
immigrants:
  environmental and
    occupational hazards of,
    100–101, *114*, 115
  health care rights of, 726–27
  improving health care, 738–39
  LBTQ, 170
  violence and abuse against,
    121, 125, 126–27, 133
immune system, 624–25
  diet and, 22, 25, 36
  HIV and, 292, 295, 296, 298,
    302, 303, 304
  T cells and, 292, 302
Implanon, 358
implants, breast, 5, 7, 613
implants, contraceptive, 358–60,
    378
  effectiveness of, 332
  switching to Vaginal Ring after,
    354
  see also Norplant
impotence, 104, 202, 205, 511
incest, 132–33, 311, 390
incisional biopsies, 603
income gap, 721, 722
incontinence, *see* urinary
    incontinence
independent midwives, *see* direct-
    entry midwives
India, RISUG in, 368
induction, of labor, 464–65
induction abortion, *395*, 401, 402
infantilization, of women, 9
infants:
  HIV and, 293, 299
  low-birth-weight, 104, 435

premature birth of, 48, 74, 104,
    289, 363
  sexual pleasure of, 197
  STIs and, 287
  see also breast-feeding;
    newborns; sudden infant
    death syndrome
infections, 618, 624
  bladder, *see* bladder infections
  chemo and, 615, 616–17
  hysterectomy and, 638
  pelvic, *see* pelvic infections
  urinary tract, *see* urinary tract
    infections
  vaginal, *see* vaginal infections
infectious diseases,
    environmental and
    occupational health and,
    104
infertility, 104, 289, 332, 364
  adoption and, 318, 320
  and assisted reproduction,
    506–24
  birth control and, 509
  causes of, 510–13, 647
  changing diagnosis and
    treatment of, 513–17
  chemo and, 616
  complementary treatments for,
    517
  defined, 508
  diagnosis of, 513–16
  emotional response to, 507–8
  endometriosis and, 628
  getting informed about,
    509–10
  in men, 511, 517
  in men vs. women, 509
  social pressures and, 507, 508
  stress during diagnostic
    workup for, 515
  support groups for, 509
  surgical treatments for, 516–17
  temporary vs. permanent,
    508–9
  treatment of, 516–17
  in women, 511–13

infertility treatments, 506–24
  ethics of, 508
  increasing social pressure and,
    508
  rise in, 509
infibulation, 643
informed consent, 702–3
injectable contraceptives, 201,
    222, 255, 330, 356–58
  effectiveness of, 332, 356
  monthly (Lunelle), 354, 356,
    378
  switching to Vaginal Ring after,
    354
  see also Depo-Provera
insemination, 510, 304, 316, 522
  see also donor insemination
insomnia, 52, 58, 83
INSTEAD softcup, *249*
insulin, 25, 26
insulin-dependent diabetes, *see*
    Type 1 diabetes
insurance, *see* health insurance
intercourse, *see* sexual intercourse
international adoptions, 317, 319
Internet, 338
  community organizations and,
    751
  dating and, 157, 171, 172–73
  evaluating information from,
    705–8
  as source of health
    information, 704–8
intersex, 143, 151, 152, 232
interstitial cystitis, 691–92
intestinal problems, diet and, 23,
    36, 41–42
intimacy:
  fear of, 162–63, 176
  in heterosexual relationships,
    160–64, 168
  in LBTQ relationships, 171,
    175–78
  sexuality and, 192–93, 194, 204
intrauterine devices, *see* IUDs
intrauterine growth restrictions,
    459

intravenous (IV) drips, 421, 463–64

intravenous (IV) drugs:
    HIV and, 292, 294, 295–96, 297
    STIs and, 281

introitus, 228, *229, 229*

inverted nipples, 481

in vitro fertilization (IVF), 516
    cost of, 521
    decision for, 519–20
    donor recruitment for, 522
    procedure, 520
    risks of, 520–21
    techniques related to, 521–23
    see also assisted reproductive
        technologies

involution, 597

iodine, 31, 662

iron, 25, 31, 32, 433–34

iron-deficiency anemia, 659

irritability, 52, 91

irritable bowel syndrome (IBS), 41–42

isolation, aging and, 560, 582

Isotretinnoin, 435

itching, STIs and, 274, 275

IUDs, *222*, 259, *325*, 329, 330, 360–65, *360, 362, 379*, 620, 625
    after abortion, *403*
    advantages of, 361
    benefits of, 363
    checking strings of, 362
    DES daughters and, 627
    disadvantages of, 361
    effectiveness of, 332, 361
    as emergency contraception, 361, 365, 374, 376, *397*
    health concerns about, 362–63
    how to use, 361–62
    medicated, 632
    PID and, 268, 328, 647
    pregnancy after use of, 364
    safety of, 332, 338, 361
    side effects of, 363–64
    skipped periods and, 362

switching to Vaginal Ring after, 354

IV drug use, *see* intravenous (IV) drugs

Jane Collective, 407–8

jaundice, 483

jaw pains, 83

jobs, 92
    being denied or loss of, 89*n*
    dangerous, 80, 98
    gender identity and sexual orientation and, 146, 150
    LBTQ dating and, 172
    secondhand smoke and, 48
    see also environmental and occupational health

joint problems, 563–64

junk food, 4, 37

juvenile diabetes, *see* Type 1 diabetes

Keeper, the, *249*, 250, 251, 252

Kegel exercises, 195, 235, 434, 535, 590, 649, 695

kidney disease, 22, 663, 682

kissing, 294

K-Y jelly, *233*, 264, 267, 335

Kytril (granisetron), 616

labia, 209, 266
    majora, 228, *230–31*
    minora, 228, *230–31*, 643

labiaplasty, 4

labor, 76
    abortion and, 401
    active, 454–55
    bathing during, 453
    beginning of, 454
    bodily changing during, 452
    body rhythms during, 462–63
    causes and signs of, 452–53
    emotional response to, 459
    environment during, 461
    fear during, 460
    having others present during, 460

induction and augmentation, 464–65

listening to body during, 461

massage during, 461–62

nourishment during, 461

phases of, 454–56

relaxation techniques during, 462–63

solace of water in, 461

spontaneous vs. induced, 453

staying active during, 461

strategies to ease, 460

see also childbirth

labor unions, 114

lactational amenorrhea method (LAM), 371–73

lactobacilli, 650

lacto-ovo vegetarian diet, 30

Lamaze classes, 438

laparoscopically assisted vaginal hysterectomy (LAVH), 641

laparoscopy, 365, 515, 595, 629

large loop excision in the transformation zone (LLETZ), 625

laryngeal nerve, 662

late luteal phase dysphoric disorder (LLPDD), *see* premenstrual dysphoric disorder

late pregnancies, childbearing loss in, 496

latex gloves, 103, 197, 206, 208, 211, 265, 266

Latinas:
    eating disorders of, 40
    grandparents raising grandchildren among, 530
    HIV/AIDS and, 293, 297
    racial barriers to health care and, 710–11
    safer sex and, 269–70
    sexuality of, 188

Law of Similars, 78

laxatives, eating disorders and, 39, 40

mycoplasma genitalium, 289
myocardial infarction (MI), *220*
    see also heart attacks
myomas, 630–32
myomectomy, 631, 638

naproxen, *222*
narcotics, *see* opioids
Native Americans:
    adoption and, 387
    diet-related illnesses of, 36
    healing practices of, 68
    personal power of, 158–59
    SIDS among, 502
Natracare tampons, *249*
natural family planning (NFP),
    370
natural methods of birth control,
    369–71, *370, 379*
naturopathic remedies, chemo
    discomfort and, 615
nausea, 49, 52, 71, 108, 201, 256,
    303
    abortion and, 396, 401, 402,
        405
    from chemo, 615, 616
    hormonal birth control and,
        349, 353, 355, 375, 376
    pregnancy and, 382, 405
neck, 83, 107
needle sharing, 52, 293–97
neoadjuvant therapy, 615
nerve deafness, 562
neuropathies, 304
newborns:
    breast-feeding difficulties of,
        480
    evaluation after childbirth of,
        457
    first hours for, 458–59
    first weeks at home with, 475
*New View of Women's Sexual
    Problems, A,* 191–93, 202
New Zealand, vasectomy in, 368
nicotine replacement, 53
night sweats, 296, 303, 532–33
911 calls, 125, 132

nipples, 231, *239, 240*
    breast-feeding and, 481
    sensitivity of, 382
noise pollution, 106, *111*
Nolvadex, 730
nongonococcal urethritis (NGU),
    289
nonmarital sex, 155
non-nucleosides (non-nukes),
    303
nonoccupational post-exposure
    prophylaxis (NPEP), 295
nonoxynol-9 (N-9), 269, 333, 343
    irritations and, 208, 268, 269,
        341, 343
    safety of, 344
nonsteroidal anti-inflammatory
    drugs (NSAIDs), 563, 620,
        661, 663–64
Norplant, *222,* 268, 346, 358, 360,
    378, 411
nose jobs, 6
noses, 6–7, 274, 294
nuclear imaging, 676
nucleosides (nukes), 303
nurse-midwives, 423
nurses, 115
nursing homes, 575–77, 581
Nutrasweet (aspartame), 35
nutrition, *see* eating well; food
nutritional supplements, 31–33
nuts, 25, 26, *27,* 28, *28*
NuvaRing, 201, *222,* 354

obesity, 21, 37
obstetric fistula, 643
obstetricians, 422–23, 426, 510
obstetrics, vs. midwifery, 425
occupational safety and health,
    see environmental and
    occupational health;
    workplace
off-pump surgery, 678
oils, 26, 28, *28*
    in sex, 207
    in USDA model, 27, *27*
Olestra (artificial fat), 35

omega-3 fatty acids, 24, 25
oophorectomy, 201, 202, 617,
    634, 637–43
    prophylactic, 635*n*
    reasons for and risks of, 639,
        640–41
    recovering from, 642–43
    and sexuality, 639–40
opiates, 54
opioids, fetal effects of, 466
opthamologist, 561, 562
optic nerve damage, 358
optometrist, 562
oral (OraSure) testing, for HIV,
    298, 300
oral contraceptives, *see* birth
    control pills
oral sex, 208, 209–10, 217
    HIV and, 294, 297
    safer sex and, 210, 262, 265–66,
        265, 267, 274, 336
    STIs and, 273, 274, 278, 288,
        336
orders of protection (restraining
    orders), 128
organic food, 23–24, 31, 37, 42
organizing for change, x, xi,
    113–16
    abortion and, 408–9, 412–14
    in the environment, 113–15
    mood-altering drugs and,
        54–55
    in the workplace, 115–16
    see also community
        organizations
orgasm, 189, 193–97, 253, 639–40
    contractions caused by, 435
    disabilities and, 216, 217–18,
        218–21
    G-spot and, 197, *234*
    Kegel exercises and, 195,
        235
    male, 205
    masturbation and, 193, 194,
        196, 197, 199, 200
    multiple, 195–96
    problems with, 196, 201

sexual intercourse and, 188, 193, 204, 205, 207
Ortho Evra, *see* patch, contraceptive
os, 228, *233, 234,* 327
osmotic dilators, 401, 402
osteoarthritis, 563, 660
osteopaths, 71–72
osteoporosis, 42, 546
   alcohol and, 47
   exercise and, 61, 64–65
   smoking and, 48
   treatments for, 564–65
ostomy, *221*
ovarian cancer, 635–37
   hormonal birth control and, 346, 347, 349, 352, 355, 356, 360
   and oophorectomy, 641
   treatments for, 636–37
ovarian cysts, 209, 346, 350, 351
ovarian reserve, evaluated for infertility workup, 514
ovaries, 104, 231, *237–38,* 590
   in menstrual cycle, 242–43, 245, 247, 367
   removal of, *see* oophorectomy
   sex hormones produced by, 238
   tumors on, 209
Ovès cap, 342
oviducts, 243
ovulation, 201, 241–48, 259, 316
   birth control pills and, 346
   monitoring in infertility workup, 514
oxytocin, 402, 463
   and breast-feeding, 458
   see also Pitocin

pads (sanitary napkins), 248, 249, *249,* 250, 252, 253, 694
pain:
   abdominal, 350, 360, 362
   in limbs, 107, 350
   vaginal penetration and, 208
   see also back pain; cramps

pain management:
   self-help for, 668
   see also chronic pain conditions
Pain Medications Preference Scale, 444
panic attacks, 49
pansexuals, 147, 148, 170
Pap smears, 590, 591–92, *592,* 594, 622–24, 634, 637, 638
   abnormal, 362
   in diagnosis of uterine bleeding, 619
   getting and understanding, 623–24
   HIV/AIDS and, 293, 302
   Liquid-Based (LB), 622
   STIs and, 277, 281, 288
ParaGard (Copper T) IUD, 361–63, *362, 364,* 365, 376, *379*
paranoia, 49
parental leave, 320–21
parents:
   caring for elder, 571
   midlife changes to relationship with, 529–30
parents, parenthood, 80, 309–21, 386
   common challenges of, 313–14
   guidelines for deciding about, 313
   nurturing positive body images and, 15
   partner considerations and, 313, 314–15
   paths to, 315–20
   pros and cons of, 311–13
   support for, 320–21
   teen birth control and, 329
   timing of, 315
   see also mothers, motherhood
Parkinson's disease, 730
"partial birth abortion" ban, 410–11

partners:
   help for new mothers from, 485–86
   loss of, 554–56
   midlife changes to relationship with, 529
   pregnancy decisions and, 385–86
passivity, body image and, 9–10, 12
pasta, 25, *27, 28,* 30
patch, contraceptive, 201, *222,* 352–53, 357, *378*
   after abortion, *403,* 405
patient advocacy, 710, 716–17
patient rights, 702–8, 716–17
patriarchy, body image and, 7
Paxil, 89, 200, 729
PCBs (polychlorinated biphenyls), 97, 98, 105
peanuts, 36
pediatrician, choosing of, 444
pelvic exams, 589–91, 623
   abortion and, 399
   bimanual, *590*
   in diagnosis of uterine bleeding, 619
   placement of speculum for, *592*
   after rape, 130
   STIs and, 277, 280
pelvic floor muscles, *see* pubococcygeus (PC) muscles
pelvic infections, 302, 638
   abortion and, 406
   IUDs and, 362, 363, 364
pelvic inflammatory disease (PID), 209, 281, 296, 640, 646–49
   causes of, 274, 289, 646–47
   cramping and, 258–59
   diagnosis and treatment of, 647–48
   hormonal birth control and, 347, 349, 350, 352, 355, 358, 360

pregnancy (*cont.*)
    unwanted and unintended, 70,
        191, 192, 247, 252, 326, 327,
        329, 338, 381–89
    violent abuse during, 446
    wellness model of, 429, 430
    withdrawal management and,
        54
    without health insurance, 427
    women's rights during, 432
    see also birth defects;
        childbirth; miscarriage;
        specific trimesters
pregnancy crisis centers
    (abortion alternatives), 383,
    390
pregnancy tests, 349, 355, 357,
    362, 382–84
    home, 383
preimplantation genetic
    diagnosis, 523
premarital sex, 155
premature birth, 48, 74, 104, 289,
    363, 435
premature ejaculation, infertility
    and, 511
premature labor, 434
premenstrual dysphoric disorder
    (PMDD), 91–92, 256
premenstrual syndrome (PMS),
    91, 253, 255
    birth control pills and, 346,
        350
    menopause and, 532
prenatal care, during first
    trimester, 432–33
prenatal diagnosis, 523
    pregnancy termination after,
        500
prenatal screening, STIs and, 281,
    287
prenatal tests:
    accuracy of, 439
    during, second trimester, 442
    information gained by, 440
    preparation for, 440–41
    reasons for, 439

risks in, 44
    see also specific tests
prenatal visits:
    examination during, 433
    miscarriages discovered at, 497
    questions for first, 432–33
Prentif cap, 342, 343
prescription drug benefits, 558
Preven, 375, 376
primary care providers, 279, 715
Primedia, 34
prisoners, 170, 298
private long-term care insurance,
    572
Probe, 264
Problem-Knowledge Couple
    (PKC) system, 704*n*
progesterone, 497
    abortion and, 395
    in birth control pills, *218*,
        345–46
    in menstrual cycle, 243–46, 345
    pregnancy and, 201, 345
    sexuality and, 200–201, *218*
progestin-only pills ("minipills"),
    222, 350–52, *378*
    as emergency contraception,
        374, 375, 376
    switching to Vaginal Ring after,
        354
progestins, in birth control,
    345–46, 347, 352, 354, 356,
    358, 360, 361, 363–64, 375,
    376
prolactin, 201, 479
proliferative phase, 244
promiscuity, body image and, 4,
    15
prophylactic mastectomy, 606,
    609
prostaglandins, 256, 258, 402, 464
    see also misoprostol
prostitution, 119, 134–35, 188
    HIV transmission and, 297–98
protease inhibitors, 70, 303
protein, 23, *23*, 25, 31, 35, 241,
    434

Prozac, 89, 91–92, 200, 729
pseudolumps, 598, 599
psychiatrists, 85, 88, 91
psychologists, 85
puberty, 241–42
pubic bone, 195, *327, 339*
pubic hair, 228, *230 260*, 241
    removal of, 4, 10
pubis symphysis, 228, *230, 231*
public health, 98
    Precautionary Priniciple of,
        100
    support for, 728
public health clinics, 279
Public Health in Complex
    Emergencies, *295*
pubococcygeus (PC) muscles
    (pelvic floor muscles), 228,
    233, 234
    Kegel exercises and, 195, 235
punch biopsies, 625
purchasing power, body image
    and, 16
purified protein derivative, 738
pushing, during childbirth,
    455–56, 465
pyelonephritis, 693

quadriplegia, *216*
queer, 143, 144, 149–52
    use of term, 147, 170
questioning, 143, 170
"Quick Start" method, 346*n*

racism, 38, 45, 80, 99, 280, 294
    as barrier to health care,
        710–11
    body image and, 4, 12
    personal power and, 159
    therapy and, 84, 87
    violence and, 121
radiation therapy, 102, 610
    for cervical cancer, 634–35
    after mastectomy or
        lumpectomy, 611, 614
    after wide excision, 609
    see also chemotherapy

saline breast implants, *see* breast
    implants
saliva, HIV and, 294, 300
salmonella, 104
salt, 31
"sandwich generation," 529–30
sanitary napkins, *see* pads
Santeria, 77
Sarafem, 91–92, 729
saturated fats, 6, 26, 27, 28, *28, 29*
scabies, 275, *286*
scar tissue, infertility and, 511
Schiller's test, 594
school food, 34
sciatic nerve, 442
scleroderma, 664
scrotum, 146, *327*, 367
Sea Pearls sea sponge, *249*
sea sponges, *249*, 250, 251
sebaceous gland, 231, *239, 240*
second trimester, 441–42
    abortion in, 394, 400–402,
      406
      bodily changes during, 441
      miscarriage during, 499–500
      prenatal care during, 441–42
secretory phase, 244
sedatives, 46, 48
sedentary lifestyle, 37, 57
selective estrogen receptor
    modulators (SERMs), 539
selective serotonin reuptake
    inhibitors (SSRIs), 89–92,
    200, *222*
self-blame, 84, 134
self-defense, 135–36
self-esteem, 54, 190
    body image and, 9, 14
    eating disorders and, 41
    weight and, 39
self-healing, capacity for, 68, 80
self-help, self-help groups, x, 325
    complementary health
      practices and, 78
    emotional well-being and, 83,
      85, 92
    for herpes, 288, *289*

mood-altering drugs and, 53,
    54
self-improvement, meaning of, 5
self-injury, 94
semen, 274, *327*, 367, 369, 373
    analysis in infertility workup,
      514
    HIV transmission and, 293,
      294, 304
sensuality, 204
sentinel node biopsies, 612
separateness, enjoying, 167
separation, 165
    during midlife, 530
sex:
    during diagnostic infertility
      workup, 515
    effect of drugs and disease on,
      543
      gender vs., 141–43, 146
      and menopause, 528, 535,
        536–37
      in midlife, 530, 535
      during pregnancy, 434–35
sex discrimination, 84, 114
sex drive, decrease in, 349, 352,
    353, 358, 364, 367
sex education, 190, 192, 202, 297
    birth control and, 330, 331
    obstacles to, 324
    about STIs, 290
sex hormones, *see* estrogen;
    progesterone; testosterone
sex industry, decriminalization
    of, 739
sexism, 38, 294
    therapy and, 84, 87, 88
sex reassignment surgery, 143,
    145, 195
sex toys and aids, 213, 266
sex trafficking, 119, 134–35
sexual abuse, 83, 268, 277, 293
    child, 84, 93, 119, 132–35, 189
    in doctor-patient relationship,
      716
    and pregnancy, 446
    sexuality and, 187, 192, 196

therapy for, 84
    of women, *see* prostitution;
      rape; sex trafficking
sexual anatomy, tour of, 227–40
    see also specific body parts
sexual assault, *see* rape
sexual dysfunction, 92, 191–92,
    196, 200, 201
    infertility and, 511
    in women, 543–45
sexual excitement stage, 194
sexual exploitation, 739–40
sexual expression, 202–13
    anal stimulation, 210–11
    celibacy and, 203
    erotica, 213
    fantasies and, 211–12
    lovemaking as, 203–6
    masturbation with a partner,
      206
    oral sex, 208, 209–10
    painful penetration, 208–9
    role-playing, sadomasochism,
      bondage and discipline,
      212–13
    vaginal intercourse, 207
    vaginal penetration, 206
    virginity and, 202–3
sexual harassment, 108, 114, 115,
    119, 120, 121, 133–34, 189
sexual imagery, male vs. female
    response to, 10
sexual intercourse, 287, 328
    birth control effectiveness and,
      331, 333
    hymen and, *233*
    male vs. female view of, 192,
      204–5
    orgasm and, 188, 193, 204, 205,
      207
    pain during, 208–9
    pregnancy and, 327
    violent, 209
sexuality, 186–224
    aging and, 541–45
    arousal and, 191, 193–94, 196,
      202, 208, 240

vegetables, 22–25, *23*, 27, *27*, 28, *28*, 29, 31, 33, 35, 37, 112
vegetarianism, 23, 30–31
venereal warts (condyloma), 296
verbal abuse, 93, 119
vestibular glands, 231, *235, 236*, 590
vestibule, 228, *230, 231*
vestibulectomy, 653
Viagra (sildenafil), 202, 205
vibrators, 197, 199
  disabilities and, *218, 219, 221*
  safer sex and, 266
violence, 93, 118–37, 152, 153
  alcohol and, 47, 126
  of anti-abortion groups, 409
  body image and, 4, 5
  common reactions to experience of, 121–22
  ending, 136–37
  homicide and, 109, 118, 119
  myths about, 120, 122, 136
  prostitution and, 119, 134–35
  race, class, prejudice and, 121
  regaining our lives after, 122
  self-defense against, 135–36
  sexuality and, 189
  therapy and, 84
  understanding, 119–21
  against women worldwide, 741–42
  at workplace, 109
  see also physical abuse; rape
virginity, 202–3, 209, 297–98
  tampons and, 249
vision, 353
  blurred, 350
  changes with age to, 548, 561
visualization, 68, 72, 76, 304
vitamin A, 25, 26, 28, 32
vitamin B$_1$ (thiamine), 22
vitamin B$_2$ (riboflavin), 22, 25
vitamin B$_6$, 25
vitamin B$_{12}$, 25, 31
vitamin C, 22–23, 28, 41, 621
vitamin D, 25, 26, 28, 42, 548
vitamin-deficiency anemia, 659

vitamin E, 25, 26, 28, 567, 621
vitamin K, 23, 26, 42
vitamins, 678
  prenatal, 316
  use during pregnancy, 436
vomiting, 251, 294, 376
  abortion and, 396, 402
  from chemo, 615, 616
  eating disorders and, 39, 40
  pregnancy and, 349, 382
von Willebrand disease (VWD), 259, 618, 619, 696
voudoun, 69, 77
vulva, 228, *230, 230*
  examination of, 589–90
  sexuality and, 194, 208
  vagina vs., *231*
vulvar cancer, 653
vulvar vestibulitis syndrome, 652
vulvitis, 651–52
vulvodynia, 209, 652–53
vulvovaginitis, 274–75

waking or basal body temperature (BBT), 245–46, *370*
walkers, 560
walking, 60, 64, 159
walking epidural, 467
warfarin, 70
warts:
  genital, *see* genital warts
  venereal (condyloma), 296
water:
  contaminated, 115
  drinking, 98, *101, 110*
  to ease labor discomfort, 461
  see also fluid retention
water sports, 266
waxing, bikini, 4
weight:
  body image and, 13, 15, 16
  comfortable, 16
  eating disorders and loss of, 38
  food allergies and, 36–37
  genetic makeup and, 36

health vs., 15, 27, 29, 37–38
loss, 5, 13, 29, 296
pathological notions about, 13
surgery for loss of, 13
see also diets, dieting
weight gain, 37
  birth control and, 349, 353, 355, 356, 357, 358, 360, 364
  during pregnancy, 432, 434, 441
"welfare reform," 310–11
Wellbutrin (bupropion), 200
wellness strategies, 83
well-woman care, *see* physical exam
wet heat, 368
white blood cells, 273
wide excision, 609
widows, 554–56
wigs, 617
Wilson's disease, 362
wire localization, 603
withdrawal (pulling out), 262, 373–74, *379*
women of color:
  abortion and, 407, 411, 413–14
  birth control for, 325
  eating disorders of, 38, 39–40
  HIV/AIDS and, 292–94
  LBTQ, 170
  as mothers, 310–11
  sex and gender of, 149–50
  sterilization of, 365
  STIs and, 280
  violence against, 121
  weight of, 37
  see also black women; Latinas
women's health:
  childbirth and risks to, 735
  in developing countries, 734–35
  disparities in, 721–22
  gender roles and, 737
  improvements in, 721
  influence of public on, 720

women's health (*cont.*)
    politics of, x, 719–47
    refugees and, 738–39
    relationship of economics and
        education to, 734–37
    worldwide, 733–34
women's rights, xiv, 13, 719–20
workplace:
    breast-feeding after return to,
        482

    organizing for change in,
        115–16
    return after childbirth to,
        487
    violence in, 109

X rays, during pregnancy, 436

yeast infections, 296, 303, 648,
    653–54

    see also candida infection;
        monilia infection
yoga, 75–76, 304
youth fixation, 16–17
yo-yo dieting, 35, 37

Zestra, 202
zinc, 25, 28, 31, 41, 621
Zofran (ondansetron), 616
Zoloft, 89, 92, 200